COLOR ATLAS OF VETERINARY ANATOMY

Volume 3

THE DOG & CAT

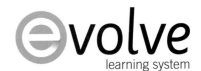

Evolve Learning Resources for Students and Lecturers:

Over 60 interactive and multiple choice questions to test your knowledge.

See the instructions and PIN code panel on the inside cover for access to the web site.

Think outside the book...evolve

DEDICATION

This volume is dedicated to the late Peter Goody

For Elsevier

Commissioning Editor: Robert Edwards
Development Editor: Lynn Watt
Project Manager: Nancy Arnott
Designer/Design Direction: George Ajayi
Illustration Manager: Merlyn Harvey
Illustrators: Jane Catherall, Samantha Elmhurst, Jenni Miller, Maurice Murphy,
          Lynda R Payne, Lee Smith, Marion Tasker

COLOR ATLAS OF VETERINARY ANATOMY

Volume 3

THE DOG & CAT

SECOND EDITION

Stanley H. Done
BA BVetMed PhD DECPHM DECVP FRCVS FRCPath
Visiting Professor of Veterinary Pathology
University of Glasgow Veterinary School
Former Lecturer in Veterinary Anatomy
Royal Veterinary College
London

The late Peter C. Goody
MSC (Ed) PhD
Former Lecturer in Veterinary Anatomy
Royal Veterinary College
London

Neil C. Stickland
BSc PhD DSc
Professor of Veterinary Anatomy
Department of Veterinary Basic Sciences
Royal Veterinary College
London

Susan A. Evans
MIScT AIMI MIAS
Former Chief Technician in Anatomy
Department of Veterinary Basic Sciences
Royal Veterinary College
London

With radiographs provided by

Elizabeth A. Baines
MA VetMB DVR DipECVDI MRCVS
Lecturer in Veterinary Radiology
Department of Veterinary Clinical Sciences
Royal Veterinary College
London

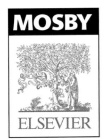

MOSBY

ELSEVIER

EDINBURGH   LONDON   NEW YORK   OXFORD   PHILADELPHIA   ST LOUIS   SYDNEY   TORONTO 2009

MOSBY
ELSEVIER

© Times Mirror International Publishers Limited 1996
© Mosby International Limited 2000
© 2002, Elsevier Science Limited.
© 2009, Elsevier Limited. All rights reserved.

First edition 1996
Second edition 2009

ISBN 9780-7234-3415-3

British Library Cataloguing in Publication Data
A catalogue record for this book is available from the British Library

Library of Congress Cataloging in Publication Data
A catalog record for this book is available from the Library of Congress

Notice

Neither the Publisher nor the Authors assume any responsibility for any loss or injury and/or damage to persons or property arising out of or related to any use of the material contained in this book. It is the responsibility of the treating practitioner, relying on independent expertise and knowledge of the patient, to determine the best treatment and method of application for the patient.

The Publisher

your source for books,
journals and multimedia
in the health sciences
www.elsevierhealth.com

Working together to grow
libraries in developing countries

www.elsevier.com | www.bookaid.org | www.sabre.org

ELSEVIER   BOOK AID International   Sabre Foundation

Printed in India

Last digit is the print number: 16

The
publisher's
policy is to use
**paper manufactured
from sustainable forests**

PREFACE

This third volume in the series, like the first two on the ruminant and horse, is primarily intended for veterinary students and practising veterinary surgeons. Nevertheless, we confidently expect it to appeal to a wider audience including dog and cat enthusiasts, research workers, comparative anatomists, premedical students, in fact anyone with a desire to appreciate the topographical anatomy of the domestic carnivores.

The book presents the important features of regional and topographical anatomy in a series of full-color photographs of detailed dissections. These structures are identified in accompanying colored and extensively labelled drawings. The nomenclature is based on that of the *Nomina Anatomica Veterinaria* (1983) with the Latin terminology used for muscles, arteries, veins, lymphatics, and nerves, but the terminology anglicised for most other structures. Captions for the photographs give additional information necessary for their interpretation, such as those structures removed or displaced to obtain the picture.

A criticism levelled at using embalmed cadavers for dissection is that they lack 'realism', normal color and form, and often bear little resemblance to organs in their natural state. This criticism indeed has some validity if one is actually doing the dissecting – embalmed material does not have the 'feel' of fresh material having lost its elasticity and pliability. However, if one is considering the topographical relationships between structures and their relative positions then much of the criticism disappears, since the embalmed cadaver is arguably better at displaying such relationships. Photographs of such embalmed specimens are also clearer and more readily interpreted than photographs of fresh material. Consequently photography of embalmed latex injected specimens was preferred in our attempts to impart an initial appreciation of regional and topographical anatomy.

The dissections and photographs have been specially prepared for this book, except for a few photographs of specimens in the Anatomy Museum collection of the Department of Veterinary Basic Sciences, The Royal Veterinary College London. The radiographs were prepared originally for teaching purposes and correspond in large measure to radiographs that practising veterinary surgeons would routinely be interpreting.

Three dogs, two bitches and two cats were dissected for this work. It was not the object of the book to consider intraspecific variation and so breed differences have been ignored in the dissections. Each animal was dissected completely through a progressive series of dissections. We therefore encountered similar problems to those facing a veterinary student dissecting the same cadaver over a period of some months with consequent deterioration.

The specimens were embalmed using methods routinely employed in the Department of Veterinary Basic Sciences at The Royal Veterinary College. Their blood vessels were subsequently injected with colored neoprene latex and they were stored in formalin (7%).

The aim of the dissections is to display the topography of the animal to, among others, the veterinary student and surgeon. Unlike the ox and horse, however, a routine clinical examination of the dog or cat is not restricted to a lateral approach with the animal in the standing position. Thus, while lateral views predominate to correspond and make comparison with the horse and ox, they are supplemented by numerous dissections from a ventral approach. Also, as with the ox and horse, we have as far as possible avoided photographs of parts removed from the body, or the use of views from unusual angles or of unusual bodily positions.

This volume differs from the first two volumes in several ways. The general introductory chapter and the inclusion of radiographs was not a feature of the earlier volumes. Radiography of the ox and horse, apart from the practical problems of obtaining good radiographs, is also of restricted value in providing topographical information. In the smaller domestic animals it is obviously easier to accomplish and provides much useful information to supplement dissections. Secondly, an additional chapter is devoted specifically to the vertebral column with special emphasis on the disposition of the epaxial musculature. Thirdly, transverse sections through the various regions are used to assist in the interpretation of three-dimensional topography, as in modern imaging methods.

A significant difference between this edition of the volume and previous editions is the addition of new radiographs, CT and MRI scans which are placed throughout the book in appropriate chapters. A second major difference is the inclusion of clinical notes at the beginning of each main chapter. These notes highlight the areas of anatomy which are of particular clinical significance. Finally, over 60 self-assessment questions are available online with this new edition to help test learning. We feel that these additions to the book add considerably to its usefulness especially to the aspiring veterinary surgeon.

ACKNOWLEDGEMENTS

Since the first edition our colleague Peter Goody has died. He was our friend, colleague and co-worker. He was a meticulous anatomist and considerable artist and his contribution to this revised edition has been greatly missed. It is therefore our pleasure to dedicate this edition to his memory and to make him first author. Without his efforts the first edition of the dog volume would never have been undertaken.

The dissections and photography for this book were carried out in the Anatomy division of the Department of Veterinary Basic Sciences at The Royal Veterinary College London. We are grateful to the department for the provision of specialised facilities without which this work would not have been possible. Whilst the dissecting was shared, sole responsibility for the photography rested with Sue Evans. In addition, with authors based in different locations, the logistics of producing the book relied heavily on her organisation. The other authors would like to take this opportunity to express the debt of gratitude they owe her for the time, trouble and attention to detail that she displayed in producing the splendid photographs, and for her consummate skill in managing the whole effort.

A number of people and organisations provided assistance during the course of producing the book. We extend our thanks to the following: Initial funding for the project was provided by Gower Medical Publishing. The task of preparing and caring for the specimens before and during the dissections was undertaken by Andrew Crook and Graham Hagger. A number of the dissections of the cat received assistance from Fay Cullingham.

Animals were loaned for photography by Mrs J. Lonsdale, Mrs V. Pritchard, Mr I. Bailey, and Mr J. Moseley.

Film processing was undertaken by Lightbox Creative Services of Camden Town – their rapid and efficient turnaround service was most appreciated. Library Services were provided by The Royal Veterinary College in Camden Town and by the Ministry of Agriculture, Fisheries and Food in Weybridge. Assistance in the interpretation of radiographs in the first edition was provided by Mr S. Dean BVetMed DVR MRCVS, to whom we are indebted. We are grateful to the Ministry of Agriculture, Fisheries and Food for the liberal interpretation of 'flexitime' working and annual leave provision without which SHD could not have found the time for dissection. We are also indebted to clinical colleagues for revising our clinical notes.

There is no doubt that without the significant contribution of Dr R. R. Ashdown to Volumes 1 and 2 of this series there would not have been an outline for us to follow or a standard to aim for in Volume 3.

The idea of producing an atlas of canine anatomy to accompany those for the ruminant and the horse resulted from discussions with Gower Medical Publishing in the early eighties. Unfortunately the project did not get underway until the early nineties, and for a variety of reasons took several years to reach fruition. During this frustrating 'stop-start' period we are very grateful to the editors, designers and illustrators (especially Jane Catherall who produced the bulk of the drawings) for bearing with us and putting up with our tardiness and individual foibles. Despite such problems Elsevier's belief in the end product has finally seen it through to completion for which we extend our thanks.

Neil Stickland
Stan Done

BIBLIOGRAPHY

Adams DR (1986) *Canine Anatomy a Systemic Study.* Ames: Iowa State University Press.

Ammann K, Seiferle E & Pelloni G. (1978) *Atlas of Topographical Surgical Anatomy of the Dog – Atlas zur Chirnrgisch-topographischen Anatomie des Hundes.* Berlin, Hamburg: Paul Parey.

Anderson W & Anderson BG (1994) *Atlas of Canine Anatomy.* Philadelphia: Lea & Febiger.

Barone R (1976) *Anatomic Compareé des Mammifères Domestiques.* 3 vols. Paris: Vigot Frères.

Baum H & Zietzschmann D. (1936) *Handbuch der Anatomie des Hundes.* 2nd edition. Berlin: Paul Parey.

Bolk L, Göppert E, Kallius E & Lubosch W. (Eds) (1931–1938) *Handbuch der vergleichenden Anatomic der Wirbeltiere.* 6 Vols. Berlin & Vienna: Urban & Schwarzenberg. (Reprinted Asher & Co: Amsterdam 1967).

Boyd JS & Patterson C. (1991) *A Colour Atlas of Clinical Anatomy of the Dog and Cat.* London: Wolfe.

Bradley DC. (1959) *Topographical Anatomy of the Dog.* 6th edition revised by T. Grahame. Edinburgh: Oliver & Boyd.

Budras K–D & Fricke W. (1991) *Atlas Anatomic des Hundes.* Lehrbuch für Tierärzte und Studierende, 3rd Edition. Hannover: Schlütersche.

Budras K–D & Fricke W. (1995) *Anatomy of the Dog: An Illustrated Text.* (Translation of 3rd Edition). London: Mosby–Wolfe.

Crouch JE. (1969) *Text-atlas of Cat Anatomy.* Philadelphia: Lea & Febiger.

deLahunta A. (1983) *Veterinary Neuroanatomy and Clinical Neurology.* 2nd Edition. Philadelphia: Saunders.

deLahunta A. & Habel RE. (1986) *Applied Veterinary Anatomy.* Philadelphia: W B Saunders.

Dyce KM, Sack WO & Wensing CJG. (1987) *Textbook of Veterinary Anatomy.* Philadelphia: W B Saunders.

Ellenberger W & Baum H. (1943) *Handbuch der vegleichenden Anatomic der Haustiere.* 18th edition. Edited by Zietzschmann O. Ackernecht E & Grau H. Berlin: Springer.

Ellenberger W, Baum H & Dittrich O. (1925) *An Atlas of Animal Anatomy for Artists.* 2nd edition revised by LS Brown, New York: Dover.

Evans HE & Christensen GC. (1979) *Miller's Anatomy of the Dog.* 2nd edition. Philadelphia: W B Saunders.

Evans HE & deLahunta A. (1988) *Miller's Guide to the Dissection of the Dog.* 3rd edition. Philadelphia: W B Saunders.

Feaney DA. (1991) *Atlas of Correlative Imaging Anatomy of the Normal Dog: Ultrasound and Computed Tomography.* Philadelphia: W B Saunders.

Field EJ & Harrison RJ. (1968) *Anatomical Terms. Their Origin and Derivation.* 3rd edition. Cambridge: Heffer.

Field HE, Taylor ME & Butterworth BB. (1969) *Atlas of Cat Anatomy.* Chicago: University of Chicago Press.

Ghoshal NG, Koch T & Popesko P. (1981) *The Venous Drainage of the Domestic Animals.* Philadelphia: W B Saunders.

Grassé PP. (Editor) (1950–1970) *Traité de Zoologie: Anatomic, Systematique. Biologic.* Vertebrates vols. 13–17. Paris: Masson.

Gilbert SG. (1975) *Pictorial Anatomy of the Cat.* Revised Edition. Seattle: University of Washington Press.

Hudson LC & Hamilton WP. (1993) *Atlas of Feline Anatomy for Veterinarians.* Philadelphia: W B Saunders.

International Committee on Veterinary Gross Anatomical Nomenclature, World Association of Veterinary Anatomists (1983) *Nomina Anatomica Veterinaria.* 3rd edition. Ithaca: International Committee on Veterinary Gross Anatomical Nomenclature.

Jayne H. (1898) *Mammalian Anatomy. Part I The Skeleton of the Cat.* Philadelphia: J B Lippincott.

McClure RC, Dallman MJ & Garrett PD. (1973) *Cat Anatomy An Atlas. Text and Dissection Guide.* Philadelphia: Lea & Febiger.

McFadyean J. (1964) *Osteology and Arthrology of the Domesticated Animals.* 4th edition. Edited by H.V. Hughes & J.W. Dransfield. London: Bailliere Tindall. Cox.

Miller ME. (1962) *Guide to the Dissection of the Dog.* 3rd edition. Ithaca: Edwards Bros.

Miller ME, Christensen GC & Evans HE. (1964) *Anatomy of the Dog.* Philadelphia: W B Saunders.

Montané L, Bourdelle E & Bressou C. (1953) *Anatomie Régionale des Animaux Domestiques.* Vol. IV – Carnivores: Chien et Chat. Paris: J–B Baillière.

Nickel R, Schummer A & Seiferle E. (1961–1967) *Lehrbuch der Anatomie der Haustiere.* Vol. 1–IV. Berlin, Hamburg: Paul Parey. (Revised and translated into English 1979–1986).

  Volume 1 (1986) *The Locomotor System of the Domestic Mammals.* 5th Edition – Revised by J. Frewein, K–H. Wille & H. Wilkens. Translated by WG Siller & WM Stokoe. Berlin, Hamburg: Paul Parey.

  Volume 2 (1979) *The Viscera of the Domestic Animals.* 2nd Edition – Translated and Revised by A. Schummer, R. Nickel & WO Sack. New York: Springer.

  Volume 3 (1981) *The Circulatory System, the Skin and the Cutaneous Organs of the Domestic Mammals.* 2nd Edition – Revised by A. Schummer, H. Wilkens, B. Vollmerhaus & K–H. Habermehl – Translated by WG Siller & PAL Wight. Berlin, Hamburg: Paul Parey.

  Volume 4 (1986) *The Nervous System, the Endocrine Glands, and the Sensory Organs of the Domestic Mammals.* 2nd Edition – Revised by E. Seiferle & G. Bohme. Berlin, Hamburg: Paul Parey.

Pierard J. (1972) *Anatomie Appliquée des Carnivores Domestiques. Chien et Chat.* Quebec: Sornabec.

Popesko P. (1977) *Atlas of Topographical Anatomy of the Domestic Animals.* 2nd edition. Philadelphia: W B Saunders.

Reighard J & Jennings HS. (1935) *Anatomy of the Cat.* 3rd edition. Edited by R Elliot. New York: Holt, Rinehart & Winston.

Schebitz H & Wilkens H. (1986) *Atlas of Radiographic Anatomy of the Dog and Cat – Atlas der Rontgenanatomie von Hund and Katze.* 4th edition revised. Berlin: Paul Parey. Philadelphia: W B Saunders.

Sisson S & Grossman JD. (1953) *The Anatomy of the Domestic Animals.* 4th edition, revised. Philadelphia: W B Saunders.

Sisson S & Grossman JD. (1975) *The Anatomy of the Domestic Animals.* Vol 2. 5th edition. Edited by R Getty. Philadelphia: W B Saunders.

Taylor JA. (1955–1970) *Regional and Applied Anatomy of the Domestic Animals.* Parts I–III. Edinburgh: Oliver & Boyd.

Vollmerhaus B & Habermehl KH. (undated) *Topographical Anatomical Diagrams of Injection Technique in Horses. Cattle, Dogs and Cats.* Marburg, Lahn: Hoechst. Behringwerke AG.

Walker WF Jr. (1967) *A Study of the Cat.* Philadelphia: W B Saunders.

CONTENTS

INTRODUCTION

Volumes 1 and 2 in this series were specifically produced to help compensate for any lack of personal dissection of the large domestic species by veterinary students. It is still the case that the bulk of a student's dissection is performed on a dog or cat cadaver, but even this may not be a complete detailed dissection of an entire specimen. Increasingly, formal dissection is not part of the curriculum as modern diagnostic techniques replace more conventional technologies. Dissection specimens have always been shared between several dissectors but nowadays, for a variety of reasons such as cost, availability and time allocation, the amount of 'hands-on' dissection that any individual student can accomplish is less than in past years. The reduced availability of material for prosection, coupled with the reduced levels of manpower to produce and maintain the prosections, means that the production of good demonstrations, as well as museum preparations of a full range of dissection stages of a specific region, is no longer feasible.

It is our sincere hope that this photographic atlas of dissections will: (a) help to compensate those students who for whatever reason are unable to carry out the detailed dissection for themselves; (b) provide a permanent reminder of what was seen, or should have been seen, by those students able to carry out their own detailed dissections.

We reiterate the plea put forward in volumes 1 and 2 that we do not want to entice students out of the dissection room, away from the specimens, and into the comfort of armchairs for their study of practical topographical anatomy. Rather, we have attempted to provide an atlas with which they can confirm and extend their own personal study of dissections of the dog and cat at times when the dissections are no longer available. However, for those of you unable to dissect for yourself or to view prosected specimens, this atlas will, we hope, provide you with the next best thing – a comprehensive selection of photographs and labelled interpretative drawings which you can examine at leisure.

The dissections presented in this volume represent complete dissection sequences from the surface inwards – a lateral sequence supplemented by a ventral sequence and a dorsal sequence. Progressive stages have been photographed at regular intervals as structures become revealed, clarified and defined, and many eventually removed. A comment is needed on the technique of dissection shown in these photographs. In many instances we have not cleaned away all of the connective tissue from the structures being displayed, although we have felt it to be necessary to clear fat from any locations in order to reveal salient features. In 'complete' dissections it is often impossible to preserve accurately the original topographical relationships of vessels and nerves. Also, such dissections encourage the student to think that textbook drawings are 'real' and that adipose, fascial and areolar tissues do not exist. We have tried to make the photographs represent the structures as they really appear during the course of an actual dissection.

Although veterinary students are the main targets for this volume it is not intended to be an atlas of applied Veterinary Anatomy. No special emphasis is given to any particular region or structure: the detail we have included will form a sound basis for any specific application.

The first chapter gives an overall general picture of the dog concentrating on its surface anatomy, the surface relationships of its internal viscera and the skeletal structure. Skeletal components are only shown as articulated units forming the bony basis of the specific region. Isolated osteological preparations have not been included as they add little to an account of topography. Each of the subsequent chapters dealing with specific regions of the body begins with photographs of regional surface features of the live animal together with complementary photographs of an articulated canine skeleton to illustrate the important palpable bony features of these regions. The bulk of each chapter then gives a detailed sequence of dissections from lateral and ventral aspects, and terminates with a series of transverse sections through the region. The thorax and abdomen include dissection sequences from both left lateral and right lateral approaches: the head and vertebral column also include sequences from a dorsal aspect. The final chapter deals with the cat and concentrates on those features which differ significantly from the dog set out in the preceding chapters.

Volumes 1 and 2 in this series assumed that readers would already have obtained the basics of systematic anatomy and were extending these to the topography of the large domestic species. This volume can make no such assumption and will undoubtedly be consulted by students at an early stage in their anatomy course or by others having scant grounding in gross anatomy. Consequently, it is felt that a few notes on the terms of position and relationship routinely used in the titles and captions is necessary. It is also necessary if the book is being consulted by a reader familiar with human anatomy in which the anatomical position of normal reference is an upright stance. Human terms of reference include anterior and posterior, superior and inferior, which are inapplicable in veterinary anatomy.

Anatomical relationships of structures will be described with the animal in a quadrupedal anatomical position – standing squarely on all four limbs with head and tail extended.

Dorsal/ventral – towards the back or upperside (dorsum)/towards the belly or underside (ventrum). In the limbs dorsal is used with reference to the front of the paws, while palmar/plantar are used for the rear (underside) of the forepaw and hindpaw respectively.

Cranial/caudal – towards the head/towards the tail. In the head itself the term rostral (towards the rostrum or muzzle) is used in preference to cranial which would be ambiguous. In the limbs the terms cranial and caudal are used to refer to the front and rear surfaces above (proximal to) the carpus and tarsus.

Medial/lateral – towards the midline (median plane)/towards the side or away from the midline. In the limbs the terms are used to refer to the inner and outer surfaces respectively.

Proximal/distal – towards the central axis of the body (or the origin of a structure)/more removed from the central axis of the body (or the origin of a structure), particularly relevant in the limbs the proximal region being closer to the trunk, the paw being the most distal part.

Axial/abaxial – close to the midline (central axis) of a limb/ structures away from this midline of a limb. In the paws this central limb axis passes between digits 3 and 4, thus the axial surface of a digit faces the axis/abaxial surface faces away from the axis.

Deep (internal)/superficial (external) – removed from the surface of the body or at the centre of a solid organ/towards the surface of the body or the surface of a solid organ.

Right/Left – determined in relation to the animal and not the observer, an important distinction when the animal is lying on its back or when a transverse section through the body is being viewed from the cranial aspect.

The head trunk and limbs have been sectioned in order to obtain some of the photographs. In this context reference is made to specific planes:

Median plane – longitudinal plane dividing the animal into equal right and left halves.

Sagittal plane – a plane parallel to the median plane.

Transverse plane – crosses body or limb at right angles to the long axis, or the long axis of an organ or body part.

With reference to the radiographs, the view is described in relation to the direction the X-rays take from point of entrance into the animal to point of exit.

It is also essential to point out that only a limited number of animals were dissected in the studies for this volume. In our many years of experience we have found considerable individual variations between animals. This is particularly so with respect to arteries and veins. Therefore variations may be found between other dissections and those described in this volume.

1. LIVE AND SKELETAL ANATOMY OF WHOLE ANIMAL

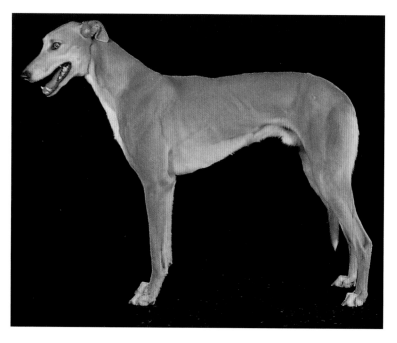

Fig. 1.1 Surface features of the dog: left lateral view. This picture is intended to show in a very basic manner the major parts of the body. Consequently the descriptive terminology used in the labelling of the drawing is deliberately kept in very general terms and in some cases colloquial terms in frequent use have been included. More detailed consideration of surface anatomy of the various parts of the body (head and neck; thorax, abdomen and pelvis; and the limbs) are shown later in this introductory chapter. Fig. 1.1A at the foot of the page shows the major topographical regions into which the body is descriptively subdivided. Viewing the body in terms of regions is especially useful for describing the position of internal organs in relation to the surface. More detailed subdivisions of these main topographical regions are illustrated later in this chapter.

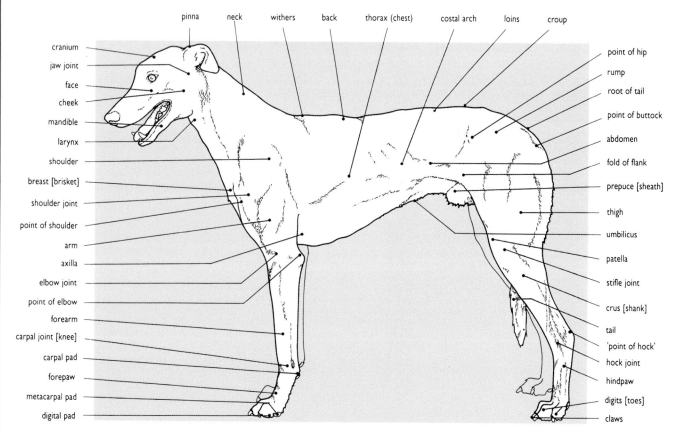

pinna · neck · withers · back · thorax (chest) · costal arch · loins · croup

cranium · jaw joint · face · cheek · mandible · larynx · shoulder · breast [brisket] · shoulder joint · point of shoulder · arm · axilla · elbow joint · point of elbow · forearm · carpal joint [knee] · carpal pad · forepaw · metacarpal pad · digital pad

point of hip · rump · root of tail · point of buttock · abdomen · fold of flank · prepuce [sheath] · thigh · umbilicus · patella · stifle joint · crus [shank] · tail · 'point of hock' · hock joint · hindpaw · digits [toes] · claws

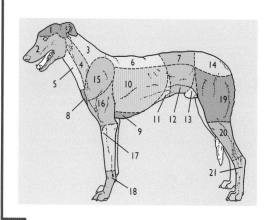

Fig. 1.1A Topographical regions of the dog: left lateral view. **1** Cranial Regions. **2** Facial Regions. **3–5** Neck Regions. **3** Dorsal Neck Region. **4** Lateral Neck Region. **5** Ventral Neck Region. **6–7** Dorsal Regions. **6** Thoracic Vertebral Region. **7** Lumbar Region. **8–10** Thoracic (Pectoral) Regions. **8** Presternal Region. **9** Sternal Region. **10** Costal Region. **11–13** Abdominal Regions. **11** Cranial Abdominal Region. **12** Middle Abdominal Region. **13** Caudal Abdominal Region. **14** Pelvic Region. **15–18** Forelimb (Thoracic Limb) Regions. **15** Scapular Region. **16** Brachial Region. **17** Antebrachial Region. **18** Forepaw (Manus) Region. **19–21** Hindlimb (Pelvic Limb) Regions. **19** Femoral Region. **20** Crural Region. **21** Hindpaw (Pes) Region.

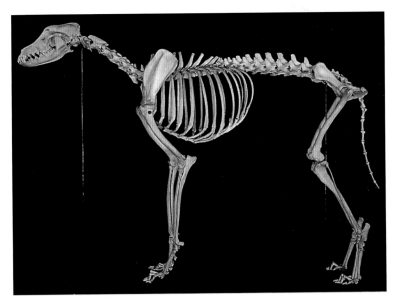

Fig. 1.2 Skeleton of the dog: left lateral view. As with the surface view on the accompanying page the drawing of the skeleton is intended to show in a very general manner the major components of the skeleton. In general terms the skeleton is divisible into two parts according to its position in the body. Axial skeleton – the skeletal basis of the head, neck, trunk and tail, consisting of the vertebral column, ribs and sternum, and the skull. Appendicular skeleton – bones of the limbs and associated girdles attaching the limb to the trunk. Absent from this skeletal preparation is the fragile hyoid apparatus, a skull component which in life suspends the tongue and larynx in the floor of the throat, and the os penis developed in the soft tissues of the free end of the penis.

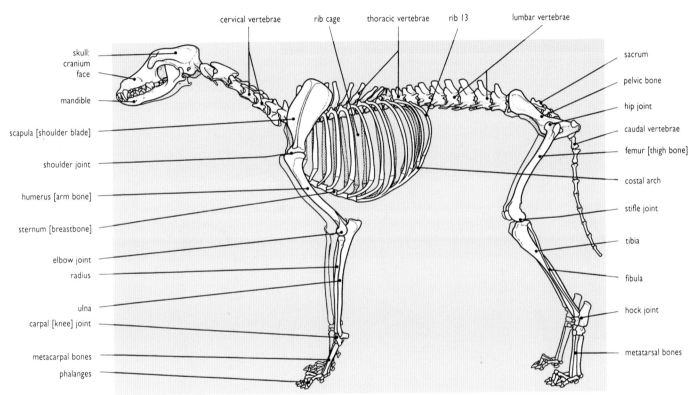

Fig. 1.2A Variation in conformation of the dog: left lateral views. The wide variation in body shape within the species is shown by three examples from the more than 300 existing breeds of domestic dog: A – Dachshund; B – Staffordshire Bull Terrier; C – Hungarian Vizla.

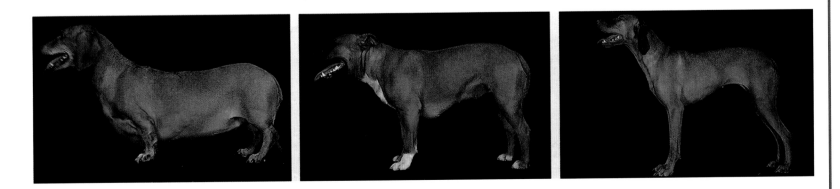

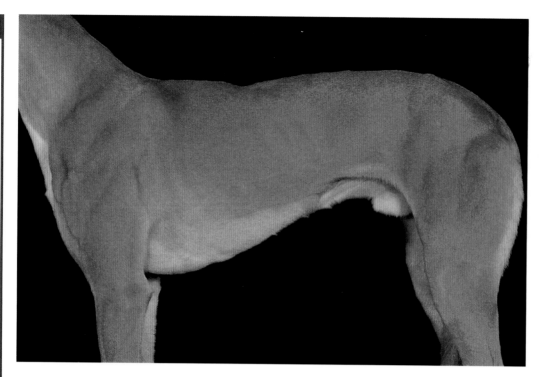

Fig. 1.3 Surface features of the thorax and abdomen: left lateral view. The major bony features of the trunk are shown. In addition the lateral surfaces of ribs 13 forwards to 5 are palpable through the overlying muscles in the normal standing position. Should the forelimb be protracted ribs 2 to 5 are also palpable, at least for some of their length. Palpation in the jugular fossa craniomedial to the shoulder joint may detect the leading edge of rib 1 at the thoracic inlet. In a standing position the cranial angle of the scapula is on a level with the tip of the spinous process of thoracic vertebral; the caudal angle level with the bodies of thoracic vertebrae 4 and 5; the shoulder joint lies lateral to the lower end of rib 1; the olecranon process of the ulna lies below the ventral end of intercostal space 5.

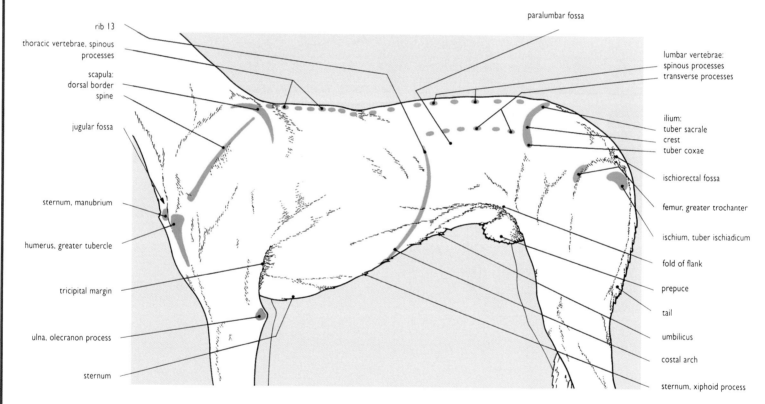

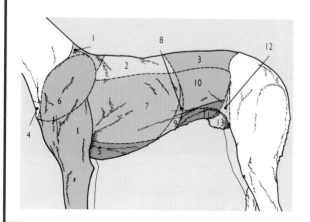

Fig. 1.3A Topographical regions of the thorax and abdomen: left lateral view. **1–3** Dorsal Regions. **1** Interscapular Region. **2** Thoracic Vertebral Region. **3** Lumbar Region. **4–7** Thoracic (Pectoral) Regions. **4** Presternal Region. **5** Sternal Region. **6** Scapular Region. **7** Costal Region. **8–9** Cranial Abdominal Region. **8** Left Hypochondriac Region. **9** Xiphoid Region. **10–11** Middle Abdominal Region. **10** Left Lateral Abdominal Region. **11** Umbilical Region. **12–13** Caudal Abdominal Region. **12** Left Inguinal Region. **13** Preputial (Pubic) Region.

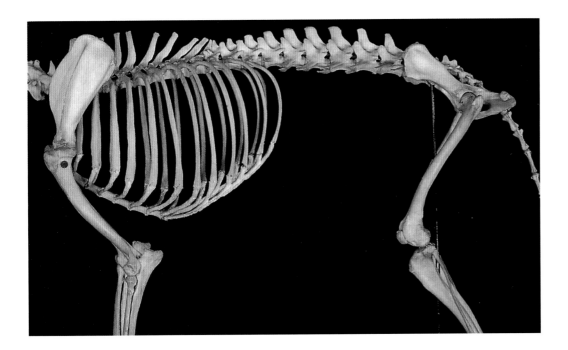

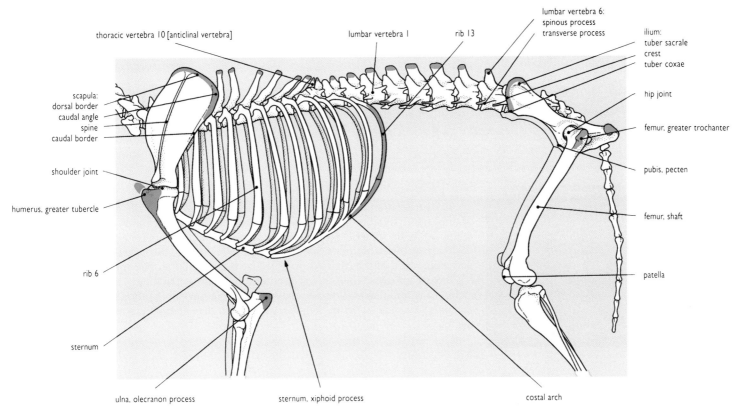

thoracic vertebra 10 [anticlinal vertebra]

lumbar vertebra 1

rib 13

lumbar vertebra 6:
spinous process
transverse process

ilium:
tuber sacrale
crest
tuber coxae

scapula:
dorsal border
caudal angle
spine
caudal border

hip joint

femur, greater trochanter

shoulder joint

humerus, greater tubercle

pubis, pecten

femur, shaft

rib 6

patella

sternum

ulna, olecranon process

sternum, xiphoid process

costal arch

Fig. 1.4 Skeleton of the thorax and abdomen: left lateral view. The palpable bony features shown in the surface view of the trunk are colored here. Rib 13, the floating rib, lies free in the abdominal wall, and occasionally remnants of additional ribs are present (see fig. 6.18 in which a small rib 14 is located on the craniodorsal part of the abdominal wall). The ribs are long and quite straight, while the costal cartilages are bent through almost a right angle to gain sternal

attachment for the first nine. The practically vertical orientation of the more cranial ribs becomes progressively more caudoventral further back. The costal arch forms the cranial boundary of the accessible abdominal wall: the caudal boundary is the pelvic inlet of which only the pubic pecten is palpable. The pelvic cavity communicates with the abdominal although it is considerably smaller and lies within the boundaries of the articulated pelvis, sacrum and caudal vertebrae.

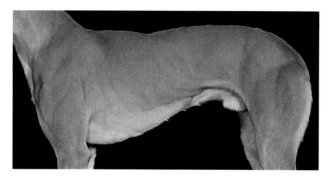

Fig. 1.5 Surface relationships of the thoracic and abdominal viscera of the dog: left lateral view. The major internal viscera in the thorax and abdomen are shown in surface projection in this and **Fig. 1.6** in lateral views. For the purposes of these drawings it is assumed that the dog is standing squarely on all four of its legs in a normal standing position. The costodiaphragmatic line of pleural reflection immediately cranial to the costal arch marks the caudal limit of the thoracic cavity. The cranial limit of the abdominal cavity is marked by the diaphragm which in the midline extends for a considerable distance cranial to the costal arch. Consequently a considerable part of the abdomen and its contents (liver and stomach primarily) lie forwards of the costal arch within the confines of the ribcage.

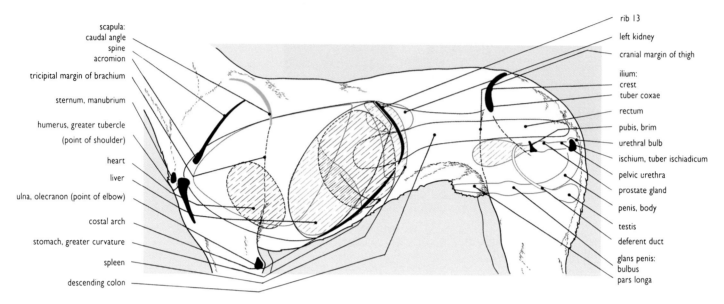

scapula:
caudal angle
spine
acromion

tricipital margin of brachium

sternum, manubrium

humerus, greater tubercle
(point of shoulder)

heart

liver

ulna, olecranon (point of elbow)

costal arch

stomach, greater curvature

spleen

descending colon

rib 13

left kidney

cranial margin of thigh

ilium:
crest
tuber coxae

rectum

pubis, brim

urethral bulb

ischium, tuber ischiadicum

pelvic urethra

prostate gland

penis, body

testis

deferent duct

glans penis:
bulbus
pars longa

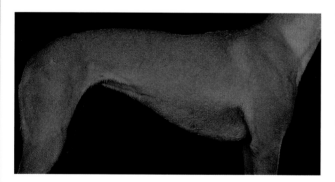

Fig. 1.6 Surface relationships of the thoracic and abdominal viscera of the bitch: lateral view. Visualization of the position of internal viscera is especially important in the thorax since palpation is inapplicable, although some verification of position can be obtained by the experienced veterinary surgeon using percussive and auscultatory techniques. In the abdomen limited palpation is possible through the muscular walls although much of the cavity is occupied by the soft and mobile coils of small intestine. Of the organs depicted in this projection some such as the kidney and the descending colon, if it contains hard faeces, may be palpable but only in thin and cooperative animals. At some stages in pregnancy fetuses in the enlarged uterine horn may also be felt.

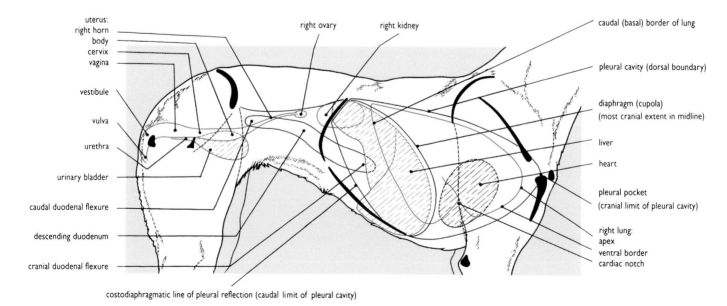

uterus:
right horn
body
cervix
vagina

vestibule

vulva

urethra

urinary bladder

caudal duodenal flexure

descending duodenum

cranial duodenal flexure

right ovary

right kidney

caudal (basal) border of lung

pleural cavity (dorsal boundary)

diaphragm (cupola)
(most cranial extent in midline)

liver

heart

pleural pocket
(cranial limit of pleural cavity)

right lung:
apex
ventral border
cardiac notch

costodiaphragmatic line of pleural reflection (caudal limit of pleural cavity)

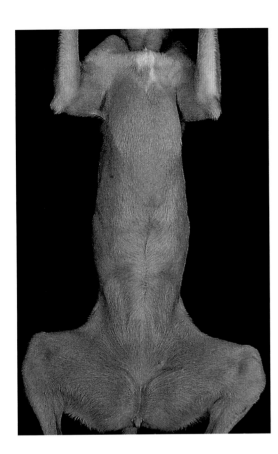

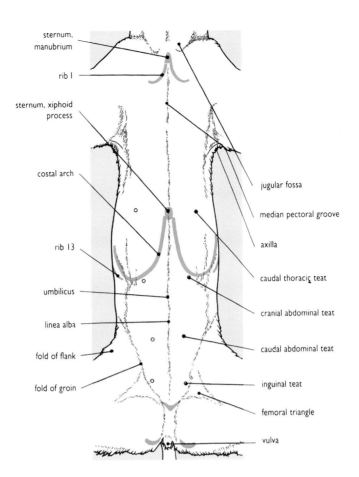

Fig. 1.7 Surface features of the thorax and abdomen of the bitch: ventral view. The major palpable features of the trunk are shown in this picture.

In Fig. 1.7, labels include:
- sternum, manubrium
- rib I
- sternum, xiphoid process
- costal arch
- rib 13
- umbilicus
- linea alba
- fold of flank
- fold of groin
- jugular fossa
- median pectoral groove
- axilla
- caudal thoracic teat
- cranial abdominal teat
- caudal abdominal teat
- inguinal teat
- femoral triangle
- vulva

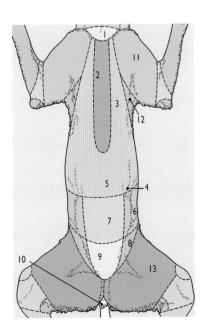

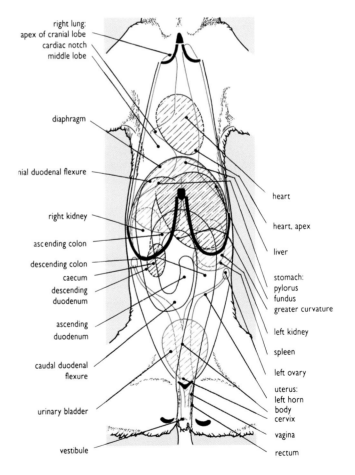

In Fig. 1.8, labels include:
- right lung: apex of cranial lobe, cardiac notch, middle lobe
- diaphragm
- cranial duodenal flexure
- right kidney
- ascending colon
- descending colon
- caecum
- descending duodenum
- ascending duodenum
- caudal duodenal flexure
- urinary bladder
- vestibule
- heart
- heart, apex
- liver
- stomach: pylorus, fundus, greater curvature
- left kidney
- spleen
- left ovary
- uterus: left horn, body, cervix
- vagina
- rectum

Fig. 1.7A Topographical regions: 1–3 Thoracic (Pectoral) Regions. **1** Presternal Region. **2** Sternal Region. **3** Costal Region. **4–9** Abdominal Regions. **4–5** Cranial Abdominal Region. **4** Left Hypochondriac Region. **5** Xiphoid Region. **6–7** Middle Abdominal Region. **6** Left Lateral Abdominal Region. **7** Umbilical Region. **8–9** Caudal Abdominal Region. **8** Left Inguinal Region. **9** Pubic Region, Pelvic Region. **10** Urogenital Component of Perineal Region. **11–12** Forelimb Regions Bordering on Trunk. **11** Brachial Region. **12** Brachial Region, Hindlimb Region Bordering on Trunk. **13** Femoral Region.

Fig. 1.8 Surface relationships of the thoracic and abdominal viscera of the bitch: ventral view. The major internal viscera are shown in surface projection in this picture. NB Surface relationships of viscera, especially thoracic, will be distinctly different when the animal is in dorsal recumbency with its forelimbs pulled forwards and hindlimbs backwards, than they are in the normal standing position and visualized from the lateral aspect.

2. THE HEAD

The head of the dog is often involved in trauma either from accidents or fighting. The position of the subcutaneous vessels is therefore important in these cases. Surgical repair of skin wounds is a common occurrence and damage to eyes, ears and mouth including the tongue is not uncommon. The tongue may also be involved in burns or electrocution. Teeth are also easily damaged by trauma, excessive chewing or foreign bodies. These foreign bodies may be trapped in the tongue, cheeks, soft palate or teeth. It is worth remembering that the oral and nasal orifices provide easy access for pathogens or excess antigens.

The mucous membranes of the mouth, eye, tongue and nose are valuable in the clinical assessment of the cardiovascular system. Paleness (pallor) may indicate anaemia, cyanosis (blue coloration) may be a result of poor oxygenation, and a yellow color indicates jaundice. There are a variety of causes some of which may originate in the liver including toxic, neoplastic and metabolic diseases. Hemorrhage (small or large) may also be seen from any of the vessels and within the mucous membranes. These may be associated with rat poisons in particular. The pulse can be obtained from the linguofacial artery and also the deep artery of the tongue (under the tip).

Most of the large blood vessels of the head and the nerves are protected by deep fascia. However, the cranial nerves V and VII supply the head. The extensive motor distribution of the facial nerve (VII) to the muscles of the head is contrasted with the less apparent distribution of sensory nerves from cranial nerve V which supply the cutaneous innervation of the skin of the head. Cranial nerve VII is easily damaged over the surface of the masseter muscle and therefore facial paralysis is not uncommon. This does not affect the upper eyelid which is supplied by branches of cranial nerve III.

The eyes are valuable in clinical diagnosis giving an impression of alertness and brightness. They are a major indicator of the state of health as retinal examination is possible. The presence of the orbital fat pad is also important. This readily dehydrates, raises the third eyelid and therefore gives a 'hooded' appearance to the eye. In cases of inanition when the orbital fat pad is reduced even further, then more of the third eyelid will be exposed. The eye is further protected laterally and caudally by the orbital ligament so the eye is retained in position. In some exophthalmic breeds, such as the Pekinese, the eye may 'pop out' and can be 'popped back' or enucleated (removed). Removal of the eyelid requires tying off of nerves and blood vessels and removal of the globe. The optic artery attaching to the back of the eye is important and in removal of the globe care should be taken not to pull too strongly or the optic chiasma may be damaged. A variety of clinical operations may be carried out on the eye including superficial keratectomy which is the removal of anterior corneal stroma. Grid keratotomy

and debridement is fairly commonly carried out. Other examples of ocular surgery include entropion, where upper and lower eyelids may turn in onto the eye producing irritation. Effectively, tissue is removed to turn the eyelid out. The opposite condition, ectropion, also occurs and is corrected by shortening the lower lid and supporting with a skin flap. The condition of districhiasis (extra hairs irritating the cornea) and ectopic cilia, can be corrected by partial tarsal plate removal; a strip of eyelid is essentially removed. In cases where the cornea is damaged or ulcerated, it is possible to use conjunctival flaps to cover the cornea to promote healing or to use contact lenses.

Where the eye becomes very dry (keratitis sicca), it is possible to transplant the parotid duct. This condition may be associated with autoimmune disease and can be treated medically (Optimmune) in many cases. It opens at the level of the carnassial tooth (4th upper premolar) on a prominent papilla. The opening of the zygomatic salivary gland is slightly posterior and nearer to the gum margin. The duct is dissected out and transplanted into the upper lateral angle of the eye, or onto the lower conjunctival sac.

In connection with the salivary glands, sometimes these ducts become blocked (mucocele) and the glands become cystic. The sublinguinal/submandibular gland complex can then be removed intact 'in toto' as they are difficult to separate. Care has to be taken to avoid the superficial maxillary vein dorsally and the linguofacial vein ventrally. Radio-opaque dyes injected into the caruncle can be used to discover patency. The mandibular salivary gland is an important structure, palpable in the angle of the jaw and easily confused with the mandibular lymph nodes.

The parotid lymph node is not normally palpable in its position close to the cartilaginous ear canal, but it may be damaged during ear surgery. The mandibular lymph nodes are larger, more important and can be identified in infectious or neoplastic disease. They are palpable just caudal to the ventral border and angle of the mandible. The linguofacial trunk and the parotid duct lie just lateral to these nodes.

The temporomandibular joint may be the seat of pain in some dogs and it can be palpated in front of the base of the ear. It can be felt when the mouth is opened and closed carefully. Dislocation may require replacement under anesthesia. Other conditions affecting the mandible include fracture of the symphysis (requires wiring together) and occasionally fracture of the ramus of the mandible may require surgical correction. This may be iatrogenic in young dogs when removing temporary teeth or lower canines. There is also the specific condition of cranial mandibular osteodystrophy.

Teeth can be vital in helping to estimate the age of dogs, as the pulp cavities narrow with increasing age. It can be more usual to rely upon the degree of tartar formation wear and general health of the gingiva. Teeth are obviously closely associated with mandible and maxillae. A malar abscess may occur around the root of the 4th (carnassial) upper premolar. It may cause swelling of the face below the eye and will eventually fistulate to the skin. It requires removal to allow drainage. It may be necessary to remove persistent temporary teeth usually the canines. Adult canine teeth have a wide root, greater than the alveolus, and require elevators or removal of lateral wall of alveolus to be able to remove a tooth. The upper and lower canine teeth have extensive roots which reach caudally beneath the roots of the first two premolars. The upper carnassial has three roots, is more difficult to remove and is easily damaged by chewing bones etc. It can easily become affected by a root granuloma or a fistula. Prosthetic dentistry is also carried out in show dogs or police dogs. The tonsil may become infected. It is usually obscured by the overlying mucosa of the crypt, but if infected, bulges from the crypt.

Tonsillectomy (removal) may then be required. The palate may be subject to two major problems. There may be the congenital abnormality of a cleft palate. Extra flaps are made by incisions and the palate is then joined to the tonsillar crypts. The soft palate does not normally extend beyond the caudal limit of the tonsillar crypts and should just contact the epiglottis which lies dorsal to the soft palate during normal breathing.

In brachycephalic breeds, the soft palate may be too long and needs to be cut back in size to fit. If cut and left long, the dog will have difficulty breathing (dyspnea) and noisy breathing will result, but if cut too short, food drips into the nasal cavity during swallowing. The endotracheal tube can be placed from oral cavity into larynx and trachea requires the soft palate to be elevated dorsally to expose the epiglottis and then the tube enters the *aditus laryngis*.

Ears can be the cause of many clinical problems; bitten, trapped and haematomas. Infection of the external ear (*otitis externa*) is the most common of all ear complaints. Infection of the inner ear can produce facial paralysis. In canines, otitis media can affect sympathetic fibers that run through the middle ear. Aural hematomas require removal of the blood and stitching flat to a matrix. There are some methods that include mattress sutures and drain placements but in many of these cases the problem recurs. A considerable amount of veterinary activity focuses on blocked auditory canals (too much hair, too much wax, foreign bodies). The problem is that there is a vertical canal which fills up, provides an excellent breeding place for pathogens, and does not self-clean easily. This is worse in flap-eared breeds with long hair such as spaniels. It has to be de-haired and cleaned by auroscope. Occasionally, this is not sufficient and has to be extended to an aural resection. In this the ventral part of the external auditory canal is ablated and this leads to increased aeration and drainage with horizontal canal opening directly to the skin. It can only be used when the horizontal canal is in good clinical condition.

The tympanic bulla is located medial to the muscular process of the mandible and great cornu of the hyoid bone. The bullae can be opened ventrally for drainage. Great care has to be taken to avoid damaging the surrounding structures including the hypoglossal nerve, internal carotid artery and internal maxillary vessels. Debris is removed and the secretory tissue as well as any inflamed tissue, and the site cleaned. It can be removed by lateral or ventral bullar osteotomy.

The last of the major clinical areas is the nostril and nasal cavity. The nasal cavity may become infected or may be the seat of trapping of foreign bodies. This is rarely done but occasionally for the treatment of conditions such as nasal aspergillosis. The nasal cavity can be examined by rhinoscopy for signs of obstruction and the nasolacrimal duct can also be checked for patency. In cases of persistent purulent nasal discharge or the occurrence of polyps, it is possible to carry out rhinectomy (removal of the conchal bones) with a midline incision from the frontal sinus to the rostral end of the nasal bones. Parallel incisions remove the central bone and the conchal bones are then removed, hemostasis applied and the skin incision stitched without the underlying bone fragment.

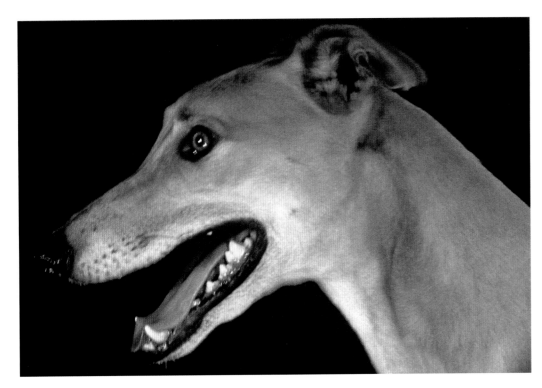

Fig. 2.1 Surface features of the head: left lateral view. The major bony features that are readily palpable and/or visible on the surface of the head are indicated in this figure. These 'points' correspond to those colored green on the bones illustrated in Fig. 2.2. Additional palpable features include the thyroid cartilage, the orbital ligament, the temporal and masseter muscles, and the mandibular lymph nodes. The position of the temporomandibular joint rostral to the base of the auricular cartilage is also readily palpable when the mouth is opened and closed carefully. Figs 2.55, 2.59 and 2.125 show the surface of the head from dorsal and ventral views and should be compared with this figure.

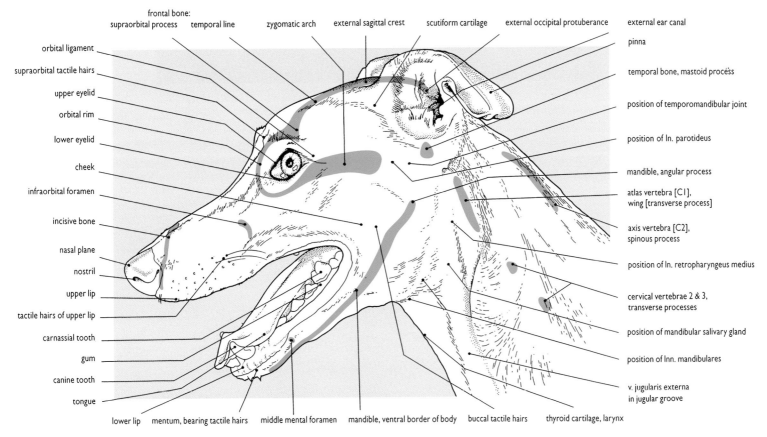

frontal bone:
supraorbital process temporal line zygomatic arch external sagittal crest scutiform cartilage external occipital protuberance external ear canal

orbital ligament
supraorbital tactile hairs
upper eyelid
orbital rim
lower eyelid
cheek
infraorbital foramen
incisive bone
nasal plane
nostril
upper lip
tactile hairs of upper lip
carnassial tooth
gum
canine tooth
tongue

pinna
temporal bone, mastoid process
position of temporomandibular joint
position of ln. parotideus
mandible, angular process
atlas vertebra [C1], wing [transverse process]
axis vertebra [C2], spinous process
position of ln. retropharyngeus medius
cervical vertebrae 2 & 3, transverse processes
position of mandibular salivary gland
position of lnn. mandibulares
v. jugularis externa in jugular groove

lower lip   mentum, bearing tactile hairs   middle mental foramen   mandible, ventral border of body   buccal tactile hairs   thyroid cartilage, larynx

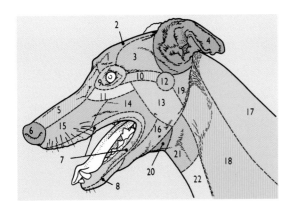

Fig. 2.1A Topographical regions of the head: left lateral view. The major topographical regions into which the head is descriptively subdivided are shown in this drawing. These regions are based upon the bones or soft tissues underlying them. **1–4** Cranial Region. **1** Frontal Region. **2** Parietal Region. **3** Temporal Region. **4** Auricular Region. **5–16** Facial Regions. **5–6** Nasal Regions. **5** Dorsal and lateral Nasal Regions. **6** Nostril Region. **7** Oral Region. **8** Mental Region. **9** Orbital Region. **10** Zygomatic Region. **11** Infraorbital Region. **12** Temporomandibular Joint Region. **13** Masseteric Region. **14** Buccal Region. **15** Maxillary Region. **16** Mandibular Region. **17–22** Neck Regions. **17** Dorsal Neck Region. **18** Lateral Neck Region. **19** Parotid Region. **20** Pharyngeal Region. **21–22** Ventral Neck Regions. **21** Laryngeal Region. **22** Tracheal Region.

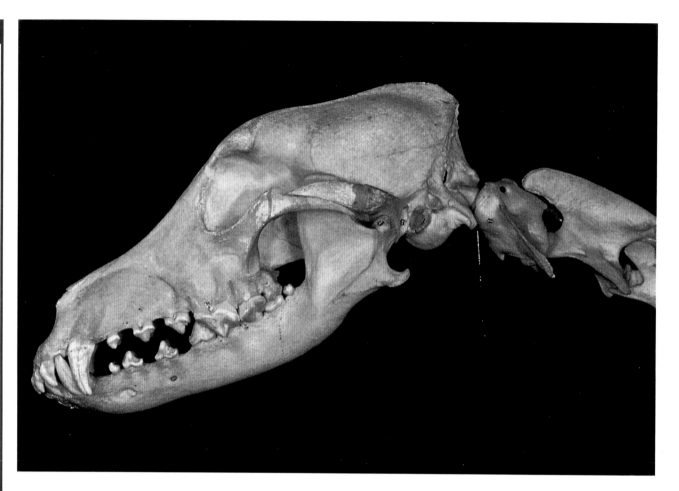

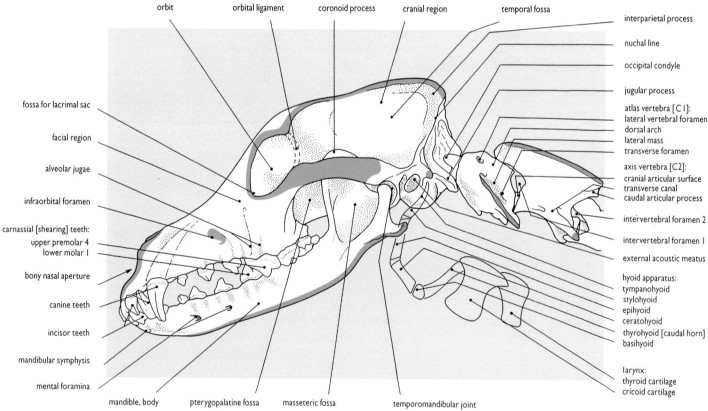

orbit   orbital ligament   coronoid process   cranial region   temporal fossa

interparietal process

nuchal line

occipital condyle

jugular process

atlas vertebra [C 1]:
lateral vertebral foramen
dorsal arch
lateral mass
transverse foramen

axis vertebra [C2]:
cranial articular surface
transverse canal
caudal articular process

intervertebral foramen 2

intervertebral foramen 1

external acoustic meatus

hyoid apparatus:
tympanohyoid
stylohyoid
epihyoid
ceratohyoid
thyrohyoid [caudal horn]
basihyoid

larynx:
thyroid cartilage
cricoid cartilage

fossa for lacrimal sac

facial region

alveolar jugae

infraorbital foramen

carnassial [shearing] teeth:
upper premolar 4
lower molar I

bony nasal aperture

canine teeth

incisor teeth

mandibular symphysis

mental foramina

mandible, body   pterygopalatine fossa   masseteric fossa   temporomandibular joint

Fig. 2.2 Skeleton of the head: left lateral view. The palpable bony features shown in Fig. 2.1 are colored green on this skull and first three cervical vertebrae. Absent from this skeletal preparation are the hyoid apparatus (the component parts and topographical position are shown in dissections of the pharyngeal region – from lateral view in Figs 2.78–2.83; from medial view in Figs 2.93 and 2.94; and from ventral view in Figs 2.129–2.133), the nasal cartilages (shown in Figs 2.99–2.106), and the auricular cartilages (shown in Figs 2.32 and 2.33, and Figs 2.61–2.67). In addition to distinct palpable 'points', large areas of bone can also be felt through the overlying musculature, particularly in the facial region.

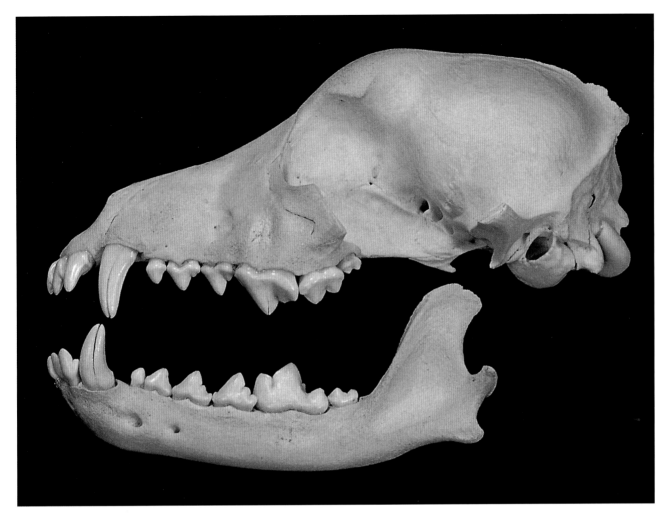

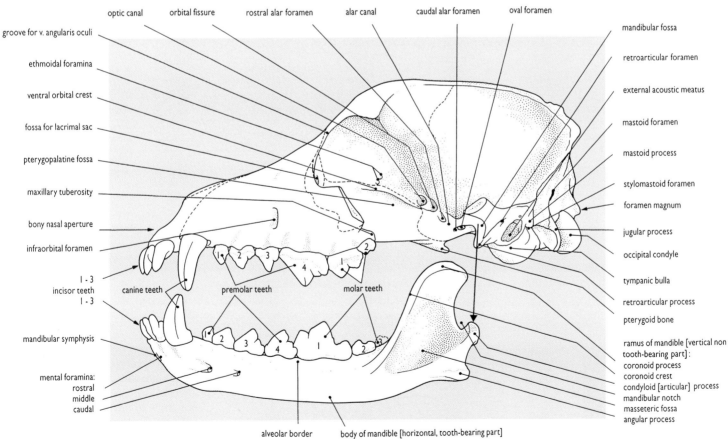

optic canal   orbital fissure   rostral alar foramen   alar canal   caudal alar foramen   oval foramen

groove for v. angularis oculi

ethmoidal foramina

ventral orbital crest

fossa for lacrimal sac

pterygopalatine fossa

maxillary tuberosity

bony nasal aperture

infraorbital foramen

I - 3
incisor teeth
I - 3

canine teeth   premolar teeth   molar teeth

mandibular symphysis

mental foramina:
rostral
middle
caudal

mandibular fossa

retroarticular foramen

external acoustic meatus

mastoid foramen

mastoid process

stylomastoid foramen

foramen magnum

jugular process

occipital condyle

tympanic bulla

retroarticular process

pterygoid bone

ramus of mandible [vertical non
tooth-bearing part] :
coronoid process
coronoid crest
condyloid [articular] process
mandibular notch
masseteric fossa
angular process

alveolar border   body of mandible [horizontal, tooth-bearing part]

Fig. 2.3 Skull after removal of the zygomatic arch and disarticulation of the lower jaw: left lateral view. The lower jaw (mandible) has been disarticulated at the temporomandibular joint and dropped ventrally and the zygomatic arch has been removed, opening the temporal and pterygopalatine fossae laterally. A number of foramina are displayed, the identification of which will provide an additional basis for interpretation of the course of the nerves and blood vessels in the detailed dissections. It should be noted that in this specimen the third lower molar tooth is absent.

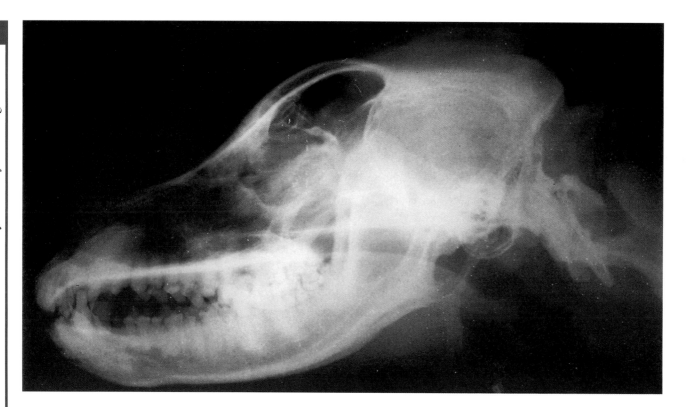

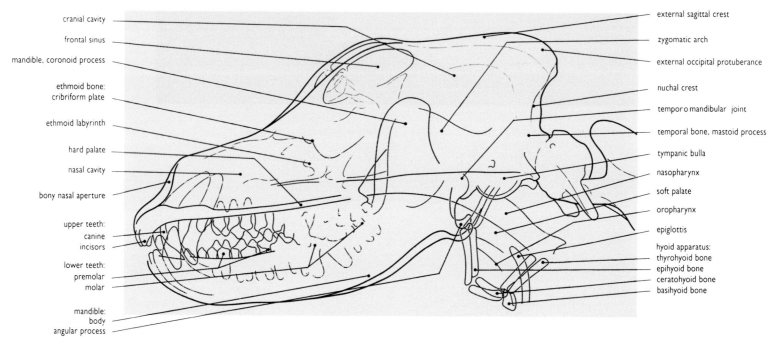

cranial cavity

frontal sinus

mandible, coronoid process

ethmoid bone:
cribriform plate

ethmoid labyrinth

hard palate

nasal cavity

bony nasal aperture

upper teeth:
canine
incisors

lower teeth:
premolar
molar

mandible:
body
angular process

external sagittal crest

zygomatic arch

external occipital protuberance

nuchal crest

temporo mandibular joint

temporal bone, mastoid process

tympanic bulla

nasopharynx

soft palate

oropharynx

epiglottis

hyoid apparatus:
thyrohyoid bone
epihyoid bone
ceratohyoid bone
basihyoid bone

Fig. 2.4 Radiograph of the head: left lateral view. The features pointed out here are primarily those palpable from the surface. Included also are such structures as the cribriform plate internally marking the boundary of cranial and nasal cavities. More detailed aspects of internal skull anatomy are specifically excluded from radiographic consideration and are dealt with osteologically later.

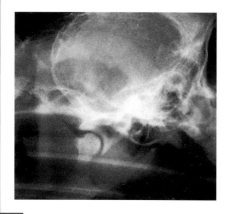

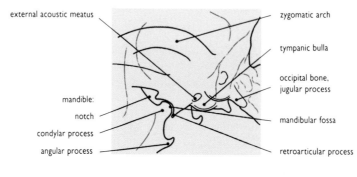

external acoustic meatus

mandible:

notch

condylar process

angular process

zygomatic arch

tympanic bulla

occipital bone,
jugular process

mandibular fossa

retroarticular process

Fig. 2.5 Radiograph of the temporomandibular joint: oblique lateral view. The jaw joint does not show to advantage in lateral radiographs because of extensive superimposition. It can be shown through using a slight alteration in the angle of view when it is projected within the air density of the nasopharynx.

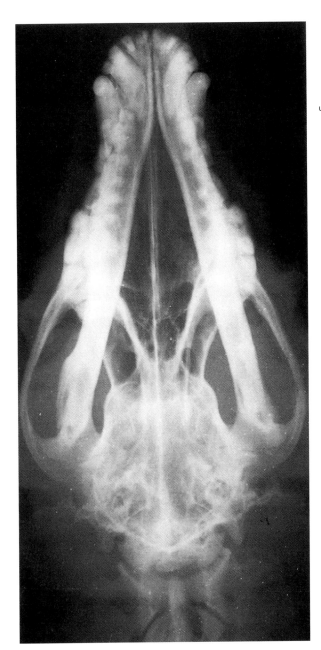

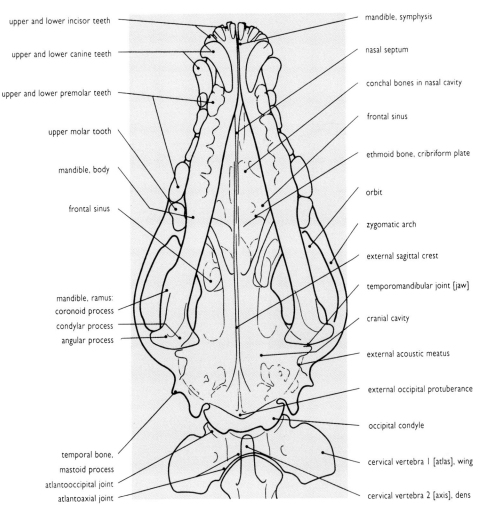

upper and lower incisor teeth

upper and lower canine teeth

upper and lower premolar teeth

upper molar tooth

mandible, body

frontal sinus

mandible, ramus:
coronoid process
condylar process
angular process

temporal bone,
mastoid process
atlantooccipital joint
atlantoaxial joint

mandible, symphysis

nasal septum

conchal bones in nasal cavity

frontal sinus

ethmoid bone, cribriform plate

orbit

zygomatic arch

external sagittal crest

temporomandibular joint [jaw]

cranial cavity

external acoustic meatus

external occipital protuberance

occipital condyle

cervical vertebra I [atlas], wing

cervical vertebra 2 [axis], dens

Fig. 2.6 Radiograph of the head: ventrodorsal view. Only the major features are pointed out here, as in fig 2.4. Of particular note is the transverse orientation of the temporomandibular joints and the somewhat narrower lower jaw and lower dental arcade. With jaw action being hinge-like the teeth of the lower dental arcade, especially the first lower molar tooth, show a shearing bite against the lingual surfaces of the teeth of the upper arcade.

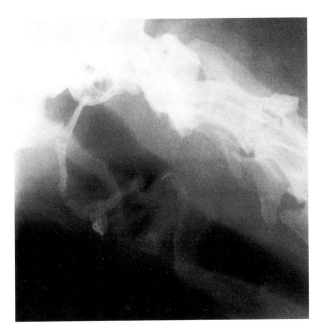

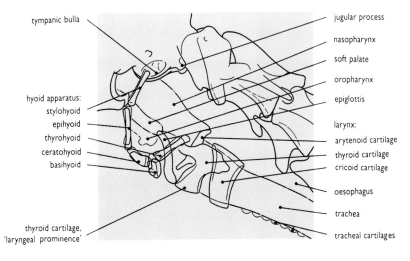

tympanic bulla

hyoid apparatus:
stylohyoid
epihyoid
thyrohyoid
ceratohyoid
basihyoid

thyroid cartilage,
'laryngeal prominence'

jugular process

nasopharynx

soft palate

oropharynx

epiglottis

larynx:
arytenoid cartilage
thyroid cartilage
cricoid cartilage

oesophagus

trachea

tracheal cartilages

Fig. 2.7 Radiograph of the hyoid apparatus and larynx: lateral view. Since the uppermost hyoid element (tympanohyoid) on either side is cartilaginous, it is radiolucent. However, the laryngeal cartilages are sufficiently dense and have some degree of calcification so that their outlines are apparent.

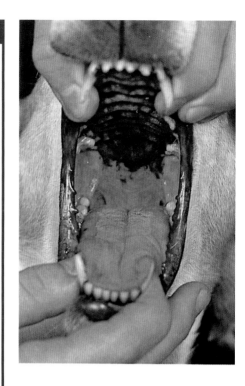

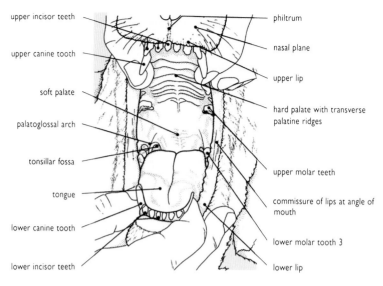

upper incisor teeth

upper canine tooth

soft palate

palatoglossal arch

tonsillar fossa

tongue

lower canine tooth

lower incisor teeth

philtrum

nasal plane

upper lip

hard palate with transverse palatine ridges

upper molar teeth

commissure of lips at angle of mouth

lower molar tooth 3

lower lip

Fig. 2.8 Surface features of the head with mouth open: rostral view. When the mouth is closed the tongue practically fills the oral cavity (see also Fig. 2.143 of the head in transverse section): an open mouth displays mucous membrane covering the tongue and palate and lining the inside of the cheeks. The length of the soft palate should be noted (see also Fig. 2.87) since in brachycephalic breeds it may interfere with air flow through the larynx.

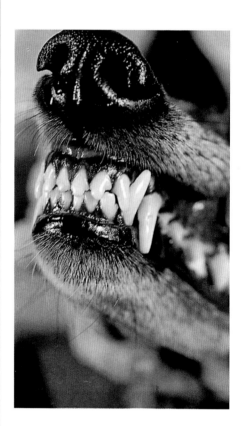

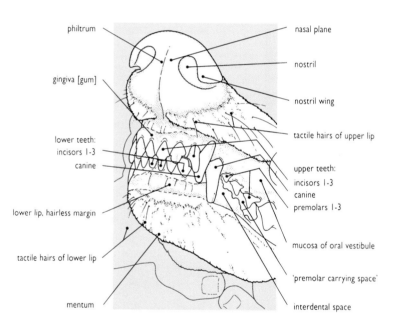

philtrum

gingiva [gum]

lower teeth:
incisors 1-3
canine

lower lip, hairless margin

tactile hairs of lower lip

mentum

nasal plane

nostril

nostril wing

tactile hairs of upper lip

upper teeth:
incisors 1-3
canine
premolars 1-3

mucosa of oral vestibule

'premolar carrying space'

interdental space

Fig. 2.9 Surface features of the muzzle: rostrolateral view. The bite between incisor and canine teeth is shown on baring the teeth. The greater normal length of the upper jaw means that upper incisors bite on the labial surfaces of the lowers. The relationship of the teeth to the lips and nostrils is also shown, the looseness of the lips and cheeks enclosing a large oral vestibule. The angle of the mouth is level with cheek tooth 3 or 4, the cheek is therefore a fairly restricted area and a wide gape is possible.

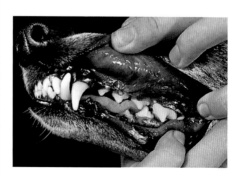

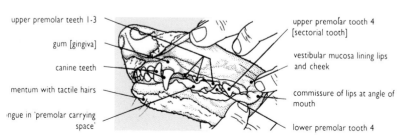

upper premolar teeth 1-3

gum [gingiva]

canine teeth

mentum with tactile hairs

tongue in 'premolar carrying space'

upper premolar tooth 4 [sectorial tooth]

vestibular mucosa lining lips and cheek

commissure of lips at angle of mouth

lower premolar tooth 4

Fig. 2.10 Teeth: left lateral view. The interlocking bite between incisor and canine teeth and the extensive overlap between shearing teeth is contrasted with the absence of occlusion between the more rostral premolars in the 'premolar carrying space'.

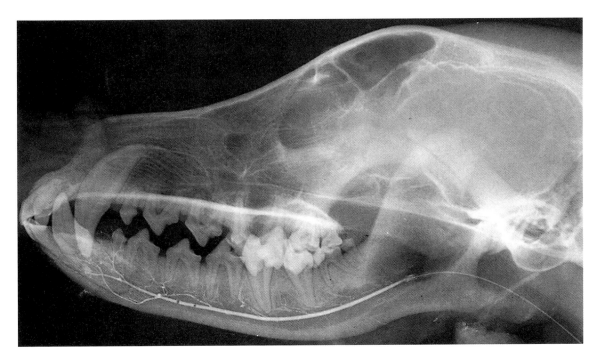

Fig. 2.11 Radiograph of the jaws and permanent teeth: lateral view. Superimposition of upper and lower jaws in a lateral view creates a confusing image of the dental arcades (see fig. 2.4). For this reason a sagittally sectioned head has been radiographed and the permanent dentition on only one side of each jaw is shown. The sectorial (carnassial) teeth – upper fourth premolar and lower first molar – have been labelled in the drawing. The permanent dental formula is:

$$2 \left(I \frac{3}{3} \quad C \frac{1}{1} \quad PM \frac{4}{4} \quad M \frac{2}{3} \right) = 42$$

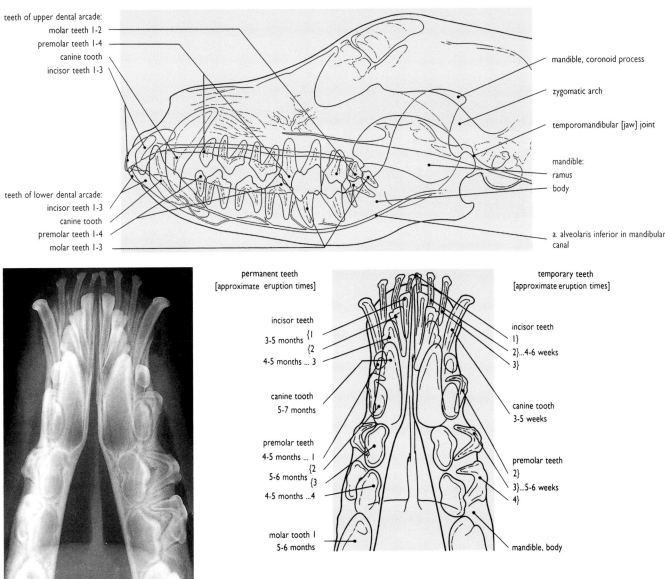

teeth of upper dental arcade:
molar teeth 1-2
premolar teeth 1-4
canine tooth
incisor teeth 1-3

mandible, coronoid process

zygomatic arch

temporomandibular [jaw] joint

mandible:
ramus
body

teeth of lower dental arcade:
incisor teeth 1-3
canine tooth
premolar teeth 1-4
molar teeth 1-3

a. alveolaris inferior in mandibular canal

permanent teeth
[approximate eruption times]

temporary teeth
[approximate eruption times]

incisor teeth
3-5 months {1
{2
4-5 months ... 3

incisor teeth
1}
2}...4-6 weeks
3}

canine tooth
5-7 months

canine tooth
3-5 weeks

premolar teeth
4-5 months ... 1
{2
5-6 months {3
4-5 months ...4

premolar teeth
2}
3}...5-6 weeks
4}

molar tooth 1
5-6 months

mandible, body

Fig. 2.12 Radiograph of the lower jaw temporary and permanent teeth: dorsoventral view. The deciduous and developing permanent teeth are shown in this radiograph. The deciduous dental formula present by two months of age is:

$$2 \left(I \frac{3}{3} \quad C \frac{1}{1} \quad PM \frac{3}{3} \right) = 28$$

Replacement begins at about 3 months of age, to be completed by about 7 months, although there is some variation in the timing of tooth eruption depending on breed and size. Premolar 1 (clearly visible) is without a deciduous precursor and erupts between 4 and 5 months.

Veterinary Anatomy: The Dog and Cat

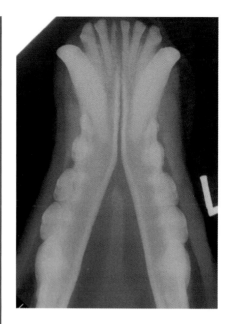

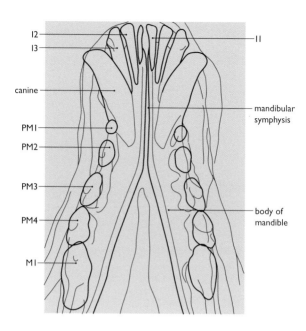

I2
I3
canine
PM1
PM2
PM3
PM4
M1
I1
mandibular symphysis
body of mandible

Fig. 2.13 Radiograph of the mandible: ventrodorsal intraoral view.

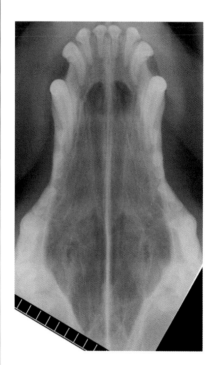

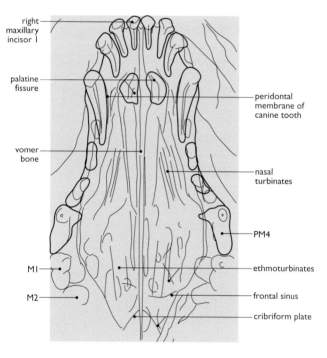

right maxillary incisor 1
palatine fissure
vomer bone
M1
M2
peridontal membrane of canine tooth
nasal turbinates
PM4
ethmoturbinates
frontal sinus
cribriform plate

Fig. 2.14 Radiograph of the maxilla and nasal chambers: dorsoventral intraoral view. The tooth roots appear foreshortened in this view as they are angled relative to the x-ray beam. The two nasal chambers can be seen without superimposition.

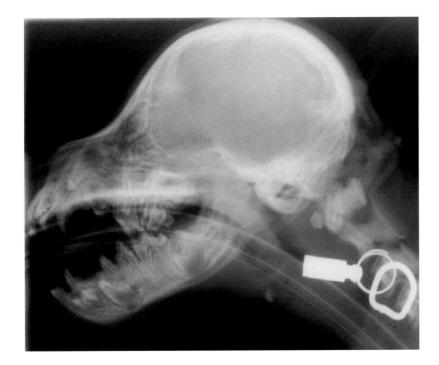

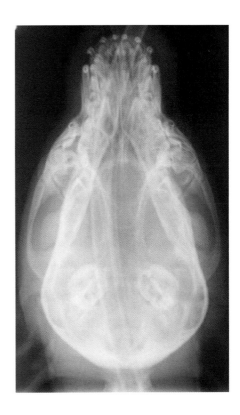

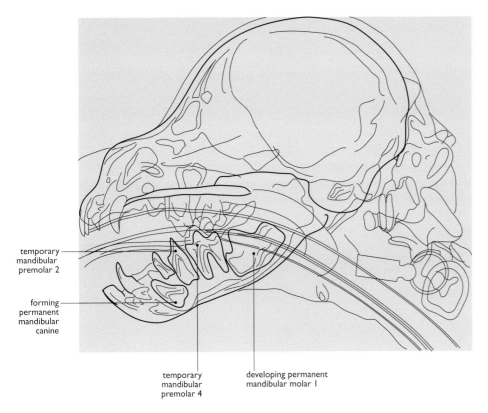

temporary mandibular premolar 2

forming permanent mandibular canine

temporary mandibular premolar 4

developing permanent mandibular molar 1

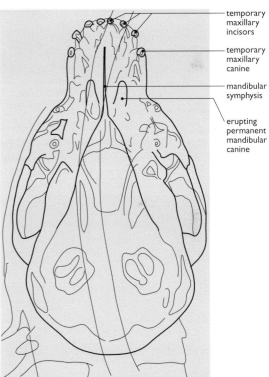

temporary maxillary incisors

temporary maxillary canine

mandibular symphysis

erupting permanent mandibular canine

Fig. 2.15 Radiograph of the head: lateral view, dentally immature dog. The developing permanent teeth can be seen within the maxilla and the mandible. The deciduous teeth, including their roots, are slender.

Fig. 2.16 Radiograph of the head: ventrodorsal view, dentally immature dog. The permanent teeth develop medial to their deciduous counterparts and grow out laterally. The suture between the zygomatic process of the temporal bone and the temporal process of the zygomatic bone is visible in this young dog.

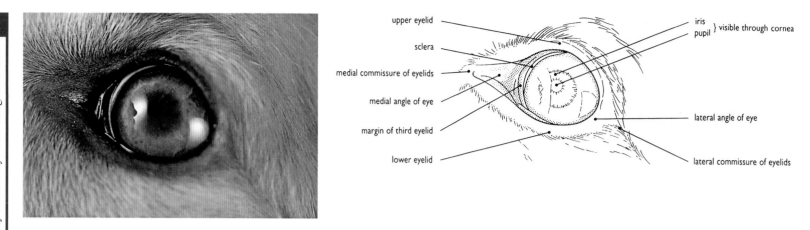

upper eyelid
sclera
medial commissure of eyelids
medial angle of eye
margin of third eyelid
lower eyelid

iris
pupil } visible through cornea

lateral angle of eye

lateral commissure of eyelids

Fig. 2.17 Surface features of the eye: left lateral view (1). The eye is shown with eyelids open. The palpable bony orbital margin is completed laterally by an orbital ligament linking the supraorbital process with the zygomatic arch (*cf.* Fig. 2.39). A dog has quite a wide field of view, in the order of 240°, and there is some measure of overlap between the fields of left and right eyes when it is looking straight ahead.

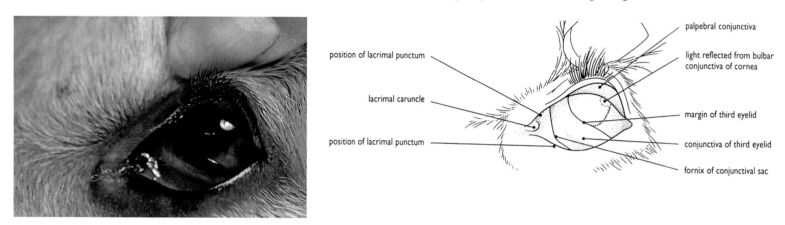

position of lacrimal punctum
lacrimal caruncle
position of lacrimal punctum

palpebral conjunctiva
light reflected from bulbar conjunctiva of cornea
margin of third eyelid
conjunctiva of third eyelid
fornix of conjunctival sac

Fig. 2.18 Surface features of the eye: left lateral view (2). The third eyelid has been exposed by manual pressure exerted through the eyelids. This procedure pushes the eyeball slightly into the orbit compressing intraorbital fat. A normal component of orbital fat is important for holding the eyeball firmly against the inner surfaces of the lids and causing it to protrude a sufficient distance beyond the orbital margin.

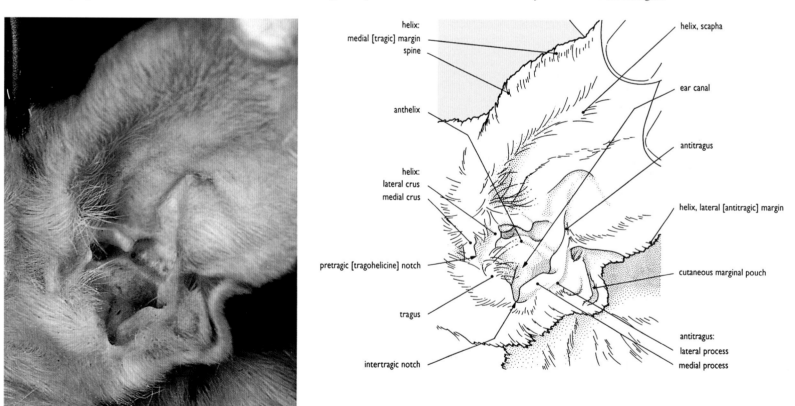

helix:
medial [tragic] margin
spine
anthelix

helix:
lateral crus
medial crus

pretragic [tragohelicine] notch

tragus

intertragic notch

helix, scapha

ear canal

antitragus

helix, lateral [antitragic] margin

cutaneous marginal pouch

antitragus:
lateral process
medial process

Fig. 2.19 Surface features of the ear: left lateral view. The helix of the pinna has been raised and held erect. From the opening visible in the picture the ear canal extends downwards almost vertically and then turns inwards and forwards at 90° towards the eardrum (see also Fig. 2.145 of the head in transverse section). Consequently lateral traction on the pinna will straighten the canal.

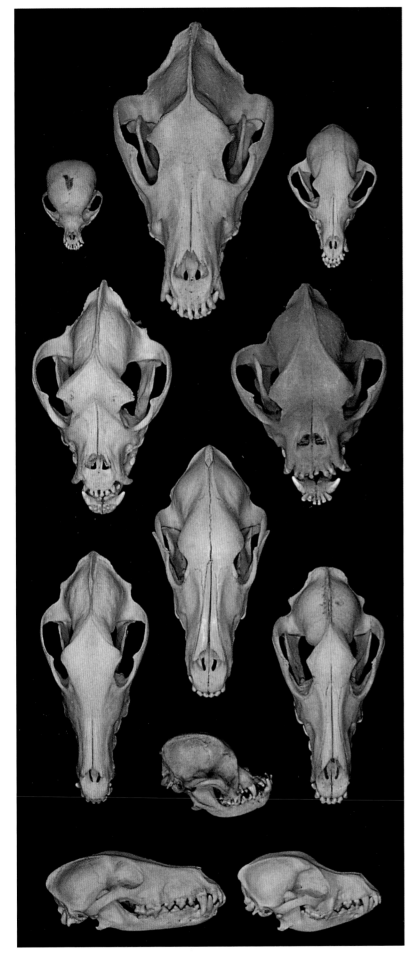

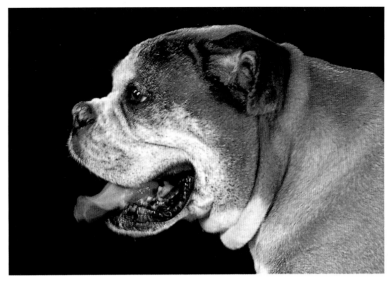

Fig. 2.20 Skeletal basis of variation in conformation of the head: dorsal and lateral views. The shape of the head is determined in large measure by the skull, and in particular the facial region. Within the spectrum of skull construction, three broad categories are generally recognized – brachycephalic, mesaticephalic and dolichocephalic. The montage of skulls in the accompanying illustration shows all three categories; e.g. bulldog (brachycephalic), basset hound (mesaticephalic), and rough collie (dolichocephalic). It is the facial part of the skull that is shortened/widened in brachycephalics, but lengthened/narrowed in dolichocephalics. These categories refer specifically to head type and say nothing about the rest of the body. This fact is demonstrated by the three lateral views at the foot of the page – brachycephalic (Pekinese), mesaticephalic (dachshund), and dolichocephalic (Sealyham terrier). The lateral views also show the difference in level between the dorsal contours of the cranium and face. Although in approximately parallel planes, the marked step down from cranial to facial level produces the nasofrontal angle or 'stop'. In brachycephalic breeds the shortened broadened face is coupled with a deepened stop and eyes that are directed more forwards. Selective breeding has also produced a discrepancy in length between upper and lower jaws – a short face is generally prognathic with an undershot lower jaw: a long face is often accompanied by a brachygnathic, receding lower jaw. The montage also demonstrates the enormous intraspecific size range, especially well displayed by the juxtaposed Chihuahua and Great Dane skulls at the top of the page. The head of a brachycephalic breed (boxer) is also displayed at the top of the page.

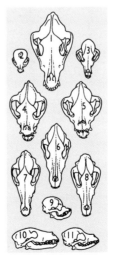

1. Great Dane

2. Chihuahua

3. Yorkshire Terrier

4. Boxer

5. Bulldog

6. Basset Hound

7. Rough Collie

8. Dobermann Pinsc

9. Pekingese

10. Sealyham Terrier

11. Dachshund

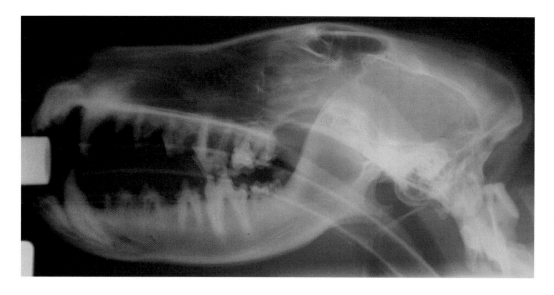

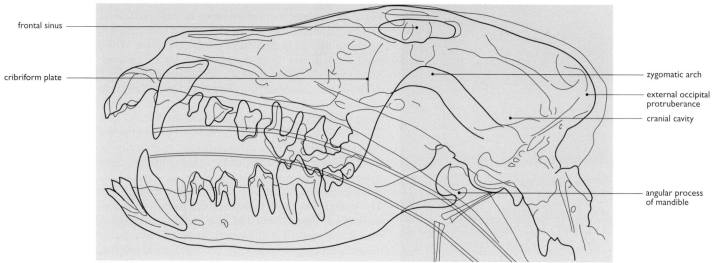

frontal sinus

cribriform plate

zygomatic arch

external occipital protruberance

cranial cavity

angular process of mandible

Fig. 2.21 Radiograph of the head: lateral view, dolichocephalic breed. The nose is elongated and there is little 'stop'. The frontal sinus is flattened dorsoventrally.

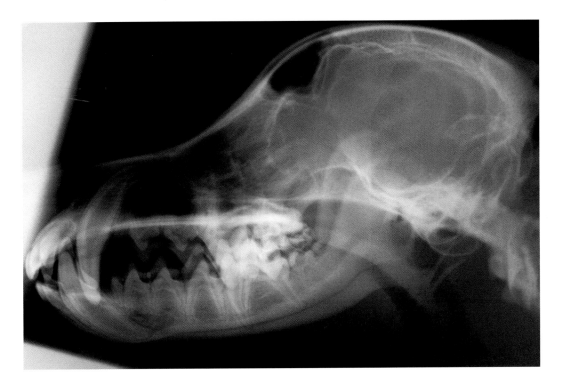

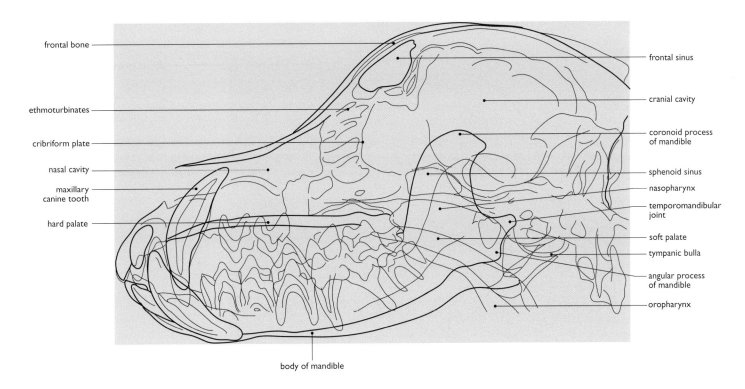

frontal bone

ethmoturbinates

cribriform plate

nasal cavity

maxillary
canine tooth

hard palate

frontal sinus

cranial cavity

coronoid process
of mandible

sphenoid sinus

nasopharynx

temporomandibular
joint

soft palate

tympanic bulla

angular process
of mandible

oropharynx

body of mandible

Fig. 2.22 Radiograph of the head: lateral view, mesaticephalic breed. The nose and cranium comprise equal proportions of the skull.

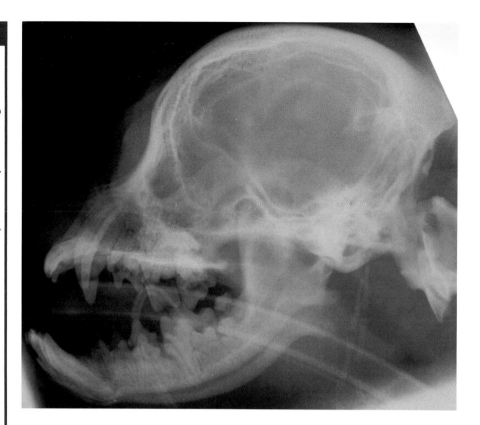

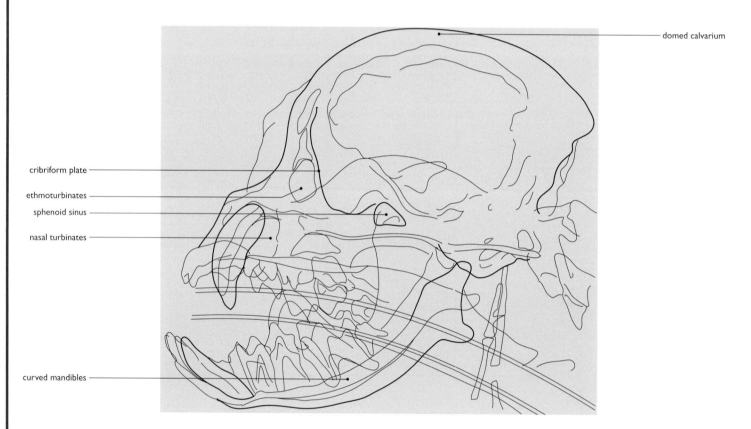

domed calvarium

cribriform plate

ethmoturbinates

sphenoid sinus

nasal turbinates

curved mandibles

Fig. 2.23 Radiograph of the head: lateral view, brachycephalic breed. The nose is markedly shortened and there is a pronounced 'stop'. The frontal sinus is virtually absent. The cranium is domed and the mandible has a convex contour. Mandibular prognathism is present.

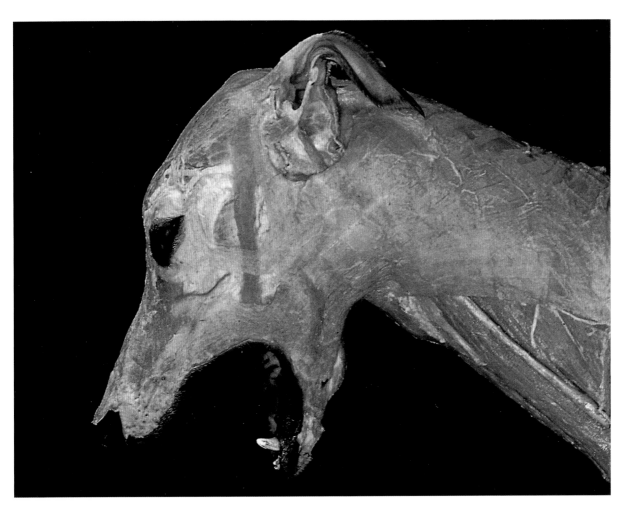

Fig. 2.24 Superficial structures of the head and cranial end of the neck: left lateral view. The skin has been removed apart from a narrow rim in the lips, around the nostril and eye, and on the distal part of the scapha of the auricular cartilage. Because the animal was embalmed with jaws open and head bent down slightly on the neck, the fat and fascia on the underside of the 'throat' was preserved as a compressed and 'waterlogged' mass. In the process of removing this mass the few delicate transverse strands of the sphincter colli superficialis muscle were removed (see Fig. 3.6). The superficial structures of the head are also shown from dorsal view in Figs 2.57 and 2.61, and from ventral view in Fig. 2.125.

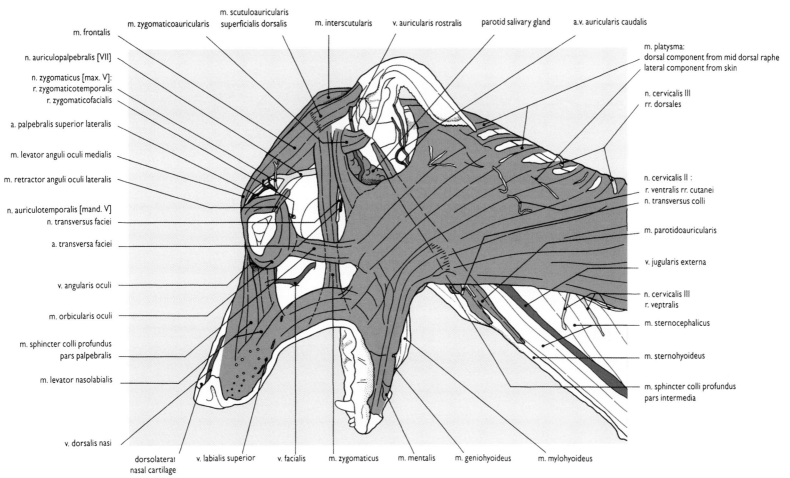

m. frontalis
n. auriculopalpebralis [VII]
n. zygomaticus [max. V]:
r. zygomaticotemporalis
r. zygomaticofacialis
a. palpebralis superior lateralis
m. levator anguli oculi medialis
m. retractor anguli oculi lateralis
n. auriculotemporalis [mand. V]
n. transversus faciei
a. transversa faciei
v. angularis oculi
m. orbicularis oculi
m. sphincter colli profundus pars palpebralis
m. levator nasolabialis
v. dorsalis nasi
dorsolateral nasal cartilage
v. labialis superior
v. facialis
m. zygomaticus
m. mentalis
m. geniohyoideus
m. mylohyoideus

m. zygomaticoauricularis
m. scutuloauricularis superficialis dorsalis
m. interscutularis
v. auricularis rostralis
parotid salivary gland
a.v. auricularis caudalis
m. platysma:
dorsal component from mid dorsal raphe
lateral component from skin
n. cervicalis III rr. dorsales
n. cervicalis II :
r. ventralis rr. cutanei
n. transversus colli
m. parotidoauricularis
v. jugularis externa
n. cervicalis III r. ventralis
m. sternocephalicus
m. sternohyoideus
m. sphincter colli profundus pars intermedia

25

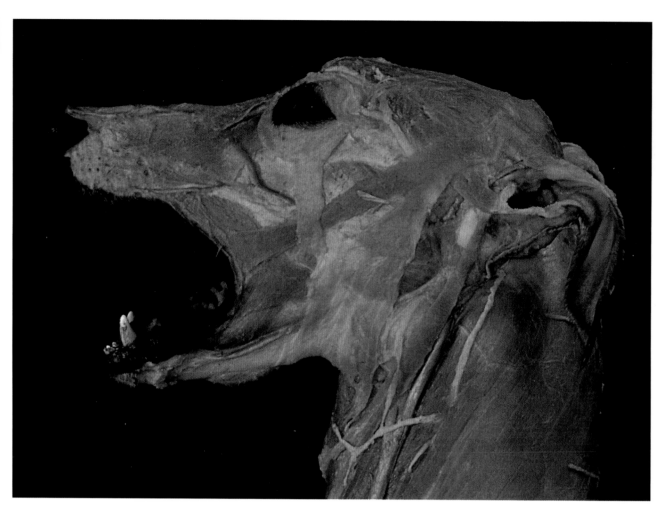

Fig. 2.25 Superficial structures of the head after removal of the platysma muscle: left lateral view. Muscle fibers from the dorsal border of the platysma are inter-mingled with those of the intermediate component so that severance of this association on platysma removal has left a 'ragged' line on the surface of the intermediate at the area labelled 'X' on the drawing. Complete removal of the orbicularis oris muscle is difficult since its fibers intermingle with those of the levator nasolabialis. Some of its place amongst the roots and follicles of the sensory tactile hairs. The mental muscle is infiltrated with fat and fibrous tissue in the mentum and therefore its limits are difficult to define.

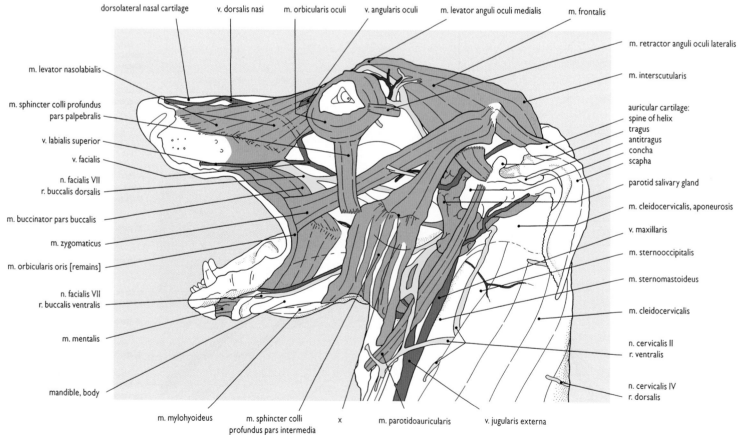

dorsolateral nasal cartilage — v. dorsalis nasi — m. orbicularis oculi — v. angularis oculi — m. levator anguli oculi medialis — m. frontalis

m. levator nasolabialis

m. sphincter colli profundus pars palpebralis

v. labialis superior

v. facialis

n. facialis VII
r. buccalis dorsalis

m. buccinator pars buccalis

m. zygomaticus

m. orbicularis oris [remains]

n. facialis VII
r. buccalis ventralis

m. mentalis

mandible, body

m. retractor anguli oculi lateralis

m. interscutularis

auricular cartilage:
spine of helix
tragus
antitragus
concha
scapha

parotid salivary gland

m. cleidocervicalis, aponeurosis

v. maxillaris

m. sternooccipitalis

m. sternomastoideus

m. cleidocervicalis

n. cervicalis II
r. ventralis

n. cervicalis IV
r. dorsalis

m. mylohyoideus — m. sphincter colli profundus pars intermedia — x — m. parotidoauricularis — v. jugularis externa

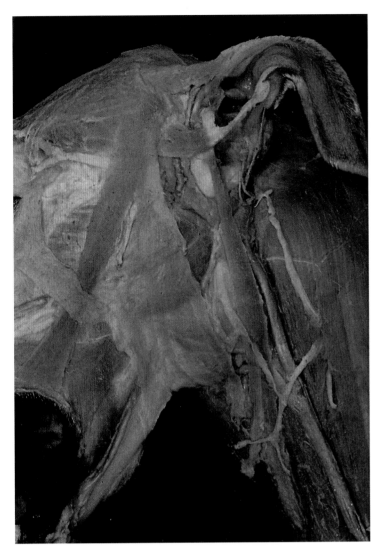

Fig. 2.26 Superficial structures of the temporal, auricular, parotid and masseteric regions after removal of the platysma muscle: left lateral view. This is a closer view of part of the dissection shown in Fig. 2.25. Some limited cleaning of superficial fascia from around the concha of the auricular cartilage exposes the parotid salivary gland and the proximal part of its duct. Cutaneous innervation of the head is through the trigeminal nerve (V), some of the branches being displayed in this dissection (see also Fig. 2.58). However, many of its terminal ramifications have been unavoidably removed along with the skin and platysma muscle so that at best only the proximal stumps of such nerves are preserved intact.

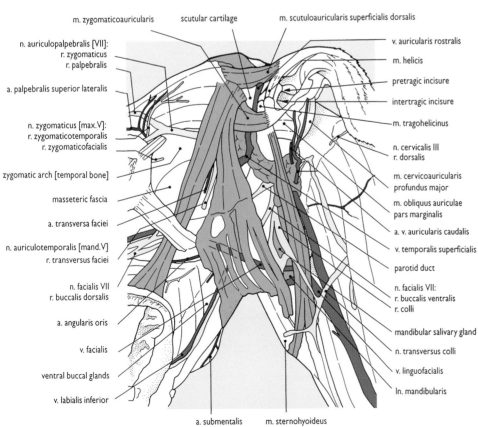

m. zygomaticoauricularis

scutular cartilage

m. scutuloauricularis superficialis dorsalis

n. auriculopalpebralis [VII]:
r. zygomaticus
r. palpebralis

a. palpebralis superior lateralis

n. zygomaticus [max.V]:
r. zygomaticotemporalis
r. zygomaticofacialis

zygomatic arch [temporal bone]

masseteric fascia

a. transversa faciei

n. auriculotemporalis [mand.V]
r. transversus faciei

n. facialis VII
r. buccalis dorsalis

a. angularis oris

v. facialis

ventral buccal glands

v. labialis inferior

a. submentalis

m. sternohyoideus

v. auricularis rostralis

m. helicis

pretragic incisure

intertragic incisure

m. tragohelicinus

n. cervicalis III
r. dorsalis

m. cervicoauricularis
profundus major

m. obliquus auriculae
pars marginalis

a. v. auricularis caudalis

v. temporalis superficialis

parotid duct

n. facialis VII:
r. buccalis ventralis
r. colli

mandibular salivary gland

n. transversus colli

v. linguofacialis

ln. mandibularis

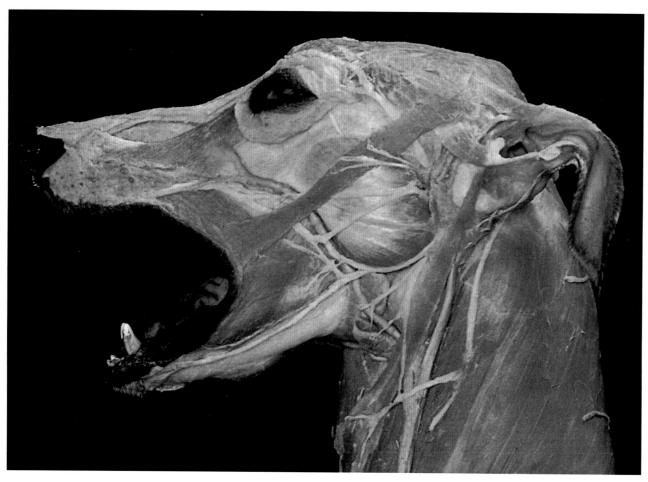

Fig. 2.27 Superficial structures of the head after removal of the platysma and sphincter colli profundus muscles: left lateral view. The intermediate component of the sphincter colli profundus and the nasofrontal part of the levator nasolabialis muscle have been removed. The extensive distribution of the facial nerve (VII) to the facial musculature is contrasted with a less apparent distribution of sensory branches of the trigeminal nerve (V). The ramifications of cutaneous nerves are generally removed with the skin. The extensive and pronounced venous drainage in the superficial fascia is in marked contrast to the more restricted distribution of arteries (see also Fig. 2.127).

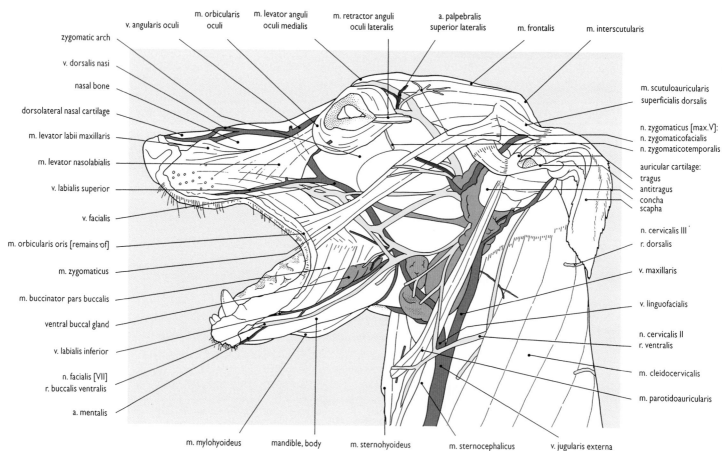

v. angularis oculi

m. orbicularis oculi

m. levator anguli oculi medialis

m. retractor anguli oculi lateralis

a. palpebralis superior lateralis

m. frontalis

m. interscutularis

zygomatic arch

v. dorsalis nasi

nasal bone

dorsolateral nasal cartilage

m. levator labii maxillaris

m. levator nasolabialis

v. labialis superior

v. facialis

m. orbicularis oris [remains of]

m. zygomaticus

m. buccinator pars buccalis

ventral buccal gland

v. labialis inferior

n. facialis [VII]
r. buccalis ventralis

a. mentalis

m. scutuloauricularis superficialis dorsalis

n. zygomaticus [max.V]:
n. zygomaticofacialis
n. zygomaticotemporalis

auricular cartilage:
tragus
antitragus
concha
scapha

n. cervicalis III
r. dorsalis

v. maxillaris

v. linguofacialis

n. cervicalis II
r. ventralis

m. cleidocervicalis

m. parotidoauricularis

m. mylohyoideus

mandible, body

m. sternohyoideus

m. sternocephalicus

v. jugularis externa

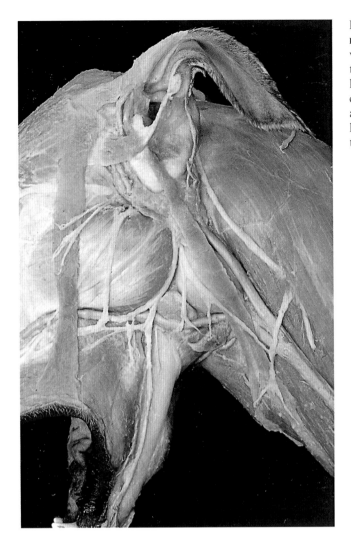

Fig. 2.28 Superficial structures of the temporal, auricular, parotid and masseteric regions after removal of the platysma and sphincter colli profundus muscles: left lateral view. This is a closer view of a part of the dissection shown in Fig. 2.27. Removal of the intermediate part of the sphincter colli profundus has exposed the mandibular lymph nodes (see also Fig. 2.127). These nodes are of considerable size when compared to the very small parotid lymph node exposed in Fig. 2.30. Lymph nodes are generally few in number and small in size (relative to body size) in the dog and lymphatic tissue is generally poorly displayed. Lymphatic vessels (apart from the thoracic duct – see Chapter 5) are not demonstrated.

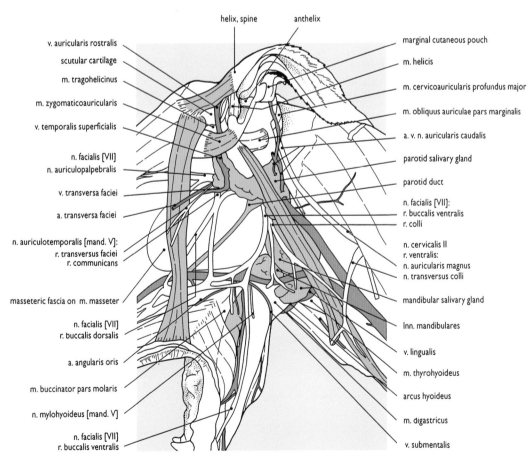

helix, spine — anthelix

v. auricularis rostralis

scutular cartilage

m. tragohelicinus

m. zygomaticoauricularis

v. temporalis superficialis

n. facialis [VII]
n. auriculopalpebralis

v. transversa faciei

a. transversa faciei

n. auriculotemporalis [mand. V]:
r. transversus faciei
r. communicans

masseteric fascia on m. masseter

n. facialis [VII]
r. buccalis dorsalis

a. angularis oris

m. buccinator pars molaris

n. mylohyoideus [mand. V]

n. facialis [VII]
r. buccalis ventralis

marginal cutaneous pouch

m. helicis

m. cervicoauricularis profundus major

m. obliquus auriculae pars marginalis

a. v. n. auricularis caudalis

parotid salivary gland

parotid duct

n. facialis [VII]:
r. buccalis ventralis
r. colli

n. cervicalis II
r. ventralis:
n. auricularis magnus
n. transversus colli

mandibular salivary gland

lnn. mandibulares

v. lingualis

m. thyrohyoideus

arcus hyoideus

m. digastricus

v. submentalis

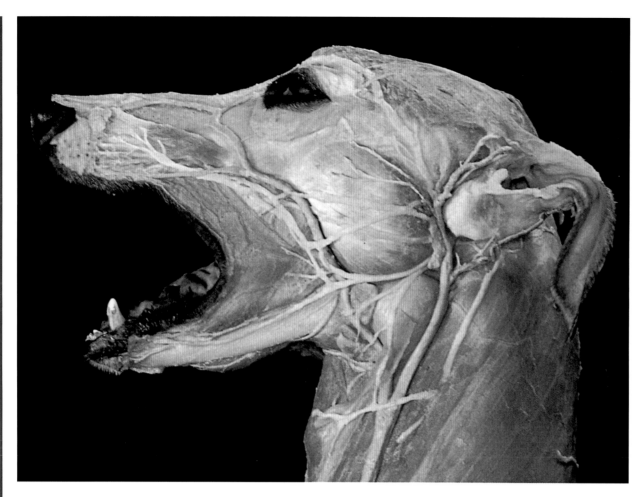

Fig. 2.29 Superficial nerves and blood vessels of the head: left lateral view. The zygomatic and zygomaticoauricular muscles, the parotidoauricular muscle in part, and the maxillary component of the levator nasolabialis muscle, have been removed. The ventral end of the parotidoauricular muscle is retained in order to leave intact the cervical branch of the facial nerve (VII) linking with the transverse cervical component of cervical nerve 2 on its surface. The parotid salivary gland has been removed 'piecemeal' until only a small component from which the duct originates remains in position.

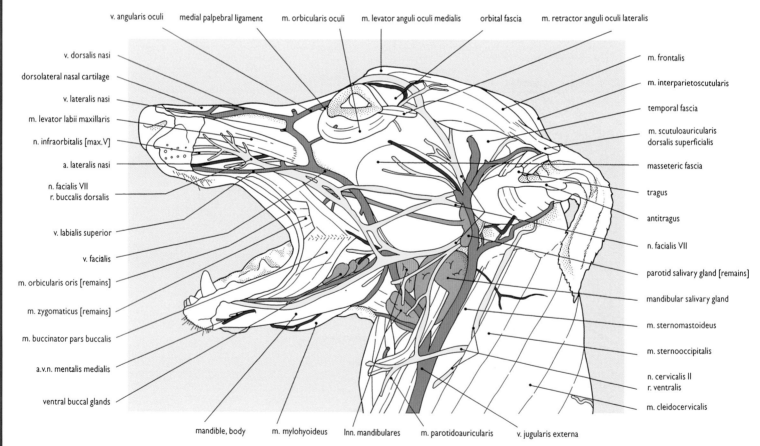

v. angularis oculi   medial palpebral ligament   m. orbicularis oculi   m. levator anguli oculi medialis   orbital fascia   m. retractor anguli oculi lateralis

v. dorsalis nasi

dorsolateral nasal cartilage

v. lateralis nasi

m. levator labii maxillaris

n. infraorbitalis [max.V]

a. lateralis nasi

n. facialis VII
r. buccalis dorsalis

v. labialis superior

v. facialis

m. orbicularis oris [remains]

m. zygomaticus [remains]

m. buccinator pars buccalis

a.v.n. mentalis medialis

ventral buccal glands

m. frontalis

m. interparietoscutularis

temporal fascia

m. scutuloauricularis dorsalis superficialis

masseteric fascia

tragus

antitragus

n. facialis VII

parotid salivary gland [remains]

mandibular salivary gland

m. sternomastoideus

m. sternooccipitalis

n. cervicalis II
r. ventralis

m. cleidocervicalis

mandible, body   m. mylohyoideus   lnn. mandibulares   m. parotidoauricularis   v. jugularis externa

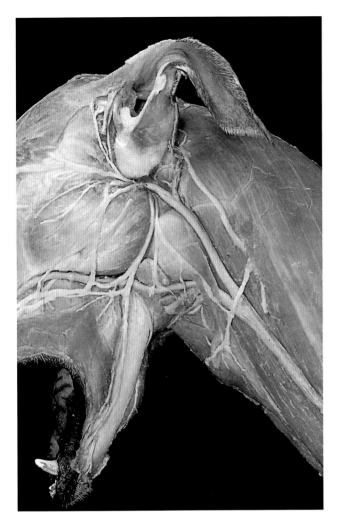

Fig. 2.30 Superficial nerves and blood vessels of the temporal, auricular, parotid and masseteric regions after removal of the facial muscles and parotid salivary glands: left lateral view. This is a closer view of a part of the dissection shown in Fig. 2.29 but with the parotid salivary gland removed, including the proximal part of its duct, and that component of the superficial temporal vein which lay embedded in parotid gland tissue also removed. The cut ends of the vein are visible as it leaves the temporal fascia dorsal to the zygomatic arch, and just before it enters the maxillary vein caudoventral to the concha of the auricular cartilage. The small parotid lymph node, now uncovered, partially obscures the communicating ramus linking the auriculotemporal branch of the trigeminal nerve (V) with the dorsal buccal branch of the facial nerve (VII).

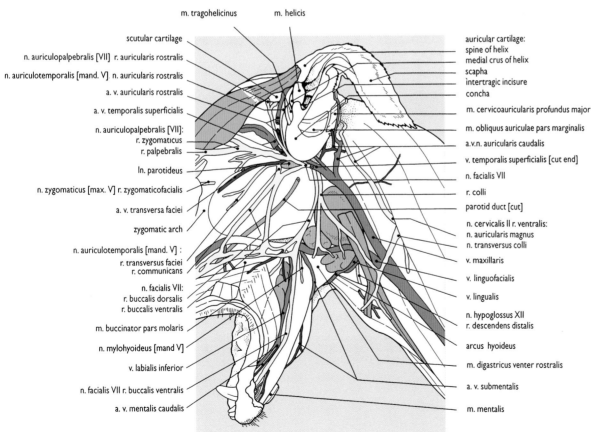

m. tragohelicinus   m. helicis

scutular cartilage

n. auriculopalpebralis [VII] r. auricularis rostralis

n. auriculotemporalis [mand. V]. n. auricularis rostralis

a. v. auricularis rostralis

a. v. temporalis superficialis

n. auriculopalpebralis [VII]:
r. zygomaticus
r. palpebralis

ln. parotideus

n. zygomaticus [max. V] r. zygomaticofacialis

a. v. transversa faciei

zygomatic arch

n. auriculotemporalis [mand. V] :
r. transversus faciei
r. communicans

n. facialis VII:
r. buccalis dorsalis
r. buccalis ventralis

m. buccinator pars molaris

n. mylohyoideus [mand V]

v. labialis inferior

n. facialis VII r. buccalis ventralis

a. v. mentalis caudalis

auricular cartilage:
spine of helix
medial crus of helix
scapha
intertragic incisure
concha

m. cervicoauricularis profundus major

m. obliquus auriculae pars marginalis

a.v.n. auricularis caudalis

v. temporalis superficialis [cut end]

n. facialis VII

r. colli

parotid duct [cut]

n. cervicalis II r. ventralis:
n. auricularis magnus
n. transversus colli

v. maxillaris

v. linguofacialis

v. lingualis

n. hypoglossus XII
r. descendens distalis

arcus hyoideus

m. digastricus venter rostralis

a. v. submentalis

m. mentalis

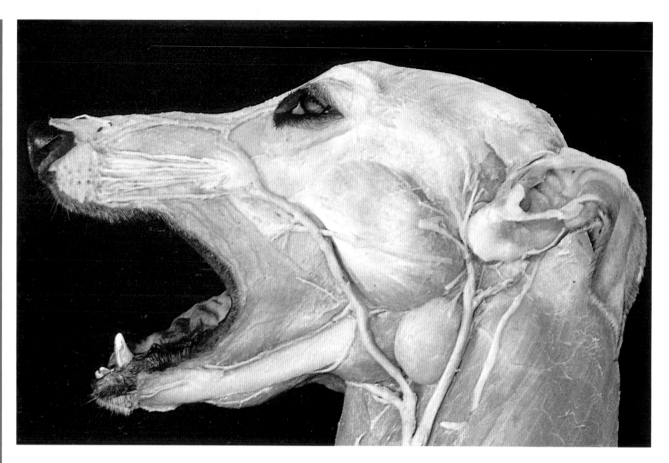

Fig. 2.31 Auricular cartilages, temporal and masseter muscles after removal of the facial muscles: left lateral view. The remaining facial muscles have been removed along with the mandibular and parotid lymph nodes and the terminal ramifications of the facial nerve (VII). Infraorbital branches of the maxillary nerve (trigeminal V) are now visible extending rostrally from the infraorbital foramen into the muzzle. Slight displacement of the facial vein away from the rostroventral border of the masseter muscle has exposed the deep facial vein, the facial artery and the mylohyoid nerve extension onto the face (see also Fig. 2.98).

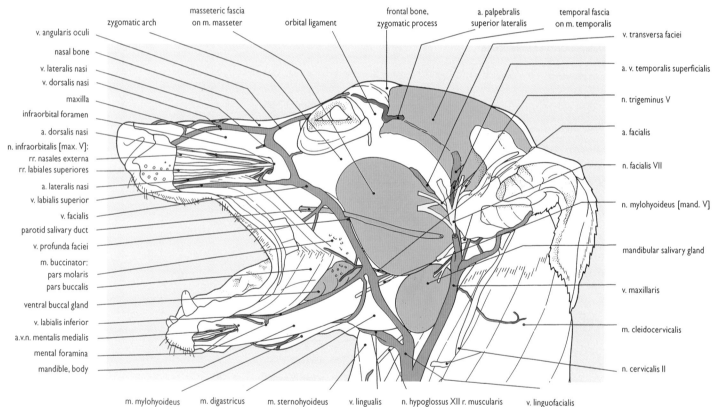

zygomatic arch — masseteric fascia on m. masseter — orbital ligament — frontal bone, zygomatic process — a. palpebralis superior lateralis — temporal fascia on m. temporalis

v. angularis oculi
nasal bone
v. lateralis nasi
v. dorsalis nasi
maxilla
infraorbital foramen
a. dorsalis nasi
n. infraorbitalis [max. V]:
rr. nasales externa
rr. labiales superiores
a. lateralis nasi
v. labialis superior
v. facialis
parotid salivary duct
v. profunda faciei
m. buccinator:
pars molaris
pars buccalis
ventral buccal gland
v. labialis inferior
a.v.n. mentalis medialis
mental foramina
mandible, body

v. transversa faciei
a. v. temporalis superficialis
n. trigeminus V
a. facialis
n. facialis VII
n. mylohyoideus [mand. V]
mandibular salivary gland
v. maxillaris
m. cleidocervicalis
n. cervicalis II

m. mylohyoideus — m. digastricus — m. sternohyoideus — v. lingualis — n. hypoglossus XII r. muscularis — v. linguofacialis

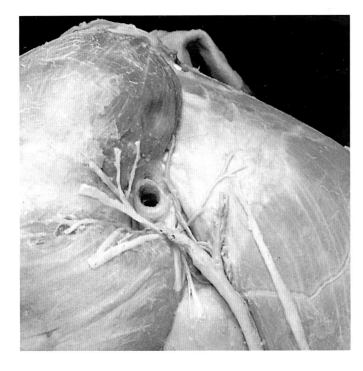

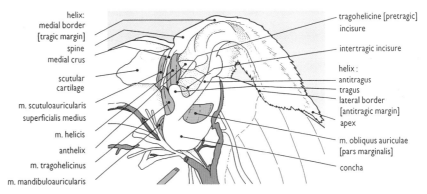

helix:
medial border
[tragic margin]
spine
medial crus

scutular
cartilage

m. scutuloauricularis
superficialis medius

m. helicis

anthelix

m. tragohelicinus

m. mandibuloauricularis

tragohelicine [pretragic]
incisure

intertragic incisure

helix:
antitragus
tragus
lateral border
[antitragic margin]
apex

m. obliquus auriculae
[pars marginalis]

concha

Fig. 2.32 Auricular and scutular cartilages after removal of the superficial muscles and parotid salivary gland: left lateral view. This enlarged view of the auricular region (Fig. 2.31) shows scutular and auricular cartilages and some intrinsic auricular muscles.

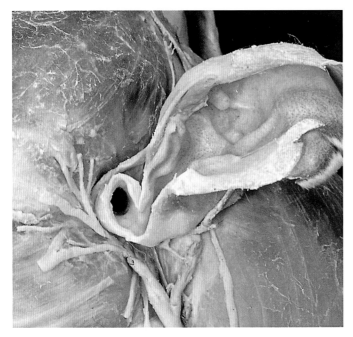

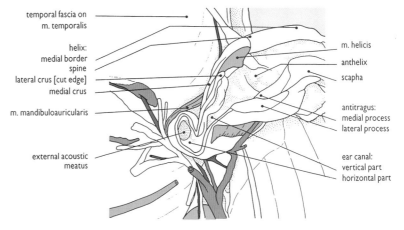

temporal fascia on
m. temporalis

helix:
medial border
spine
lateral crus [cut edge]
medial crus

m. mandibuloauricularis

external acoustic
meatus

m. helicis

anthelix

scapha

antitragus:
medial process
lateral process

ear canal:
vertical part
horizontal part

Fig. 2.33 Auricular cartilage and external acoustic canal following tragic resection: left lateral view. The ear canal is opened to demonstrate its right-angled bend before the external acoustic meatus and tympanic membrane are reached (see also sections, Figs 2.145 and 2.146).

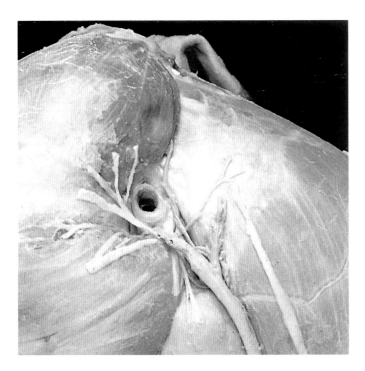

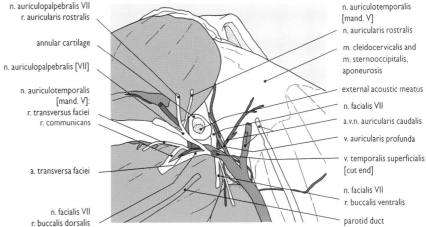

n. auriculopalpebralis VII
r. auricularis rostralis

annular cartilage

n. auriculopalpebralis [VII]

n. auriculotemporalis
[mand. V]:
r. transversus faciei
r. communicans

a. transversa faciei

n. facialis VII
r. buccalis dorsalis

n. auriculotemporalis
[mand. V]

n. auricularis rostralis

m. cleidocervicalis and
m. sternooccipitalis,
aponeurosis

external acoustic meatus

n. facialis VII

a.v.n. auricularis caudalis

v. auricularis profunda

v. temporalis superficialis
[cut end]

n. facialis VII
r. buccalis ventralis

parotid duct

Fig. 2.34 Temporal, parotid, auricular and masseteric regions and the external acoustic canal following removal of the auricular cartilage: left lateral view. The facial nerve (VII) emerges from the stylomastoid foramen caudal to the meatus (see Fig. 2.3) and practically encircles it.

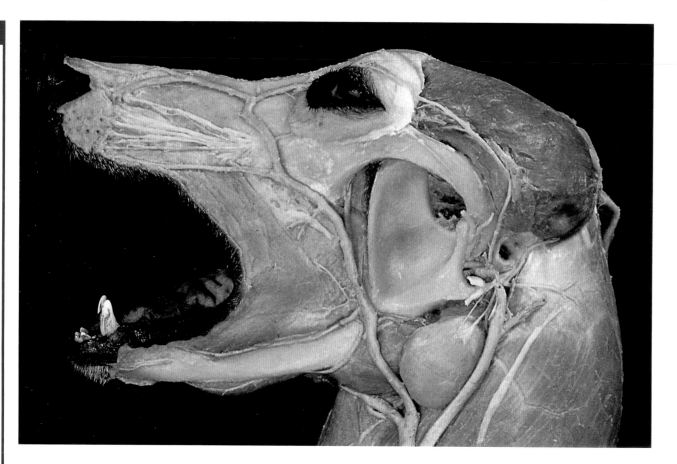

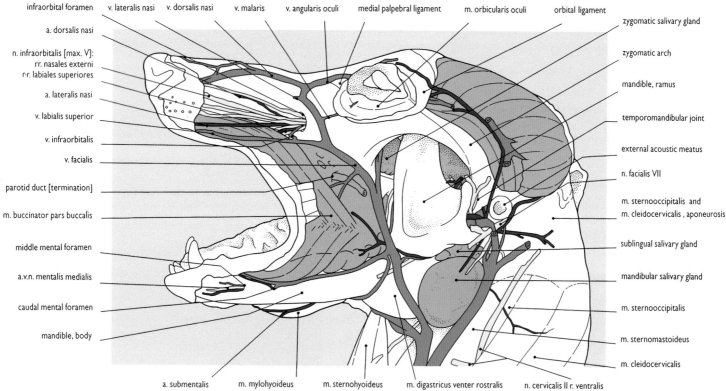

infraorbital foramen   v. lateralis nasi   v. dorsalis nasi   v. malaris   v. angularis oculi   medial palpebral ligament   m. orbicularis oculi   orbital ligament

a. dorsalis nasi

n. infraorbitalis [max. V]:
rr. nasales externi
rr. labiales superiores

a. lateralis nasi

v. labialis superior

v. infraorbitalis

v. facialis

parotid duct [termination]

m. buccinator pars buccalis

middle mental foramen

a.v.n. mentalis medialis

caudal mental foramen

mandible, body

zygomatic salivary gland

zygomatic arch

mandible, ramus

temporomandibular joint

external acoustic meatus

n. facialis VII

m. sternooccipitalis and
m. cleidocervicalis , aponeurosis

sublingual salivary gland

mandibular salivary gland

m. sternooccipitalis

m. sternomastoideus

m. cleidocervicalis

a. submentalis   m. mylohyoideus   m. sternohyoideus   m. digastricus venter rostralis   n. cervicalis II r. ventralis

Fig. 2.35 Mandibular ramus and temporal muscle after removal of the masseter muscle and temporal fascia: left lateral view (1). Removal of the auricular and scutular cartilages exposed the stout temporal fascia which was subsequently removed. Some 'ragged' areas of the temporal muscle surface show where numerous fibers took origin from the internal face of the temporal fascia itself. Removal of the masseter muscle has involved further cutting back of superficial components of both the trigeminal (V) and facial (VII) nerves. The cut stumps of these nerves are visible above and below the maxillary artery and vein, lateral to the temporomandibular joint.

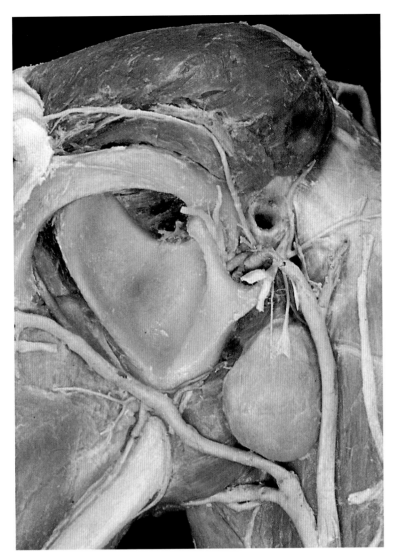

Fig. 2.36 Mandibular ramus and temporal muscle after removal of the masseter muscle and temporal fascia: left lateral view (2). This is a closer view of the temporal and masseteric regions of the dissection shown in Fig. 2.35. It displays the deep facial vein leaving the pterygopalatine fossa and embedded to some extent in the zygomatic salivary gland. The buccal nerve from the mandibular branch of the trigeminal nerve (V) appears in the cheek immediately rostral to the coronoid process of the mandibular ramus. Caudal to the external acoustic meatus the remains of the caudal auricular vessels and nerve have been displaced caudally after removal of the auricular cartilage. They are spread out on the aponeurosis of the cleidocervical and sterno-occipital muscles in the region of the atlas wing.

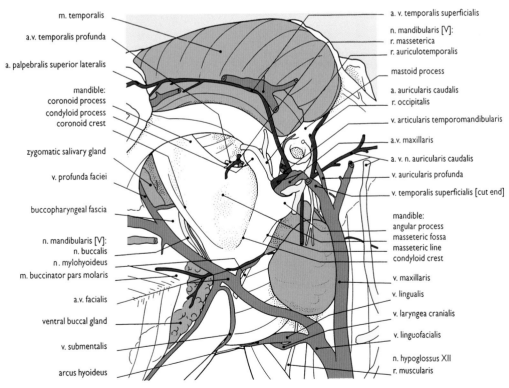

m. temporalis	a. v. temporalis superficialis
a.v. temporalis profunda	n. mandibularis [V]:
	r. masseterica
a. palpebralis superior lateralis	r. auriculotemporalis
	mastoid process
mandible:	a. auricularis caudalis
coronoid process	r. occipitalis
condyloid process	
coronoid crest	v. articularis temporomandibularis
zygomatic salivary gland	a.v. maxillaris
	a. v. n. auricularis caudalis
v. profunda faciei	v. auricularis profunda
	v. temporalis superficialis [cut end]
buccopharyngeal fascia	mandible:
	angular process
n. mandibularis [V]:	masseteric fossa
n. buccalis	masseteric line
n . mylohyoideus	condyloid crest
m. buccinator pars molaris	v. maxillaris
a.v. facialis	v. lingualis
	v. laryngea cranialis
ventral buccal gland	v. linguofacialis
v. submentalis	n. hypoglossus XII
arcus hyoideus	r. muscularis

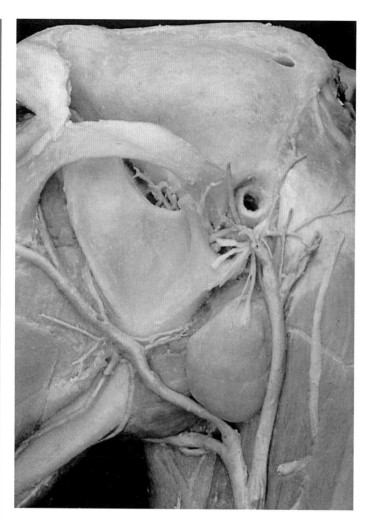

Fig. 2.37 Temporal fossa and mandibular ramus after removal of the temporal and masseter muscles: left lateral view. 'Piecemeal' removal of the temporal muscle has left its nerve and blood supply intact and visible through the mandibular notch (see also Figs 2.69 and 2.70). In the process of temporal muscle removal the isolation of orbital structures within the periorbita was clearly apparent: temporal fascia fuses with the orbital ligament whereas the temporal muscle itself merely butts onto but does not attach to the periorbita (see also Fig. 2.70). Likewise, separation of the temporal muscle from the maxillary nerve and blood vessels and buccal nerve in the pterygopalatine fossa ventral to it was readily accomplished (see also Fig. 2.72). The hole in the cranium at the point labelled 'X' was made to allow the insertion of a hook to support the head following embalming of the cadaver.

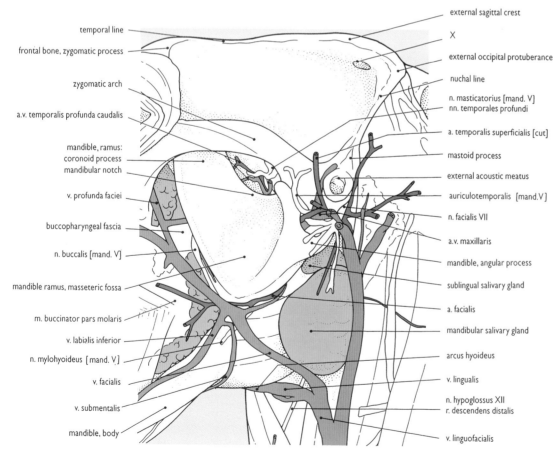

temporal line

frontal bone, zygomatic process

zygomatic arch

a.v. temporalis profunda caudalis

mandible, ramus:
coronoid process
mandibular notch

v. profunda faciei

buccopharyngeal fascia

n. buccalis [mand. V]

mandible ramus, masseteric fossa

m. buccinator pars molaris

v. labialis inferior

n. mylohyoideus [mand. V]

v. facialis

v. submentalis

mandible, body

external sagittal crest

X

external occipital protuberance

nuchal line

n. masticatorius [mand. V]
nn. temporales profundi

a. temporalis superficialis [cut]

mastoid process

external acoustic meatus

auriculotemporalis [mand. V]

n. facialis VII

a.v. maxillaris

mandible, angular process

sublingual salivary gland

a. facialis

mandibular salivary gland

arcus hyoideus

v. lingualis

n. hypoglossus XII
r. descendens distalis

v. linguofacialis

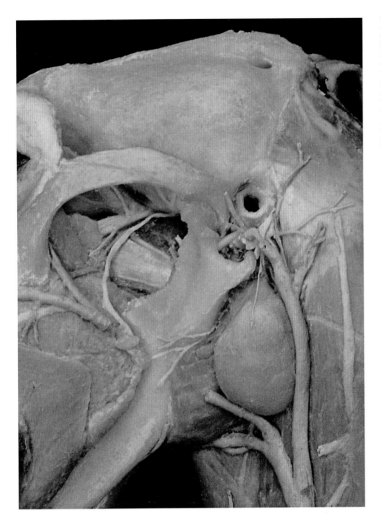

Fig. 2.38 Temporal and pterygopalatine fossae after removal of the coronoid process of the mandible: left lateral view. The coronoid process of the mandible has been sawn through and removed, opening the pterygopalatine fossa from a lateral aspect. Fat and fascia were cleaned from around the deep facial vein and the zygomatic salivary gland, and from the underlying buccopharyngeal fascia rostral to the medial pterygoid muscle. A short section of facial vein where it crosses the mandible has also been removed so that the cheek with its muscular basis of buccinator muscle is traceable for a short distance caudally, internal to the mandibular ramus.

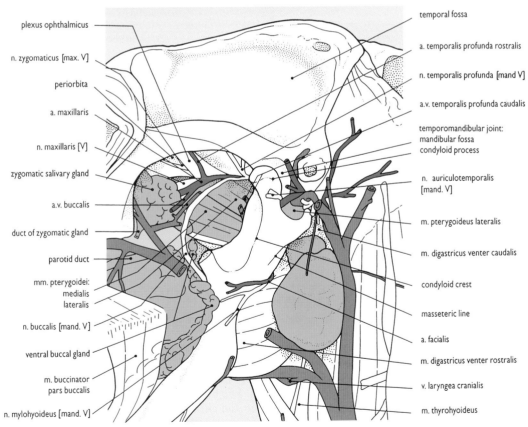

Labels (left side):
- plexus ophthalmicus
- n. zygomaticus [max. V]
- periorbita
- a. maxillaris
- n. maxillaris [V]
- zygomatic salivary gland
- a.v. buccalis
- duct of zygomatic gland
- parotid duct
- mm. pterygoidei: medialis lateralis
- n. buccalis [mand. V]
- ventral buccal gland
- m. buccinator pars buccalis
- n. mylohyoideus [mand. V]

Labels (right side):
- temporal fossa
- a. temporalis profunda rostralis
- n. temporalis profunda [mand V]
- a.v. temporalis profunda caudalis
- temporomandibular joint: mandibular fossa condyloid process
- n. auriculotemporalis [mand. V]
- m. pterygoideus lateralis
- m. digastricus venter caudalis
- condyloid crest
- masseteric line
- a. facialis
- m. digastricus venter rostralis
- v. laryngea cranialis
- m. thyrohyoideus

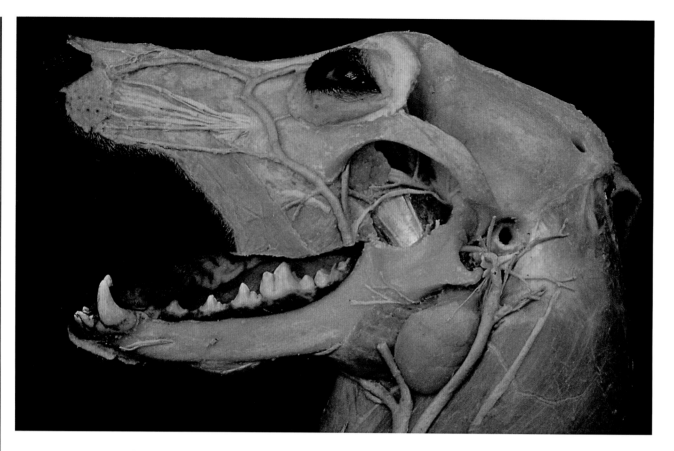

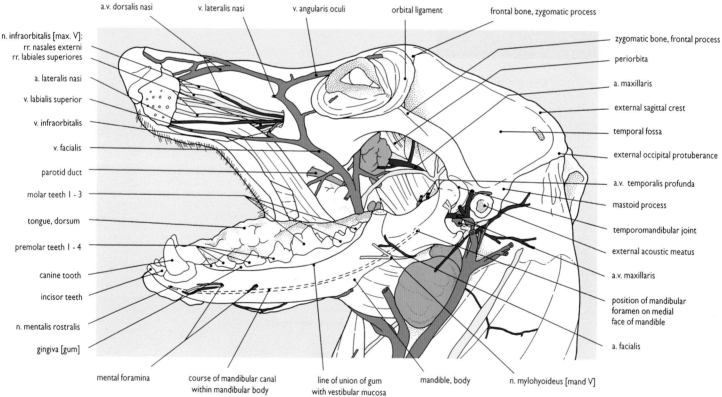

a.v. dorsalis nasi · v. lateralis nasi · v. angularis oculi · orbital ligament · frontal bone, zygomatic process

n. infraorbitalis [max. V]:
rr. nasales externi
rr. labiales superiores

a. lateralis nasi

v. labialis superior

v. infraorbitalis

v. facialis

parotid duct

molar teeth I - 3

tongue, dorsum

premolar teeth I - 4

canine tooth

incisor teeth

n. mentalis rostralis

gingiva [gum]

zygomatic bone, frontal process

periorbita

a. maxillaris

external sagittal crest

temporal fossa

external occipital protuberance

a.v. temporalis profunda

mastoid process

temporomandibular joint

external acoustic meatus

a.v. maxillaris

position of mandibular
foramen on medial
face of mandible

a. facialis

mental foramina · course of mandibular canal within mandibular body · line of union of gum with vestibular mucosa · mandible, body · n. mylohyoideus [mand V]

Fig. 2.39 Lower jaw after removal of the masseter muscle, ventral part of the cheek and lower lip: left lateral view. The lower jaw (mandible) has been exposed by removing the lower part of the cheek. From the angle of the mouth a cut was made caudally through the buccinator muscle and buccal fascia to the mandibular ramus at the level at which the coronoid process was removed (see Fig. 2.38). The buccinator muscle was cut from the mandible and the buccal mucosa was severed at its line of reflection from the internal surface of the lip and cheek onto the mandible.

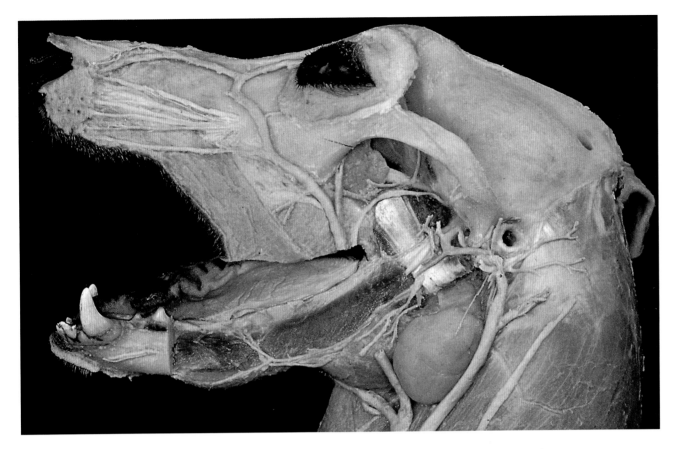

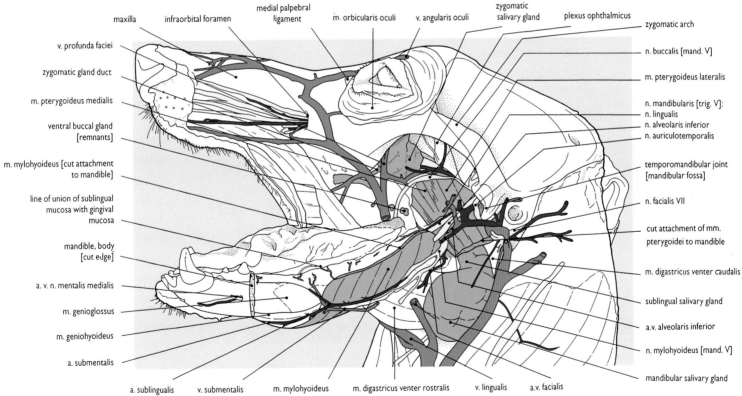

maxilla   infraorbital foramen   medial palpebral ligament   m. orbicularis oculi   v. angularis oculi   zygomatic salivary gland   plexus ophthalmicus   zygomatic arch

v. profunda faciei

zygomatic gland duct

m. pterygoideus medialis

ventral buccal gland [remnants]

m. mylohyoideus [cut attachment to mandible]

line of union of sublingual mucosa with gingival mucosa

mandible, body [cut edge]

a. v. n. mentalis medialis

m. genioglossus

m. geniohyoideus

a. submentalis

n. buccalis [mand. V]

m. pterygoideus lateralis

n. mandibularis [trig. V]:
n. lingualis
n. alveolaris inferior
n. auriculotemporalis

temporomandibular joint [mandibular fossa]

n. facialis VII

cut attachment of mm. pterygoidei to mandible

m. digastricus venter caudalis

sublingual salivary gland

a.v. alveolaris inferior

n. mylohyoideus [mand. V]

mandibular salivary gland

a. sublingualis   v. submentalis   m. mylohyoideus   m. digastricus venter rostralis   v. lingualis   a.v. facialis

Fig. 2.40 Pterygopalatine fossa and lower jaw after removal of the mandible: left lateral view. The remaining part of the left mandible has been removed by: making a vertical saw cut through the mandibular body caudal to lower premolar tooth 2; disarticulating the temporomandibular joint; severing the digastric, medial pterygoid, lateral pterygoid, mylohyoid, geniohyoid and genioglossal muscles at their attachments; cutting the mandibular alveolar vessels and nerve at their entry into the mandibular canal (see Fig. 2.98); severing sublingual mucosa in the floor of the mouth at its line of reflection onto the internal face of the mandible.

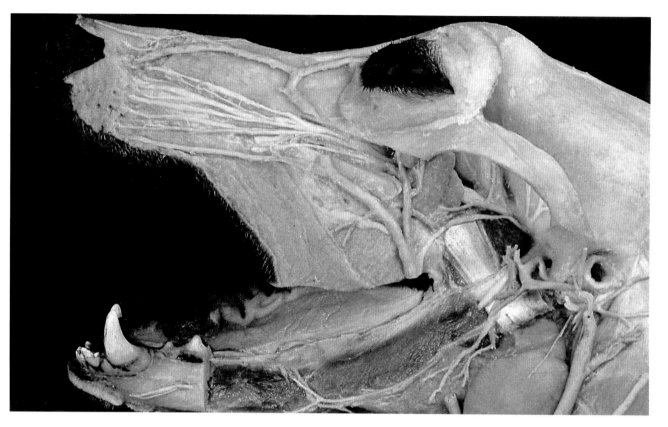

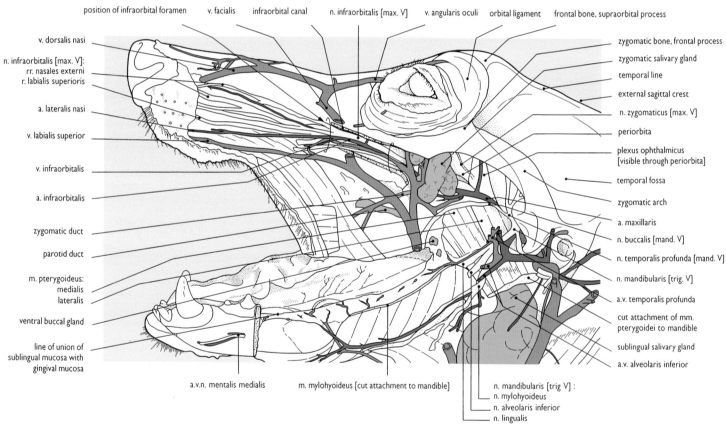

Fig. 2.41 Upper jaw and pterygopalatine fossa after removal of the wall of the infraorbital canal: left lateral view. The infraorbital canal has been opened by making parallel saw cuts through the maxillary bone from the dorsal and ventral boundaries of the infraorbital foramen. Caudally the saw cuts pass through the zygomatic bone and have opened up the rostral part of the pterygopalatine fossa below the orbit. The ventral saw cut has also exposed the roots of the cheek teeth (upper PM4 and M1), whilst the dorsal saw cut has broken through the medial wall of the canal and entered the maxillary recess (see also Figs 2.99, 2.100 and 2.141).

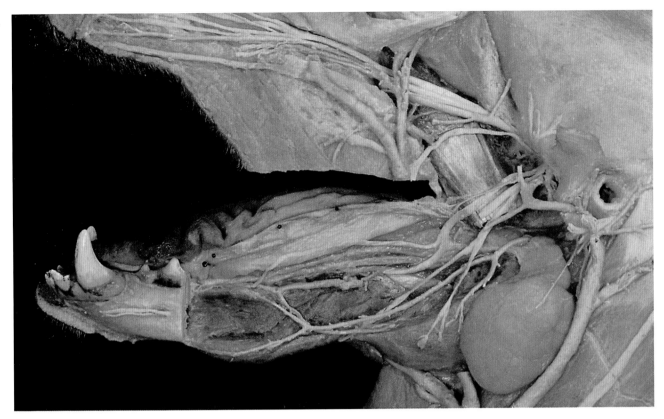

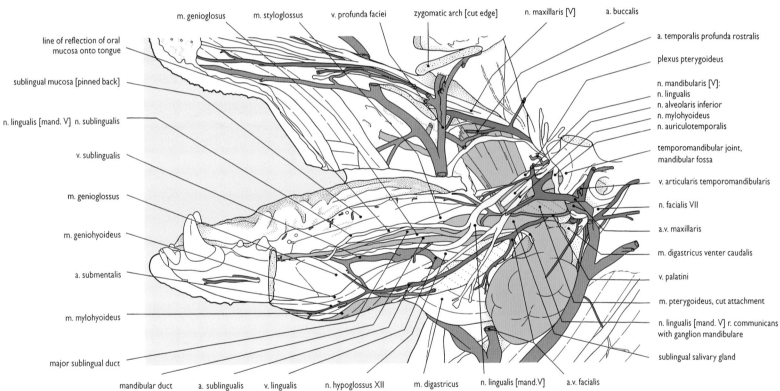

m. genioglosus   m. styloglossus   v. profunda faciei   zygomatic arch [cut edge]   n. maxillaris [V]   a. buccalis

line of reflection of oral mucosa onto tongue

sublingual mucosa [pinned back]

n. lingualis [mand. V] n. sublingualis

v. sublingualis

m. genioglossus

m. geniohyoideus

a. submentalis

m. mylohyoideus

major sublingual duct

a. temporalis profunda rostralis

plexus pterygoideus

n. mandibularis [V]:
n. lingualis
n. alveolaris inferior
n. mylohyoideus
n. auriculotemporalis

temporomandibular joint, mandibular fossa

v. articularis temporomandibularis

n. facialis VII

a.v. maxillaris

m. digastricus venter caudalis

v. palatini

m. pterygoideus, cut attachment

n. lingualis [mand. V] r. communicans with ganglion mandibulare

sublingual salivary gland

mandibular duct   a. sublingualis   v. lingualis   n. hypoglossus XII   m. digastricus   n. lingualis [mand.V]   a.v. facialis

Fig. 2.42 Lower jaw – lingual nerve, mandibular and sublingual salivary glands and ducts: left lateral view. The thinner, almost vertically oriented component of the mylohyoid muscle has been removed. The mucosa of the floor of the mouth between the cut gingival margin and the tongue encompasses the sublingual fold of mucosa. In order to display the sublingual nerve and major and minor salivary gland ducts the mucosal fold is gathered up and pinned against the lateral surface of the tongue. Some further cutting back of the severed ends of the pterygoid muscles exposes the full extent of the monostomatic part of the sublingual salivary gland.

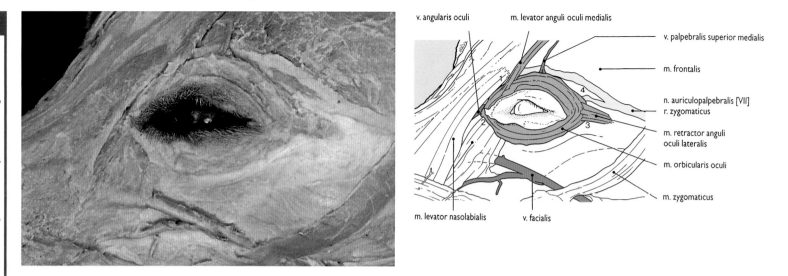

Fig. 2.43 Superficial structures of the eye and orbital region (1). Musculature of the eyelids: left lateral view. The skin has been removed and the superficial fascia cleaned. Cutaneous branches of the trigeminal nerve (V) were removed with the skin. Their positions are indicated at the points labelled: 1) frontal branch and 2) infratrochlear branch of the ophthalmic nerve; 3) zygomaticofacial branch and 4) zygomaticotemporal branch of the maxillary nerve.

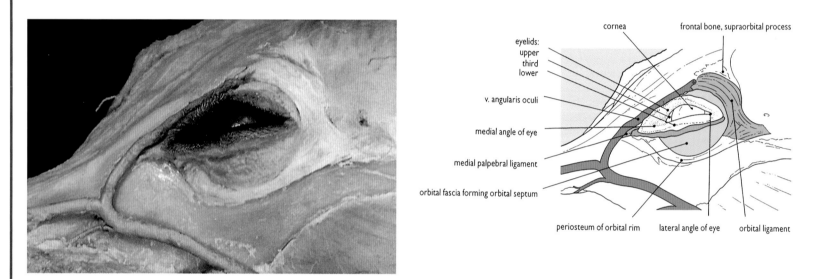

Fig. 2.44 Superficial structures of the eye and orbital region (2). Orbital fascia and orbital ligament: left lateral view. The superficial muscles have been removed and the orbicularis muscle has been trimmed to expose the orbital ligament. Removal of the levator nasolabialis muscle has exposed the angularis oculi vein and the medial palpebral ligament which anchors the medial angle of the eye.

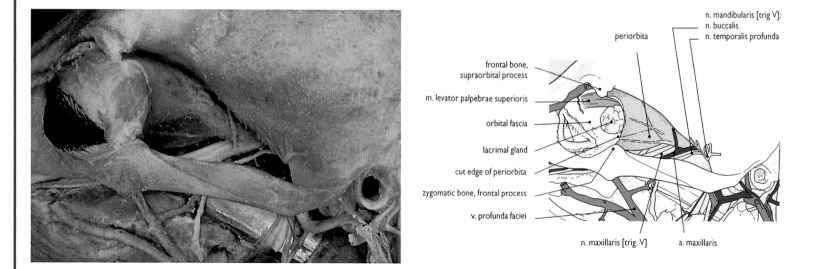

Fig. 2.45 Orbit and temporal fossa after removal of the temporal muscle and orbital ligament: left dorsolateral view. The temporal and masseter muscles have been removed, exposing the periorbita surrounding and confining orbital 'contents'. The orbital ligament has also been removed, opening the orbital rim dorsolaterally and displaying the cut edge of the periorbita which blended with it.

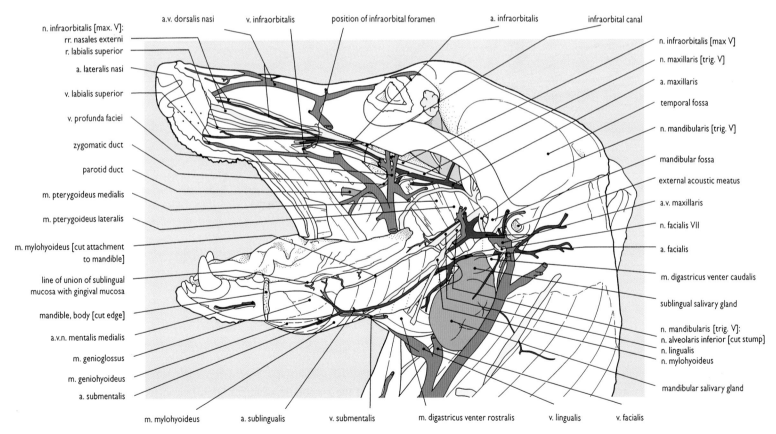

n. infraorbitalis [max. V]:
rr. nasales externi
r. labialis superior

a. lateralis nasi

v. labialis superior

v. profunda faciei

zygomatic duct

parotid duct

m. pterygoideus medialis

m. pterygoideus lateralis

m. mylohyoideus [cut attachment
to mandible]

line of union of sublingual
mucosa with gingival mucosa

mandible, body [cut edge]

a.v.n. mentalis medialis

m. genioglossus

m. geniohyoideus

a. submentalis

a.v. dorsalis nasi   v. infraorbitalis   position of infraorbital foramen   a. infraorbitalis   infraorbital canal

n. infraorbitalis [max V]

n. maxillaris [trig. V]

a. maxillaris

temporal fossa

n. mandibularis [trig. V]

mandibular fossa

external acoustic meatus

a.v. maxillaris

n. facialis VII

a. facialis

m. digastricus venter caudalis

sublingual salivary gland

n. mandibularis [trig. V]:
n. alveolaris inferior [cut stump]
n. lingualis
n. mylohyoideus

mandibular salivary gland

m. mylohyoideus   a. sublingualis   v. submentalis   m. digastricus venter rostralis   v. lingualis   v. facialis

Fig. 2.46 Upper jaw, maxillary artery and nerve and deep facial vein after opening of the infraorbital canal: left lateral view. The point reached in the dissection of the orbit illustrated in Fig. 2.45 is an enlarged view of this stage of the dissection of the head overall. Through removal of the orbital ligament the orbit is now opened dorsolaterally into the temporal fossa as well as ventrally into the pterygopalatine fossa (see also Fig. 2.71 of this stage in dorsal view). The zygomatic salivary gland has been removed, a straightforward procedure since it is not firmly fixed in position and does not have a well developed capsule. It was eased out from the pterygopalatine fossa around the branches of the deep facial vein.

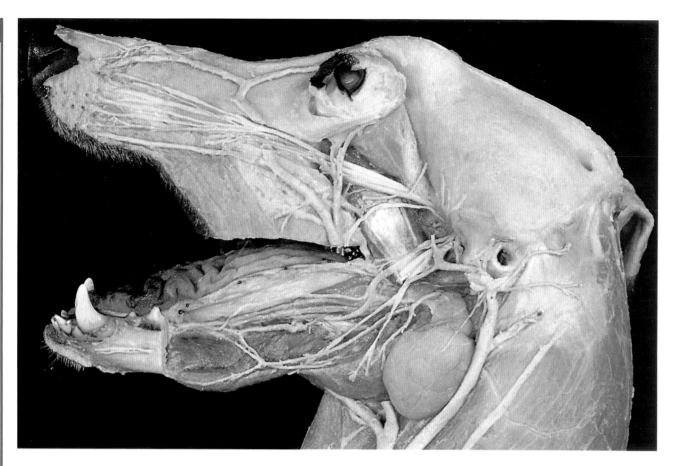

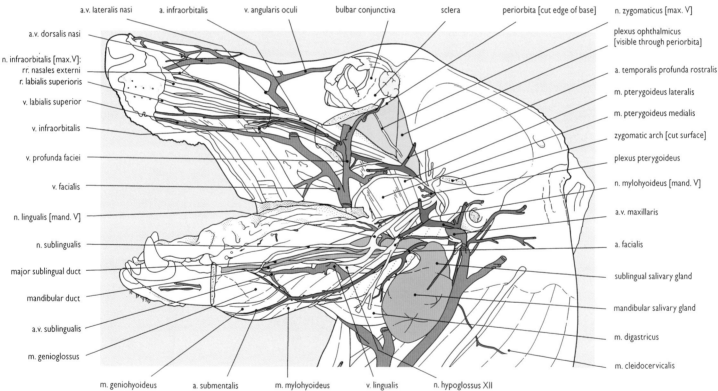

a.v. lateralis nasi   a. infraorbitalis   v. angularis oculi   bulbar conjunctiva   sclera   periorbita [cut edge of base]   n. zygomaticus [max. V]

a.v. dorsalis nasi

n. infraorbitalis [max.V]:
rr. nasales externi
r. labialis superioris

v. labialis superior

v. infraorbitalis

v. profunda faciei

v. facialis

n. lingualis [mand. V]

n. sublingualis

major sublingual duct

mandibular duct

a.v. sublingualis

m. genioglossus

plexus ophthalmicus
[visible through periorbita]

a. temporalis profunda rostralis

m. pterygoideus lateralis

m. pterygoideus medialis

zygomatic arch [cut surface]

plexus pterygoideus

n. mylohyoideus [mand. V]

a.v. maxillaris

a. facialis

sublingual salivary gland

mandibular salivary gland

m. digastricus

m. cleidocervicalis

m. geniohyoideus   a. submentalis   m. mylohyoideus   v. lingualis   n. hypoglossus XII

Fig. 2.47 Upper jaw, maxillary artery and nerve and deep facial vein after removal of the zygomatic arch: left lateral view. Removal of the orbicularis oculi muscle and the orbital ligament begins the deep dissection of the orbit by 'opening' the periorbital sac at its base. Removal of the zygomatic salivary gland from around the deep facial vein in the pterygopalatine fossa exposes the periorbita and demonstrates how the fascial sheath confines orbital 'contents'. Two of the major tributaries of the deep facial vein are exposed intact: an anastomotic connection with the ventral ophthalmic vein through the periorbita (see Fig. 2.142); and a connection with the superficial temporal vein.

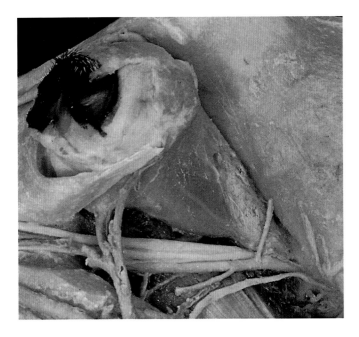
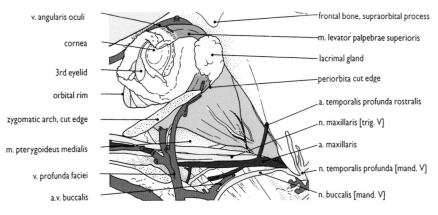

v. angularis oculi
cornea
3rd eyelid
orbital rim
zygomatic arch, cut edge
m. pterygoideus medialis
v. profunda faciei
a.v. buccalis

frontal bone, supraorbital process
m. levator palpebrae superioris
lacrimal gland
periorbita cut edge
a. temporalis profunda rostralis
n. maxillaris [trig. V]
a. maxillaris
n. temporalis profunda [mand. V]
n. buccalis [mand. V]

Fig. 2.48 Orbit and pterygopalatine fossa after removal of the zygomatic arch: left lateral view. This is an enlarged view of the orbit and pterygopalatine fossa of Fig. 2.47. The lateral halves of upper and lower eyelids and the palpebral conjunctiva have been removed. The orbital septum has also been removed from the lateral and ventral aspect of the eyeball.

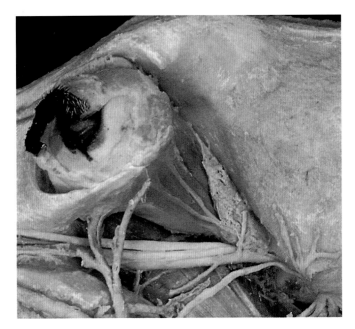
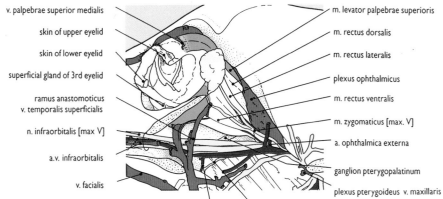

v. palpebrae superior medialis
skin of upper eyelid
skin of lower eyelid
superficial gland of 3rd eyelid
ramus anastomoticus v. temporalis superficialis
n. infraorbitalis [max V]
a.v. infraorbitalis
v. facialis

m. levator palpebrae superioris
m. rectus dorsalis
m. rectus lateralis
plexus ophthalmicus
m. rectus ventralis
m. zygomaticus [max. V]
a. ophthalmica externa
ganglion pterygopalatinum
plexus pterygoideus v. maxillaris

Fig. 2.49 Orbit and pterygopalatine fossa after removal of the periorbita: left lateral view. The periorbita has been removed from around the orbital contents and some intraperiorbital fat has been taken out from the ventral margin of the orbit exposing the superficial gland of the third eyelid.

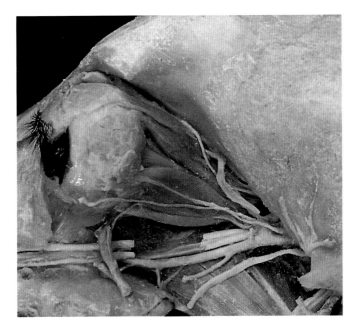
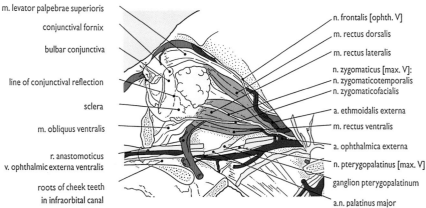

m. levator palpebrae superioris
conjunctival fornix
bulbar conjunctiva
line of conjunctival reflection
sclera
m. obliquus ventralis
r. anastomoticus v. ophthalmic externa ventralis
roots of cheek teeth in infraorbital canal

n. frontalis [ophth. V]
m. rectus dorsalis
m. rectus lateralis
n. zygomaticus [max. V]:
n. zygomaticotemporalis
n. zygomaticofacialis
a. ethmoidalis externa
m. rectus ventralis
a. ophthalmica externa
n. pterygopalatinus [max. V]
ganglion pterygopalatinum
a.n. palatinus major

Fig. 2.50 Orbit and pterygopalatine fossa after removal of the ventral boundary of the orbital rim: left lateral view. The remnant of the zygomatic arch has been removed as has the ophthalmic venous plexus and the fat infiltrated between the extrinsic eyeball muscles giving a more detailed exposure of the orbital contents.

Veterinary Anatomy: The Dog and Cat

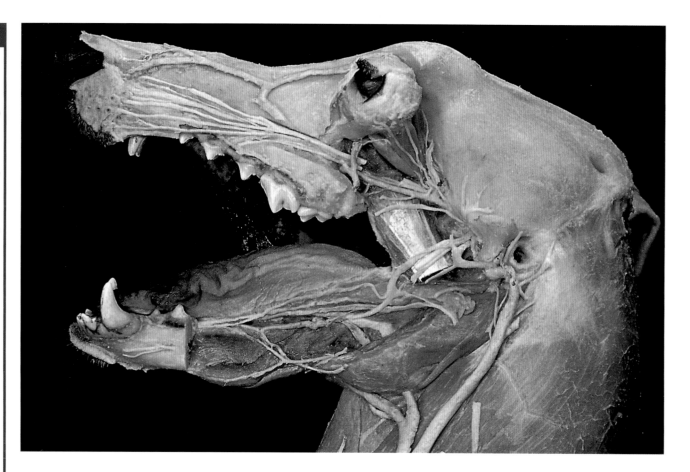

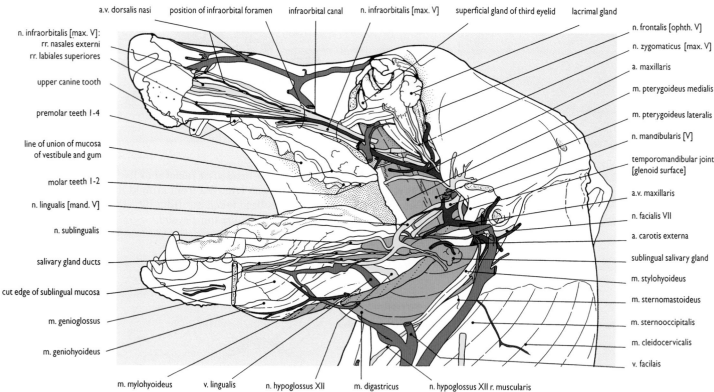

a.v. dorsalis nasi   position of infraorbital foramen   infraorbital canal   n. infraorbitalis [max. V]   superficial gland of third eyelid   lacrimal gland

n. infraorbitalis [max. V]:
rr. nasales externi
rr. labiales superiores

upper canine tooth

premolar teeth 1-4

line of union of mucosa
of vestibule and gum

molar teeth 1-2

n. lingualis [mand. V]

n. sublingualis

salivary gland ducts

cut edge of sublingual mucosa

m. genioglossus

m. geniohyoideus

n. frontalis [ophth. V]

n. zygomaticus [max. V]

a. maxillaris

m. pterygoideus medialis

m. pterygoideus lateralis

n. mandibularis [V]

temporomandibular joint
[glenoid surface]

a.v. maxillaris

n. facialis VII

a. carotis externa

sublingual salivary gland

m. stylohyoideus

m. sternomastoideus

m. sternooccipitalis

m. cleidocervicalis

v. facilais

m. mylohyoideus   v. lingualis   n. hypoglossus XII   m. digastricus   n. hypoglossus XII r. muscularis

Fig. 2.51 Upper jaw, maxillary nerve and artery after removal of the dorsal part of the cheek and upper lip: left lateral view. The upper part of the cheek and the upper lip have been partially removed as far rostrally as upper premolar tooth I so that the upper lip ramifications of the maxillary component of the trigeminal nerve (V) remain displayed. The buccal mucosa lining the oral vestibule was severed at its line of reflection from the internal surface of the lip and cheek onto the surface of the maxilla. The remaining part of the zygomatic arch has been removed from below the orbit and the periorbita is removed along with the ophthalmic plexus.

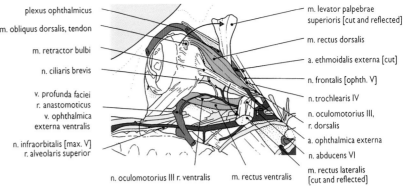

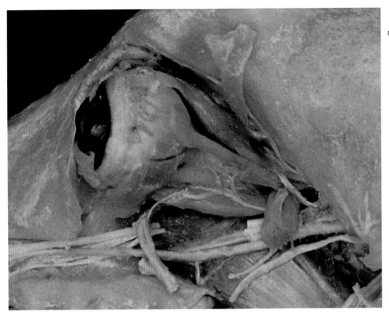

Fig. 2.52 Orbital contents and pterygopalatine ganglion: left lateral view. The levator muscle of the upper eyelid and the lateral rectus muscle have both been cut and reflected away from the eyeball. A section of maxillary nerve has been removed from the pterygopalatine fossa exposing the pterygopalatine ganglion and its connections with the pterygopalatine and greater palatine branches of the maxillary nerve (trigeminal V).

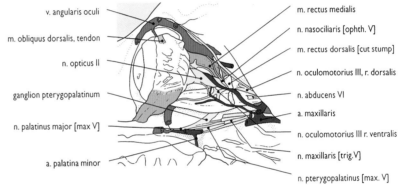

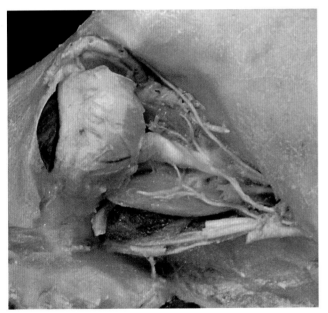

Fig. 2.53 Orbital contents – external ophthalmic artery and oculomotor nerve: left lateral view. The dorsal rectus muscle, the levator of the upper eyelid and two parts of the bulbar retractor muscle have been removed from the orbit. In the pterygopalatine fossa the infraorbital artery and nerve, the deep facial vein and much of the medial pterygoid muscle have been removed.

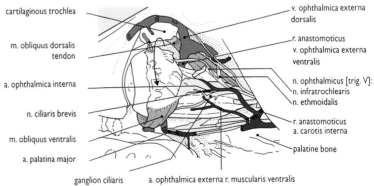

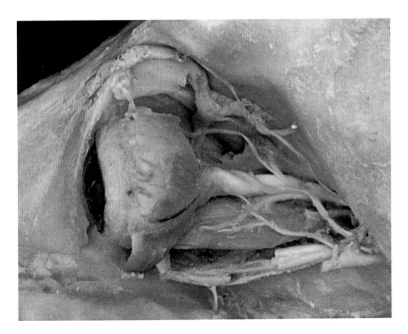

Fig. 2.54 Orbital contents – oblique muscles, frontal and nasociliary nerves: left lateral view. Lateral rotation of the eyeball has exposed the cartilaginous trochlear plate with its associated dorsal oblique muscle and tendon and has allowed part of the medial rectus muscle to be removed. Removal of the stumps of the dorsal and lateral rectus muscles and the bulbar retractor reveals the ciliary ganglion, a short ciliary nerve and the external ophthalmic artery accompanying the optic nerve (II).

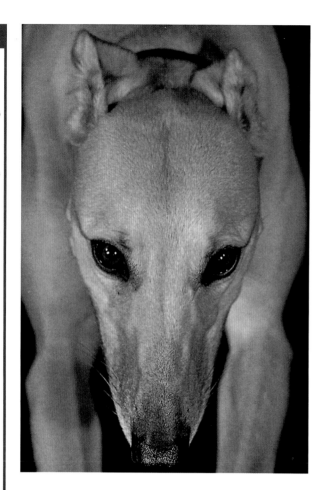

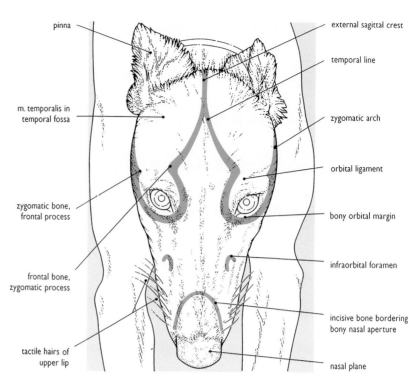

pinna

external sagittal crest

temporal line

m. temporalis in temporal fossa

zygomatic arch

orbital ligament

zygomatic bone, frontal process

bony orbital margin

infraorbital foramen

frontal bone, zygomatic process

incisive bone bordering bony nasal aperture

tactile hairs of upper lip

nasal plane

Fig. 2.55 Surface features of the head: dorsal view. The major bony features that are readily palpable and/or visible on the surface of the head are indicated. These 'points' correspond to those colored on the bones illustrated below (Fig. 2.56). Compare with the surface views from lateral (Fig. 2.1) and ventral (Fig. 2.125) aspects.

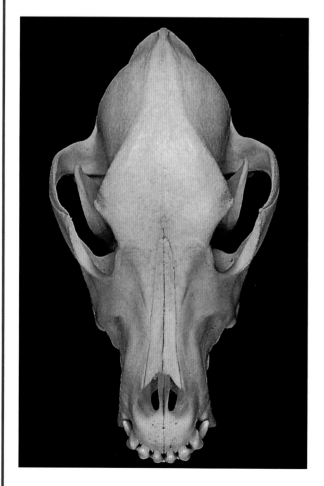

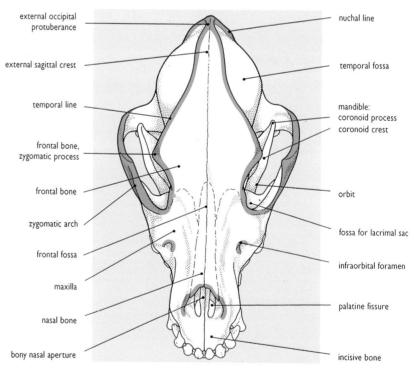

external occipital protuberance

nuchal line

external sagittal crest

temporal fossa

temporal line

mandible: coronoid process coronoid crest

frontal bone, zygomatic process

frontal bone

orbit

zygomatic arch

fossa for lacrimal sac

frontal fossa

infraorbital foramen

maxilla

palatine fissure

nasal bone

bony nasal aperture

incisive bone

Fig. 2.56 Skull: dorsal view. The palpable bony features shown in the surface view above (Fig. 2.55) are colored on this skull. In addition to the palpable 'points' large areas of bone can also be felt through the overlying musculature.

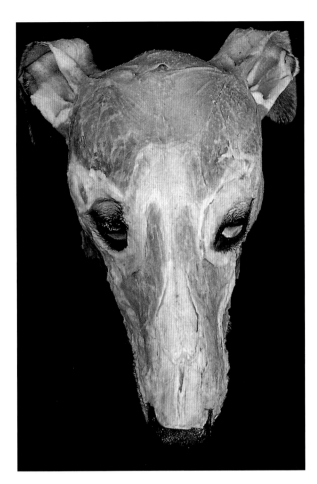

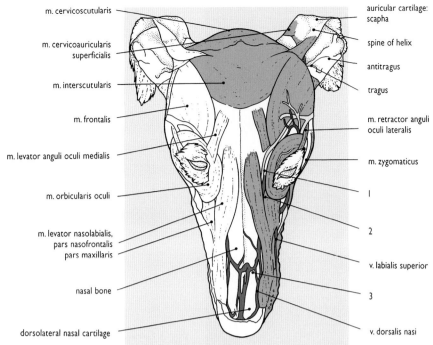

m. cervicoscutularis

m. cervicoauricularis superficialis

m. interscutularis

m. frontalis

m. levator anguli oculi medialis

m. orbicularis oculi

m. levator nasolabialis, pars nasofrontalis pars maxillaris

nasal bone

dorsolateral nasal cartilage

auricular cartilage: scapha

spine of helix

antitragus

tragus

m. retractor anguli oculi lateralis

m. zygomaticus

1

2

v. labialis superior

3

v. dorsalis nasi

Fig. 2.57 Superficial structures of the cranial and facial regions: dorsal view (1). The skin has been removed from the head leaving a narrow rim of skin in the lip, around the nostrils and eyes, and on the scapha of the auricular cartilage. On the dorsum and side of the muzzle cutaneous ramifications of the ophthalmic branch of the trigeminal nerve (V) have not been identified. 1) Frontal nerve; 2) Infratrochlear nerve; 3) External nasal nerve.

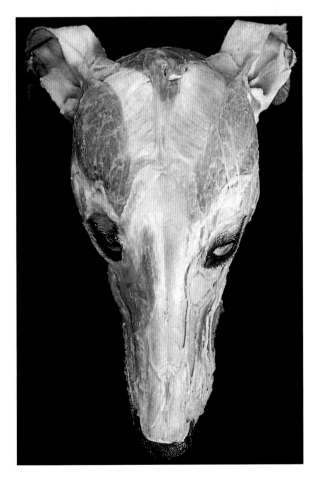

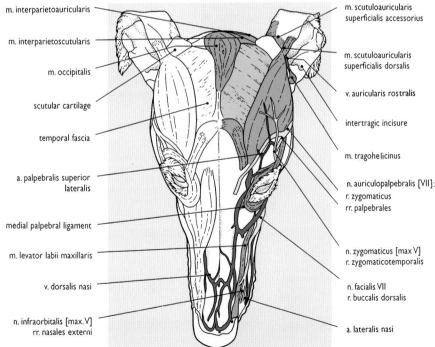

m. interparietoauricularis

m. interparietoscutularis

m. occipitalis

scutular cartilage

temporal fascia

a. palpebralis superior lateralis

medial palpebral ligament

m. levator labii maxillaris

v. dorsalis nasi

n. infraorbitalis [max. V] rr. nasales externi

m. scutuloauricularis superficialis accessorius

m. scutuloauricularis superficialis dorsalis

v. auricularis rostralis

intertragic incisure

m. tragohelicinus

n. auriculopalpebralis [VII]: r. zygomaticus rr. palpebrales

n. zygomaticus [max V] r. zygomaticotemporalis

n. facialis VII r. buccalis dorsalis

a. lateralis nasi

Fig. 2.58 Superficial structures of the cranial and facial regions: dorsal view (2). The interscutular and the levator nasolabialis muscle of the left side have been removed and the orbicularis oculi has been trimmed. Some cleaning and removal of nasofrontal fascia has exposed the bones of the dorsum of the face. Because neighbouring muscles in the superficial sheets intermingle to considerable extents at their margins, precise demarcation of individual facial muscles is often difficult and to some extent arbitrary.

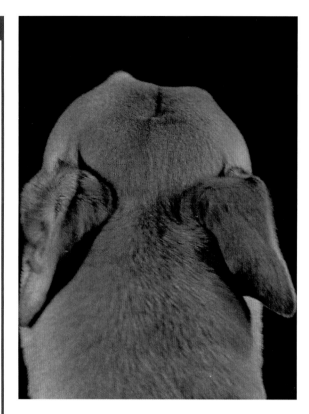

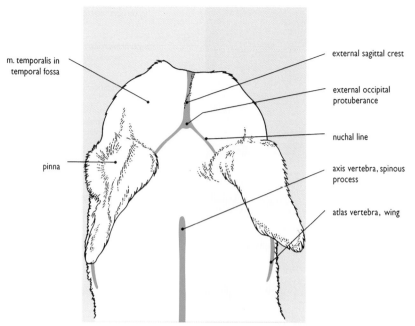

Fig. 2.59 Surface features of the head and cranial end of the neck: dorsal view. The major bony features that are readily palpable and/or visible on the surface of this region are indicated. These 'points' correspond to those colored on the bones illustrated in Fig. 2.60. The surface of the head is shown from lateral view in Fig. 2.1.

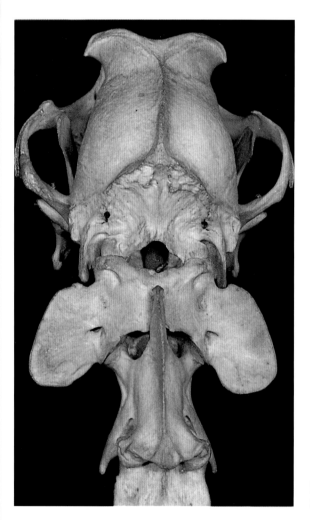

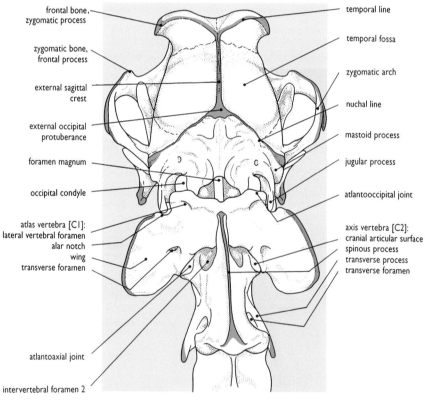

Fig. 2.60 Skeleton of the head and cranial end of the neck: dorsal view. The palpable bony features shown in the surface view in Fig. 2.59 are colored on this drawing.

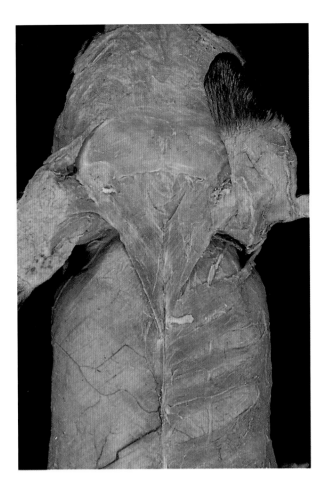

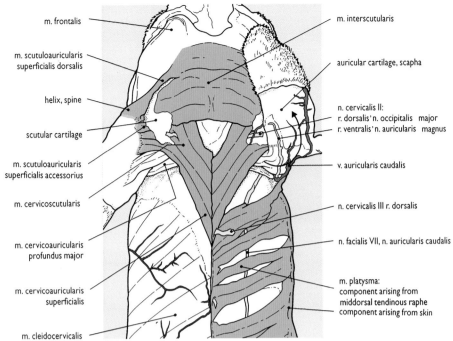

m. frontalis

m. scutuloauricularis
superficialis dorsalis

helix, spine

scutular cartilage

m. scutuloauricularis
superficialis accessorius

m. cervicoscutularis

m. cervicoauricularis
profundus major

m. cervicoauricularis
superficialis

m. cleidocervicalis

m. interscutularis

auricular cartilage, scapha

n. cervicalis II:
r. dorsalis'n. occipitalis major
r. ventralis'n. auricularis magnus

v. auricularis caudalis

n. cervicalis III r. dorsalis

n. facialis VII, n. auricularis caudalis

m. platysma:
component arising from
middorsal tendinous raphe
component arising from skin

Fig. 2.61 Superficial structures of the cranial, auricular and retroauricular regions (1). Dorsal auricular and platysma muscles: dorsal view. The skin has been removed along with some limited cleaning of superficial fascia to display superficial structures. On the right side the pinna has been reflected rostrally to show the caudal nerves and blood vessels of the ear, and the continuation of the caudal auricular branch of the facial nerve (VII) to supply the platysma muscle (see also Fig. 3.7).

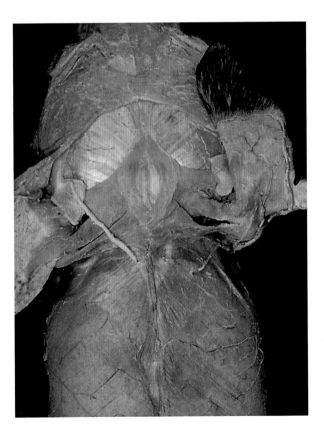

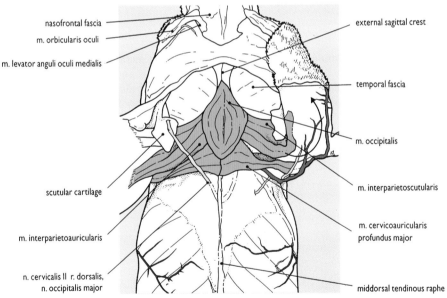

nasofrontal fascia

m. orbicularis oculi

m. levator anguli oculi medialis

scutular cartilage

m. interparietoauricularis

n. cervicalis II r. dorsalis,
n. occipitalis major

external sagittal crest

temporal fascia

m. occipitalis

m. interparietoscutularis

m. cervicoauricularis
profundus major

middorsal tendinous raphe

Fig. 2.62 Superficial structures of the cranial, auricular and retroauricular regions (2). Deep dorsal auricular muscles and scutular cartilage: dorsal view. The interscutular, cervicoscutular and superficial cervicoauricular muscles have been removed, exposing the interparietoscutular and interparietoauricular muscles (middle levators of the pinna) and the deep cervicoauricular muscles major and minor (long and short outward rotators of the pinna).

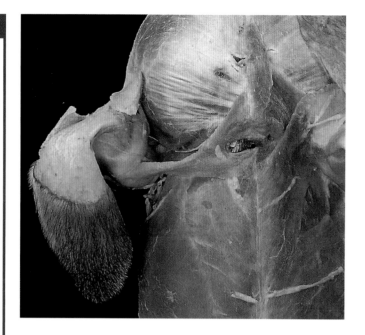

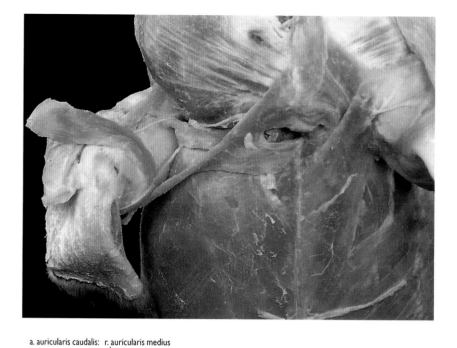

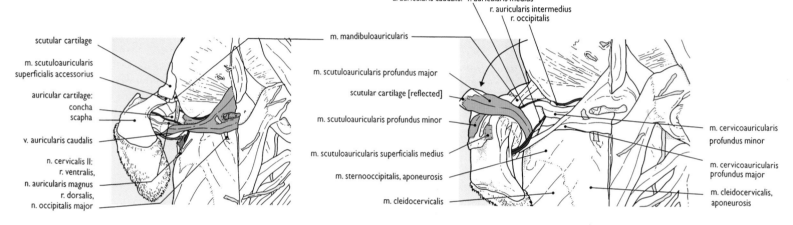

a. auricularis caudalis: r. auricularis medius
r. auricularis intermedius
r. occipitalis

m. mandibuloauricularis

m. scutuloauricularis profundus major

scutular cartilage [reflected]

m. scutuloauricularis profundus minor

m. scutuloauricularis superficialis medius

m. sternooccipitalis, aponeurosis

m. cleidocervicalis

m. cervicoauricularis profundus minor

m. cervicoauricularis profundus major

m. cleidocervicalis, aponeurosis

scutular cartilage

m. scutuloauricularis superficialis accessorius

auricular cartilage:
concha
scapha

v. auricularis caudalis

n. cervicalis II:
r. ventralis,
n. auricularis magnus
r. dorsalis,
n. occipitalis major

Fig. 2.63 Auricular and scutular cartilages of the left side (1). Caudal auricular vessels and nerve: dorsal view. The interparietoscutular and interparietoauricular muscles of the left side have been removed along with the dorsal superficial scutuloauricular component of the frontal muscle. After removal of these scutular components the scutular cartilage has been displaced slightly ventrally.

Fig. 2.64 Auricular and scutular cartilages of the left side (2). Deep intrinsic muscles after scutular reflection: dorsal view. The scutular cartilage has been reflected caudolaterally from the surface of the temporal fascia exposing the prominent scutuloauricularis profundus major muscle (the large conchal rotator) on its underside. Dissection of the cartilages and deep muscles of the pinna involves removing a cushion of fat deep to the scutular cartilage and around the base of the auricular cartilage.

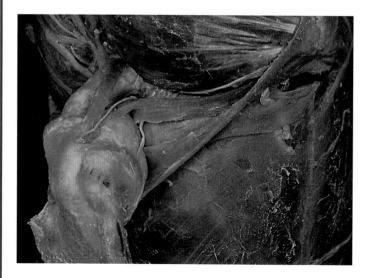

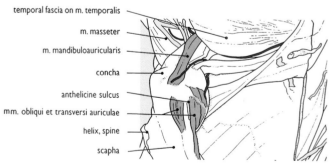

temporal fascia on m. temporalis

m. masseter

m. mandibuloauricularis

concha

anthelicine sulcus

mm. obliqui et transversi auriculae

helix, spine

scapha

Fig. 2.65 Auricular cartilage of the left side – mandibuloauricular muscle after scutular cartilage removal: dorsolateral view. The shallow anthelicine sulcus underlies the anthelix on the concave auricular surface (see also Figs 2.32 and 2.33) and marks the distinction between concha and scapha.

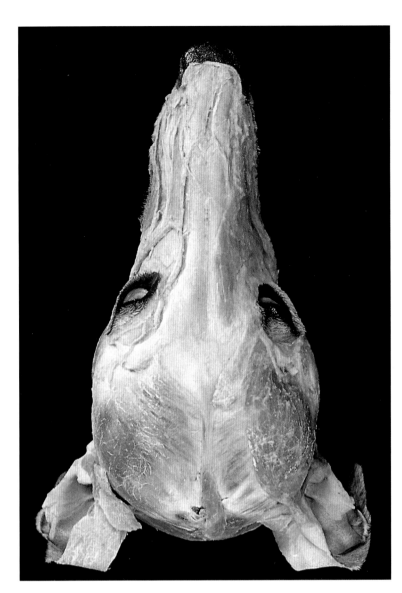

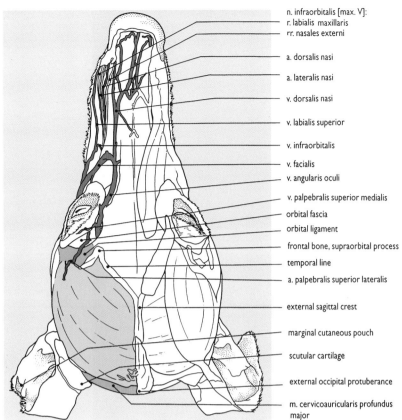

n. infraorbitalis [max. V]:
r. labialis maxillaris
rr. nasales externi

a. dorsalis nasi

a. lateralis nasi

v. dorsalis nasi

v. labialis superior

v. infraorbitalis

v. facialis

v. angularis oculi

v. palpebralis superior medialis

orbital fascia

orbital ligament

frontal bone, supraorbital process

temporal line

a. palpebralis superior lateralis

external sagittal crest

marginal cutaneous pouch

scutular cartilage

external occipital protuberance

m. cervicoauricularis profundus major

Fig. 2.66 Cranial and facial regions after removal of the superficial muscles: dorsal view. Practically all of the superficial muscles have been removed from the surface of the head along with the terminal branches of the facial nerve (VII). The isolated auricular and scutular cartilages of the left side remain in position on the temporal fascia.

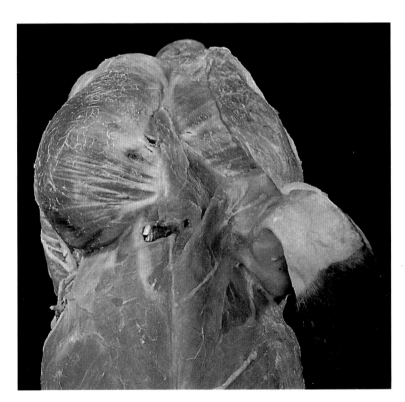

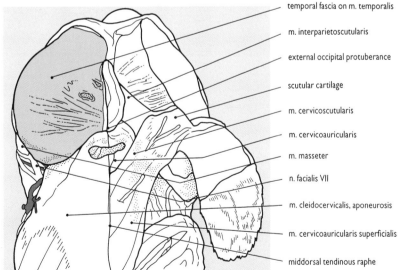

temporal fascia on m. temporalis

m. interparietoscutularis

external occipital protuberance

scutular cartilage

m. cervicoscutularis

m. cervicoauricularis

m. masseter

n. facialis VII

m. cleidocervicalis, aponeurosis

m. cervicoauricularis superficialis

middorsal tendinous raphe

Fig. 2.67 Cranial, auricular and retroauricular regions – temporal muscle after removal of the auricular and scutular cartilages: dorsal view. The auricular cartilage of the left side has been removed along with the remaining auricular muscles to expose the surface of the temporal muscle covered with temporal fascia.

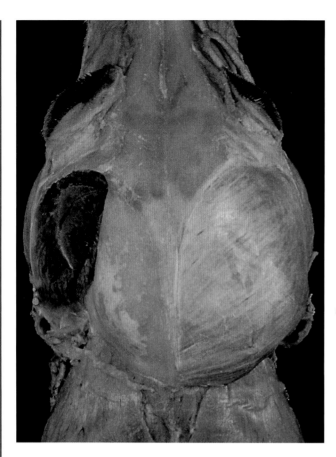

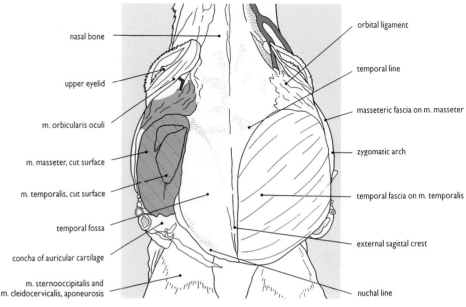

nasal bone

upper eyelid

m. orbicularis oculi

m. masseter, cut surface

m. temporalis, cut surface

temporal fossa

concha of auricular cartilage

m. sternooccipitalis and
m. cleidocervicalis, aponeurosis

orbital ligament

temporal line

masseteric fascia on m. masseter

zygomatic arch

temporal fascia on m. temporalis

external sagittal crest

nuchal line

Fig. 2.68 Temporal fossa of the left side following removal of the temporal muscle: dorsal view. The temporal fascia has been removed from the left side of the head and the underlying temporal muscle has been largely removed. The terminal part of the muscle attaching to the coronoid process is still in position and the process is as yet hidden. Medial to the zygomatic arch the masseter muscle blends to some extent with the temporal.

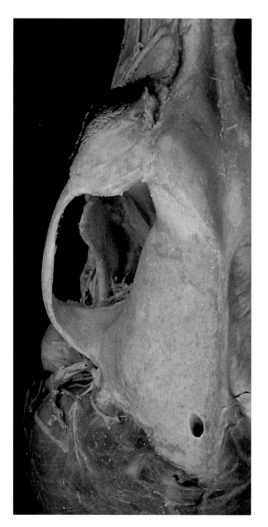

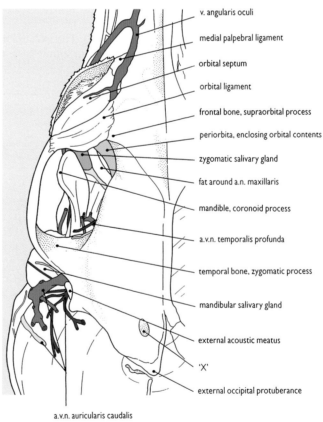

v. angularis oculi

medial palpebral ligament

orbital septum

orbital ligament

frontal bone, supraorbital process

periorbita, enclosing orbital contents

zygomatic salivary gland

fat around a.n. maxillaris

mandible, coronoid process

a.v.n. temporalis profunda

temporal bone, zygomatic process

mandibular salivary gland

external acoustic meatus

'X'

external occipital protuberance

a.v.n. auricularis caudalis

Fig. 2.69 Orbit, pterygopalatine and temporal fossae of the left side after removal of the temporal and masseter muscles: dorsal view. The temporal and masseter muscles have been removed exposing the entire dorsal surface of the cranium. This view clearly demonstrates how removal of the temporal muscle in no way disturbs orbital contents which are confined within the periorbita. NB The hole in the cranium at the point labelled 'X' in the drawing was made in order for a hook to be inserted for support of the embalmed dog.

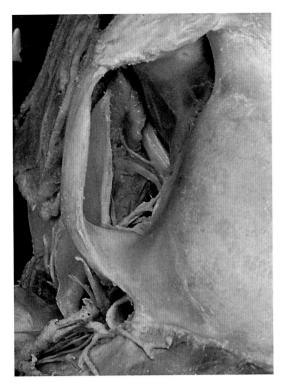

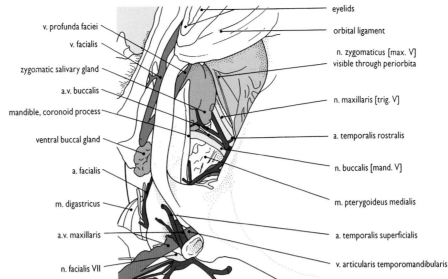

eyelids
orbital ligament

v. profunda faciei
v. facialis

n. zygomaticus [max. V]
visible through periorbita

zygomatic salivary gland

a.v. buccalis

n. maxillaris [trig. V]

mandible, coronoid process

a. temporalis rostralis

ventral buccal gland

n. buccalis [mand. V]

a. facialis

m. pterygoideus medialis

m. digastricus

a.v. maxillaris

a. temporalis superficialis

n. facialis VII

v. articularis temporomandibularis

Fig. 2.70 Pterygopalatine fossa of the left side – zygomatic gland and coronoid process of the mandible: dorsolateral view. This is a closer view of the specimen illustrated in Fig. 2.69 but viewed from a slightly more lateral angle. A limited amount of cleaning of fat and fascia from the floor of the pterygopalatine fossa has displayed the zygomatic gland together with the maxillary artery and nerve lying on the surface of the medial pterygoid muscle.

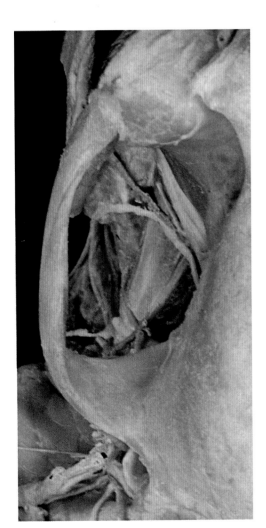

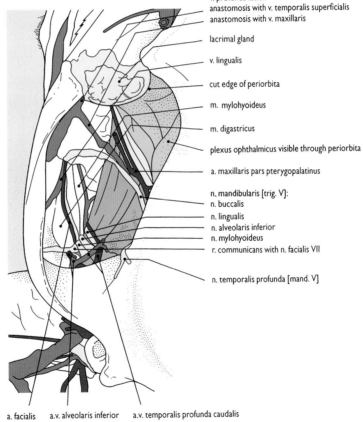

v. profunda faciei:
anastomosis with v. temporalis superficialis
anastomosis with v. maxillaris

lacrimal gland

v. lingualis

cut edge of periorbita

m. mylohyoideus

m. digastricus

plexus ophthalmicus visible through periorbita

a. maxillaris pars pterygopalatinus

n. mandibularis [trig. V]:
n. buccalis
n. lingualis
n. alveolaris inferior
n. mylohyoideus
r. communicans with n. facialis VII

n. temporalis profunda [mand. V]

a. facialis   a.v. alveolaris inferior   a.v. temporalis profunda caudalis

Fig. 2.71 Pterygopalatine and infratemporal fossae of the left side – maxillary and mandibular components of the trigeminal nerve: dorsal view. The orbital ligament has been removed opening the orbital rim and exposing the lacrimal gland. The cut edge of the periorbita is exposed where it blended with the orbital ligament 'sealing' the periorbital cone at its base. Removal of the lower jaw has allowed the zygomatic gland to be dissected out of the pterygopalatine fossa and orbital floor.

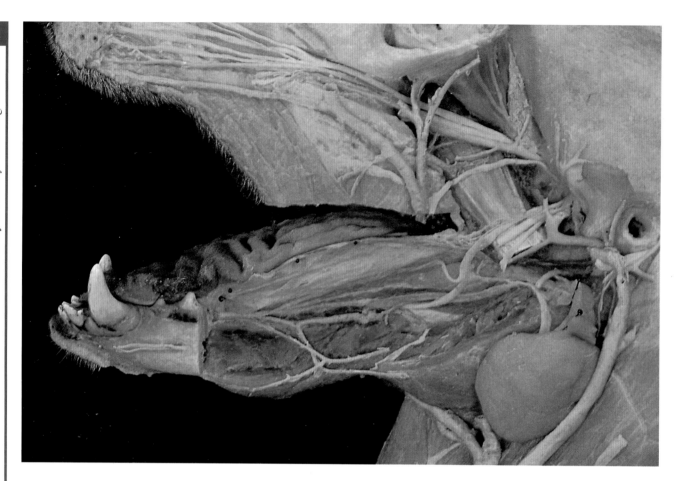

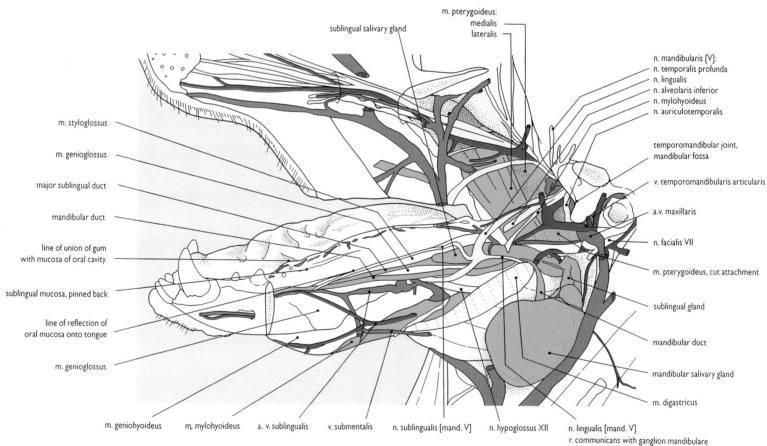

sublingual salivary gland

m. pterygoideus:
medialis
lateralis

n. mandibularis [V]:
n. temporalis profunda
n. lingualis
n. alveolaris inferior
n. mylohyoideus
n. auriculotemporalis

m. styloglossus

m. genioglossus

major sublingual duct

mandibular duct

line of union of gum
with mucosa of oral cavity

sublingual mucosa, pinned back

line of reflection of
oral mucosa onto tongue

m. genioglossus

temporomandibular joint,
mandibular fossa

v. temporomandibularis articularis

a.v. maxillaris

n. facialis VII

m. pterygoideus, cut attachment

sublingual gland

mandibular duct

mandibular salivary gland

m. digastricus

m. geniohyoideus   m. mylohyoideus   a. v. sublingualis   v. submentalis   n. sublingualis [mand. V]   n. hypoglossus XII   n. lingualis [mand. V]
r. communicans with ganglion mandibulare

Fig. 2.72 Pterygopalatine fossa and lower jaw – mandibular and sublingual salivary glands and ducts: left lateral view. This deep dissection has involved removal of the temporal and masseter muscles, and the zygomatic arch and mandible. In the pterygopalatine fossa and orbit both zygomatic gland and periorbita are removed and the pterygoid muscles have been trimmed back further. In the lower jaw the mylohyoid nerve and facial artery have been removed and the cut mandibular attachments of both digastric and mylohyoid muscles have been additionally trimmed. The sublingual salivary gland has been displaced and pinned out of the way to expose the mandibular duct.

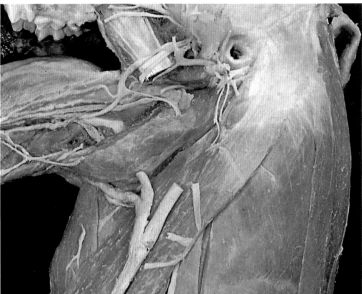

Fig. 2.73 Pharyngeal and laryngeal regions (1). Digastric muscle after removal of the mandibular salivary gland: left lateral view. The initial part of the sublingual gland and the whole of the mandibular salivary gland have been removed, along with that part of the maxillary vein bordering the mandibular gland. Since this specimen was embalmed with its mouth wide open and its head bent down on its neck, the digastric and sterno-occipital muscles are approximated and obscure the structures in the pharyngeal region which would be more clearly visible were the mouth closed (see also Figs 3.17–3.21). This region at the boundary between neck and head is dealt with to some extent in Chapter 3.

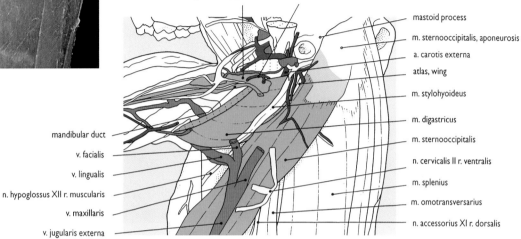

sublingual salivary gland — a. facialis — mastoid process — m. sternooccipitalis, aponeurosis — a. carotis externa — atlas, wing — m. stylohyoideus — m. digastricus — m. sternooccipitalis — n. cervicalis II r. ventralis — m. splenius — m. omotransversarius — n. accessorius XI r. dorsalis

mandibular duct — v. facialis — v. lingualis — n. hypoglossus XII r. muscularis — v. maxillaris — v. jugularis externa

Fig. 2.74 Pharyngeal and laryngeal regions (2). Medial retropharyngeal lymph node after reflection of the mastoid muscles: left lateral view. The external jugular vein and the sterno-occipital component of the sternocephalic muscle have been removed; the sternomastoid and cleidomastoid muscles have been cut and reflected. The medial retropharyngeal lymph node is exposed to a limited extent although it is exposed to greater advantage in Figs 3.14–3.20 and in section in Figs 3.35 and 3.36.

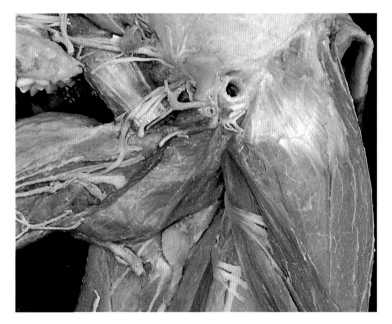

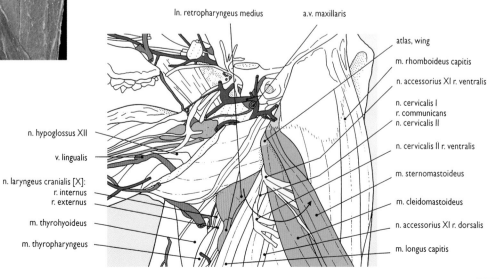

ln. retropharyngeus medius — a.v. maxillaris — atlas, wing — m. rhomboideus capitis — n. accessorius XI r. ventralis — n. cervicalis I r. communicans — n. cervicalis II — n. cervicalis II r. ventralis — m. sternomastoideus — m. cleidomastoideus — n. accessorius XI r. dorsalis — m. longus capitis

n. hypoglossus XII — v. lingualis — n. laryngeus cranialis [X]: r. internus, r. externus — m. thyrohyoideus — m. thyropharyngeus

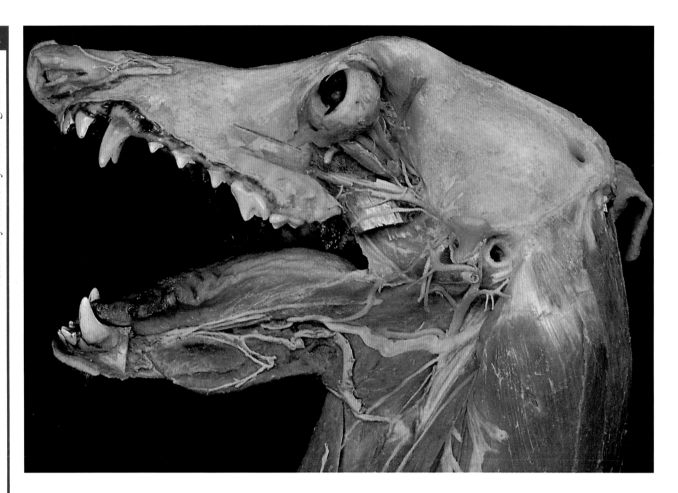

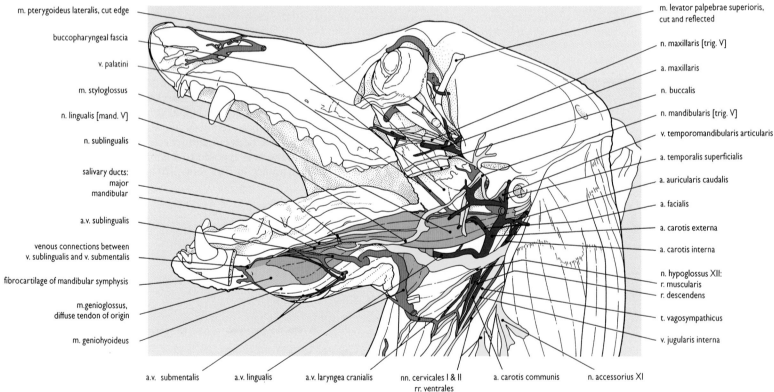

m. pterygoideus lateralis, cut edge

buccopharyngeal fascia

v. palatini

m. styloglossus

n. lingualis [mand. V]

n. sublingualis

salivary ducts:
major
mandibular

a.v. sublingualis

venous connections between
v. sublingualis and v. submentalis

fibrocartilage of mandibular symphysis

m.genioglossus,
diffuse tendon of origin

m. geniohyoideus

m. levator palpebrae superioris,
cut and reflected

n. maxillaris [trig. V]

a. maxillaris

n. buccalis

n. mandibularis [trig. V]

v. temporomandibularis articularis

a. temporalis superficialis

a. auricularis caudalis

a. facialis

a. carotis externa

a. carotis interna

n. hypoglossus XII:
r. muscularis
r. descendens

t. vagosympathicus

v. jugularis interna

a.v. submentalis   a.v. lingualis   a.v. laryngea cranialis   nn. cervicales I & II   a. carotis communis   n. accessorius XI
rr. ventrales

Fig. 2.75 Pharynx and tongue (1). Hypoglossal nerve, external carotid artery and styloglossal muscle: left lateral view. The pharyngeal region and the root of the tongue have been exposed by removal of the digastric, stylohyoid, sternomastoid and cleidomastoid muscles, the sublingual salivary gland and the medial retropharyneal lymph node. An extremely delicate hypoglossal loop is visible on the surface of the common carotid artery although a muscular branch from the hypoglossal nerve to the sternohyoid muscle, passing beneath the cranial laryngeal vein, is a considerably more substantial structure.

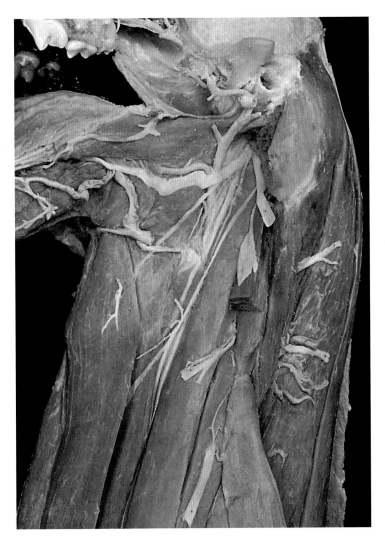

Fig. 2.76 Pharynx and tongue (2). Hypoglossal nerve, accessory nerve and ventral ramus of cervical nerve 1: left ventrolateral view. This picture shows essentially the same stage of pharyngeal dissection as that in Fig. 2.75, but from a slightly different angle. In the nasopharyngeal region the proximal part of the mandibular branch of trigeminal nerve (V) and the underlying pterygoid muscles have been removed. The more distal part of the nerve, the lingual component, remains on the styloglossal muscle but it is displaced dorsally to demonstrate its entry into the tongue ventral to the muscle. Removal of the pterygoid muscles has exposed the palatine and pterygoid bones where they form the medial boundary of the pterygopalatine fossa and the lateral wall of the nasopharynx (shown in section, Fig. 2.143). Dorsally in the neck, the splenius, rhomboideus and omotransverse muscles have been removed, except for a stump of the omotransverse attached to the atlas wing. For details of this part of the neck see Chapters 3 and 9.

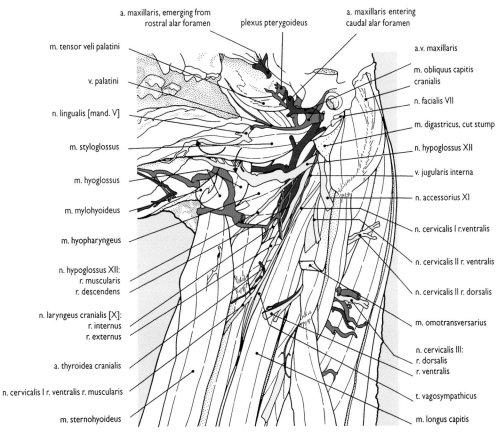

a. maxillaris, emerging from rostral alar foramen

plexus pterygoideus

a. maxillaris entering caudal alar foramen

m. tensor veli palatini

v. palatini

n. lingualis [mand. V]

m. styloglossus

m. hyoglossus

m. mylohyoideus

m. hyopharyngeus

n. hypoglossus XII:
r. muscularis
r. descendens

n. laryngeus cranialis [X]:
r. internus
r. externus

a. thyroidea cranialis

n. cervicalis I r. ventralis r. muscularis

m. sternohyoideus

a.v. maxillaris

m. obliquus capitis cranialis

n. facialis VII

m. digastricus, cut stump

n. hypoglossus XII

v. jugularis interna

n. accessorius XI

n. cervicalis I r.ventralis

n. cervicalis II r. ventralis

n. cervicalis II r. dorsalis

m. omotransversarius

n. cervicalis III:
r. dorsalis
r. ventralis

t. vagosympathicus

m. longus capitis

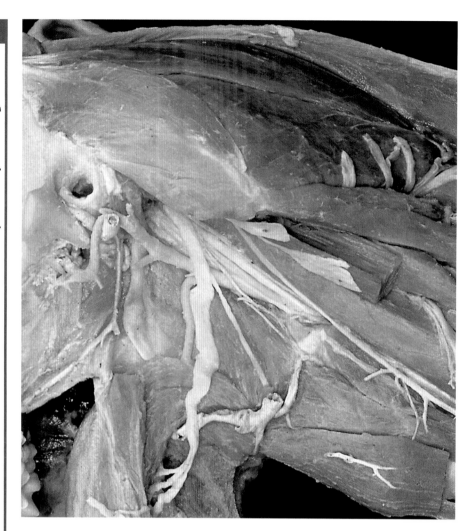

Fig. 2.77 Pharynx and tongue (3). Cranial horn of the hyoid and root of the tongue: left lateral view. The proximal part of the styloglossal muscle has been removed to expose the stylohyoid and epihyoid bones. Displacement of the hypoglossal nerve (XII) and the remnant of the lingual nerve demonstrates the entry of the hyoglossal muscle into the tongue between the lingual artery and vein. Rostral to the hyoid horn some further clearing of external pharyngeal fascia reveals both tensor and levator muscles of the palatine veil and the pterygopharyngeal muscle. Dorsally the splenius muscle has been removed, displaying the oblique capital muscles and muscular branches of the dorsal rami of cervical nerves 2 and 3.

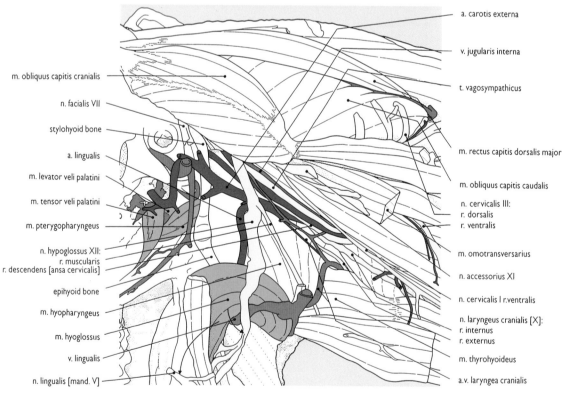

m. obliquus capitis cranialis

n. facialis VII

stylohyoid bone

a. lingualis

m. levator veli palatini

m. tensor veli palatini

m. pterygopharyngeus

n. hypoglossus XII:
r. muscularis
r. descendens [ansa cervicalis]

epihyoid bone

m. hyopharyngeus

m. hyoglossus

v. lingualis

n. lingualis [mand. V]

a. carotis externa

v. jugularis interna

t. vagosympathicus

m. rectus capitis dorsalis major

m. obliquus capitis caudalis

n. cervicalis III:
r. dorsalis
r. ventralis

m. omotransversarius

n. accessorius XI

n. cervicalis I r.ventralis

n. laryngeus cranialis [X]:
r. internus
r. externus

m. thyrohyoideus

a.v. laryngea cranialis

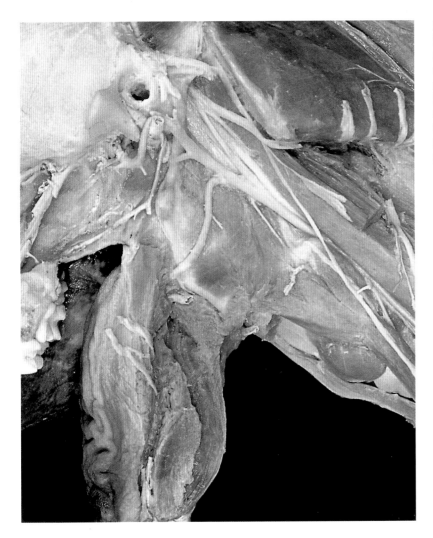

Fig. 2.78 Pharynx and tongue (4). Hyoid apparatus and carotid arterial branching: left lateral view. The hypoglossal nerve (XII) has been reflected along with the remains of the lingual nerve. The lingual vein and hyoglossal muscle have also been removed, although their cut stumps remain in position. In the pharyngeal region removal of veins has clarified the limits of pharyngeal muscles caudal to the lingual artery. Dorsally in the neck removal of the cranial capital oblique and the rectus capitis lateralis muscles has exposed the accessory nerve (XI), the ventral ramus of cervical nerve 1, and the continuations of the internal carotid and occipital arteries.

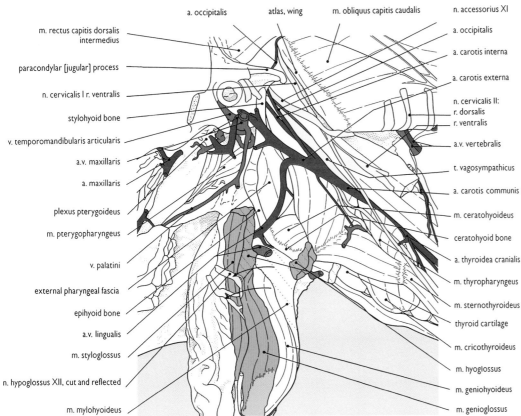

a. occipitalis   atlas, wing   m. obliquus capitis caudalis   n. accessorius XI

m. rectus capitis dorsalis intermedius

paracondylar [jugular] process

n. cervicalis I r. ventralis

stylohyoid bone

v. temporomandibularis articularis

a.v. maxillaris

a. maxillaris

plexus pterygoideus

m. pterygopharyngeus

v. palatini

external pharyngeal fascia

epihyoid bone

a.v. lingualis

m. styloglossus

n. hypoglossus XII, cut and reflected

m. mylohyoideus

a. occipitalis

a. carotis interna

a. carotis externa

n. cervicalis II:
r. dorsalis
r. ventralis

a.v. vertebralis

t. vagosympathicus

a. carotis communis

m. ceratohyoideus

ceratohyoid bone

a. thyroidea cranialis

m. thyropharyngeus

m. sternothyroideus

thyroid cartilage

m. cricothyroideus

m. hyoglossus

m. geniohyoideus

m. genioglossus

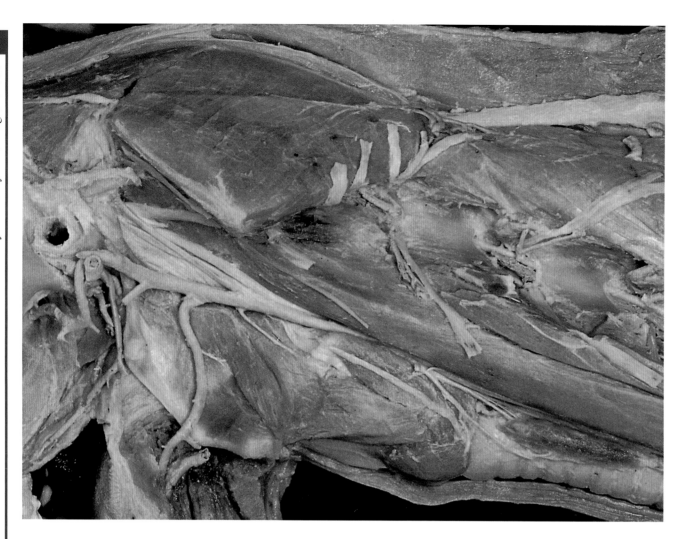

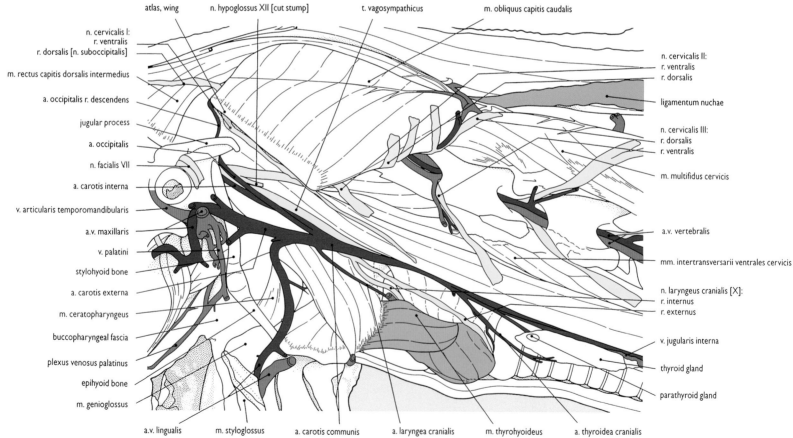

atlas, wing   n. hypoglossus XII [cut stump]   t. vagosympathicus   m. obliquus capitis caudalis

n. cervicalis I:
r. ventralis
r. dorsalis [n. suboccipitalis]

m. rectus capitis dorsalis intermedius

a. occipitalis r. descendens

jugular process

a. occipitalis

n. facialis VII

a. carotis interna

v. articularis temporomandibularis

a.v. maxillaris

v. palatini

stylohyoid bone

a. carotis externa

m. ceratopharyngeus

buccopharyngeal fascia

plexus venosus palatinus

epihyoid bone

m. genioglossus

n. cervicalis II:
r. ventralis
r. dorsalis

ligamentum nuchae

n. cervicalis III:
r. dorsalis
r. ventralis

m. multifidus cervicis

a.v. vertebralis

mm. intertransversarii ventrales cervicis

n. laryngeus cranialis [X]:
r. internus
r. externus

v. jugularis interna

thyroid gland

parathyroid gland

a.v. lingualis   m. styloglossus   a. carotis communis   a. laryngea cranialis   m. thyrohyoideus   a. thyroidea cranialis

Fig. 2.79 Pharynx and larynx (1). Hyoid apparatus and extrinsic laryngeal muscles: left lateral view. This picture and the following six show progressive stages in the exposure of the larynx and musculature of the palate and pharynx. Their innervation through branches from glossopharyngeal (IX) and vagus (X) nerves and the sympathetic system is shown. Laryngeal structure is also shown from ventral view in Figs 2.131 and 2.135, and in cross section in Chapter 3. Removal of the sternohyoid and sternothyroid muscles begins laryngeal exposure. The remains of the omotransverse, biventer, complexus, longissimus and intertransverse muscles have all been removed, exposing cervical vertebrae 3 and 4 with vertebral vessels (see Chapter 3).

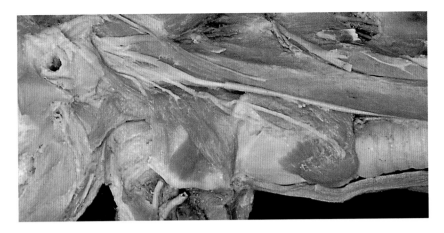

Fig. 2.80 Pharynx and larynx (2). Palatine and pharyngeal muscles and innervation of the larynx: left lateral view. The palatine and pharyngeal muscles and the pharyngeal and laryngeal nerve supply have been exposed by removing: the terminal branching of the common carotid artery; the remains of the maxillary vein and its tributaries; a section of the cranial hyoid horn; external pharyngeal fascia; the thyrohyoid muscle. Removal of the thyroid gland has also exposed the caudal laryngeal nerve (X).

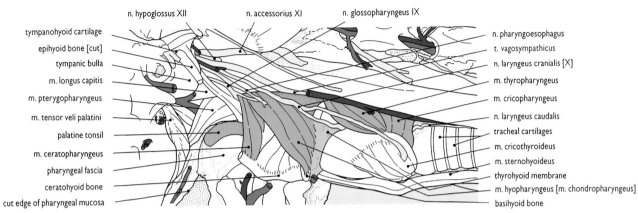

n. hypoglossus XII — n. accessorius XI — n. glossopharyngeus IX

tympanohyoid cartilage
epihyoid bone [cut]
tympanic bulla
m. longus capitis
m. pterygopharyngeus
m. tensor veli palatini
palatine tonsil
m. ceratopharyngeus
pharyngeal fascia
ceratohyoid bone
cut edge of pharyngeal mucosa

n. pharyngoesophagus
t. vagosympathicus
n. laryngeus cranialis [X]
m. thyropharyngeus
m. cricopharyngeus
n. laryngeus caudalis
tracheal cartilages
m. cricothyroideus
m. sternohyoideus
thyrohyoid membrane
m. hyopharyngeus [m. chondropharyngeus]
basihyoid bone

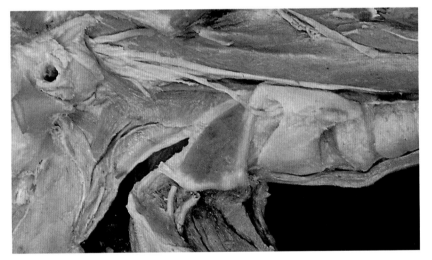

Fig. 2.81 Pharynx and larynx (3). Soft palate, pharyngeal nerves and muscles, and laryngeal cartilages: left lateral view. Further dissection has involved removing: the ceratopharyngeal, hyopharyngeal, thyropharyngeal, cricopharyngeal and cricothyroid muscles; the palatine tonsil and palatine fascia; and some oropharyngeal mucosa from the palatoglossal arch caudally. The full extent of the palatopharyngeal and stylopharyngeal muscles is exposed in the nasopharyngeal wall (see also Figs 2.91 and 2.92 from a medial view).

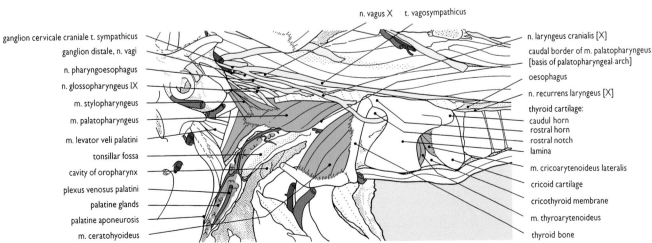

n. vagus X — t. vagosympathicus

ganglion cervicale craniale t. sympathicus
ganglion distale, n. vagi
n. pharyngoesophagus
n. glossopharyngeus IX
m. stylopharyngeus
m. palatopharyngeus
m. levator veli palatini
tonsillar fossa
cavity of oropharynx
plexus venosus palatini
palatine glands
palatine aponeurosis
m. ceratohyoideus

n. laryngeus cranialis [X]
caudal border of m. palatopharyngeus [basis of palatopharyngeal arch]
oesophagus
n. recurrens laryngeus [X]
thyroid cartilage:
caudul horn
rostral horn
rostral notch
lamina
m. cricoarytenoideus lateralis
cricoid cartilage
cricothyroid membrane
m. thyroarytenoideus
thyroid bone

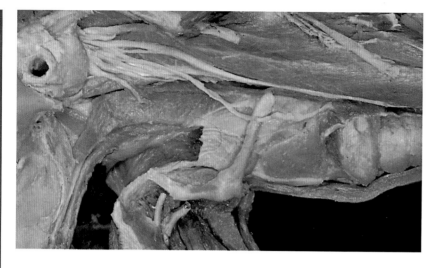

Fig. 2.82 Pharynx and larynx (4). Intrinsic laryngeal muscles, laryngeal ventricle and laryngeal innervation: left lateral view. The glandular and venous tissue of the soft palate have been removed to expose the longitudinal palatine muscle. The thyroid lamina has been removed, exposing intrinsic laryngeal muscles and the sac-like laryngeal ventricle. At the base of the tongue removal of the ceratohyoid muscle exposes geniohyoid, mylohyoid and tongue muscles converging on the basihyoid and ceratohyoid bones.

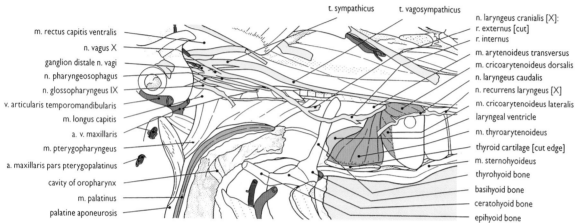

Fig. 2.83 Pharynx and larynx (5). Intrinsic laryngeal muscles and interior of the larynx: left lateral view. This picture completes the dissection from a left lateral aspect with the thyrohyoid bone, thyroarytenoid muscle and laryngeal ventricle having been removed from the larynx. Removal of pharyngeal mucosa also reveals the epiglottis, its apex related to the caudal border of the soft palate marked by the termination of the palatopharyngeal muscle at the palatopharyngeal arch.

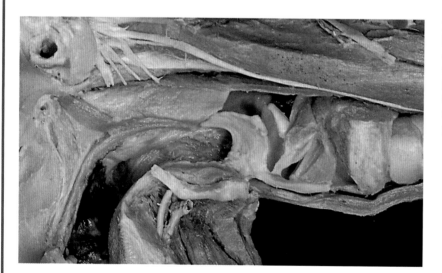

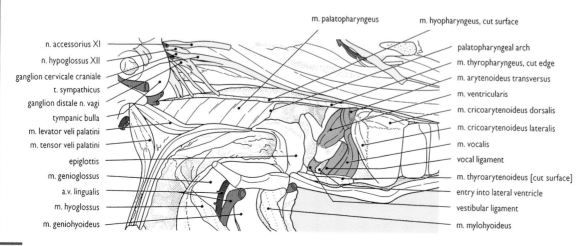

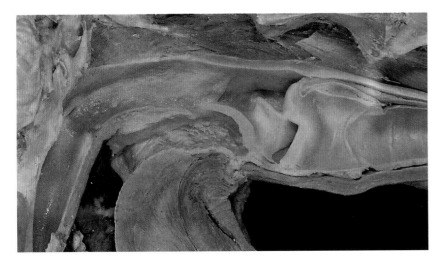

Fig. 2.84 Pharynx, larynx and root of tongue in median section: medial view of right half. The pharynx, larynx and the root of the tongue have been sectioned in the median plane to give a medial view of the right half of the pharynx and larynx. The approximate extent of the lateral ventricle is indicated on the drawing by a broken line.

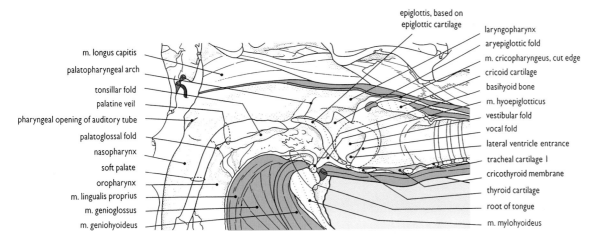

epiglottis, based on epiglottic cartilage

m. longus capitis
palatopharyngeal arch
tonsillar fold
palatine veil
pharyngeal opening of auditory tube
palatoglossal fold
nasopharynx
soft palate
oropharynx
m. lingualis proprius
m. genioglossus
m. geniohyoideus

laryngopharynx
aryepiglottic fold
m. cricopharyngeus, cut edge
cricoid cartilage
basihyoid bone
m. hyoepiglotticus
vestibular fold
vocal fold
lateral ventricle entrance
tracheal cartilage I
cricothyroid membrane
thyroid cartilage
root of tongue
m. mylohyoideus

Fig. 2.85 Pharyngeal and laryngeal muscles of the right side: medial view. On stripping the lining mucosa from the wall of the pharynx and larynx the epiglottis came free from its fibrous connections with the thyroid cartilage and basihyoid bone and has been pinned back into its approximate position. The structure of the larynx is also shown in Fig. 2.134 and in Chapter 3.

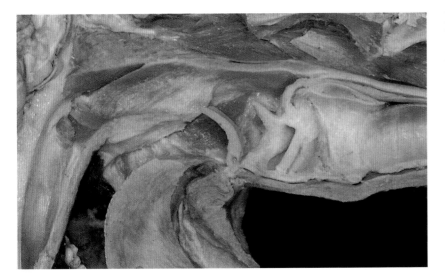

m. ceratohyoideus   thyrohyoid bone

m. palatopharyngeus
m. pterygopharyngeus
m. levator veli palatini
m. tensor veli palatini
palatine tonsil
pterygoid
sphenoid bone
m. styloglossus
palatine aponeurosis
m. ceratopharyngeus
m. hyoglossus
v. n. sublingualis

laryngeal ventricle
arytenoid cartilage:
corniculate process
cuneiform process
articular process
oesophagus
cricotracheal ligament
arytenoid cartilage, vocal process
m. cricoarytenoideus lateralis
m. cricothyroideus
m. vocalis
vocal ligament
vestibular ligament

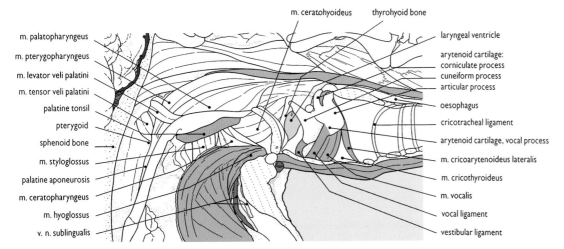

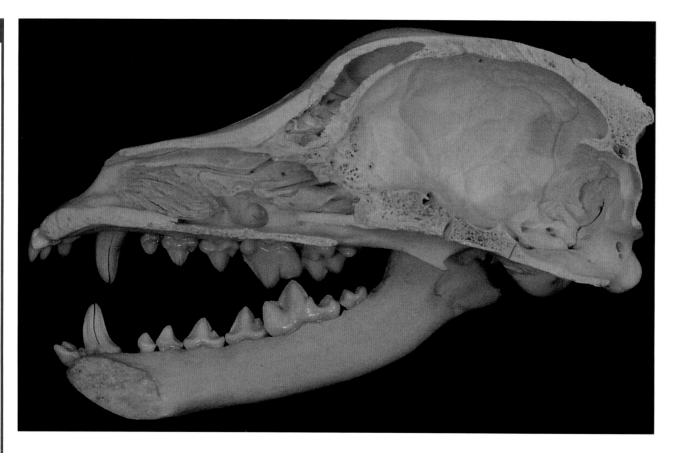

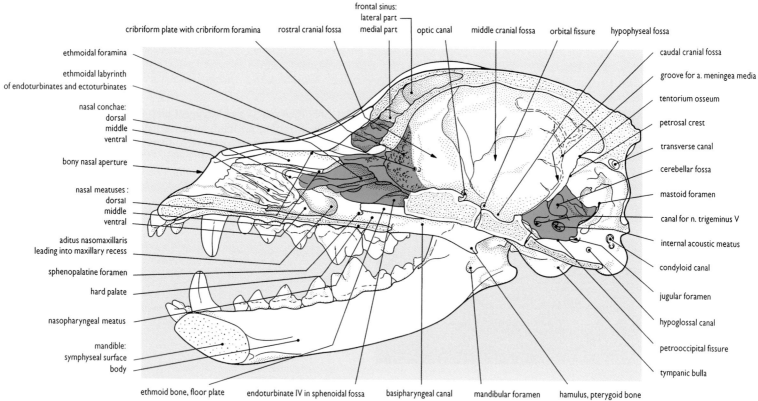

frontal sinus:
lateral part
medial part

cribriform plate with cribriform foramina · rostral cranial fossa · optic canal · middle cranial fossa · orbital fissure · hypophyseal fossa

ethmoidal foramina

ethmoidal labyrinth
of endoturbinates and ectoturbinates

nasal conchae:
dorsal
middle
ventral

bony nasal aperture

nasal meatuses :
dorsal
middle
ventral

aditus nasomaxillaris
leading into maxillary recess

sphenopalatine foramen

hard palate

nasopharyngeal meatus

mandible:
symphyseal surface
body

caudal cranial fossa

groove for a. meningea media

tentorium osseum

petrosal crest

transverse canal

cerebellar fossa

mastoid foramen

canal for n. trigeminus V

internal acoustic meatus

condyloid canal

jugular foramen

hypoglossal canal

petrooccipital fissure

tympanic bulla

ethmoid bone, floor plate · endoturbinate IV in sphenoidal fossa · basipharyngeal canal · mandibular foramen · hamulus, pterygoid bone

Fig. 2.86 Skull in median section: medial view of right half. This picture is included to provide a basis for interpretation of many of the next 30 pictures. After sectioning, the septal processes of the frontal and nasal bones were removed, opening the frontal sinus of the right side. Its medial compartment contains turbinate extensions from the ethmoidal labyrinth (see also Fig. 2.105). The internasal septum has also been removed, opening the right nasal fossa. For clarification the ethmoid bone and the complex petrous temporal bone (pyramid) are colored in the drawing (see Figs 2.115 and 2.116).

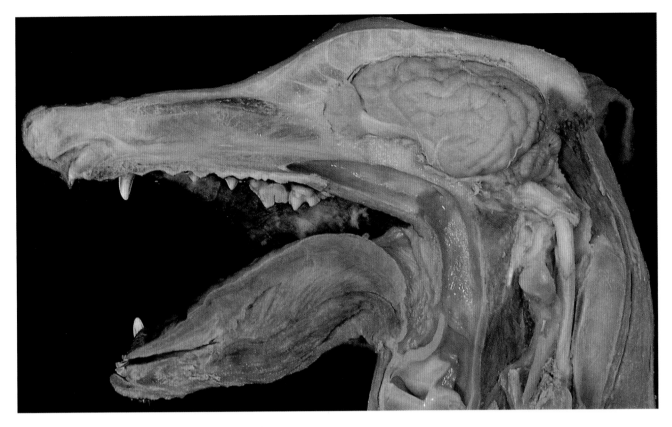

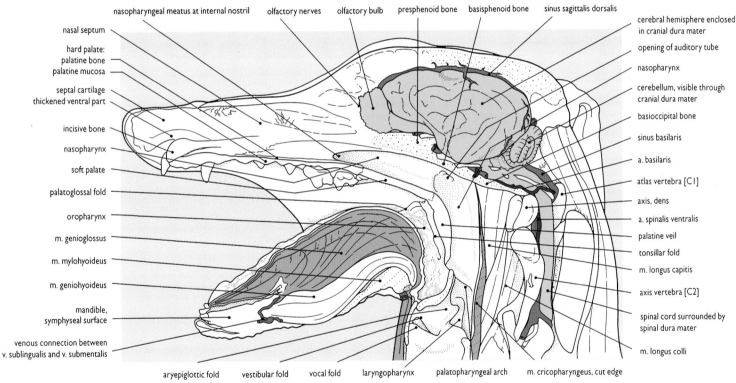

nasopharyngeal meatus at internal nostril   olfactory nerves   olfactory bulb   presphenoid bone   basisphenoid bone   sinus sagittalis dorsalis

nasal septum

hard palate:
palatine bone
palatine mucosa

septal cartilage
thickened ventral part

incisive bone

nasopharynx

soft palate

palatoglossal fold

oropharynx

m. genioglossus

m. mylohyoideus

m. geniohyoideus

mandible,
symphyseal surface

venous connection between
v. sublingualis and v. submentalis

cerebral hemisphere enclosed
in cranial dura mater

opening of auditory tube

nasopharynx

cerebellum, visible through
cranial dura mater

basioccipital bone

sinus basilaris

a. basilaris

atlas vertebra [C1]

axis, dens

a. spinalis ventralis

palatine veil

tonsillar fold

m. longus capitis

axis vertebra [C2]

spinal cord surrounded by
spinal dura mater

m. longus colli

aryepiglottic fold   vestibular fold   vocal fold   laryngopharynx   palatopharyngeal arch   m. cricopharyngeus, cut edge

Fig. 2.87 Nasal cavity, tongue, pharynx and larynx in median section: medial view of right half. The midline section of the nasal region exposes the nasal septum (shown in more detail in Fig. 2.103). The tongue in median section begins a sequence continued in Figs 2.89–2.94. The pharynx and larynx in median section are continued in Figs 2.91–2.94. The brain was left intact within its meninges when the cranial bones were removed 'piecemeal' and is shown in more detail in Figs 2.109–2.115 and Figs 2.118–2.121. The atlas has been sectioned in the midline but the axis has only had the lateral wall of its arch removed.

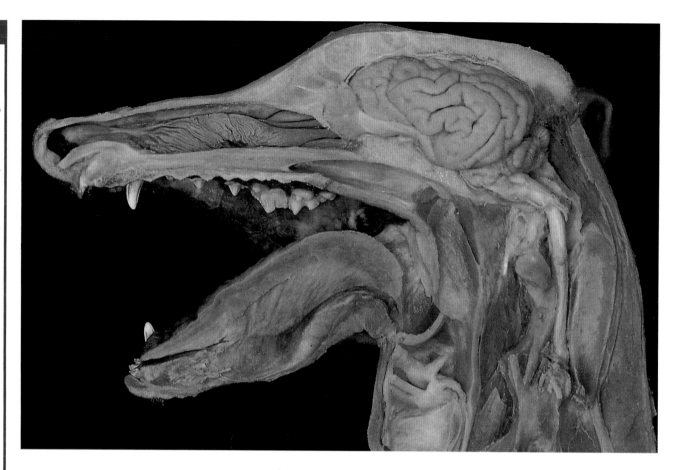

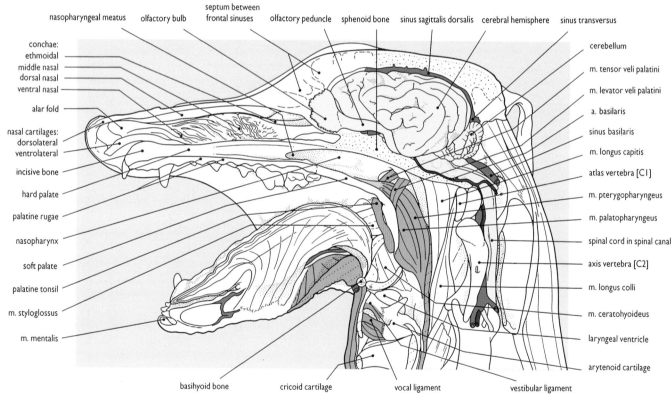

nasopharyngeal meatus   olfactory bulb   septum between frontal sinuses   olfactory peduncle   sphenoid bone   sinus sagittalis dorsalis   cerebral hemisphere   sinus transversus

conchae:
ethmoidal
middle nasal
dorsal nasal
ventral nasal

alar fold

nasal cartilages:
dorsolateral
ventrolateral

incisive bone

hard palate

palatine rugae

nasopharynx

soft palate

palatine tonsil

m. styloglossus

m. mentalis

cerebellum

m. tensor veli palatini

m. levator veli palatini

a. basilaris

sinus basilaris

m. longus capitis

atlas vertebra [C1]

m. pterygopharyngeus

m. palatopharyngeus

spinal cord in spinal canal

axis vertebra [C2]

m. longus colli

m. ceratohyoideus

laryngeal ventricle

arytenoid cartilage

basihyoid bone   cricoid cartilage   vocal ligament   vestibular ligament

Fig. 2.88 Nasal cavity, tongue, pharynx and larynx of the right side: medial view. Removal of the nasal septum opening the nasal fossa begins the dissection of the right side of the nose (enlarged in Fig. 2.104). In the tongue removal of the geniohyoid muscle begins the exposure of vessels and nerves continued in the dissections shown in Figs 2.89 and 2.90.

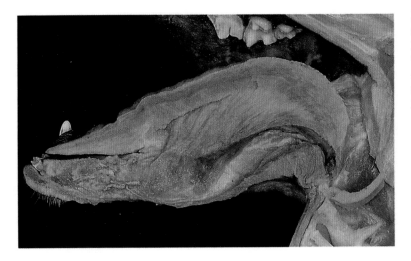

Fig. 2.89 Tongue (1). Muscles of the right side: medial view. This is an enlarged view of the tongue shown in Fig. 2.88. The geniohyoid muscle has been removed and the genioglossal muscle spreading fan-like into the body of the tongue is exposed. Removal of oropharyngeal mucosa caudal to the palatoglossal fold has exposed the styloglossal muscle. The structure of the tongue is shown from a ventral view in Figs 2.129 and 2.130, and its internal structure in section in Figs 2.139–2.145.

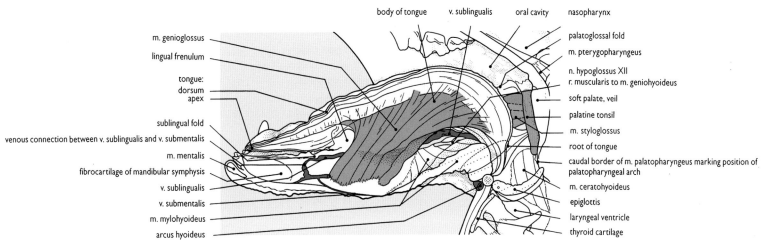

Fig. 2.90 Tongue (2). Blood and nerve supply to the right side: medial view. Removal of the genioglossal muscle has allowed the tongue to be raised, stretching the sublingual mucosa and exposing the salivary ducts, sublingual vessels and nerve (see also sections, Figs 2.139–2.142). Raising the tongue has rotated its root caudally displacing the epiglottic cartilage – much as would happen during normal deglutition.

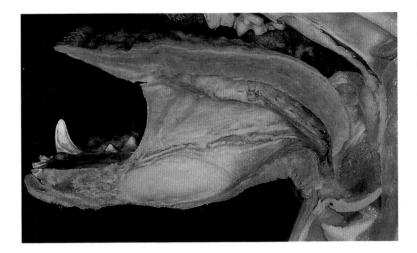

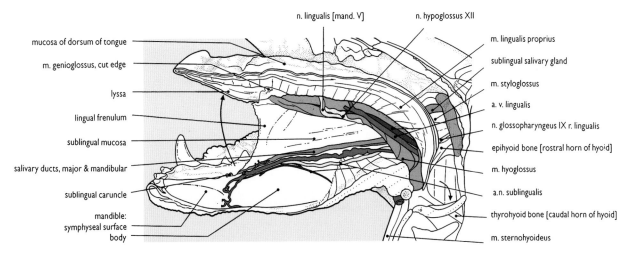

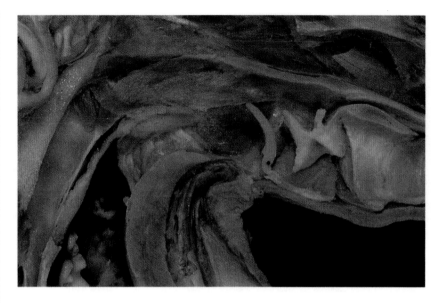

Fig. 2.91 Pharynx and larynx (1). Pharyngeal muscles and palatine tonsil of the right side and root of the tongue: medial view. This picture continues the stage reached in Fig. 2.85. Removal of the genioglossal and geniohyoid muscles exposes nerves and blood vessels displayed more fully in Fig. 2.90. The vocal and vestibular ligaments and the vocal muscle have been removed, exposing the arytenoid cartilage (see also Figs 2.78–2.81 in lateral view).

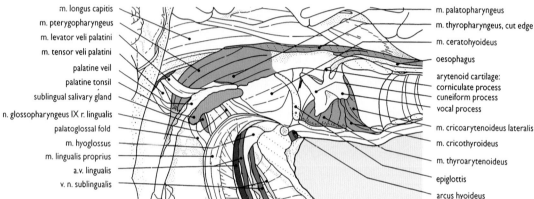

m. longus capitis
m. pterygopharyngeus
m. levator veli palatini
m. tensor veli palatini
palatine veil
palatine tonsil
sublingual salivary gland
n. glossopharyngeus IX r. lingualis
palatoglossal fold
m. hyoglossus
m. lingualis proprius
a.v. lingualis
v. n. sublingualis

m. palatopharyngeus
m. thyropharyngeus, cut edge
m. ceratohyoideus
oesophagus
arytenoid cartilage:
corniculate process
cuneiform process
vocal process
m. cricoarytenoideus lateralis
m. cricothyroideus
m. thyroarytenoideus
epiglottis
arcus hyoideus

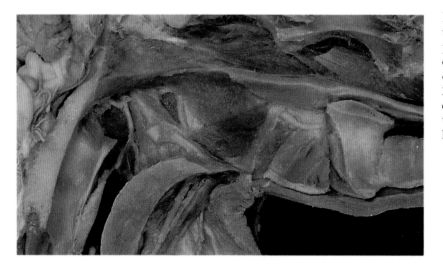

Fig. 2.92 Pharynx and larynx (2). Pharyngeal and hyoid muscles of the right side and root of the tongue: medial view. Removal of the palatine tonsil, palatine veil and palatine muscles has broken down the division between oro- and nasopharynx (the structure of the soft palate is also shown in ventral view in Figs 2.135 and 2.136 and in section in Figs 2.143–2.145). Removal of the epiglottis and arytenoid cartilages and the upper ends of the first two tracheal cartilages has exposed the cranial and caudal laryngeal nerves.

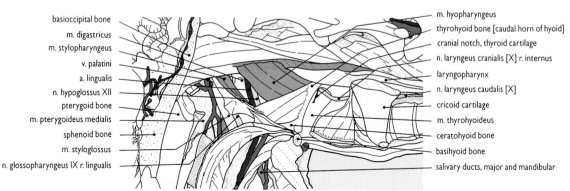

basioccipital bone
m. digastricus
m. stylopharyngeus
v. palatini
a. lingualis
n. hypoglossus XII
pterygoid bone
m. pterygoideus medialis
sphenoid bone
m. styloglossus
n. glossopharyngeus IX r. lingualis

m. hyopharyngeus
thyrohyoid bone [caudal horn of hyoid]
cranial notch, thyroid cartilage
n. laryngeus cranialis [X] r. internus
laryngopharynx
n. laryngeus caudalis [X]
cricoid cartilage
m. thyrohyoideus
ceratohyoid bone
basihyoid bone
salivary ducts, major and mandibular

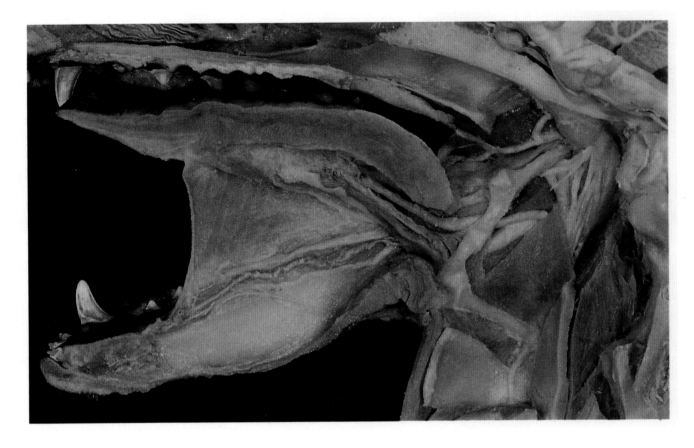

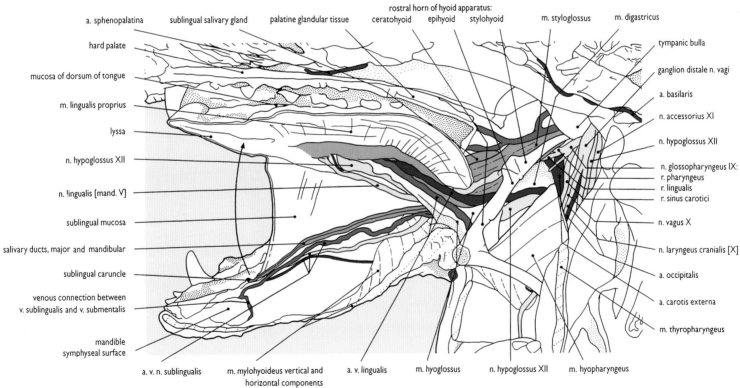

a. sphenopalatina | sublingual salivary gland | palatine glandular tissue | rostral horn of hyoid apparatus: ceratohyoid | epihyoid | stylohyoid | m. styloglossus | m. digastricus

hard palate

tympanic bulla

mucosa of dorsum of tongue

ganglion distale n. vagi

m. lingualis proprius

a. basilaris

n. accessorius XI

lyssa

n. hypoglossus XII

n. hypoglossus XII

n. glossopharyngeus IX:
r. pharyngeus
r. lingualis
r. sinus carotici

n. lingualis [mand. V]

sublingual mucosa

n. vagus X

salivary ducts, major and mandibular

n. laryngeus cranialis [X]

sublingual caruncle

a. occipitalis

venous connection between
v. sublingualis and v. submentalis

a. carotis externa

m. thyropharyngeus

mandible
symphyseal surface

a. v. n. sublingualis | m. mylohyoideus vertical and horizontal components | a. v. lingualis | m. hyoglossus | n. hypoglossus XII | m. hyopharyngeus

Fig. 2.93 Hyoid apparatus, blood vessels and nerves bordering the right side of the pharynx: medial view (1). Removal of the ceratohyoid, stylopharyngeal and longus capitis muscles has exposed nerves and blood vessels bordering the pharynx as well as both hyoid horns (see also Figs 2.132 and 2.133). The attachment of the intrinsic tongue muscles to the hyoid has been severed and a portion removed, allowing the lingual artery and vein and the lingual branch of the glossopharyngeal nerve to be traced into the tongue.

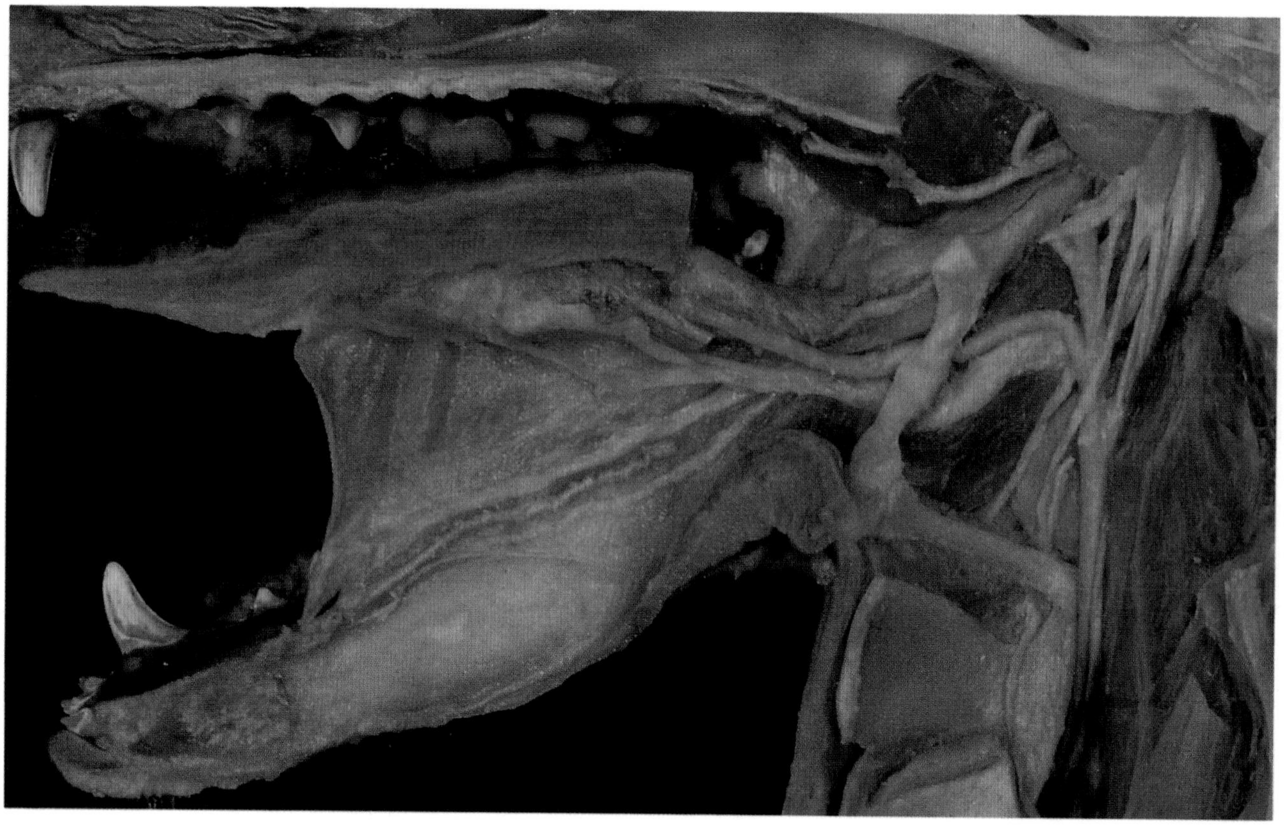

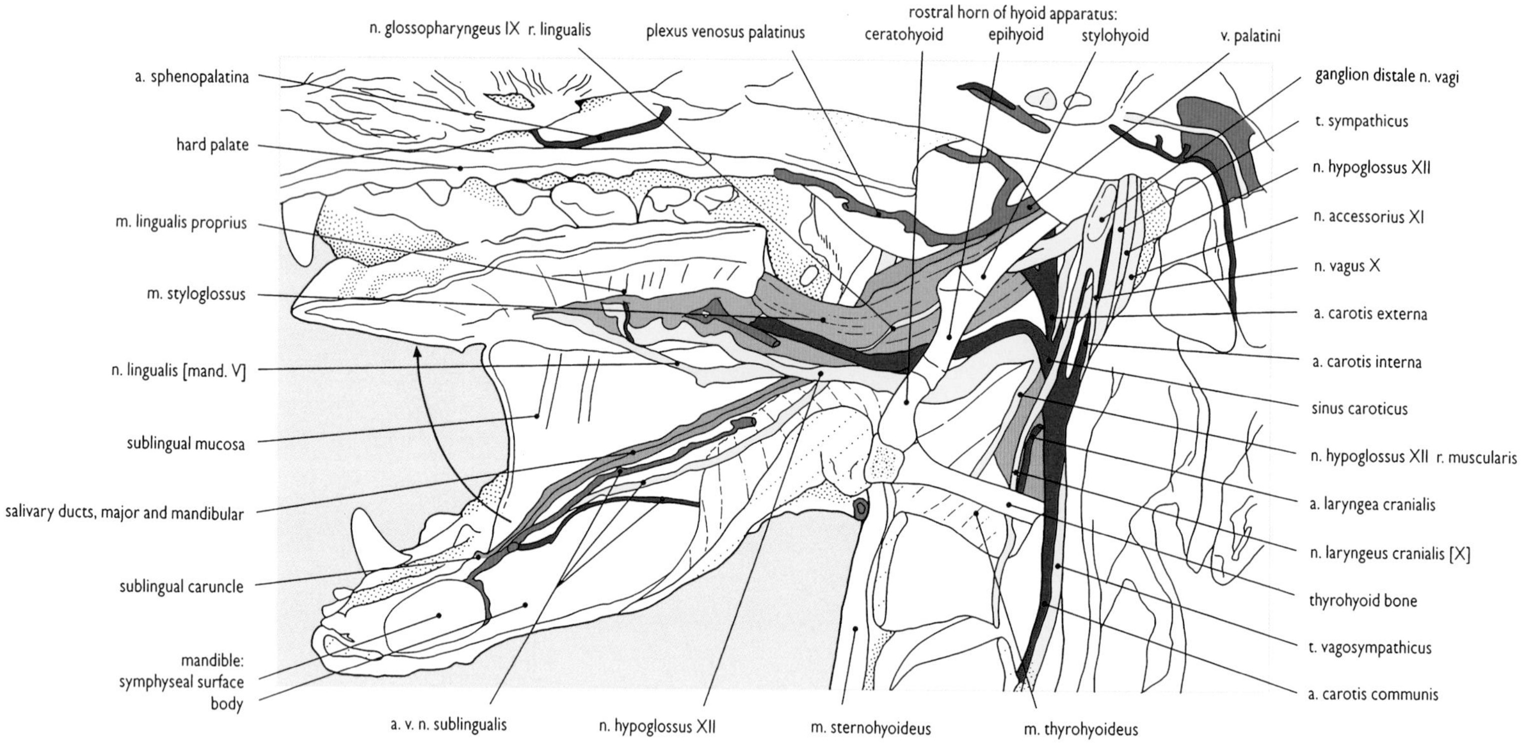
n. glossopharyngeus IX r. lingualis
plexus venosus palatinus
rostral horn of hyoid apparatus:
ceratohyoid
epihyoid
stylohyoid
v. palatini
a. sphenopalatina
hard palate
m. lingualis proprius
m. styloglossus
n. lingualis [mand. V]
sublingual mucosa
salivary ducts, major and mandibular
sublingual caruncle
mandible:
symphyseal surface
body
ganglion distale n. vagi
t. sympathicus
n. hypoglossus XII
n. accessorius XI
n. vagus X
a. carotis externa
a. carotis interna
sinus caroticus
n. hypoglossus XII r. muscularis
a. laryngea cranialis
n. laryngeus cranialis [X]
thyrohyoid bone
t. vagosympathicus
a. carotis communis
a. v. n. sublingualis
n. hypoglossus XII
m. sternohyoideus
m. thyrohyoideus

Fig. 2.94 Hyoid apparatus, blood vessels and nerves bordering the right side of the pharynx: medial view (2). Removal of the hyopharyngeal muscle completes the exposure of the nerves and arteries bordering the pharynx. The hyoglossal muscle has been removed, along with a large section of intrinsic tongue muscle exposing the styloglossal muscle. The lingual and proximal part of the sublingual vein have been removed so that the passage of the hypoglossal nerve (XII) into the tongue is exposed. The remains of the palatine muscles and palatine glandular tissue have been removed and some buccal mucosa behind lower molar tooth 3 has been stripped away.

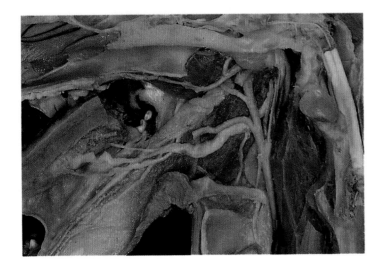

Fig. 2.95 Mandibular nerve, sublingual salivary gland and mylohyoid muscle of the right side: medial view. The sublingual salivary gland and the mandibular duct have been exposed following removal of the cranial hyoid horn and the styloglossal muscle. Removal of the vagus (X) and glossopharyngeal (IX) nerves and the sympathetic trunk has uncovered the occipital (incompletely filled with colored latex) and internal carotid arteries.

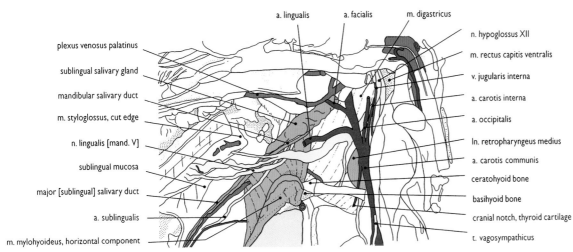

a. lingualis   a. facialis   m. digastricus

plexus venosus palatinus

sublingual salivary gland

mandibular salivary duct

m. styloglossus, cut edge

n. lingualis [mand. V]

sublingual mucosa

major [sublingual] salivary duct

a. sublingualis

m. mylohyoideus, horizontal component

n. hypoglossus XII

m. rectus capitis ventralis

v. jugularis interna

a. carotis interna

a. occipitalis

ln. retropharyngeus medius

a. carotis communis

ceratohyoid bone

basihyoid bone

cranial notch, thyroid cartilage

t. vagosympathicus

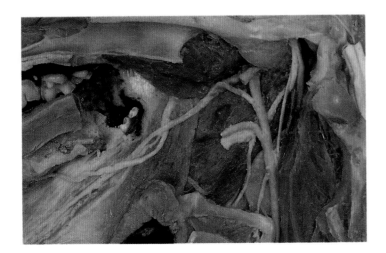

Fig. 2.96 Pterygoid and digastric muscles of the right side: medial view. Removal of the sublingual salivary gland, a part of the hypoglossal nerve (XII) and the veins draining the palatine plexus, has exposed the medial pterygoid, digastric and mylohyoid muscles. Removal of the glossopharyngeal (IX) and vagus (X) nerves exposes the proximal parts of the hypoglossal (XII) and accessory (XI) nerves (shown in lateral view in Figs 2.75–2.77).

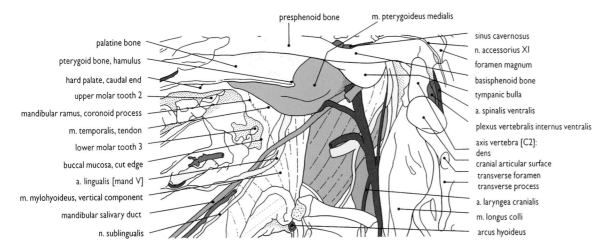

presphenoid bone   m. pterygoideus medialis

palatine bone

pterygoid bone, hamulus

hard palate, caudal end

upper molar tooth 2

mandibular ramus, coronoid process

m. temporalis, tendon

lower molar tooth 3

buccal mucosa, cut edge

a. lingualis [mand V]

m. mylohyoideus, vertical component

mandibular salivary duct

n. sublingualis

sinus cavernosus

n. accessorius XI

foramen magnum

basisphenoid bone

tympanic bulla

a. spinalis ventralis

plexus vertebralis internus ventralis

axis vertebra [C2]:
dens
cranial articular surface
transverse foramen
transverse process

a. laryngea cranialis

m. longus colli

arcus hyoideus

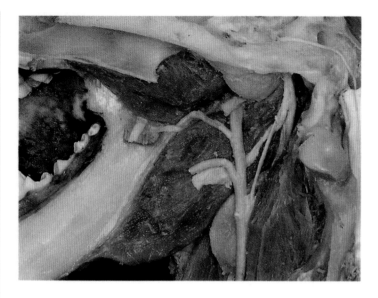

Fig. 2.97 External carotid artery, medial retropharyngeal lymph node and digastric muscle of the right side: medial view. The remaining parts of the tongue have been removed, as have the mylohyoid muscle, the lingual nerve and the mandibular salivary duct. The mandible is exposed with the digastric muscle attaching to its lower border. The mylohyoid nerve and the sublingual branch from the facial artery run together in the region of this attachment (see also Fig. 2.40 in lateral view and Fig. 2.143 in section).

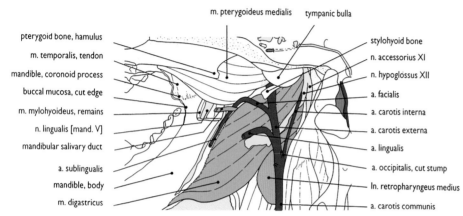

pterygoid bone, hamulus —   m. pterygoideus medialis   tympanic bulla

pterygoid bone, hamulus
m. temporalis, tendon
mandible, coronoid process
buccal mucosa, cut edge
m. mylohyoideus, remains
n. lingualis [mand. V]
mandibular salivary duct
a. sublingualis
mandible, body
m. digastricus

stylohyoid bone
n. accessorius XI
n. hypoglossus XII
a. facialis
a. carotis interna
a. carotis externa
a. lingualis
a. occipitalis, cut stump
ln. retropharyngeus medius
a. carotis communis

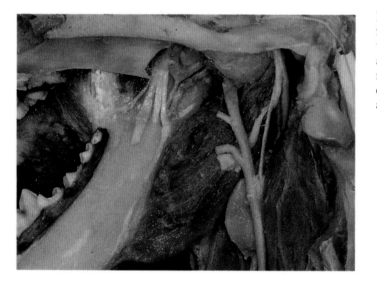

Fig. 2.98 Mandibular alveolar nerve and vessels entering the mandibular foramen of the right half of the mandible: medial view. 'Piecemeal' removal of the medial pterygoid muscle has exposed the mandibular nerve (trigeminal V) and its three main branches which cross the dorsal and lateral surfaces of the muscle (see also Figs 2.46 and 2.47). Some buccal mucosa has been removed, exposing the masseter muscle lying immediately rostral to the coronoid attachment of the temporal muscle.

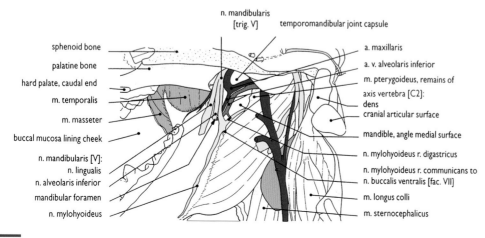

n. mandibularis [trig. V]   temporomandibular joint capsule

sphenoid bone
palatine bone
hard palate, caudal end
m. temporalis
m. masseter
buccal mucosa lining cheek
n. mandibularis [V]:
n. lingualis
n. alveolaris inferior
mandibular foramen
n. mylohyoideus

a. maxillaris
a. v. alveolaris inferior
m. pterygoideus, remains of
axis vertebra [C2]:
dens
cranial articular surface
mandible, angle medial surface
n. mylohyoideus r. digastricus
n. mylohyoideus r. communicans to
n. buccalis ventralis [fac. VII]
m. longus colli
m. sternocephalicus

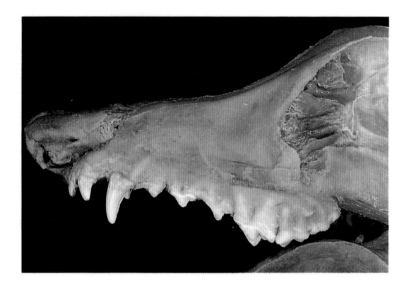

Fig. 2.99 Nasal cavity (1). Ethmoid labyrinth, nasal fundus and frontal sinus: left lateral view. To begin this sequence of nasal cavity dissections the nasal fundus and frontal sinus of the left side have been opened by removing the medial orbital wall down into the pterygopalatine fossa as far as the sphenopalatine foramen. The distinction between olfactory and air-conditioning mucosa is indicated by the extensive submucosal vasculature of the latter which has been filled with blue latex.

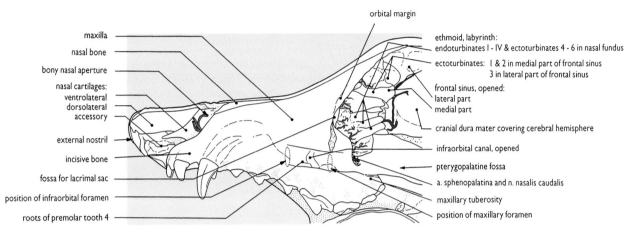

orbital margin

maxilla

nasal bone

bony nasal aperture

nasal cartilages:
ventrolateral
dorsolateral
accessory

external nostril

incisive bone

fossa for lacrimal sac

position of infraorbital foramen

roots of premolar tooth 4

ethmoid, labyrinth:
endoturbinates I - IV & ectoturbinates 4 - 6 in nasal fundus

ectoturbinates: 1 & 2 in medial part of frontal sinus
3 in lateral part of frontal sinus

frontal sinus, opened:
lateral part
medial part

cranial dura mater covering cerebral hemisphere

infraorbital canal, opened

pterygopalatine fossa

a. sphenopalatina and n. nasalis caudalis

maxillary tuberosity

position of maxillary foramen

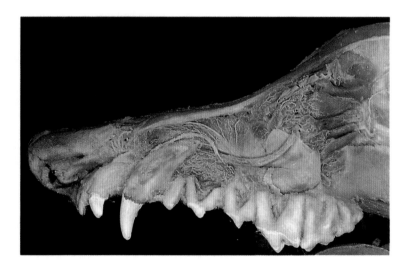

Fig. 2.100 Nasal cavity (2). Lacrimal canal and interior of the nasal fossa: left lateral view. The lateral nasal wall has been removed, except for part of the internal lamina of the maxilla where it carries the nasolacrimal duct. The course of the duct is indicated by the blue latex which has infiltrated into the submucosal lining of the lacrimal canal. The roots of the teeth are exposed, although those of upper premolar 4 were sawn through when the infraorbital canal was opened (see Fig. 2.41). The position of the uncinate process of the ethmoid in the nasomaxillary opening is indicated by a band of latex-impregnated mucosa visible through the maxilla where it forms the medial wall of the infraorbital canal.

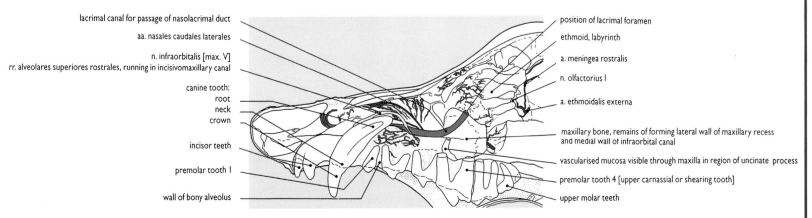

lacrimal canal for passage of nasolacrimal duct

aa. nasales caudales laterales

n. infraorbitalis [max. V]
rr. alveolares superiores rostrales, running in incisivomaxillary canal

canine tooth:
root
neck
crown

incisor teeth

premolar tooth I

wall of bony alveolus

position of lacrimal foramen

ethmoid, labyrinth

a. meningea rostralis

n. olfactorius I

a. ethmoidalis externa

maxillary bone, remains of forming lateral wall of maxillary recess
and medial wall of infraorbital canal

vascularised mucosa visible through maxilla in region of uncinate process

premolar tooth 4 [upper carnassial or shearing tooth]

upper molar teeth

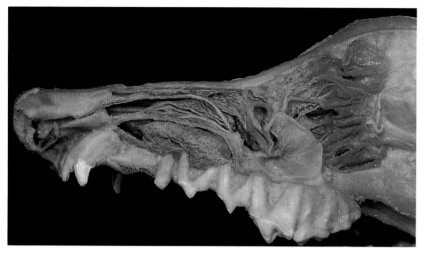

Fig. 2.101 Nasal cavity (3). Maxillary recess and blood vessels of the nasal conchae: left lateral view. Complete maxillary removal has opened the maxillary recess exposing the lateral (orbital) lamina of the ethmoid which forms its medial wall. The position of the nasomaxillary opening into the recess is marked by the uncinate process of the ethmoid. The nasal vestibule is opened after much of the ventrolateral nasal cartilage has been removed, exposing the alar fold.

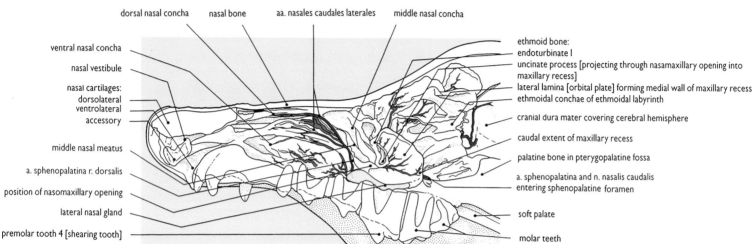

dorsal nasal concha — nasal bone — aa. nasales caudales laterales — middle nasal concha

ethmoid bone:
endoturbinate I
uncinate process [projecting through nasamaxillary opening into maxillary recess]
lateral lamina [orbital plate] forming medial wall of maxillary recess
ethmoidal conchae of ethmoidal labyrinth
cranial dura mater covering cerebral hemisphere
caudal extent of maxillary recess
palatine bone in pterygopalatine fossa
a. sphenopalatina and n. nasalis caudalis
entering sphenopalatine foramen
soft palate
molar teeth

ventral nasal concha
nasal vestibule
nasal cartilages:
dorsolateral
ventrolateral
accessory
middle nasal meatus
a. sphenopalatina r. dorsalis
position of nasomaxillary opening
lateral nasal gland
premolar tooth 4 [shearing tooth]

Fig. 2.102 Nasal cavity (4). Nasal septum and vomeronasal organ: left lateral view. The nasal cavity and palate have been sectioned slightly to the left of the midline, and the left parts removed. The mucosa covering the nasal septum is exposed and in the nasal vestibule the loss of pigmentation indicates the transition from surface to nasal epithelium. Caudal to the incisive bone the section passes through the palatine fissure of the left side (see also Fig. 2.126).

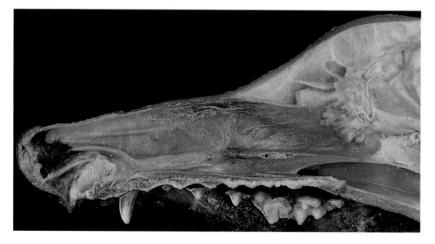

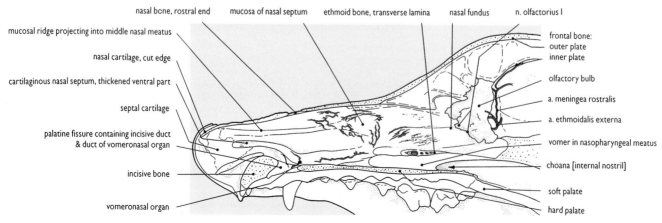

nasal bone, rostral end — mucosa of nasal septum — ethmoid bone, transverse lamina — nasal fundus — n. olfactorius I

mucosal ridge projecting into middle nasal meatus
nasal cartilage, cut edge
cartilaginous nasal septum, thickened ventral part
septal cartilage
palatine fissure containing incisive duct & duct of vomeronasal organ
incisive bone
vomeronasal organ

frontal bone:
outer plate
inner plate
olfactory bulb
a. meningea rostralis
a. ethmoidalis externa
vomer in nasopharyngeal meatus
choana [internal nostril]
soft palate
hard palate

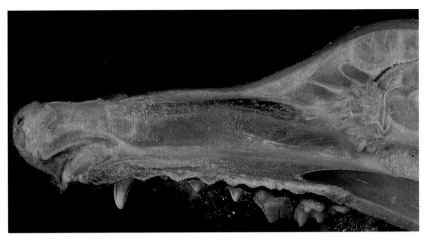

Fig. 2.103 Nasal cavity (5). In median section: medial view of the right half. The left half of the nasal cavity and palate have been removed and the nasal cavity is displayed in median section. However, the nasal septum and its covering mucosa remain intact and the various contributions to the septum are distinguishable.

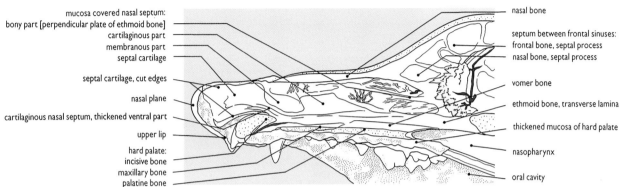

Fig. 2.104 Nasal cavity (6). Nasal fossa and nasal conchae of the right side: medial view. The nasal septum has been removed, except for the vomer, opening the right nasal fossa and displaying the nasal conchae. The alar fold continuing the ventral concha is a prominent feature occupying much of the nasal vestibule (see Fig. 2.138).

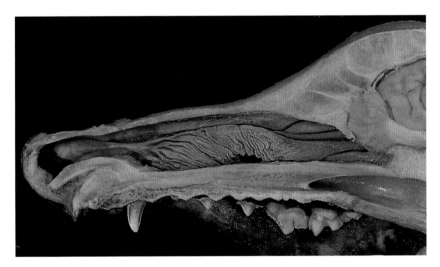

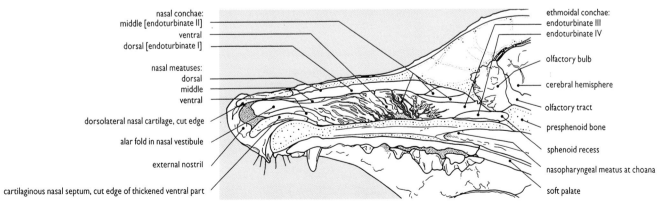

Nasal conchae and frontal sinus of the right

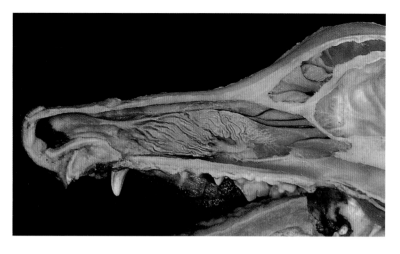

Fig. 2.105 Nasal cavity (7). Nasal conchae and frontal sinus of the right side: medial view. Following removal of the vomer and the transverse lamina of the ethmoid, the position of the longitudinal nasal meatuses are displayed (see Figs 2.139–2.142). The sphenoid recess has been opened with its contained endoturbinate; the frontal sinus has been opened after removal of the septal process of the frontal bone.

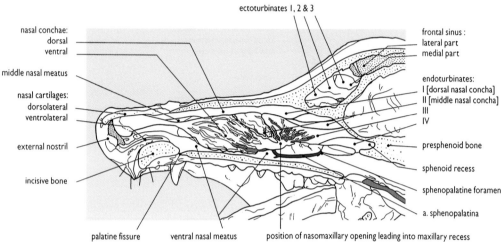

Fig. 2.106 Nasal cavity (8). Maxillary recess and wall of the nasal fossa of the right side: medial view. Nasal conchae, bar the dorsal, have been removed, exposing the lateral lamina of the ethmoid in the nasal fundus forming the medial wall of the maxillary recess. The nasomaxillary opening into the recess is visible ventrolateral to the uncinate process of the dorsal nasal concha.

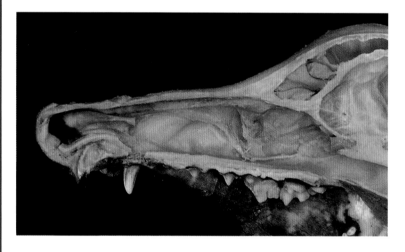

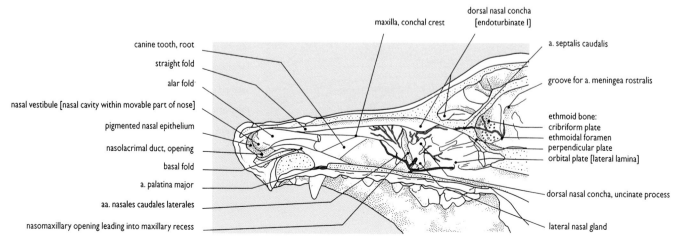

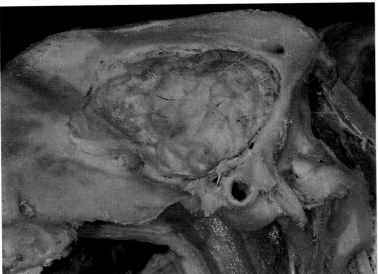

Fig. 2.107 Cranium and cranial dura mater: left lateral view. To begin the sequence of brain dissections the cranial wall has been removed from the ethmoid foramen in the medial orbital wall back to the nuchal crest. Ventrally the mandibular fossa of the jaw joint has also been removed. 'Piecemeal' removal of the bone ensured that the cranial dura mater remained intact and it is exposed with its venous sinuses. The temporal sinus left the skull through the retroauricular foramen to become the temporomandibular articular vein (see Fig. 2.42). Removal of the rectus capitis dorsalis muscle has exposed the occipital condyle where it enters into the atlanto-occipital joint.

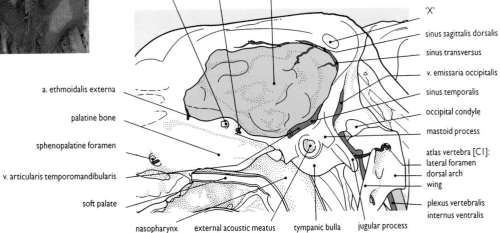

Fig. 2.108 Cranial dura mater, dural venous sinuses and internal carotid artery: left lateral view. The cranial wall has been removed to the midline dorsally and caudally. Ventrolaterally much of the temporal bone has been removed and the internal carotid artery is displayed since the carotid canal of the temporal bone has been opened following removal of the tympanic bulla. Rostrally the orbital wall is removed lateral to the nasal fundus and frontal sinus. The area labelled 'X' in this and the previous picture marks the damage made by a hook inserted to support the head during preservation.

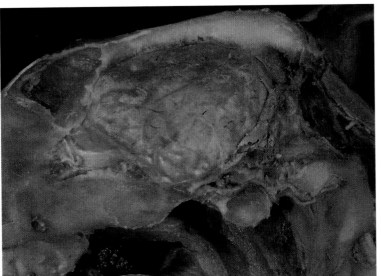

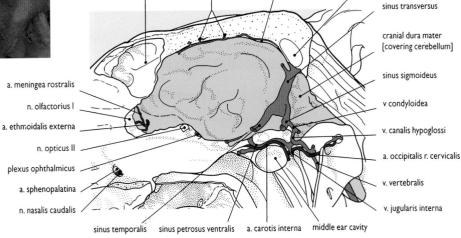

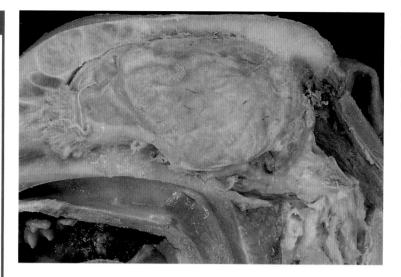

Fig. 2.109 Cranial and spinal dura mater, olfactory bulb and olfactory nerve: left lateral view. The cranial bones have all been sectioned in the midline, as has the atlas. Dural venous sinuses have been removed and the continuity of the cranial and spinal dura is evident at the foramen magnum. The olfactory bulb and numerous filaments of the olfactory nerve (1) which have been preserved after removal of the left half of the cribriform plate are displayed.

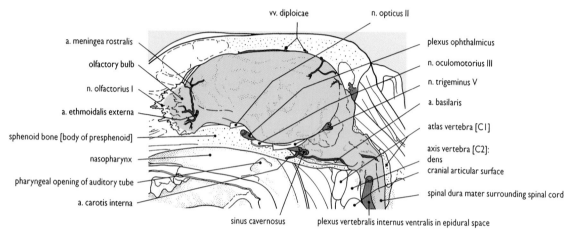

vv. diploicae — n. opticus II

a. meningea rostralis
olfactory bulb
n. olfactorius I
a. ethmoidalis externa
sphenoid bone [body of presphenoid]
nasopharynx
pharyngeal opening of auditory tube
a. carotis interna

plexus ophthalmicus
n. oculomotorius III
n. trigeminus V
a. basilaris
atlas vertebra [C1]
axis vertebra [C2]:
dens
cranial articular surface
spinal dura mater surrounding spinal cord

sinus cavernosus — plexus vertebralis internus ventralis in epidural space

Fig. 2.110 Brain *in situ* after removal of the cranial meninges: left lateral view. Removal of the dura mater along with some cleaning of the underlying pia/arachnoid has exposed the brain. The cerebral hemisphere is marked by sulci and gyri and there is a broad topographical subdivision into four lobes: frontal, parietal, temporal and occipital. A fifth lobe, the piriform, has continuity with the olfactory bulb through the olfactory peduncle (see Fig. 2.124 of the isolated brain).

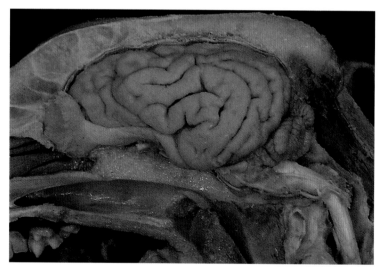

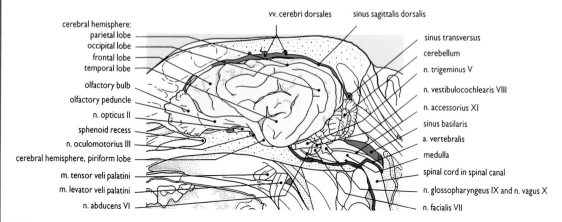

vv. cerebri dorsales — sinus sagittalis dorsalis

cerebral hemisphere:
parietal lobe
occipital lobe
frontal lobe
temporal lobe
olfactory bulb
olfactory peduncle
n. opticus II
sphenoid recess
n. oculomotorius III
cerebral hemisphere, piriform lobe
m. tensor veli palatini
m. levator veli palatini
n. abducens VI

sinus transversus
cerebellum
n. trigeminus V
n. vestibulocochlearis VIII
n. accessorius XI
sinus basilaris
a. vertebralis
medulla
spinal cord in spinal canal
n. glossopharyngeus IX and n. vagus X
n. facialis VII

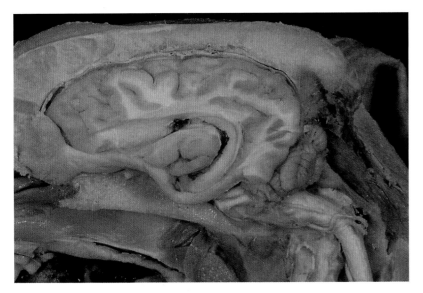

Fig. 2.111 Brain (1). Lateral ventricle and hippocampus: left lateral view. A large part of the left cerebral hemisphere has been removed by extending a sagittal cut down from the dorsal surface through the corpus callosum into the cavity of the lateral ventricle. Removal of cerebral hemisphere lateral to the incision has opened the ventricle by removing its roof and lateral wall. The rostral end of the choroid plexus marks the position of the interventricular foramen.

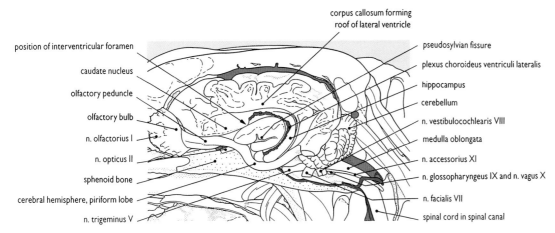

corpus callosum forming
roof of lateral ventricle

position of interventricular foramen

caudate nucleus

olfactory peduncle

olfactory bulb

n. olfactorius I

n. opticus II

sphenoid bone

cerebral hemisphere, piriform lobe

n. trigeminus V

pseudosylvian fissure

plexus choroideus ventriculi lateralis

hippocampus

cerebellum

n. vestibulocochlearis VIII

medulla oblongata

n. accessorius XI

n. glossopharyngeus IX and n. vagus X

n. facialis VII

spinal cord in spinal canal

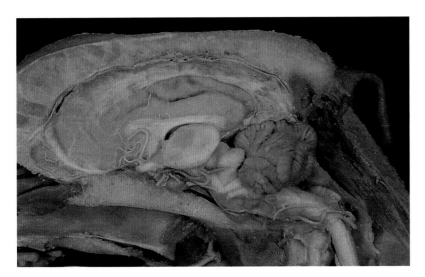

Fig. 2.112 Brain (2). Brainstem, cerebellum and falx cerebri: left lateral view. The left cerebral hemisphere has been removed by severing the thalamus rostral to the optic tract, and the corpus callosum, fornix, rostral commissure, lamina terminalis, epithalamus and caudal commissure all in the midline. In the midline the falx cerebri extends ventrally, obscuring much of the right hemisphere from view. The blood vessels of the base of the brain are shown to greater advantage in the isolated brain, Fig. 2.124.

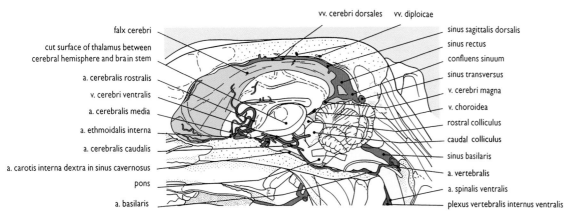

vv. cerebri dorsales   vv. diploicae

falx cerebri

cut surface of thalamus between
cerebral hemisphere and brain stem

a. cerebralis rostralis

v. cerebri ventralis

a. cerebralis media

a. ethmoidalis interna

a. cerebralis caudalis

a. carotis interna dextra in sinus cavernosus

pons

a. basilaris

sinus sagittalis dorsalis

sinus rectus

confluens sinuum

sinus transversus

v. cerebri magna

v. choroidea

rostral colliculus

caudal colliculus

sinus basilaris

a. vertebralis

a. spinalis ventralis

plexus vertebralis internus ventralis

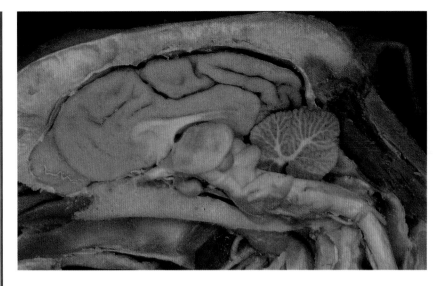

Fig. 2.113 Brain (3). Brainstem and right cerebral hemisphere: left lateral view. The falx cerebri, tentorium cerebelli and associated venous sinuses have been removed to expose the right cerebral hemisphere from medial view. Blood vessels at the base of the brain have been removed from the left side exposing the hypophysis which they encircled (see Fig. 2.144 in section). The cerebellum has been sectioned in the midline and the left half removed by severing the cerebellar peduncles.

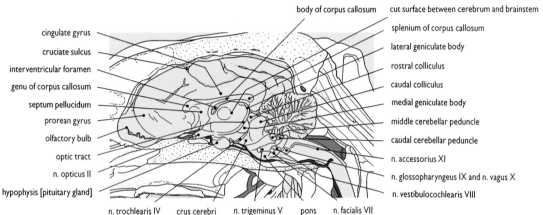

body of corpus callosum — cut surface between cerebrum and brainstem

cingulate gyrus — splenium of corpus callosum

cruciate sulcus — lateral geniculate body

interventricular foramen — rostral colliculus

genu of corpus callosum — caudal colliculus

septum pellucidum — medial geniculate body

prorean gyrus — middle cerebellar peduncle

olfactory bulb — caudal cerebellar peduncle

optic tract — n. accessorius XI

n. opticus II — n. glossopharyngeus IX and n. vagus X

hypophysis [pituitary gland] — n. vestibulocochlearis VIII

n. trochlearis IV   crus cerebri   n. trigeminus V   pons   n. facialis VII

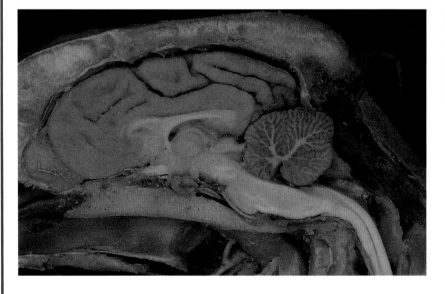

Fig. 2.114 Brain (4). In median section: medial view of right half. The brain has been sectioned in the median plane. The ventricular system is displayed except for the lateral ventricle of the right side, although the interventricular foramen is visible. The interthalamic adhesion is cut through in the midline and below it in the floor of the third ventricle the optic chiasm, hypophysis and mammillary body are all sectioned.

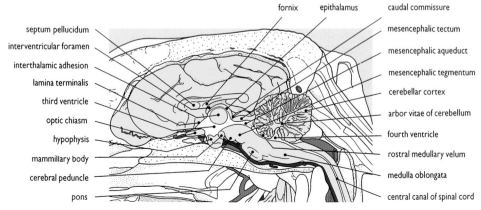

fornix   epithalamus   caudal commissure

septum pellucidum — mesencephalic tectum

interventricular foramen — mesencephalic aqueduct

interthalamic adhesion — mesencephalic tegmentum

lamina terminalis — cerebellar cortex

third ventricle — arbor vitae of cerebellum

optic chiasm — fourth ventricle

hypophysis — rostral medullary velum

mammillary body — medulla oblongata

cerebral peduncle — central canal of spinal cord

pons

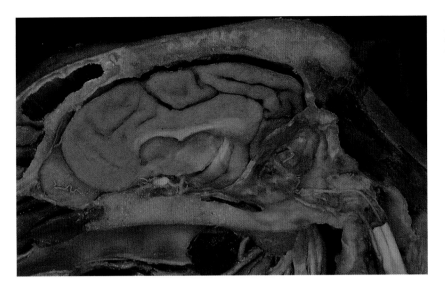

Fig. 2.115 Brain (5). Right cerebral hemisphere *in situ* after removal of the cerebellum and brain stem: medial view. The brainstem and remaining cerebellum have been removed by severing the thalamus of the right side and the roots of the cranial nerves. From the medial surface of the right cerebral hemisphere the rostral column of the fornix has been removed rostral to the interventricular foramen along with the septum pellucidum opening the lateral ventricle.

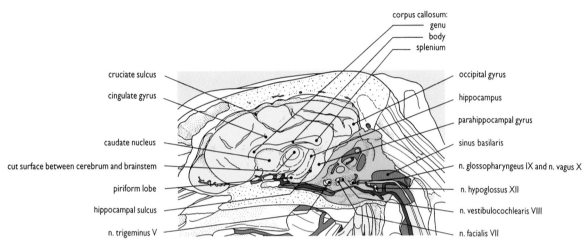

corpus callosum:
genu
body
splenium

cruciate sulcus
cingulate gyrus
caudate nucleus
cut surface between cerebrum and brainstem
piriform lobe
hippocampal sulcus
n. trigeminus V

occipital gyrus
hippocampus
parahippocampal gyrus
sinus basilaris
n. glossopharyngeus IX and n. vagus X
n. hypoglossus XII
n. vestibulocochlearis VIII
n. facialis VII

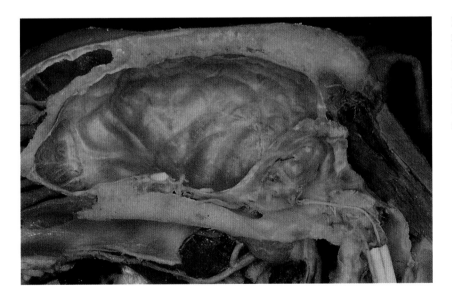

Fig. 2.116 Dura mater and dural sinuses of the right side after removal of the brain: medial view. The right cerebral hemisphere has been removed from the rostral and middle cranial fossae leaving the cranial dura mater in place where it forms the periosteum of the cranial bones. The sigmoid and temporal sinuses are visible in relation to the pyramid of the temporal bone, while in the braincase floor the cavernous and ventral petrosal sinuses are displayed (cf. Figs 2.86 and 2.122).

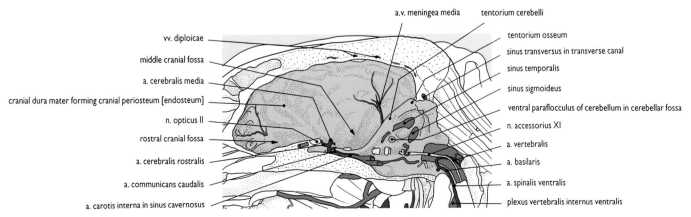

a.v. meningea media   tentorium cerebelli

vv. diploicae
middle cranial fossa
a. cerebralis media
cranial dura mater forming cranial periosteum [endosteum]
n. opticus II
rostral cranial fossa
a. cerebralis rostralis
a. communicans caudalis
a. carotis interna in sinus cavernosus

tentorium osseum
sinus transversus in transverse canal
sinus temporalis
sinus sigmoideus
ventral paraflocculus of cerebellum in cerebellar fossa
n. accessorius XI
a. vertebralis
a. basilaris
a. spinalis ventralis
plexus vertebralis internus ventralis

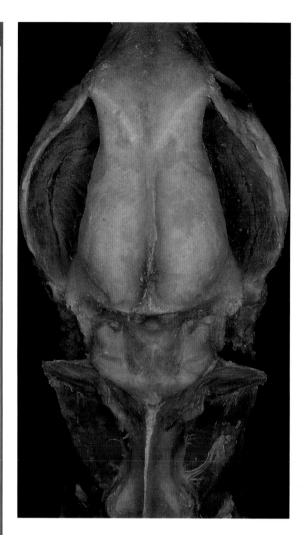

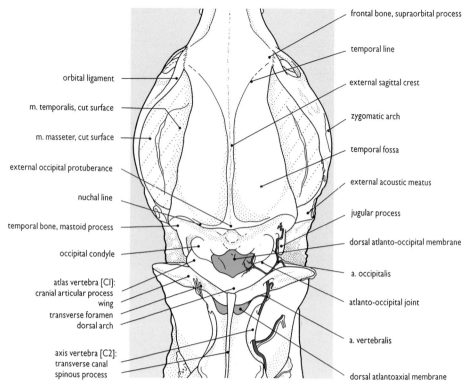

frontal bone, supraorbital process

temporal line

external sagittal crest

zygomatic arch

temporal fossa

external acoustic meatus

jugular process

dorsal atlanto-occipital membrane

a. occipitalis

atlanto-occipital joint

a. vertebralis

dorsal atlantoaxial membrane

orbital ligament

m. temporalis, cut surface

m. masseter, cut surface

external occipital protuberance

nuchal line

temporal bone, mastoid process

occipital condyle

atlas vertebra [CI]:
cranial articular process
wing
transverse foramen
dorsal arch

axis vertebra [C2]:
transverse canal
spinous process

Fig. 2.117 Cranium after removal of the temporal and dorsal neck muscles: dorsal view. The temporal muscles of both sides and the dorsal neck muscles which attached to the rear of the skull and to the axis and atlas have been removed. The occipital condyles and the atlanto-occipital joints are exposed and the dorsal atlanto-occipital membrane is stretched. On the right side the vertebral artery anastomosis with the occipital artery is displayed in the atlantal fossa.

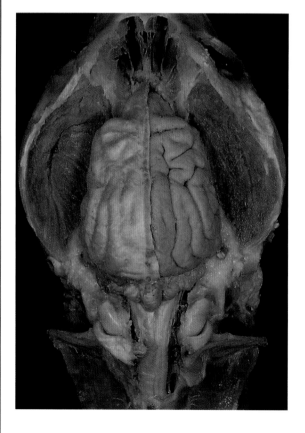

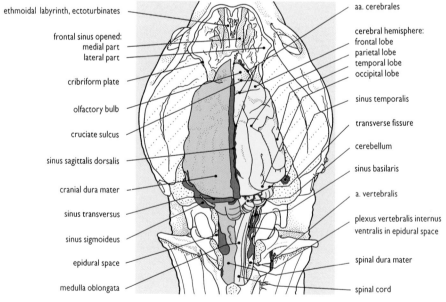

ethmoidal labyrinth, ectoturbinates

frontal sinus opened:
medial part
lateral part

cribriform plate

olfactory bulb

cruciate sulcus

sinus sagittalis dorsalis

cranial dura mater

sinus transversus

sinus sigmoideus

epidural space

medulla oblongata

aa. cerebrales

cerebral hemisphere:
frontal lobe
parietal lobe
temporal lobe
occipital lobe

sinus temporalis

transverse fissure

cerebellum

sinus basilaris

a. vertebralis

plexus vertebralis internus
ventralis in epidural space

spinal dura mater

spinal cord

Fig. 2.118 Brain (1). Cerebrum, cranial dura mater and dural venous sinuses: dorsal view. The roof and rear wall of the cranium have been removed, as have the dorsal arch of the atlas and the cranial end of the spinous process and arch of the axis. On the left the dura mater has been left in position; on the right it has been removed. Dural venous sinuses are consequently visible on the left through the periosteal dural layer. On the right side the basilar sinus is continued at the foramen magnum by the ventral vertebral venous plexus in the epidural space.

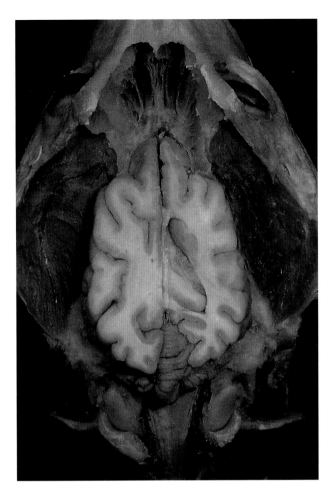

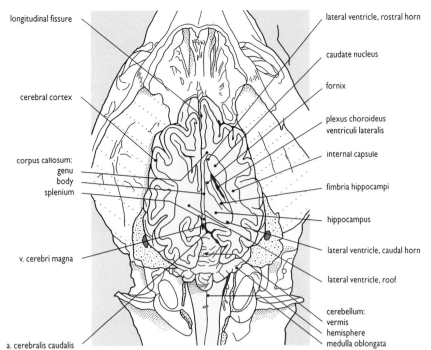

longitudinal fissure

lateral ventricle, rostral horn

caudate nucleus

cerebral cortex

fornix

plexus choroideus
ventriculi lateralis

corpus callosum:
genu
body
splenium

internal capsule

fimbria hippocampi

hippocampus

lateral ventricle, caudal horn

v. cerebri magna

lateral ventricle, roof

cerebellum:
vermis
hemisphere
medulla oblongata

a. cerebralis caudalis

Fig. 2.119 Brain (2). Cerebral cortex, corpus callosum and lateral ventricle: dorsal view. Both cerebral hemispheres have been sectioned horizontally: on the left down almost to the corpus callosum; on the right the sectioning has removed the corpus callosum opening the lateral ventricle. In the midline a strip of corpus callosum remains in position from its splenium to its genu. Sectioning has removed considerable parts of the occipital lobes of the cerebrum uncovering more of the vermis of the cerebellum in the midline (see Fig. 2.111).

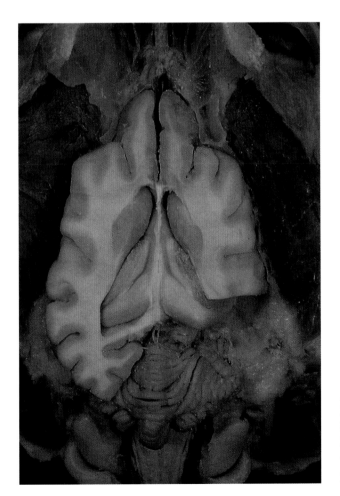

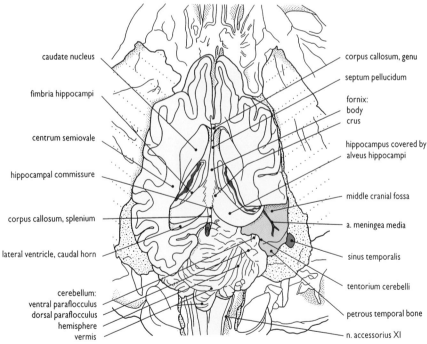

caudate nucleus

corpus callosum, genu

septum pellucidum

fimbria hippocampi

fornix:
body
crus

centrum semiovale

hippocampus covered by
alveus hippocampi

hippocampal commissure

middle cranial fossa

corpus callosum, splenium

a. meningea media

lateral ventricle, caudal horn

sinus temporalis

tentorium cerebelli

cerebellum:
ventral paraflocculus
dorsal paraflocculus
hemisphere
vermis

petrous temporal bone

n. accessorius XI

Fig. 2.120 Brain (3). Hippocampus, fornix and cerebellum: dorsal view. The left cerebral hemisphere has been sectioned down to the same level as the right side opening the lateral ventricle. On the right side the remains of the occipital lobe and part of the temporal lobe of the cerebral hemisphere have been removed through a vertical cut. The cerebellar tentorium is exposed where it separated cerebral from cerebellar hemisphere and a branch of the middle meningeal artery is visible on it (see Fig. 2.115).

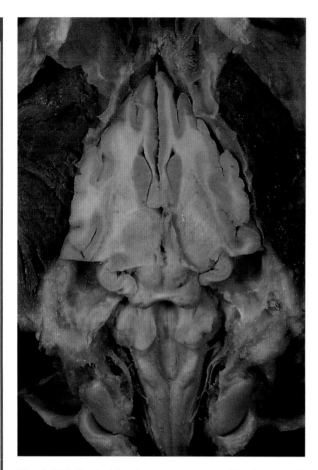

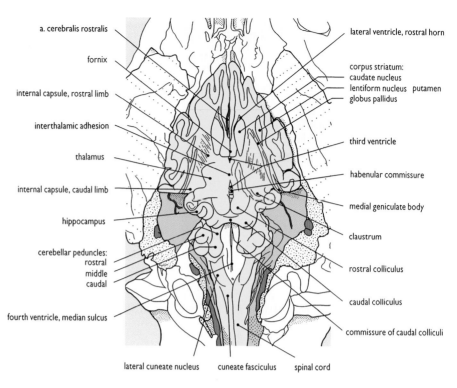

a. cerebralis rostralis
fornix
internal capsule, rostral limb
interthalamic adhesion
thalamus
internal capsule, caudal limb
hippocampus
cerebellar peduncles:
rostral
middle
caudal
fourth ventricle, median sulcus

lateral ventricle, rostral horn
corpus striatum:
caudate nucleus
lentiform nucleus putamen
globus pallidus
third ventricle
habenular commissure
medial geniculate body
claustrum
rostral colliculus
caudal colliculus
commissure of caudal colliculi

lateral cuneate nucleus   cuneate fasciculus   spinal cord

Fig. 2.121 Brain (4). Corpus striatum and brainstem: dorsal view. Horizontal sectioning of the cerebral hemispheres has been continued. The fornix and hippocampi are removed bar their caudoventral parts which lay in the caudal horns of the lateral ventricles. Removal of the cerebellum has exposed the medulla oblongata, the cavity of the fourth ventricle, and the corpora quadrigemina. On the right side the cerebellar tentorium has been cut back slightly to the level of the petrosal crest, the cerebellar fossa of the petrous temporal bone is therefore exposed (see Figs 2.115 and 2.116).

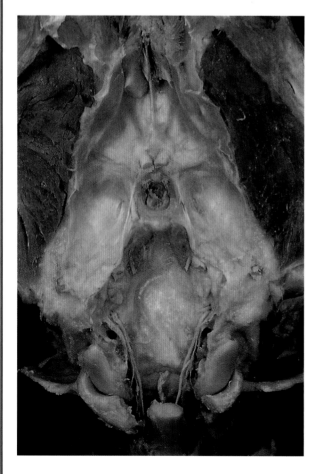

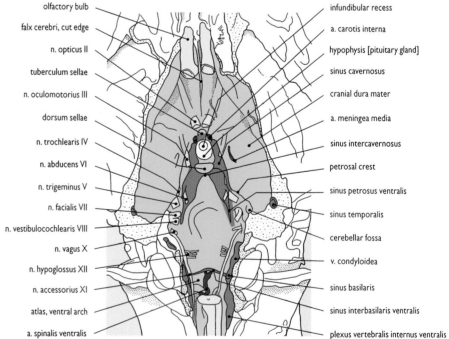

olfactory bulb
falx cerebri, cut edge
n. opticus II
tuberculum sellae
n. oculomotorius III
dorsum sellae
n. trochlearis IV
n. abducens VI
n. trigeminus V
n. facialis VII
n. vestibulocochlearis VIII
n. vagus X
n. hypoglossus XII
n. accessorius XI
atlas, ventral arch
a. spinalis ventralis

infundibular recess
a. carotis interna
hypophysis [pituitary gland]
sinus cavernosus
cranial dura mater
a. meningea media
sinus intercavernosus
petrosal crest
sinus petrosus ventralis
sinus temporalis
cerebellar fossa
v. condyloidea
sinus basilaris
sinus interbasilaris ventralis
plexus vertebralis internus ventralis

Fig. 2.122 Dura mater and dural venous sinuses of the cranial floor after brain removal: dorsal view. The remains of the brain have been removed by severing the olfactory bulbs, the spinal cord, and the cranial nerve roots. The arterial supply to the brain was poorly injected with latex and was removed with the brain (see Fig. 2.124), the severed ends of the internal carotid arteries are visible where they penetrate the meningeal dura mater rostral to the hypophysis. The dural venous sinuses in the cranial floor are distinguishable through the meningeal dura.

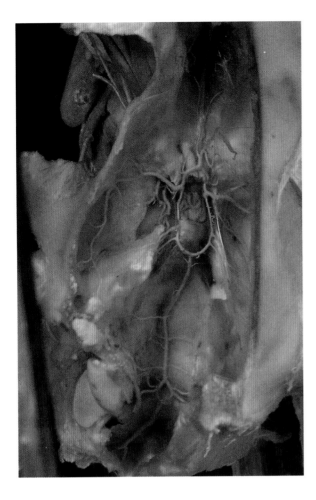

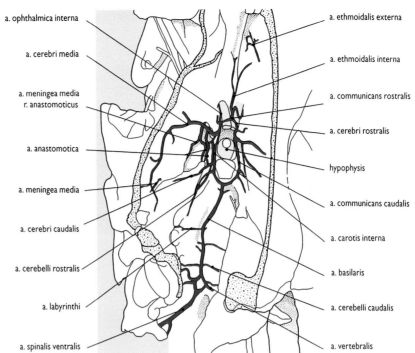

a. ophthalmica interna

a. cerebri media

a. meningea media
r. anastomoticus

a. anastomotica

a. meningea media

a. cerebri caudalis

a. cerebelli rostralis

a. labyrinthi

a. spinalis ventralis

a. ethmoidalis externa

a. ethmoidalis interna

a. communicans rostralis

a. cerebri rostralis

hypophysis

a. communicans caudalis

a. carotis interna

a. basilaris

a. cerebelli caudalis

a. vertebralis

Fig. 2.123 Blood supply to the brain (1). Cerebral arteries *in situ* after brain removal: dorsal view. In this dissection the brain was removed leaving the arteries in the cranial floor. The arterial circle surrounds the hypophysis and dorsum sellae and the rostral, middle and caudal cerebral arteries arising from it are clearly shown on the left side lying dorsal to the cavernous sinus. The meningeal dura has been removed, opening the sinus and displaying the internal carotid artery medially.

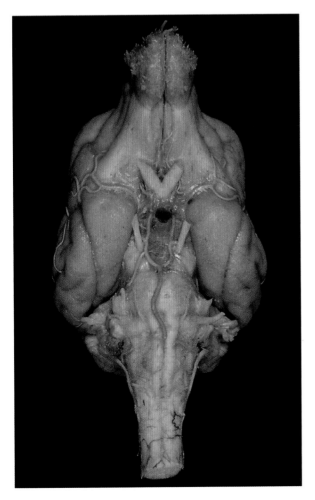

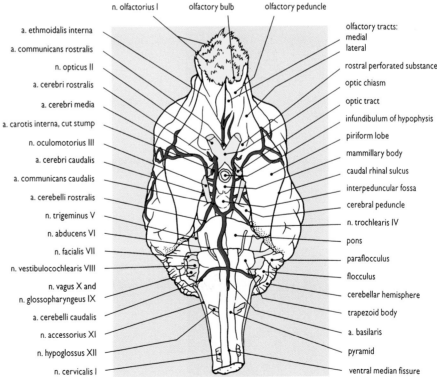

n. olfactorius I   olfactory bulb   olfactory peduncle

a. ethmoidalis interna

a. communicans rostralis

n. opticus II

a. cerebri rostralis

a. cerebri media

a. carotis interna, cut stump

n. oculomotorius III

a. cerebri caudalis

a. communicans caudalis

a. cerebelli rostralis

n. trigeminus V

n. abducens VI

n. facialis VII

n. vestibulocochlearis VIII

n. vagus X and
n. glossopharyngeus IX

a. cerebelli caudalis

n. accessorius XI

n. hypoglossus XII

n. cervicalis I

olfactory tracts:
medial
lateral

rostral perforated substance

optic chiasm

optic tract

infundibulum of hypophysis

piriform lobe

mammillary body

caudal rhinal sulcus

interpeduncular fossa

cerebral peduncle

n. trochlearis IV

pons

paraflocculus

flocculus

cerebellar hemisphere

trapezoid body

a. basilaris

pyramid

ventral median fissure

Fig. 2.124 Blood supply to the brain (2). Isolated brain: ventral view. In this dissection the brain has been removed from the cranium with its blood vessels remaining in position on its ventral and lateral surfaces. After removal some limited cleaning of the leptomeninges on the brain surface has revealed the arteries more distinctly, but has also revealed all of the cranial nerve roots at their attachments to the brain.

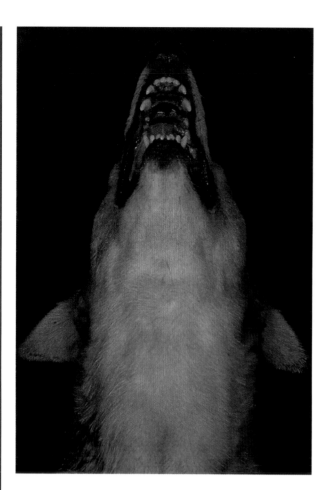

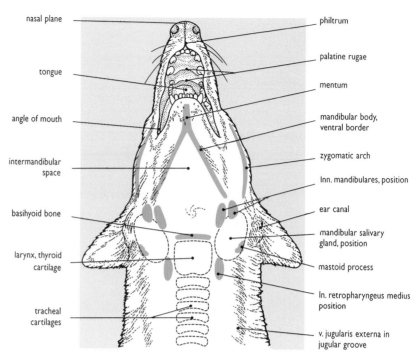

nasal plane

tongue

angle of mouth

intermandibular space

basihyoid bone

larynx, thyroid cartilage

tracheal cartilages

philtrum

palatine rugae

mentum

mandibular body, ventral border

zygomatic arch

lnn. mandibulares, position

ear canal

mandibular salivary gland, position

mastoid process

ln. retropharyngeus medius position

v. jugularis externa in jugular groove

Fig. 2.125 Surface features of the head: ventral view. The major bony features that are readily palpable and/or visible on the underside of the head and cranial end of the neck are indicated in this figure. These 'points' correspond to those colored on the bones illustrated in Fig. 2.126. Figures 2.1, 2.55 and 2.59 show surface views of the head from lateral and dorsal aspects and should be viewed in conjunction with this figure.

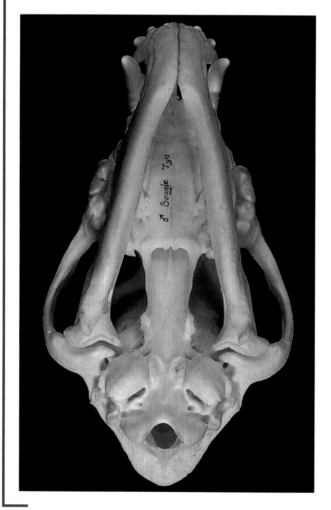

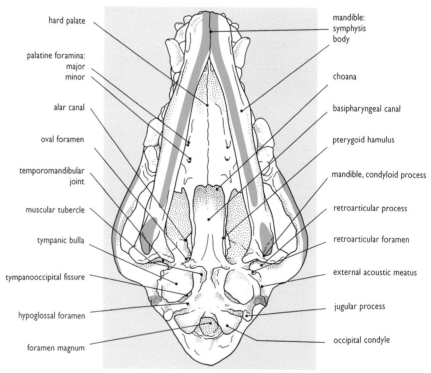

hard palate

palatine foramina:
major
minor

alar canal

oval foramen

temporomandibular joint

muscular tubercle

tympanic bulla

tympanooccipital fissure

hypoglossal foramen

foramen magnum

mandible:
symphysis
body

choana

basipharyngeal canal

pterygoid hamulus

mandible, condyloid process

retroarticular process

retroarticular foramen

external acoustic meatus

jugular process

occipital condyle

Fig. 2.126 Skull: ventral view. The palpable bony features shown in the surface view in Fig. 2.125 are colored on this skull. Absent from this skeletal preparation are the hyoid components suspending the larynx. Figures 2.132 and 2.133 show these structures in position following further dissection.

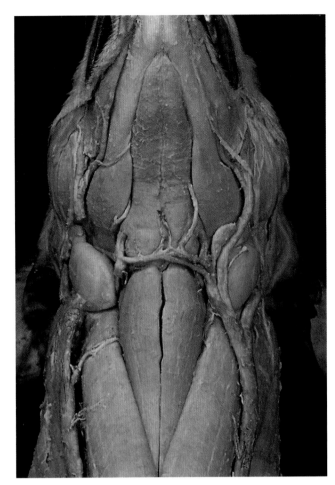

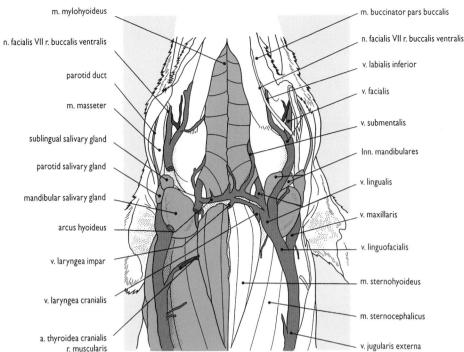

m. mylohyoideus

n. facialis VII r. buccalis ventralis

parotid duct

m. masseter

sublingual salivary gland

parotid salivary gland

mandibular salivary gland

arcus hyoideus

v. laryngea impar

v. laryngea cranialis

a. thyroidea cranialis
r. muscularis

m. buccinator pars buccalis

n. facialis VII r. buccalis ventralis

v. labialis inferior

v. facialis

v. submentalis

lnn. mandibulares

v. lingualis

v. maxillaris

v. linguofacialis

m. sternohyoideus

m. sternocephalicus

v. jugularis externa

Fig. 2.127 Superficial structures of the head after removal of the superficial fascia and facial muscles: ventral view. The skin, superficial fascia and cutaneous muscles have been removed from the ventral surface of the head and neck. On the right, parts of the facial, lingual and linguofacial veins and the mandibular lymph nodes have also been removed. This view gives a clear indication of the variable nature of superficial venous distribution with a hyoid venous arch single on one side and doubled on the other.

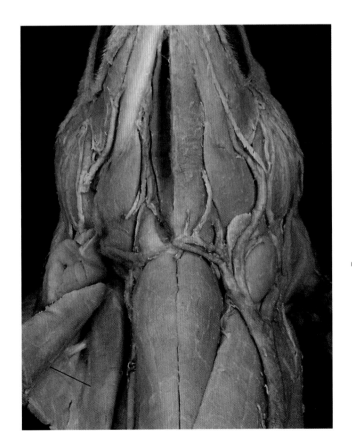

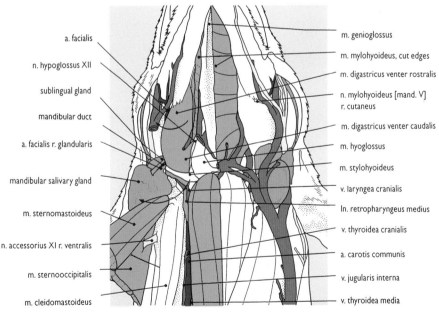

a. facialis

n. hypoglossus XII

sublingual gland

mandibular duct

a. facialis r. glandularis

mandibular salivary gland

m. sternomastoideus

n. accessorius XI r. ventralis

m. sternooccipitalis

m. cleidomastoideus

m. genioglossus

m. mylohyoideus, cut edges

m. digastricus venter rostralis

n. mylohyoideus [mand. V]
r. cutaneus

m. digastricus venter caudalis

m. hyoglossus

m. stylohyoideus

v. laryngea cranialis

ln. retropharyngeus medius

v. thyroidea cranialis

a. carotis communis

v. jugularis interna

v. thyroidea media

Fig. 2.128 Extrinsic tongue muscles, mandibular and sublingual salivary glands: ventral view. The dissection of the right side is continued by: removal of the remaining superficial veins and lateral displacement of the cut end of the facial vein; removal of the horizontal component of the mylohyoid muscle (see also Fig. 2.144, in section) and the geniohyoid muscle; lateral displacement of the mandibular salivary gland and sternomastoid muscle. The 'line' visible on the surface of the digastric muscle is the sole indication of its division into rostral and caudal parts.

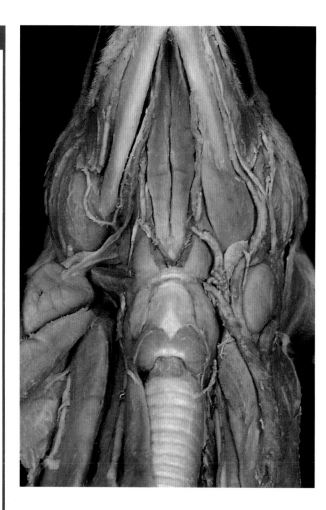

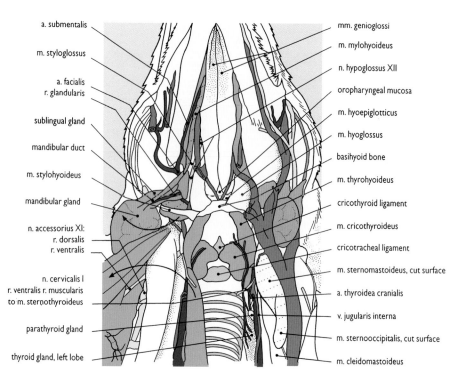

a. submentalis
m. styloglossus
a. facialis
r. glandularis
sublingual gland
mandibular duct
m. stylohyoideus
mandibular gland
n. accessorius XI:
r. dorsalis
r. ventralis
n. cervicalis I
r. ventralis r. muscularis
to m. sternothyroideus
parathyroid gland
thyroid gland, left lobe

mm. genioglossi
m. mylohyoideus
n. hypoglossus XII
oropharyngeal mucosa
m. hyoepiglotticus
m. hyoglossus
basihyoid bone
m. thyrohyoideus
cricothyroid ligament
m. cricothyroideus
cricotracheal ligament
m. sternomastoideus, cut surface
a. thyroidea cranialis
v. jugularis interna
m. sternooccipitalis, cut surface
m. cleidomastoideus

Fig. 2.129 Tongue, hyoid and larynx: ventral view (1). On the right side the rostral belly of the digastric muscle has been removed; on the left side the horizontal component of the mylohyoid muscle and the geniohyoid muscle. On the left side also the ventral part of the sternocephalic muscle has been cut through on a level with the ventral border of the external jugular vein and removed. The sternohyoid muscles of both sides have been removed, along with the sternothyroid muscle of the left side.

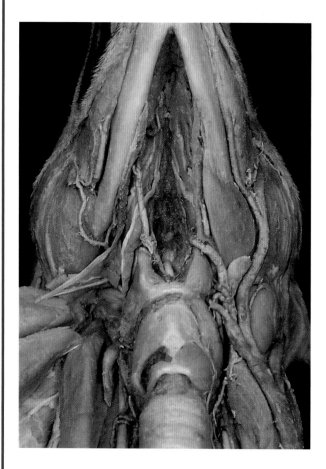

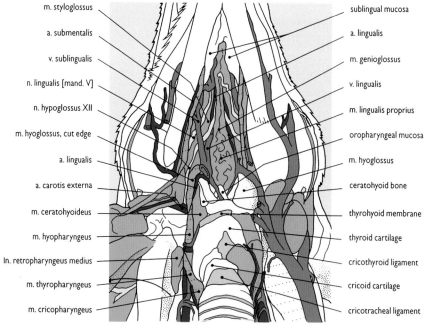

m. styloglossus
a. submentalis
v. sublingualis
n. lingualis [mand. V]
n. hypoglossus XII
m. hyoglossus, cut edge
a. lingualis
a. carotis externa
m. ceratohyoideus
m. hyopharyngeus
ln. retropharyngeus medius
m. thyropharyngeus
m. cricopharyngeus

sublingual mucosa
a. lingualis
m. genioglossus
v. lingualis
m. lingualis proprius
oropharyngeal mucosa
m. hyoglossus
ceratohyoid bone
thyrohyoid membrane
thyroid cartilage
cricothyroid ligament
cricoid cartilage
cricotracheal ligament

Fig. 2.130 Tongue, hyoid and larynx: ventral view (2). The genioglossal muscles of both sides have been removed along with the rostral part of the hyoglossal muscle and the caudal belly of the digastric of the right side. Also on the right side, removal of thyrohyoid and cricothyroid muscles has exposed more of the hyoid arch and laryngeal cartilages. A clearer appreciation of the musculature of the hyoid, pharynx and larynx is obtained from lateral (Figs 2.79–2.81) and medial (Figs 2.91–2.94) views.

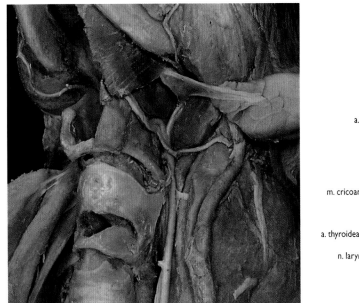

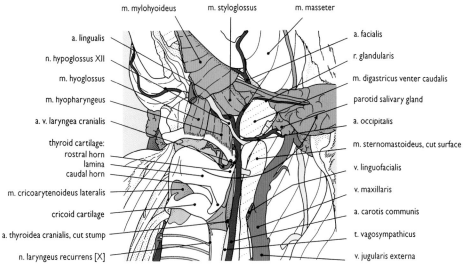

m. mylohyoideus   m. styloglossus   m. masseter

a. lingualis
n. hypoglossus XII
m. hyoglossus
m. hyopharyngeus
a. v. laryngea cranialis
thyroid cartilage:
rostral horn
lamina
caudal horn
m. cricoarytenoideus lateralis
cricoid cartilage
a. thyroidea cranialis, cut stump
n. laryngeus recurrens [X]

a. facialis
r. glandularis
m. digastricus venter caudalis
parotid salivary gland
a. occipitalis
m. sternomastoideus, cut surface
v. linguofacialis
v. maxillaris
a. carotis communis
t. vagosympathicus
v. jugularis externa

Fig. 2.131 Larynx and hyoid: left ventrolateral view (1). The superficial veins and mandibular lymph nodes of the left side have been removed, allowing lateral reflection of the mandibular salivary gland. Additional removals include the rostral belly of the digastric muscle, the cricothyroid and thyrohyoid muscles, more of the sternomastoid muscle, the attachments to the larynx of the thyropharyngeal and cricopharyngeal muscles, and the thyroid gland.

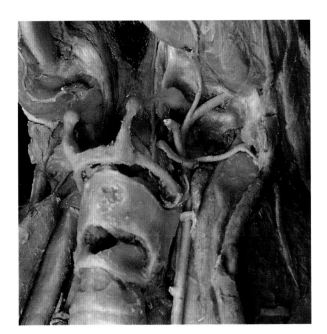

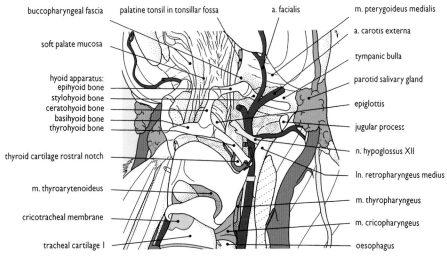

buccopharyngeal fascia   palatine tonsil in tonsillar fossa   a. facialis   m. pterygoideus medialis

soft palate mucosa

hyoid apparatus:
epihyoid bone
stylohyoid bone
ceratohyoid bone
basihyoid bone
thyrohyoid bone

thyroid cartilage rostral notch

m. thyroarytenoideus

cricotracheal membrane

tracheal cartilage I

a. carotis externa
tympanic bulla
parotid salivary gland
epiglottis
jugular process
n. hypoglossus XII
ln. retropharyngeus medius
m. thyropharyngeus
m. cricopharyngeus
oesophagus

Fig. 2.132 Larynx and hyoid: left ventrolateral view (2). The remnants of the tongue and floor of the mouth have been removed by: severing the hyoid attachments of the hyoglossal and styloglossal muscles and the hypoglossal nerve and lingual artery; removing the salivary glands and ducts, the remains of the mylohyoid, digastric, hyopharyngeal and ceratohyoid muscles; cutting the mucosal lining of the floor of the mouth and walls of the oropharynx back to the base of the epiglottis.

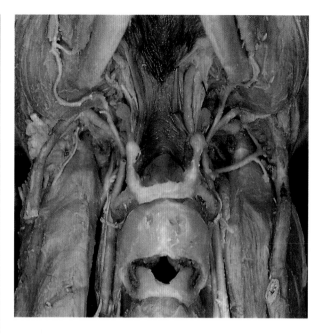
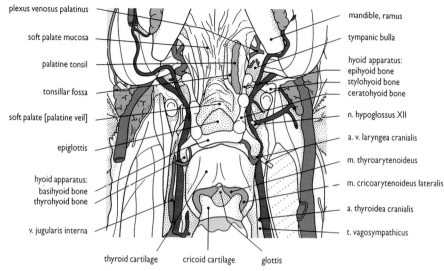

plexus venosus palatinus — mandible, ramus
soft palate mucosa — tympanic bulla
palatine tonsil — hyoid apparatus:
  epihyoid bone
  stylohyoid bone
tonsillar fossa — ceratohyoid bone
soft palate [palatine veil] — n. hypoglossus XII
epiglottis — a. v. laryngea cranialis
  — m. thyroarytenoideus
hyoid apparatus:
  basihyoid bone — m. cricoarytenoideus lateralis
  thyrohyoid bone — a. thyroidea cranialis
v. jugularis interna — t. vagosympathicus

thyroid cartilage   cricoid cartilage   glottis

Fig. 2.133 Larynx, hyoid, tonsil and soft palate: ventral view. This is a different view of the dissection shown in Fig. 2.132 with the addition that the palatine tonsil of the left side has been exposed more fully by pinning back the margins of its fossa. Lateral to the tonsil the mucosa has been removed from the underside of the medial pterygoid muscle.

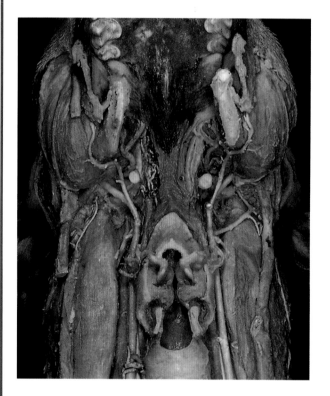
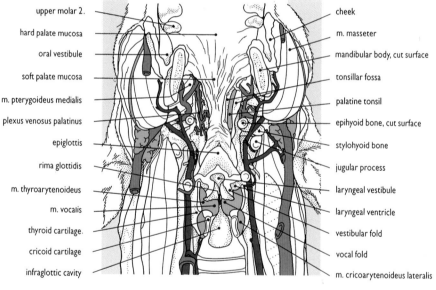

upper molar 2. — cheek
hard palate mucosa — m. masseter
oral vestibule — mandibular body, cut surface
soft palate mucosa — tonsillar fossa
m. pterygoideus medialis — palatine tonsil
plexus venosus palatinus — epihyoid bone, cut surface
epiglottis — stylohyoid bone
rima glottidis — jugular process
m. thyroarytenoideus — laryngeal vestibule
m. vocalis — laryngeal ventricle
thyroid cartilage. — vestibular fold
cricoid cartilage — vocal fold
infraglottic cavity — m. cricoarytenoideus lateralis

Fig. 2.134 Soft palate, palatine tonsil and interior of the larynx: ventral view. The lower jaw has been removed by cutting back on either side from the angle of the mouth through the cheek and body of the mandible. Much of the hyoid has been removed by severing the epihyoid and thyrohyoid bones on both sides. Continued removal of mucosa from the soft palate and roof of the mouth reveals the ramifications of the palatine plexus. The larynx has been sectioned horizontally although the trachea remains intact.

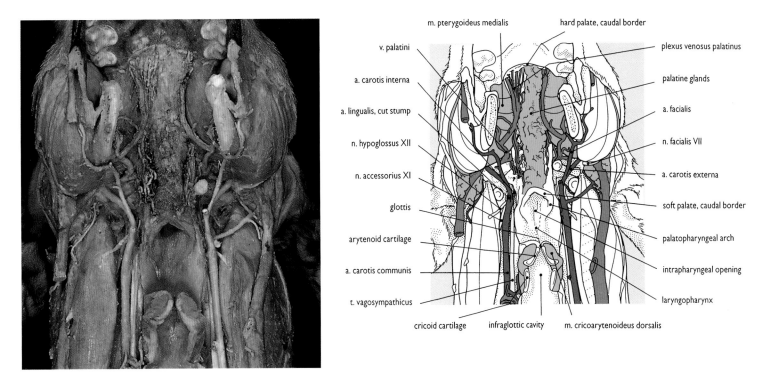

m. pterygoideus medialis   hard palate, caudal border

v. palatini

a. carotis interna

a. lingualis, cut stump

n. hypoglossus XII

n. accessorius XI

glottis

arytenoid cartilage

a. carotis communis

t. vagosympathicus

plexus venosus palatinus

palatine glands

a. facialis

n. facialis VII

a. carotis externa

soft palate, caudal border

palatopharyngeal arch

intrapharyngeal opening

laryngopharynx

cricoid cartilage   infraglottic cavity   m. cricoarytenoideus dorsalis

Fig. 2.135 Soft palate (1). Palatine glands, palatine plexus and laryngopharynx: ventral view. Complete removal of the mucosa of the soft palate and some clearing of the palatine plexus on the left side exposes the dense mass of palatine glandular tissue. A clear indication of the substantial 'depth' of the soft palate is also shown in section (Figs 2.144 and 2.145). Further horizontal sectioning of the larynx has removed the thyroid cartilage and epiglottis, leaving the arytenoid cartilages articulated with the leading edge of the cricoid.

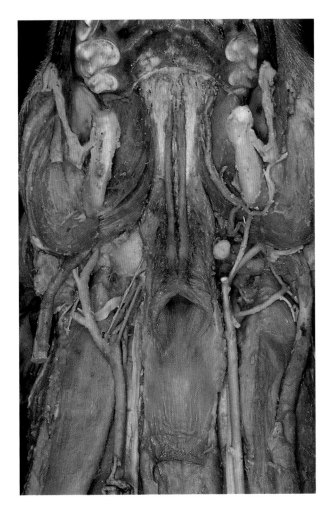

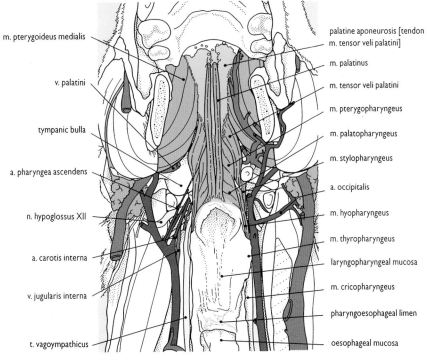

m. pterygoideus medialis

v. palatini

tympanic bulla

a. pharyngea ascendens

n. hypoglossus XII

a. carotis interna

v. jugularis interna

t. vagoympathicus

palatine aponeurosis [tendon m. tensor veli palatini]

m. palatinus

m. tensor veli palatini

m. pterygopharyngeus

m. palatopharyngeus

m. stylopharyngeus

a. occipitalis

m. hyopharyngeus

m. thyropharyngeus

laryngopharyngeal mucosa

m. cricopharyngeus

pharyngoesophageal limen

oesophageal mucosa

Fig. 2.136 Soft palate (2). Palatine and pharyngeal muscles and carotid arterial branches: ventral view. The glandular tissue and venous plexus of the palate are removed. On the right side the stylohyoid has been removed and the facial and external carotid arteries have been displaced laterally. The remaining parts of the larynx have been removed and the demarcation between laryngopharynx and esophagus is visible.

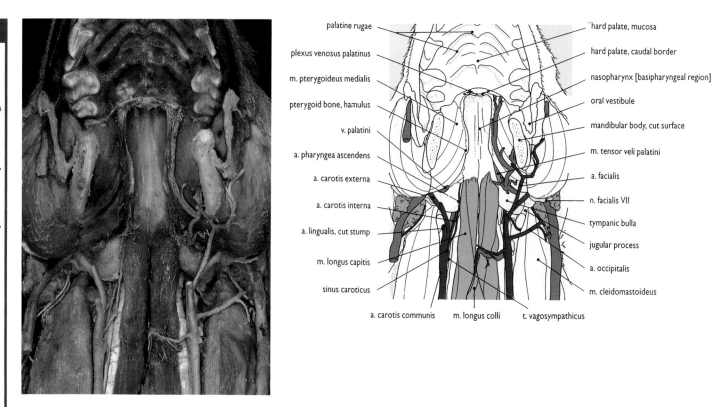

Fig. 2.137 Nasopharynx, tympanic bullae and longus capitis muscles: ventral view. The soft palate and its muscles have been removed, opening the nasopharynx in the basipharyngeal canal of the skull (see Fig. 2.126). The caudal border of the hard palate marks the position of the choanae (internal nostrils). The remaining mucosa and muscles of the roof of the laryngopharynx and esophagus are also removed and the long strap-like longus capitis muscles are exposed attached to the braincase floor between the tympanic bullae.

Fig. 2.138–2.146 Transverse sections 1–9 through the head: rostral views. The transverse sections through the head begin a sequence of sections through the entire body and limbs. The sections through the head are all viewed from the rostral aspect and the accompanying sketch shows the approximate levels at which the sections were taken.

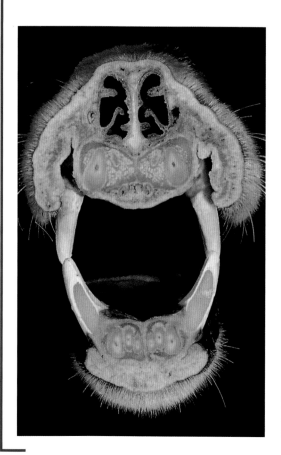

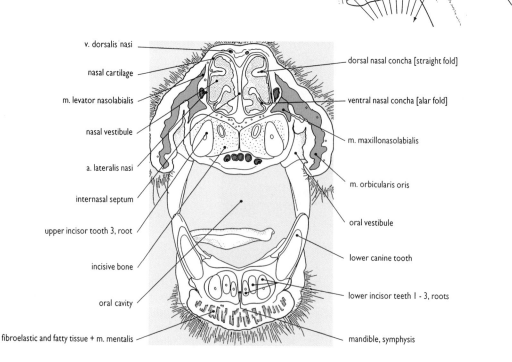

Fig. 2.138 Transverse section (1). Through the nasal vestibule and lower jaw at the level of the canine teeth: rostral view. This first section is through the nasal vestibule and shows the cartilaginous framework of their movable part of the nose.

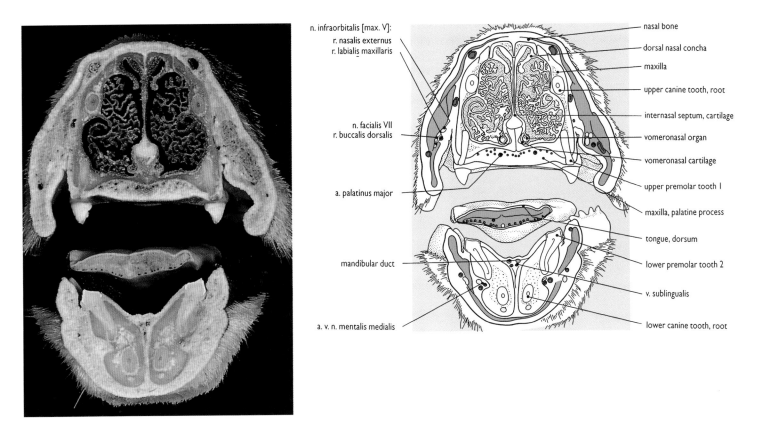

Fig. 2.139 Transverse section (2). Through the nasal cavity at the level of upper premolar tooth 1 and the lower jaw at lower premolar tooth 2: rostral view. This section is through the nasal cavity proper and demonstrates the complex branching of the ventral nasal concha (maxilloturbinate) and the extensive vascularity of the submucosal tissues lining the nasal cavity (cf. Figs 2.101 and 2.102). The vomeronasal organs and their associated vomeronasal cartilages are visible on either side of the base of the nasal septum (cf. Fig. 2.102).

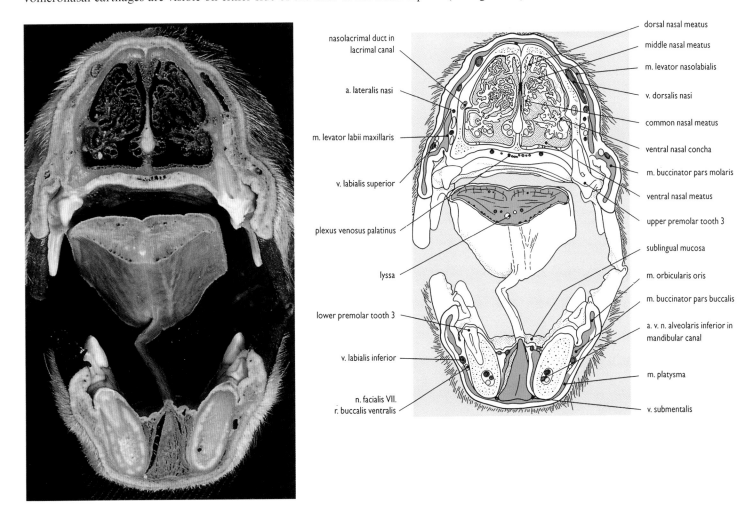

Fig. 2.140 Transverse section (3). Through the nasal cavity, tongue and lower jaw at the level of upper and lower premolar teeth 3: rostral view. This section through the nasal cavity demonstrates how the nasal mucosa on its supporting framework of conchal bones fills practically the entire nasal cavity. Longitudinal nasal meatuses are consequently indistinct except for the ventral. The mandibular symphysis is shown to advantage in Fig. 2.139 while in this section the genioglossal and geniohyoid muscles are shown at their origins immediately caudal to the symphysis.

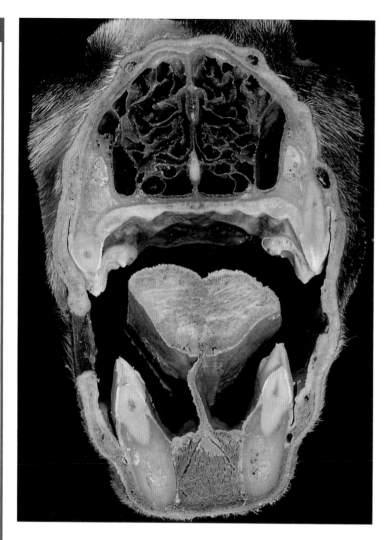

Fig. 2.141 Transverse section (4). Through the nasal cavity, tongue and lower jaw at the level of upper premolar tooth 4 and lower molar tooth 1: rostral view. This section passes through the shearing (carnassial) teeth on a level with the angle of the mouth. Within the nasal cavity the section passes through the rostral part of the ethmoidal labyrinth demonstrating both ectoturbinate and endoturbinate bones supporting olfactory mucosa (see Figs 2.104 and 2.105). The frenulum of the tongue contains bilateral extensions from the genioglossal muscles passing into the tongue between rostrally running elements of the hyoglossal muscles. The bulk of the tongue is made up of various bundles of intrinsic muscles, of particular note are perpendicular and transverse fibers. The extrinsic tongue muscles are shown to advantage in lateral (Fig. 2.77) and especially medial (Figs 2.87–2.94) views.

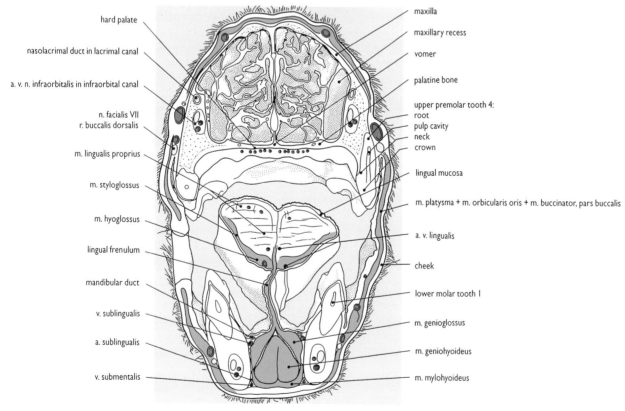

Labels (left side):
- hard palate
- nasolacrimal duct in lacrimal canal
- a. v. n. infraorbitalis in infraorbital canal
- n. facialis VII
  r. buccalis dorsalis
- m. lingualis proprius
- m. styloglossus
- m. hyoglossus
- lingual frenulum
- mandibular duct
- v. sublingualis
- a. sublingualis
- v. submentalis

Labels (right side):
- maxilla
- maxillary recess
- vomer
- palatine bone
- upper premolar tooth 4:
  root
  pulp cavity
  neck
  crown
- lingual mucosa
- m. platysma + m. orbicularis oris + m. buccinator, pars buccalis
- a. v. lingualis
- cheek
- lower molar tooth 1
- m. genioglossus
- m. geniohyoideus
- m. mylohyoideus

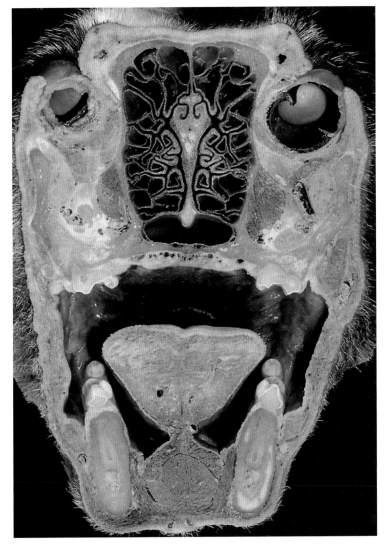

Fig. 2.142 Transverse section (5). Through the nasal cavity, orbits, pterygopalatine fossae, tongue and lower jaw: rostral view. This section passes through the orbits and the pterygopalatine fossae. The eyeball is sectioned, as are the extrinsic muscles and the confining periorbital layer. On the left side the periorbita is perforated by the connection linking the ventral external ophthalmic vein with the deep facial vein (see Figs 2.48 and 2.52). The maxillary artery and nerve are just visible prior to their entry into the infraorbital canal at the maxillary foramen. The presence of the zygomatic salivary gland and the fat obscures these structures to some extent. Spanning the intermandibular space the mylohyoid muscle is clearly shown forming a 'diaphragm' across the floor of the mouth.

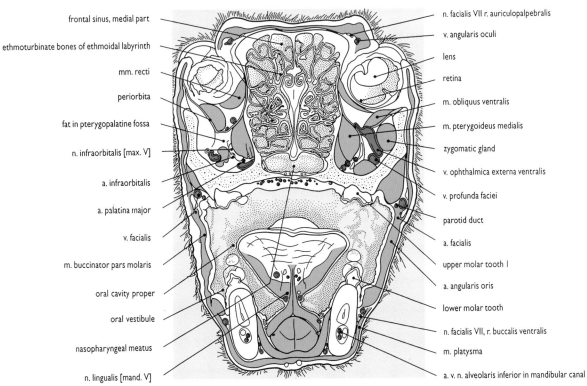

frontal sinus, medial part

ethmoturbinate bones of ethmoidal labyrinth

mm. recti

periorbita

fat in pterygopalatine fossa

n. infraorbitalis [max. V]

a. infraorbitalis

a. palatina major

v. facialis

m. buccinator pars molaris

oral cavity proper

oral vestibule

nasopharyngeal meatus

n. lingualis [mand. V]

n. facialis VII r. auriculopalpebralis

v. angularis oculi

lens

retina

m. obliquus ventralis

m. pterygoideus medialis

zygomatic gland

v. ophthalmica externa ventralis

v. profunda faciei

parotid duct

a. facialis

upper molar tooth I

a. angularis oris

lower molar tooth

n. facialis VII, r. buccalis ventralis

m. platysma

a. v. n. alveolaris inferior in mandibular canal

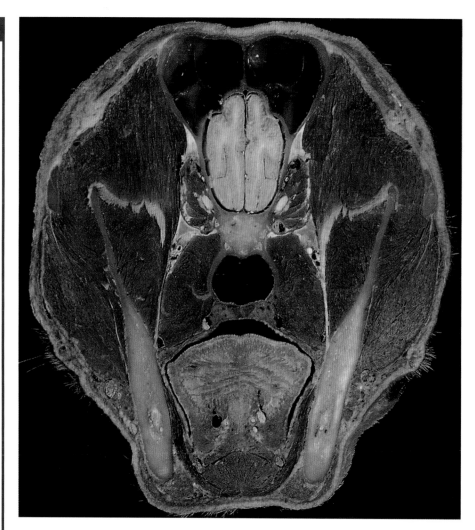

Fig. 2.143 Transverse section (6). Through the frontal sinuses, the rostral end of the cranial cavity, the nasopharynx, body of the tongue and the mandibular rami: rostral view. The orbits and the pterygopalatine fossae are still represented in this section, although the orbit is sectioned close to the apex of the periorbital 'cone'. Extrinsic ocular muscles and orbital nerves are visible but the section passes caudal to the emergence of the optic nerve (see Figs 2.48–2.54). The oropharynx is practically obliterated by the bulk of the tongue. In its lateral walls the sublingual salivary glands lie against the medial face of the mandible and the mylohyoid muscle. Frontal lobes of the cerebral hemispheres are identified in the cranial cavity below the lateral compartment of the frontal sinus. Figures 2.110–2.115 and 2.118–2.121 show details of the gross internal structure of the brain, from lateral and dorsal views respectively.

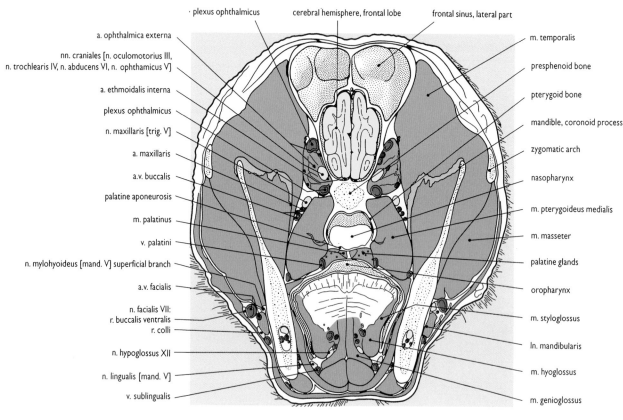

· plexus ophthalmicus

cerebral hemisphere, frontal lobe

frontal sinus, lateral part

a. ophthalmica externa

nn. craniales [n. oculomotorius III, n. trochlearis IV, n. abducens VI, n. ophthamicus V]

a. ethmoidalis interna

plexus ophthalmicus

n. maxillaris [trig. V]

a. maxillaris

a.v. buccalis

palatine aponeurosis

m. palatinus

v. palatini

n. mylohyoideus [mand. V] superficial branch

a.v. facialis

n. facialis VII:
r. buccalis ventralis
r. colli

n. hypoglossus XII

n. lingualis [mand. V]

v. sublingualis

m. temporalis

presphenoid bone

pterygoid bone

mandible, coronoid process

zygomatic arch

nasopharynx

m. pterygoideus medialis

m. masseter

palatine glands

oropharynx

m. styloglossus

ln. mandibularis

m. hyoglossus

m. genioglossus

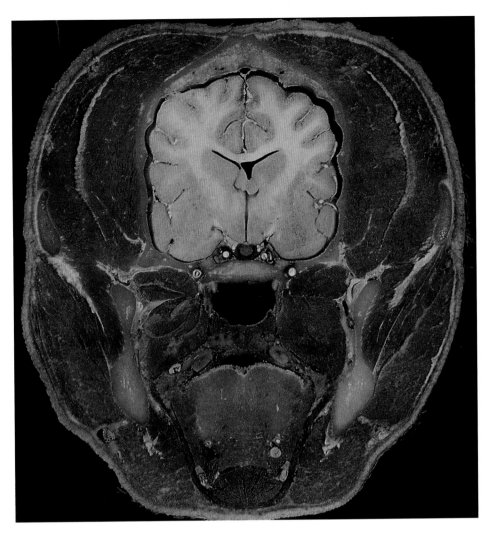

Fig. 2.144 Transverse section (7). Through the cerebral hemispheres, pituitary gland, nasopharynx, palatine tonsils and the root of the tongue: rostral view. In this section a number of structures are evident flanking the pituitary gland, notably the cerebral arterial circle and the internal carotid artery running within the cavernous sinus (see Figs 2.113, 2.115, 2.123 and 2.124). Lateral to this on the outer surface of the braincase the maxillary artery is visible at its entry into the alar canal of the sphenoid bone (see Figs 2.3 and 2.82). The lower jaw is sectioned through the mandibular notch rostral to the jaw joint (see Fig. 2.3) but caudal to the mandibular foramen. The mandibular alveolar artery, vein and nerve appear from between medial and lateral pterygoid muscles *en route* for the foramen (Fig. 2.98).

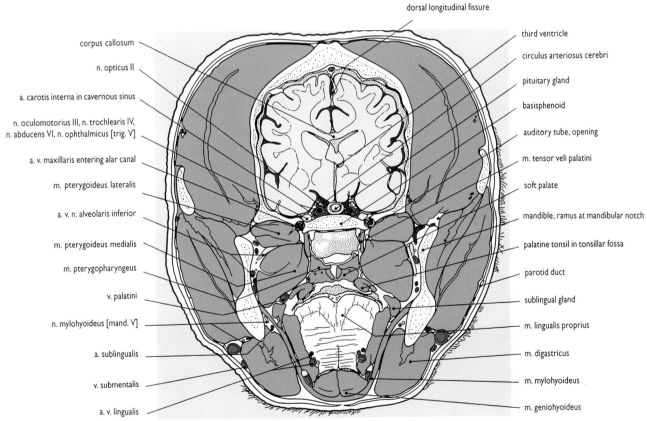

dorsal longitudinal fissure

corpus callosum

n. opticus II

a. carotis interna in cavernous sinus

n. oculomotorius III, n. trochlearis IV, n. abducens VI, n. ophthalmicus [trig. V]

a. v. maxillaris entering alar canal

m. pterygoideus lateralis

a. v. n. alveolaris inferior

m. pterygoideus medialis

m. pterygopharyngeus

v. palatini

n. mylohyoideus [mand. V]

a. sublingualis

v. submentalis

a. v. lingualis

third ventricle

circulus arteriosus cerebri

pituitary gland

basisphenoid

auditory tube, opening

m. tensor veli palatini

soft palate

mandible, ramus at mandibular notch

palatine tonsil in tonsillar fossa

parotid duct

sublingual gland

m. lingualis proprius

m. digastricus

m. mylohyoideus

m. geniohyoideus

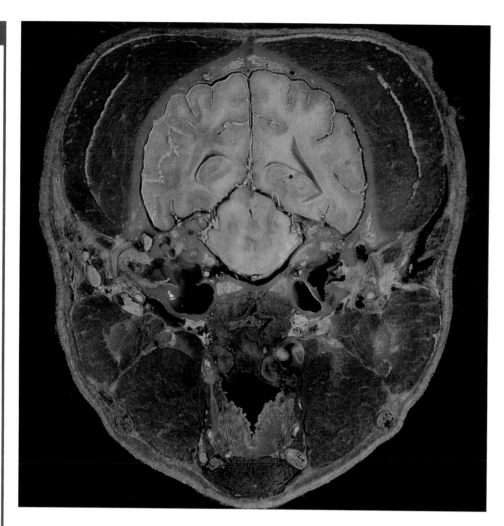

Fig. 2.145 Transverse section (8). Through the cerebral hemispheres, midbrain, tympanic membranes, middle ear cavities, palatine tonsils and oropharynx: rostral view. On the right side of this section two of the three auditory ossicles (incus and malleus) as well as the tensor tympani muscle and the tympanic membrane are shown, and the external acoustic meatus is partially sectioned. The close relationship of maxillary artery and vein and facial nerve (VII) to the meatus is apparent, these structures lying deep to the parotid salivary gland (see Figs 2.39 and 2.45). The lower jaw is just represented by the angular processes, but masseter, pterygoid and digastric muscles remain prominent masses.

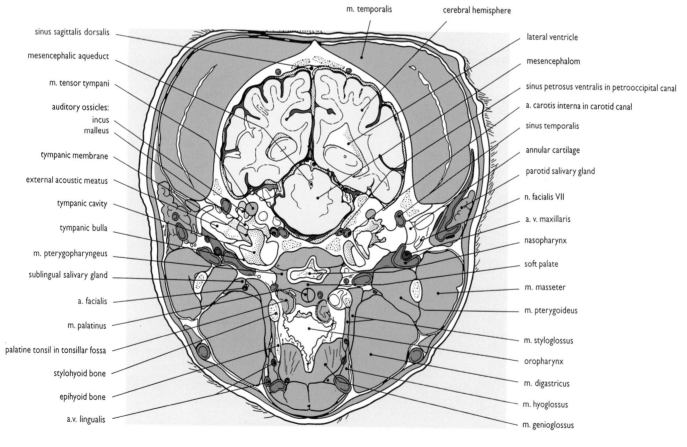

m. temporalis — cerebral hemisphere

sinus sagittalis dorsalis

mesencephalic aqueduct

m. tensor tympani

auditory ossicles:
incus
malleus

tympanic membrane

external acoustic meatus

tympanic cavity

tympanic bulla

m. pterygopharyngeus

sublingual salivary gland

a. facialis

m. palatinus

palatine tonsil in tonsillar fossa

stylohyoid bone

epihyoid bone

a.v. lingualis

lateral ventricle

mesencephalom

sinus petrosus ventralis in petrooccipital canal

a. carotis interna in carotid canal

sinus temporalis

annular cartilage

parotid salivary gland

n. facialis VII

a. v. maxillaris

nasopharynx

soft palate

m. masseter

m. pterygoideus

m. styloglossus

oropharynx

m. digastricus

m. hyoglossus

m. genioglossus

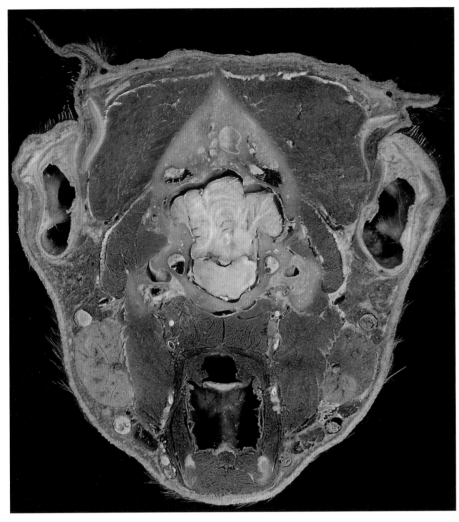

Fig. 2.146 Transverse section (9). Through the occipital region, cerebellum, hindbrain, and parotid and mandibular salivary glands: rostral view. Ventral to the atlanto-occipital joint in this section several cranial nerves (X, XI and XII) and the internal and external carotid arteries are sectioned where they lie between the digastric muscle laterally and the longus capitis muscle medially (see Figs 2.78–2.82 and 2.92–2.95). The section passes through the pharynx just caudal to the free border of the soft palate so that the apex of the epiglottic cartilage is just apparent in the plane of the section. Within the oropharyngeal cavity the oral surface of the epiglottis is identifiable.

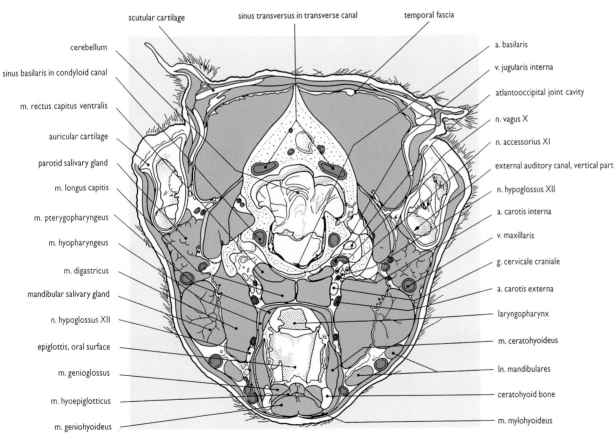

scutular cartilage

sinus transversus in transverse canal

temporal fascia

cerebellum

sinus basilaris in condyloid canal

m. rectus capitus ventralis

auricular cartilage

parotid salivary gland

m. longus capitis

m. pterygopharyngeus

m. hyopharyngeus

m. digastricus

mandibular salivary gland

n. hypoglossus XII

epiglottis, oral surface

m. genioglossus

m. hyoepiglotticus

m. geniohyoideus

a. basilaris

v. jugularis interna

atlantooccipital joint cavity

n. vagus X

n. accessorius XI

external auditory canal, vertical part

n. hypoglossus XII

a. carotis interna

v. maxillaris

g. cervicale craniale

a. carotis externa

laryngopharynx

m. ceratohyoideus

ln. mandibulares

ceratohyoid bone

m. mylohyoideus

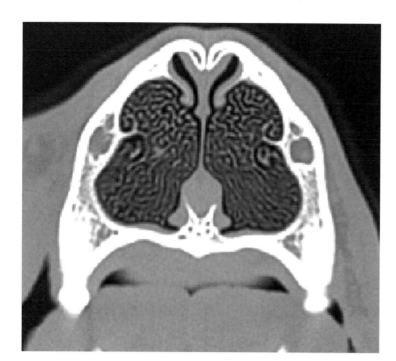

Fig. 2.147 Computed tomography image of the nose: transverse plane, level of 1st premolar.

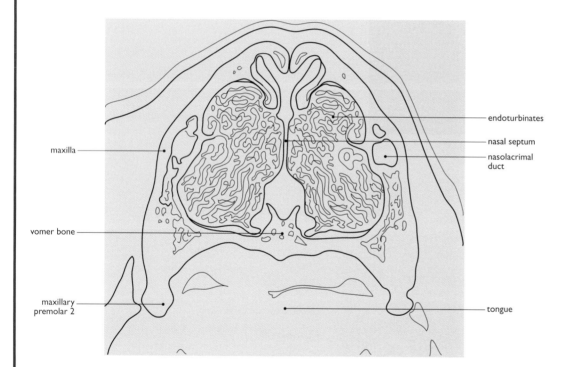

endoturbinates

nasal septum

nasolacrimal duct

maxilla

vomer bone

maxillary premolar 2

tongue

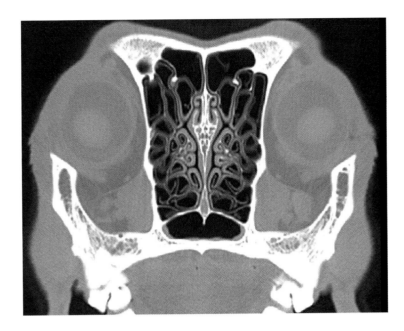

Fig. 2.148 Computed tomography image of the nose: transverse plane, level of orbits.

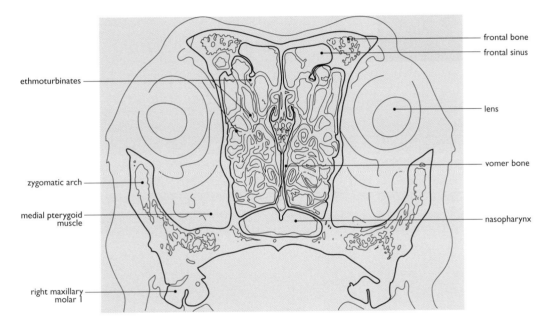

frontal bone
frontal sinus

ethmoturbinates

lens

vomer bone

zygomatic arch

medial pterygoid muscle

nasopharynx

right maxillary molar 1

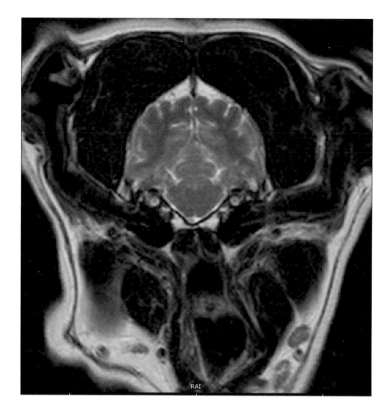

Fig. 2.149 Magnetic resonance image of the head: transverse plane, at the level of the tympanic bullae, T₂ weighted image.

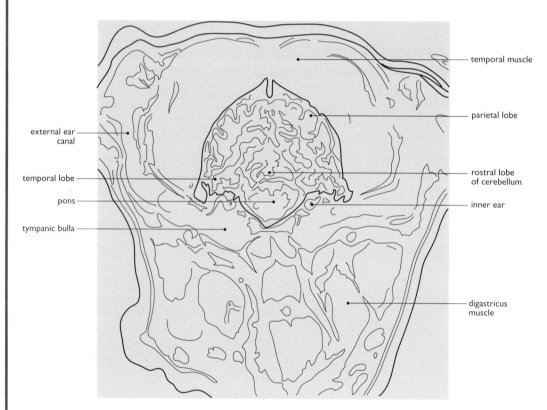

temporal muscle

parietal lobe

external ear canal

rostral lobe of cerebellum

temporal lobe

pons

inner ear

tympanic bulla

digastricus muscle

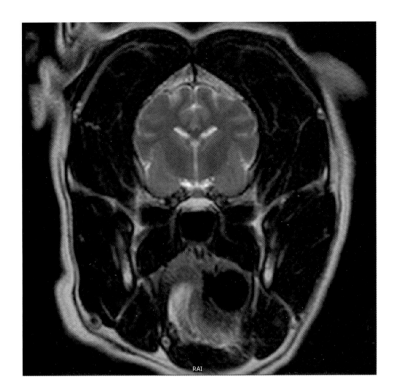

Fig. 2.150 Magnetic resonance image of the head: transverse plane, at the level of the pituitary, T$_2$ weighted image.

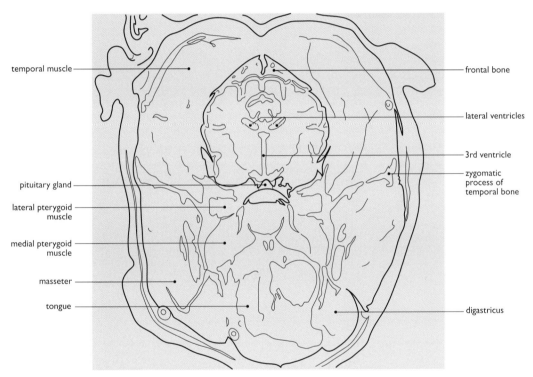

temporal muscle

frontal bone

lateral ventricles

3rd ventricle

pituitary gland

zygomatic process of temporal bone

lateral pterygoid muscle

medial pterygoid muscle

masseter

tongue

digastricus

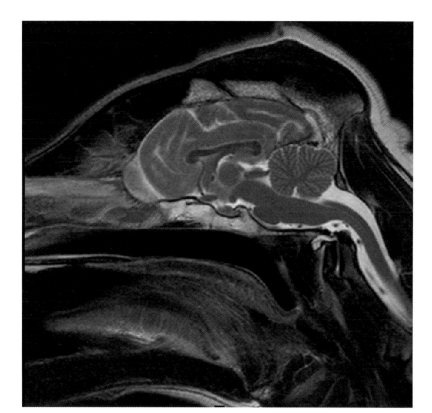

Fig. 2.151 Magnetic resonance image of the head: sagittal plane, midline, T$_2$ weighted image.

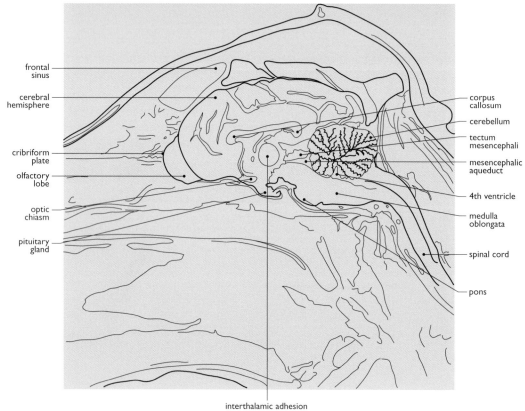

frontal
sinus

cerebral
hemisphere

cribriform
plate

olfactory
lobe

optic
chiasm

pituitary
gland

corpus
callosum

cerebellum

tectum
mesencephali

mesencephalic
aqueduct

4th ventricle

medulla
oblongata

spinal cord

pons

interthalamic adhesion

3. THE NECK

The neck has three regions: the parotid region, the ventral margin of the neck and the prescapular region. Many conditions link the head and the neck and one of the most important is the brachycephalic dog that has upper airway syndrome due to distortion of the face.

The neck is often injured in fights with damage to superficial nerves and vessels. In the dorsal part of the neck, which does not contain the delicate structures, there are few vital structures to damage so injury is to skin, subcutis and muscles. The most important landmark is the thyroid cartilage of the larynx (laryngeal prominence) caudal to the basihyoid bone. The important clinical structures are the thyroid, larynx, trachea, esophagus and cervical vertebrae.

The thyroid gland is not palpable in the healthy dog. Palpable enlargements called goiter do occur, but are quite rare. The thyroid gland occupies the position over the 5th to 9th tracheal cartilages. There are two parathyroid glands within each lobe of the thyroid. The internal is at the caudal pole of the thyroid and the other two are found in the foramina cranial to each of the thyroid lobules. Thyroidectomy must leave the parathyroid glands intact. This is particularly important in cats. Clinically, it is important to note that the epiglottis lies dorsal to the soft palate.

One of the common clinical conditions seen in dogs is difficulty in swallowing or dysphagia. This has three phases: esophageal, pharyngeal and gastro-esophageal. In cases of mega-esophagus, which is a dilated esophagus, a distended fluid-filled esophagus may be rarely palpable. Surgical access to this region is usually in the middle third of the neck. Persistent right aortic arch is quite an interesting anatomical problem leading to mega-esophagus Surgery to the esophagus requires care to locate and protect the carotid artery and vago-sympathetic trunk and if moving the esophagus it should be done carefully to avoid damage to the left recurrent laryngeal nerve. This lies between the esophagus and trachea on the left of the midline. The usual site for surgery in the neck is the midline ventral fibrous raphe with the animal in dorsal recumbency. Incisions are made through this line to minimize trauma to the surrounding tissues and reduce hemorrhage. The ventral strap muscles can then be spread laterally. This site is used for tracheal, esophageal, thyroid and disc surgery.

A relatively common condition in older dogs, tracheal collapse, is particularly common in Yorkshire terriers and is also repaired through the midline raphe about 2 to 3 cm caudal to the larynx in the midline. In this condition, there is degeneration of the tracheal cartilage and repair consists of tightening the tracheal ligament to reconstitute the round shape of the trachea.

Ventral cervical disc fenestration is used to relieve the damage to the intervertebral discs, which occurs in the cervical region of small dogs in particular. The nucleus pulposus of the disc either prolapses laterally or dorsally which produces pressure on the spinal cord and the resulting pain produces muscular spasm. This correction procedure is also carried out in dorsal recumbency.

An understanding of the structure of the larynx is essential to ensure successful endotracheal intubation. Several other clinical conditions involving the larynx and pharynx are also treated surgically. Vocal cords can be removed surgically if necessary. Arytenoid lateralization is used to treat laryngeal paralysis and in this the arytenoid cartilages are dislocated from the underlying cricoid cartilage and are attached more posteriorly to the ipsilateral wing of the thyroid cartilage, thus abducting the attached vocal cords. Cricopharyngeal myotomy is used to treat cricopharyngeal achalasia, in which the cricopharyngeal sphincter cannot relax and does not allow passage of food from pharynx to esophagus. In this case, part of the cricopharyngeal muscle mass is removed.

Pharyngeal intubation allows a tube to be placed *in situ* and down the esophagus and assists repair of esophageal wounds and pharyngeal paralysis. It is possible to collect cerebrospinal fluid (CSF) from a site halfway between the occipital protuberances and a line joining the wings of the atlas. There is very little CSF in the dog.

There are two other important structures in the neck. The first of these is the superficial cervical lymph node or chain of lymph nodes. This is not normally palpable in the dog unless pathologically infected with either tumours or infectious disease. Enlargement of the cervical lymph nodes will not normally be palpable.

The second is the jugular vein which runs ventrolaterally and is accessible for venepuncture for a variety of reasons (blood sampling, anaesthesia, drug administration etc) and it can be raised by pressure at the caudal limit of the neck. The cephalic vein is located in the pectoral sulcus. Both the cephalic vein and the superficial cervical vein empty into the external jugular vein in the jugular fossa. The omobrachial vein also drains into the external jugular vein.

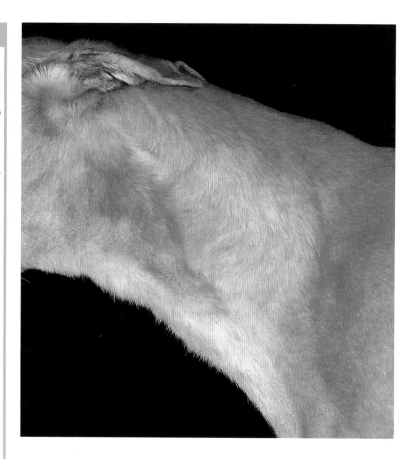

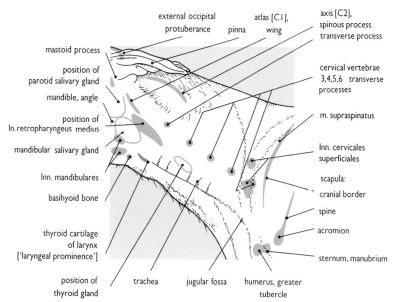

Fig. 3.1 Surface features: left lateral view. The palpable bony 'landmarks' of the neck are shown. The hyoid, larynx and trachea are clearly palpable on the underside of the neck. Soft structures which are occasionally palpable include the mandibular and superficial cervical lymph nodes. The external jugular vein may be raised by pressure in the jugular fossa at the thoracic inlet.

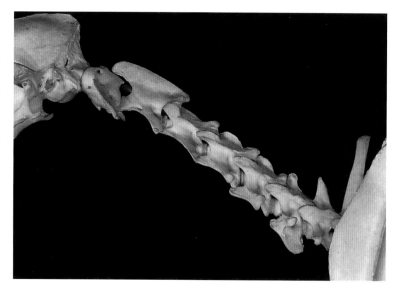

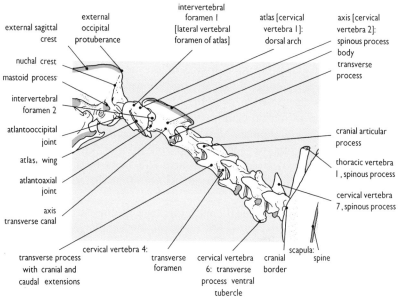

Fig. 3.2 Skeleton: left lateral view. The palpable bony features shown in Fig. 3.1 are colored green on this diagram for reference. However, any features of cervical vertebrae 3 to 7 are, even in thin dogs, only palpable with difficulty, and not at all in larger breeds.

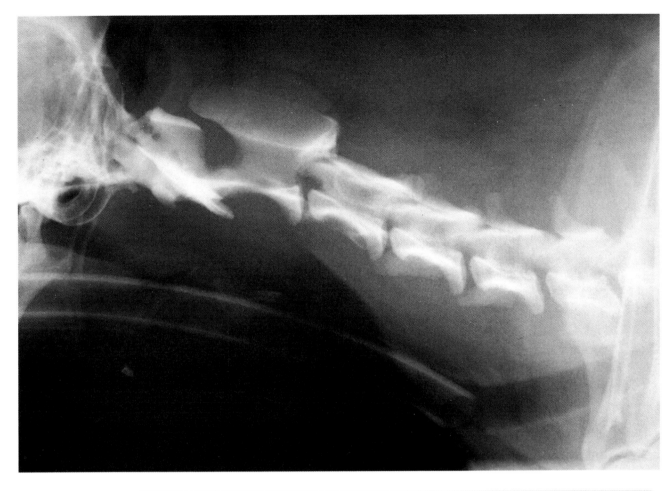

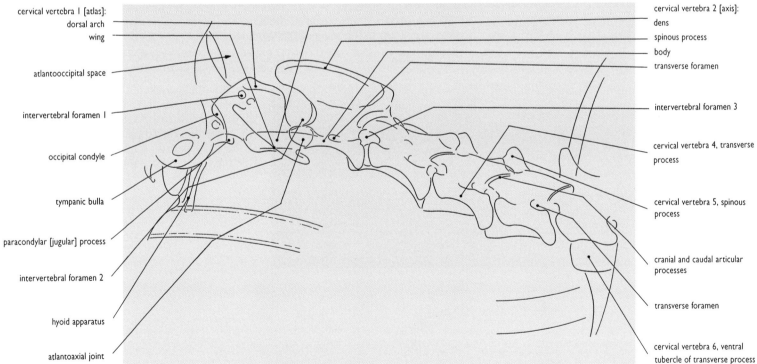

cervical vertebra 1 [atlas]:
dorsal arch
wing

atlantooccipital space

intervertebral foramen 1

occipital condyle

tympanic bulla

paracondylar [jugular] process

intervertebral foramen 2

hyoid apparatus

atlantoaxial joint

cervical vertebra 2 [axis]:
dens
spinous process
body
transverse foramen

intervertebral foramen 3

cervical vertebra 4, transverse
process

cervical vertebra 5, spinous
process

cranial and caudal articular
processes

transverse foramen

cervical vertebra 6, ventral
tubercle of transverse process

Fig. 3.3 Radiograph of the neck: left lateral view. The major structural features of the neck are shown in this and the following radiograph. Both give clear views of the vertebral canal housing the spinal cord. The atlanto-occipital space extends inwards to the atlanto-occipital membrane spanning the gap between the dorsal arch of the atlas and the dorsal border of the foramen magnum. The space is enlarged when the head is bent down on the neck providing access to the vertebral canal through the atlanto-occipital membrane.

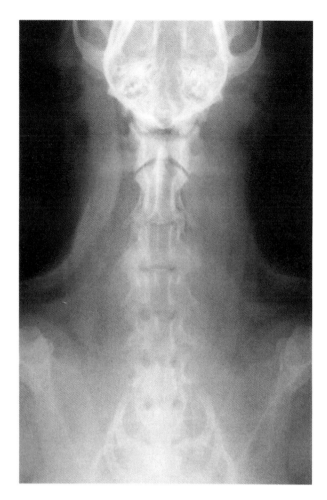

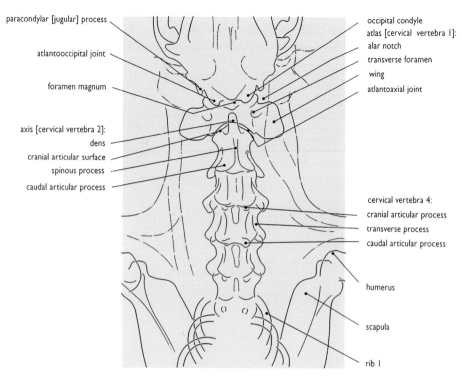

paracondylar [jugular] process

atlantooccipital joint

foramen magnum

axis [cervical vertebra 2]:
dens
cranial articular surface
spinous process
caudal articular process

occipital condyle
atlas [cervical vertebra 1]:
alar notch
transverse foramen
wing
atlantoaxial joint

cervical vertebra 4:
cranial articular process
transverse process
caudal articular process

humerus

scapula

rib I

Fig. 3.4 Radiograph of the neck: ventrodorsal view. This radiograph shows the position of transverse processes, especially the readily palpable wings of the atlas. It also demonstrates the variety of joints providing the extensive mobility of the head and neck – (i) overlapping synovial joints between articular processes of contiguous vertebrae; (ii) cartilaginous (radiolucent) intervertebral discs between vertebral bodies; (iii) atlanto-occipital joint at the occipital condyles allowing up and down movements of the head on the neck; (iv) atlantoaxial joint based on the pivotal peg of the dens allowing rotational movement of the head on the neck. The absence of a clavicle is clearly apparent in this view of the shoulder.

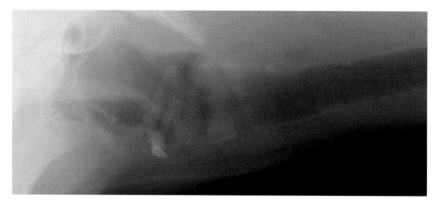

Fig. 3.5 Radiograph of the larynx: lateral view.
The laryngeal cartilages are poorly visible as ill-defined soft tissue opacities highlighted by the air within the larynx. The tympanohyoid bone is cartilaginous and so not visible against the retropharyngeal soft tissues.

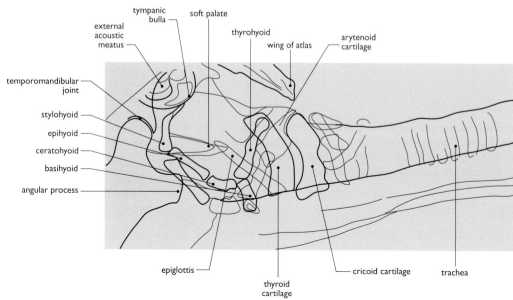

external
acoustic
meatus

tympanic
bulla

soft palate

thyrohyoid

wing of atlas

arytenoid
cartilage

temporomandibular
joint

stylohyoid

epihyoid

ceratohyoid

basihyoid

angular process

epiglottis

thyroid
cartilage

cricoid cartilage

trachea

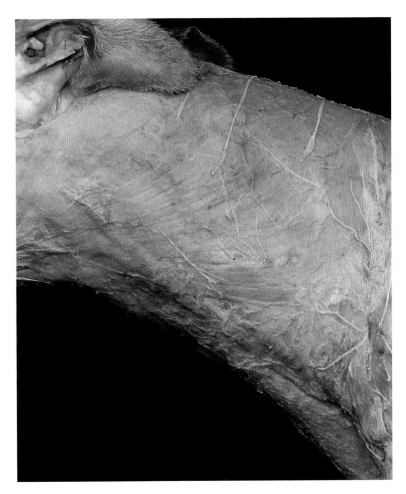

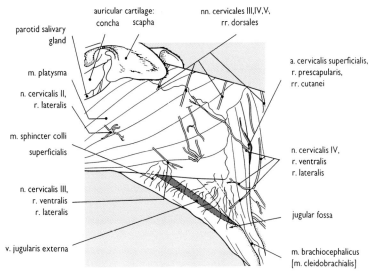

Fig. 3.6 Superficial structures (1). Superficial fascia, cutaneous muscles and cutaneous nerves: left lateral view. The superficial fascia of the neck is exposed following removal of the skin. It continues cranially (over temporal, parotid and masseteric regions) as the superficial fascia of the head, and caudally as the superficial brachial and pectoral fascia. Exposed are the prominent platysma muscle and some isolated strands of the superficial sphincter colli muscle.

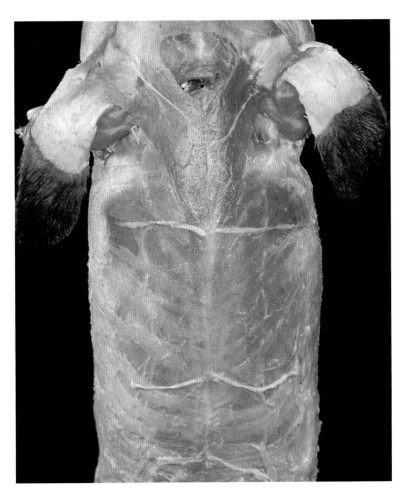

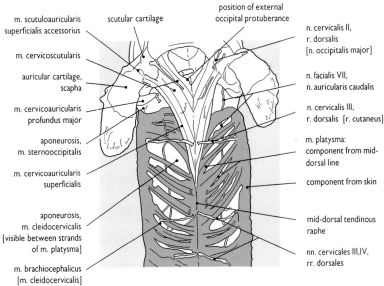

Fig. 3.7 Superficial structures (2). Cutaneous muscles and cutaneous nerves: dorsal view. The two components of the platysma muscle can be seen as a number of separate strands originating from the mid-dorsal line of the neck, and as a more substantial component arising from the internal surface of the skin itself. The two join dorsolaterally on the neck. The cutaneous branches from the dorsal rami of the cervical spinal nerves appear close to the mid-dorsal line and spread over the platysma surface.

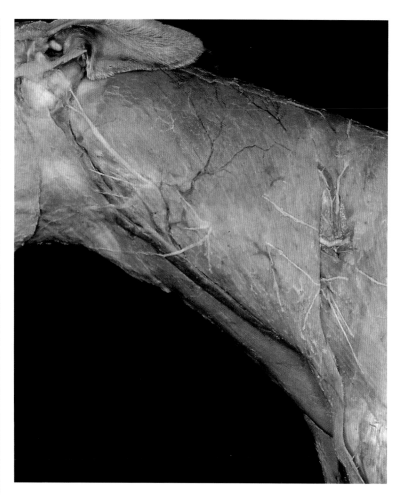

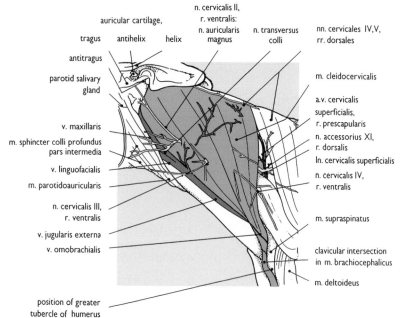

n. cervicalis II,
r. ventralis:

auricular cartilage,

n. auricularis magnus

n. transversus colli

nn. cervicales IV,V, rr. dorsales

tragus   antihelix   helix

antitragus

parotid salivary gland

m. cleidocervicalis

a.v. cervicalis superficialis, r. prescapularis

v. maxillaris

m. sphincter colli profundus pars intermedia

n. accessorius XI, r. dorsalis

ln. cervicalis superficialis

v. linguofacialis

n. cervicalis IV, r. ventralis

m. parotidoauricularis

n. cervicalis III, r. ventralis

m. supraspinatus

v. jugularis externa

clavicular intersection in m. brachiocephalicus

v. omobrachialis

m. deltoideus

position of greater tubercle of humerus

Fig. 3.8 Superficial structures (3). Cutaneous nerves and external jugular vein: left lateral view. The platysma muscle has been removed, and the superficial fascia cleared, to expose the underlying muscles, and isolate cutaneous ramifications of cervical nerves 2, 3 and 4. Cervical nerve 5 lacks lateral cutaneous branches, whilst cervical nerves 6, 7 and 8 contribute to the brachial plexus (see Fig. 3.19). Cutaneous branches from cervical nerve 4 distribute to the base of the neck.

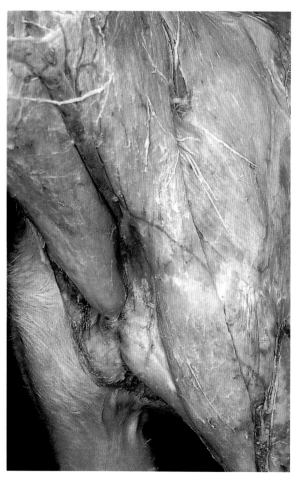

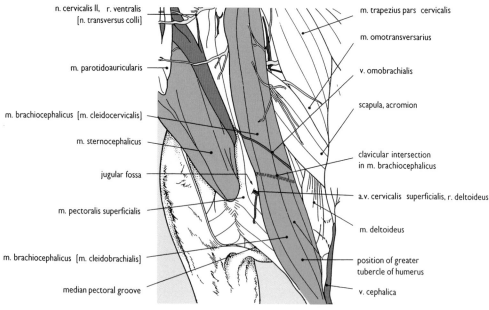

n. cervicalis II, r. ventralis [n. transversus colli]

m. trapezius pars cervicalis

m. omotransversarius

m. parotidoauricularis

v. omobrachialis

scapula, acromion

m. brachiocephalicus [m. cleidocervicalis]

m. sternocephalicus

clavicular intersection in m. brachiocephalicus

jugular fossa

a.v. cervicalis superficialis, r. deltoideus

m. pectoralis superficialis

m. deltoideus

m. brachiocephalicus [m. cleidobrachialis]

position of greater tubercle of humerus

median pectoral groove

v. cephalica

Fig. 3.9 Superficial structures (4). Cutaneous nerves, external jugular vein and jugular fossa: left craniolateral view. This clearly demonstrates the jugular fossa at the base of the neck and the deep and somewhat triangular depression bounded by sternocephalic, brachiocephalic and superficial pectoral muscles (see also Fig. 3.41). Also evident is the clavicular intersection within the brachiocephalic muscle, denoted by an indistinct fascial line lateral to the jugular fossa.

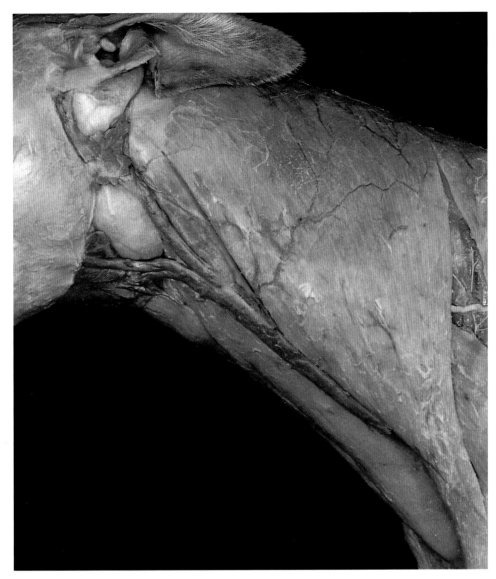

Fig. 3.10 Superficial musculature: left lateral view. The loose superficial fascia in the prescapular region and the retromandibular fossa has been cleaned, and the cutaneous muscles removed. This has exposed the mandibular and parotid salivary glands, the mandibular lymph nodes, and the main tributaries of the external jugular vein.

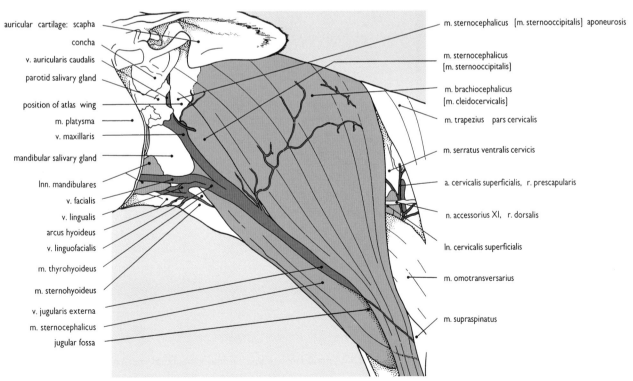

auricular cartilage: scapha
concha
v. auricularis caudalis
parotid salivary gland
position of atlas wing
m. platysma
v. maxillaris
mandibular salivary gland
lnn. mandibulares
v. facialis
v. lingualis
arcus hyoideus
v. linguofacialis
m. thyrohyoideus
m. sternohyoideus
v. jugularis externa
m. sternocephalicus
jugular fossa

m. sternocephalicus [m. sternooccipitalis] aponeurosis
m. sternocephalicus [m. sternooccipitalis]
m. brachiocephalicus [m. cleidocervicalis]
m. trapezius pars cervicalis
m. serratus ventralis cervicis
a. cervicalis superficialis, r. prescapularis
n. accessorius XI, r. dorsalis
ln. cervicalis superficialis
m. omotransversarius
m. supraspinatus

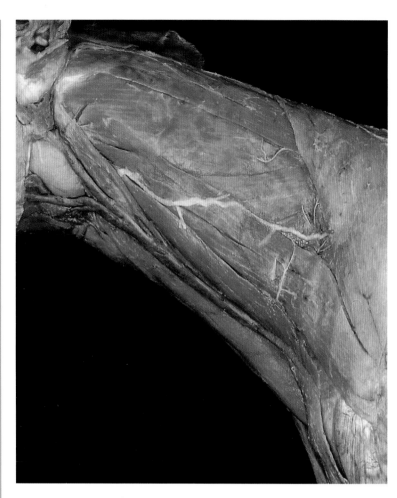

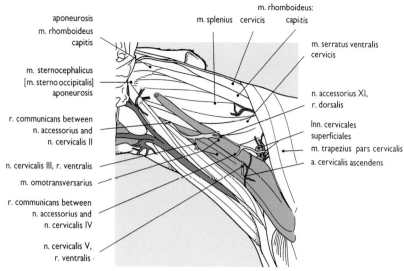

aponeurosis
m. rhomboideus
capitis

m. sternocephalicus
[m. sterno occipitalis]
aponeurosis

r. communicans between
n. accessorius and
n. cervicalis II

n. cervicalis III, r. ventralis

m. omotransversarius

r. communicans between
n. accessorius and
n. cervicalis IV

n. cervicalis V,
r. ventralis

m. rhomboideus:
m. splenius   cervicis   capitis

m. serratus ventralis
cervicis

n. accessorius XI,
r. dorsalis

lnn. cervicales
superficiales

m. trapezius pars cervicalis

a. cervicalis ascendens

Fig. 3.11 Omotransverse muscle and dorsal ramus of the accessory nerve: left lateral view. The pinna of the ear has been pulled forwards onto the head to expose the craniodorsal part of the neck. The cervicoauricular and cervicoscutular muscles have been cut from their attachments in the dorsal midline of the neck. The cleidocervical muscle has been removed from the lateral surface of the neck by cutting through its belly on a line with the dorsal border of the external jugular vein. This has exposed the full extent of the dorsal branch of the accessory nerve (XI) to the trapezius muscle.

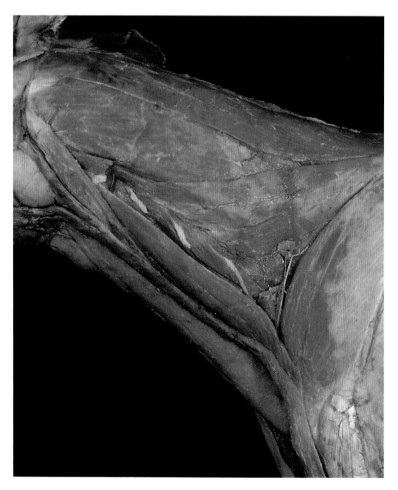

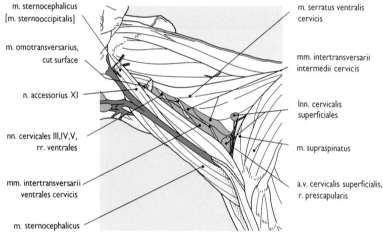

m. sternocephalicus
[m. sternooccipitalis]

m. omotransversarius,
cut surface

n. accessorius XI

nn. cervicales III,IV,V,
rr. ventrales

mm. intertransversarii
ventrales cervicis

m. sternocephalicus

m. serratus ventralis
cervicis

mm. intertransversarii
intermedii cervicis

lnn. cervicalis
superficiales

m. supraspinatus

a.v. cervicalis superficialis,
r. prescapularis

Fig. 3.12 Ventral serrate muscle and superficial cervical lymph nodes: left lateral view. The omotransverse muscle and the cervical part of the trapezius muscle have been removed along with the dorsal branch of the accessory nerve (XI) which innervates them, exposing the ventral serrate muscle.

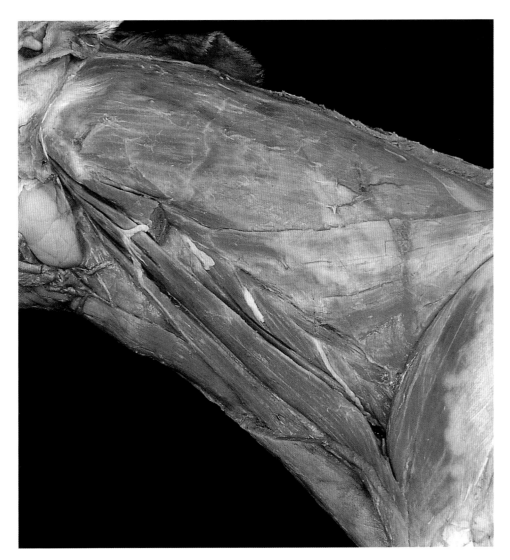

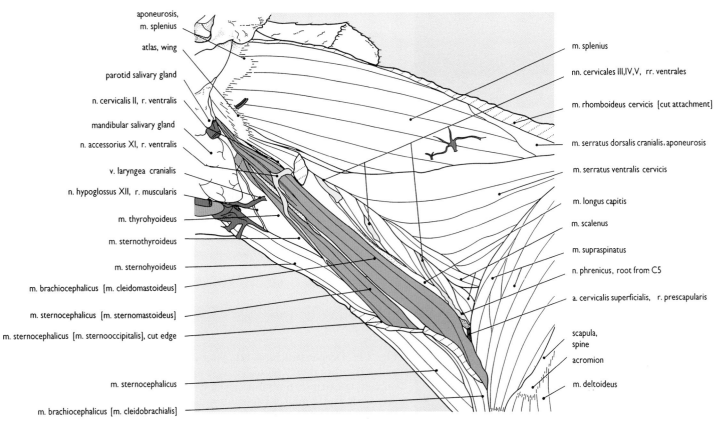

Fig. 3.13 Sternomastoid and cleidomastoid muscles and the ventral ramus of the accessory nerve: left lateral view. The external jugular vein and the sterno-occipital component of the sternocephalic muscle have been removed to expose the full length of the sternomastoid and cleidomastoid muscles.

aponeurosis, m. splenius
atlas, wing
parotid salivary gland
n. cervicalis II, r. ventralis
mandibular salivary gland
n. accessorius XI, r. ventralis
v. laryngea cranialis
n. hypoglossus XII, r. muscularis
m. thyrohyoideus
m. sternothyroideus
m. sternohyoideus
m. brachiocephalicus [m. cleidomastoideus]
m. sternocephalicus [m. sternomastoideus]
m. sternocephalicus [m. sternooccipitalis], cut edge
m. sternocephalicus
m. brachiocephalicus [m. cleidobrachialis]

m. splenius
nn. cervicales III,IV,V, rr. ventrales
m. rhomboideus cervicis [cut attachment]
m. serratus dorsalis cranialis, aponeurosis
m. serratus ventralis cervicis
m. longus capitis
m. scalenus
m. supraspinatus
n. phrenicus, root from C5
a. cervicalis superficialis, r. prescapularis
scapula, spine
acromion
m. deltoideus

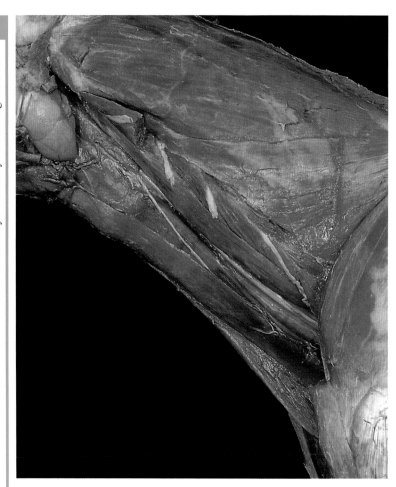

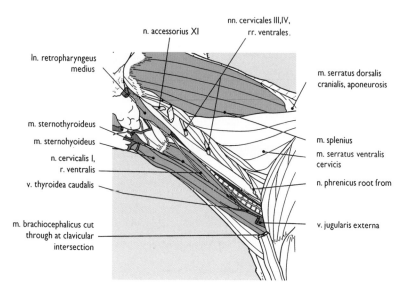

n. accessorius XI

nn. cervicales III,IV,
rr. ventrales.

ln. retropharyngeus
medius

m. serratus dorsalis
cranialis, aponeurosis

m. sternothyroideus

m. sternohyoideus

m. splenius

m. serratus ventralis
cervicis

n. cervicalis I,
r. ventralis

v. thyroidea caudalis

n. phrenicus root from

m. brachiocephalicus cut
through at clavicular
intersection

v. jugularis externa

Fig. 3.14 Deeper structures (1). Sternohyoid and sternothyroid muscles and the medial retropharyngeal lymph node: left lateral view. The remains of the sternocephalic muscle have been removed caudally to its origin from the sternal manubrium. The cleidomastoid muscle, and the remains of the cleidocervical components of the brachiocephalic muscle, have also been removed by cutting through at the clavicular intersection (see Fig. 3.9).

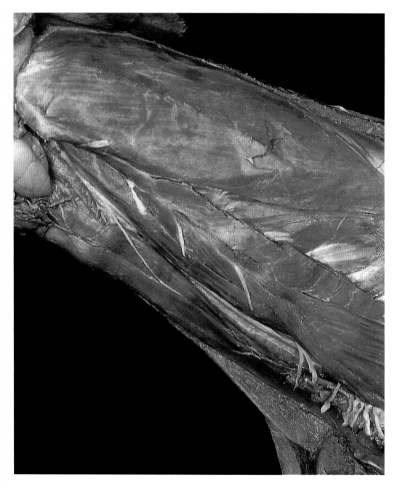

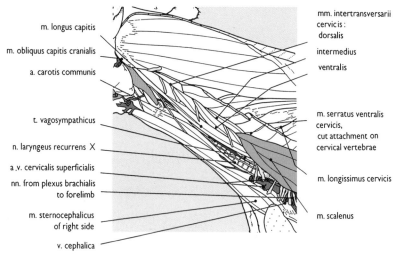

m. longus capitis

mm. intertransversarii
cervicis:
dorsalis

m. obliquus capitis cranialis

intermedius

a. carotis communis

ventralis

t. vagosympathicus

m. serratus ventralis
cervicis,
cut attachment on
cervical vertebrae

n. laryngeus recurrens X

a .v. cervicalis superficialis

nn. from plexus brachialis
to forelimb

m. longissimus cervicis

m. sternocephalicus
of right side

m. scalenus

v. cephalica

Fig. 3.15 Deeper structures (2). After removal of the forelimb: left lateral view. The rhomboid, ventral serrate and pectoral muscles (i.e. the remaining extrinsic limb muscles) have been severed and the forelimb removed. The prominent splenius muscle and the scalene muscles bridging the area between thorax and neck are now exposed, as are the cervical viscera in the ventral part of the neck. A selection of severed forelimb nerves and blood vessels appear from beneath the scalene muscles.

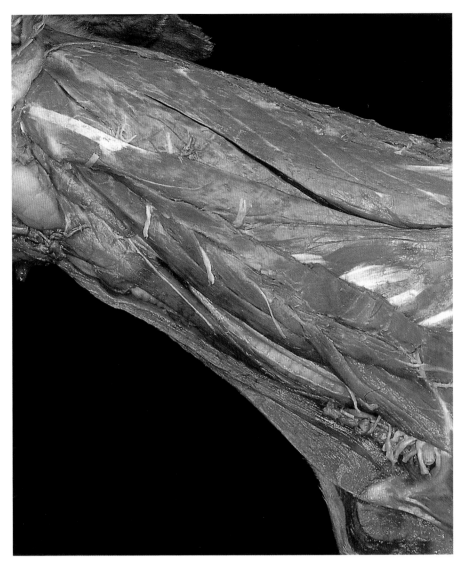

Fig. 3.16 Deeper structures (3). Longissimus muscles: left lateral view. The splenius muscle has been removed to expose the two components of the semispinalis capitis muscle, the biventer cervicis and the complexus, and the two components, cervical and capital, of the longissimus muscle.

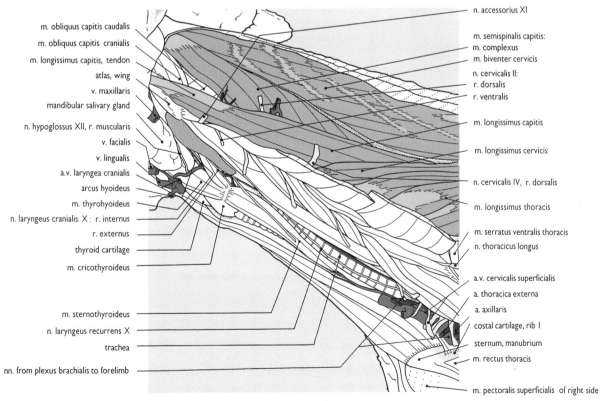

Labels (left): m. obliquus capitis caudalis; m. obliquus capitis cranialis; m. longissimus capitis, tendon; atlas, wing; v. maxillaris; mandibular salivary gland; n. hypoglossus XII, r. muscularis; v. facialis; v. lingualis; a.v. laryngea cranialis; arcus hyoideus; m. thyrohyoideus; n. laryngeus cranialis X: r. internus; r. externus; thyroid cartilage; m. cricothyroideus; m. sternothyroideus; n. laryngeus recurrens X; trachea; nn. from plexus brachialis to forelimb

Labels (right): n. accessorius XI; m. semispinalis capitis:; m. complexus; m. biventer cervicis; n. cervicalis II:; r. dorsalis; r. ventralis; m. longissimus capitis; m. longissimus cervicis; n. cervicalis IV, r. dorsalis; m. longissimus thoracis; m. serratus ventralis thoracis; n. thoracicus longus; a.v. cervicalis superficialis; a. thoracica externa; a. axillaris; costal cartilage, rib I; sternum, manubrium; m. rectus thoracis; m. pectoralis superficialis of right side

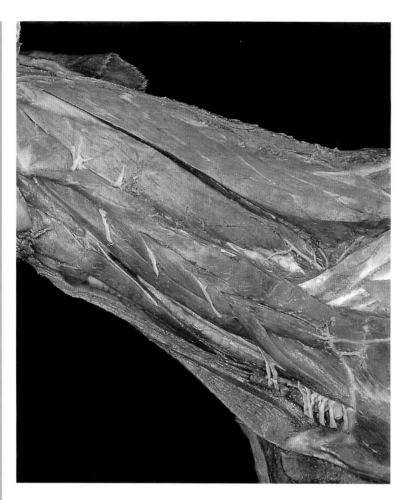

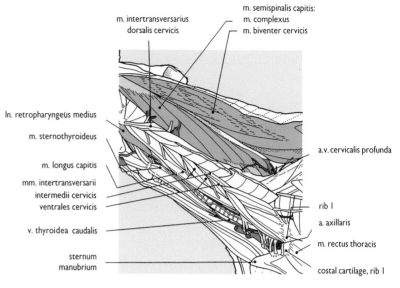

m. intertransversarius
dorsalis cervicis

m. semispinalis capitis:
m. complexus
m. biventer cervicis

ln. retropharyngeus medius

m. sternothyroideus

m. longus capitis

mm. intertransversarii
intermedii cervicis
ventrales cervicis

v. thyroidea caudalis

sternum
manubrium

a.v. cervicalis profunda

rib I

a. axillaris

m. rectus thoracis

costal cartilage, rib I

Fig. 3.17 Deep structures (1). Biventer and complexus muscles: left lateral view. The capital and cervical components of the longissimus muscle have been removed to expose the biventer cervicis and complexus muscles (the semispinalis capitis components). Some ramifications of the deep cervical artery are exposed caudodorsally whilst, cranially, branches are displayed from the dorsal rami of cervical spinal nerves 2 and 3. Removal of the middle and dorsal parts of the scalene muscle reveals rib 1.

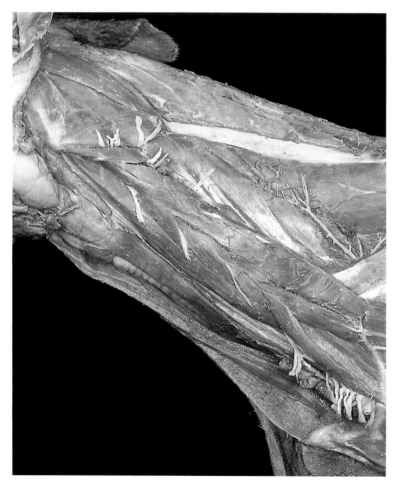

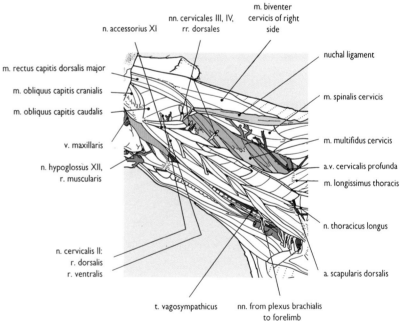

n. accessorius XI

nn. cervicales III, IV,
rr. dorsales

m. biventer
cervicis of right
side

nuchal ligament

m. rectus capitis dorsalis major

m. obliquus capitis cranialis

m. obliquus capitis caudalis

v. maxillaris

n. hypoglossus XII,
r. muscularis

n. cervicalis II:
r. dorsalis
r. ventralis

t. vagosympathicus

m. spinalis cervicis

m. multifidus cervicis

a.v. cervicalis profunda

m. longissimus thoracis

n. thoracicus longus

a. scapularis dorsalis

nn. from plexus brachialis
to forelimb

Fig. 3.18 Deep structures (2). Deep cervical vessels, multifidus, rectus capitis and obliquus muscles: left lateral view. The biventer cervicis and complexus muscles have been removed, exposing the midline nuchal ligament attached to the spine of the axis and the multifidi and spinalis cervicis muscles ventrally.

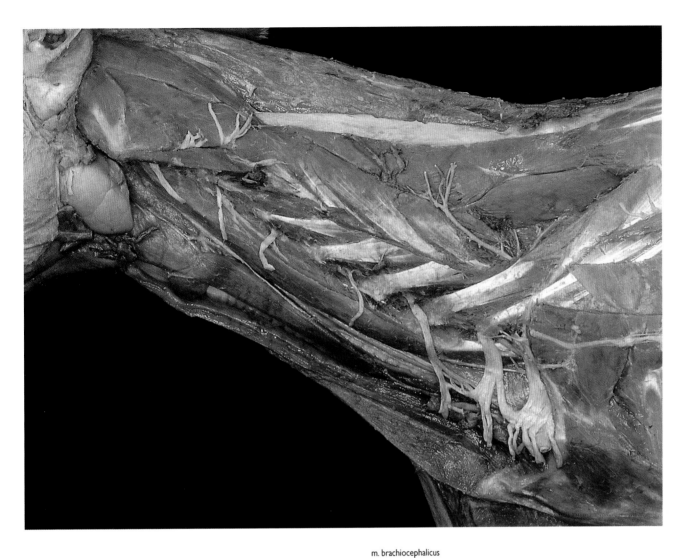

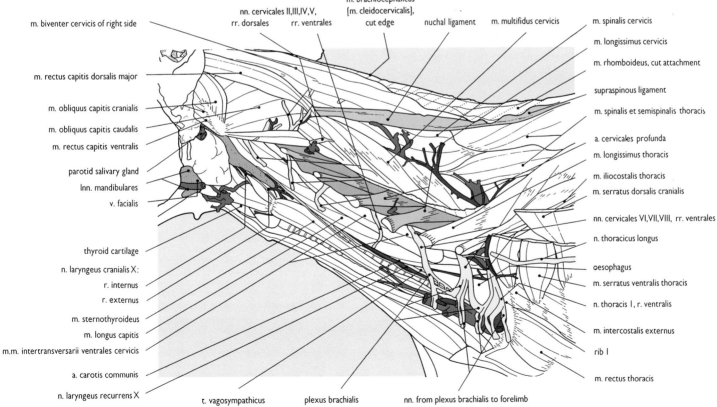

m. biventer cervicis of right side

m. rectus capitis dorsalis major

m. obliquus capitis cranialis

m. obliquus capitis caudalis

m. rectus capitis ventralis

parotid salivary gland

lnn. mandibulares

v. facialis

thyroid cartilage

n. laryngeus cranialis X:

r. internus

r. externus

m. sternothyroideus

m. longus capitis

m.m. intertransversarii ventrales cervicis

a. carotis communis

n. laryngeus recurrens X

nn. cervicales II,III,IV,V,
rr. dorsales   rr. ventrales

m. brachiocephalicus
[m. cleidocervicalis],
cut edge   nuchal ligament   m. multifidus cervicis

t. vagosympathicus   plexus brachialis   nn. from plexus brachialis to forelimb

m. spinalis cervicis

m. longissimus cervicis

m. rhomboideus, cut attachment

supraspinous ligament

m. spinalis et semispinalis thoracis

a. cervicales profunda

m. longissimus thoracis

m. iliocostalis thoracis

m. serratus dorsalis cranialis

nn. cervicales VI,VII,VIII, rr. ventrales

n. thoracicus longus

oesophagus

m. serratus ventralis thoracis

n. thoracis I, r. ventralis

m. intercostalis externus

rib I

m. rectus thoracis

Fig. 3.19 Deep structures (3). Nuchal ligament: left lateral view. The remaining parts of the ventral serrate muscle in the neck have been removed, along with the dorsal and intermediate components of the intertransverse muscles and the remaining part of the scalene muscle attached to rib 1. The attachments to cervical vertebrae of the cervical longissimus muscle are displayed. Cervical nerves 2 to 5 are shown in sequence and the formation of the brachial plexus from the ventral rami of cervical nerves 6, 7, 8 and thoracic nerve 1 is exposed.

Veterinary Anatomy: The Dog and Cat

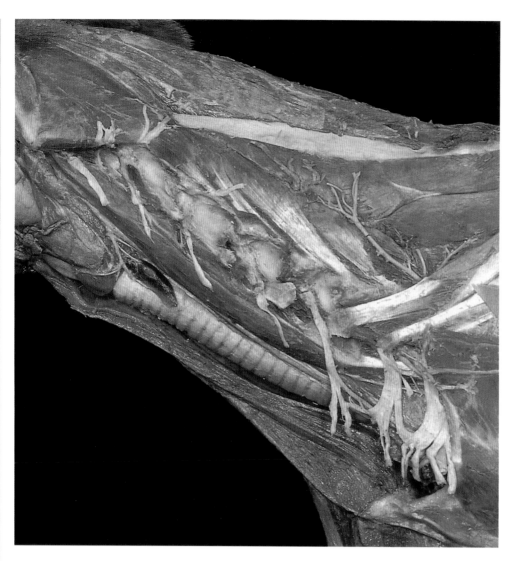

Fig. 3.20 Deep structures (4). Medial retropharyngeal lymph node, thyroid gland and viscera: left lateral view. The cut attachments of the cervical longissimus muscle have been removed to expose the arches and transverse processes of cervical vertebrae 3 to 6. Cervical spinal nerves are now exposed in series along the neck, although most of the dorsal primary rami of the nerves have been removed with the epaxial musculature in which they ramified. The removal of both sternohyoid and sternothyroid muscles from the ventral surface of the neck has exposed the manubrium of the sternum and the costal cartilage of rib 1 at the thoracic inlet, and the trachea along much of the neck.

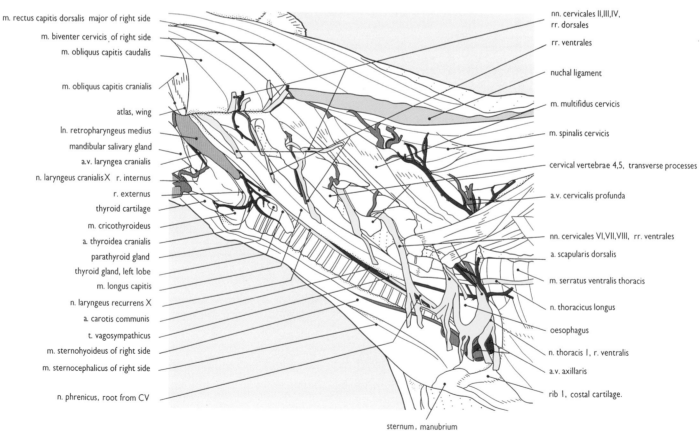

m. rectus capitis dorsalis major of right side

m. biventer cervicis of right side

m. obliquus capitis caudalis

m. obliquus capitis cranialis

atlas, wing

ln. retropharyngeus medius

mandibular salivary gland

a.v. laryngea cranialis

n. laryngeus cranialis X r. internus

r. externus

thyroid cartilage

m. cricothyroideus

a. thyroidea cranialis

parathyroid gland

thyroid gland, left lobe

m. longus capitis

n. laryngeus recurrens X

a. carotis communis

t. vagosympathicus

m. sternohyoideus of right side

m. sternocephalicus of right side

n. phrenicus, root from CV

nn. cervicales II,III,IV, rr. dorsales

rr. ventrales

nuchal ligament

m. multifidus cervicis

m. spinalis cervicis

cervical vertebrae 4,5, transverse processes

a.v. cervicalis profunda

nn. cervicales VI,VII,VIII, rr. ventrales

a. scapularis dorsalis

m. serratus ventralis thoracis

n. thoracicus longus

oesophagus

n. thoracis I, r. ventralis

a.v. axillaris

rib 1, costal cartilage.

sternum, manubrium

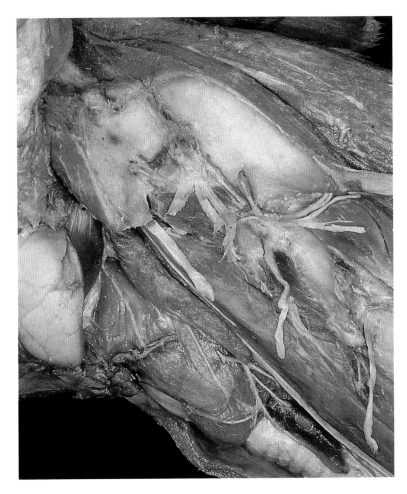

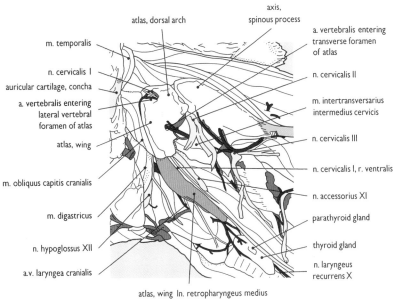

atlas, dorsal arch — axis, spinous process

m. temporalis

n. cervicalis I

auricular cartilage, concha

a. vertebralis entering lateral vertebral foramen of atlas

atlas, wing

m. obliquus capitis cranialis

m. digastricus

n. hypoglossus XII

a.v. laryngea cranialis

a. vertebralis entering transverse foramen of atlas

n. cervicalis II

m. intertransversarius intermedius cervicis

n. cervicalis III

n. cervicalis I, r. ventralis

n. accessorius XI

parathyroid gland

thyroid gland

n. laryngeus recurrens X

atlas, wing   ln. retropharyngeus medius

Fig. 3.21 Deep structures at the cranial end of the neck (1). Atlas and axis vertebrae, medial retropharyngeal lymph node and thyroid gland: left lateral view. The oblique capital muscles have been removed exposing the atlas (C1) and axis (C2) vertebrae, and cervical spinal nerve 2, leaving the second intervertebral foramen between them. Cervical spinal nerve 1 and the vertebral vessels are visible in the lateral vertebral foramen of the atlas.

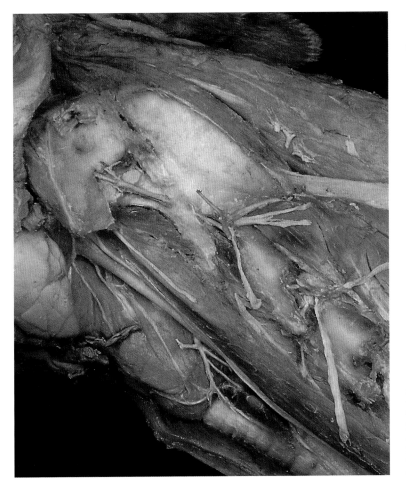

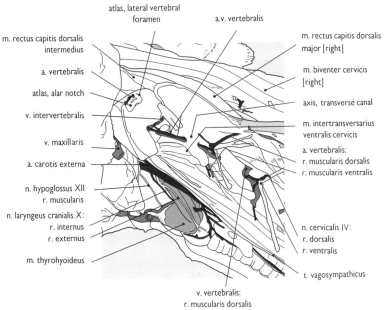

atlas, lateral vertebral foramen   a.v. vertebralis

m. rectus capitis dorsalis intermedius

a. vertebralis

atlas, alar notch

v. intervertebralis

v. maxillaris

a. carotis externa

n. hypoglossus XII r. muscularis

n. laryngeus cranialis X: r. internus r. externus

m. thyrohyoideus

m. rectus capitis dorsalis major [right]

m. biventer cervicis [right]

axis, transverse canal

m. intertransversarius ventralis cervicis

a. vertebralis: r. muscularis dorsalis r. muscularis ventralis

n. cervicalis IV: r. dorsalis r. ventralis

t. vagosympathicus

v. vertebralis: r. muscularis dorsalis

Fig. 3.22 Deep structures at the cranial end of the neck (2). Vertebral artery and vein, larynx and common carotid artery: left lateral view. The medial retropharyngeal lymph node has been removed exposing the pharyngeal region with the common carotid artery, and the cranial laryngeal nerves and vessels entering the larynx between the thyrohyoid and thyropharyngeal muscles (see Chapter 2).

121

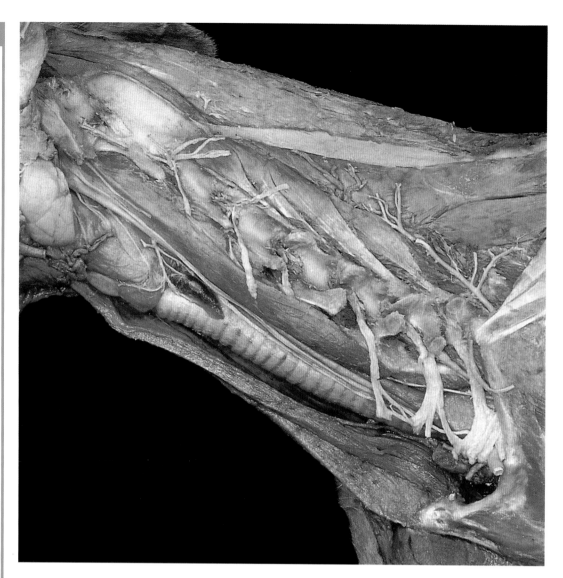

Fig. 3.23 Deep structures (5). Cervical spinal nerves and brachial plexus: left lateral view. The cervical vertebral column has now been almost completely exposed by the removal of the remaining ventral intertransverse muscles, the element of the thoracic longissimus muscle onto cervical vertebra 6 and the cervical continuation of the iliocostalis thoracis muscle onto cervical vertebrae 7. The vertebral artery and vein are exposed at the base of the neck.

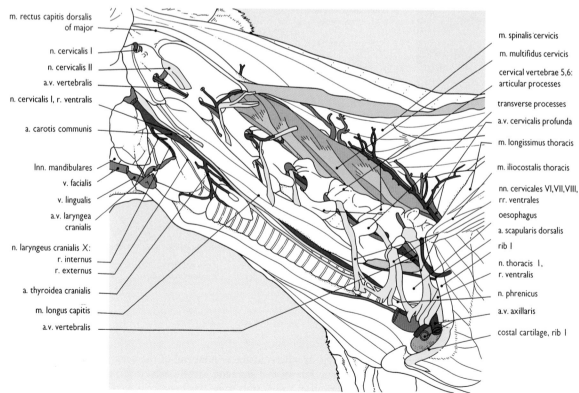

m. rectus capitis dorsalis of major

n. cervicalis I

n. cervicalis II

a.v. vertebralis

n. cervicalis I, r. ventralis

a. carotis communis

lnn. mandibulares

v. facialis

v. lingualis

a.v. laryngea cranialis

n. laryngeus cranialis X:
r. internus
r. externus

a. thyroidea cranialis

m. longus capitis

a.v. vertebralis

m. spinalis cervicis

m. multifidus cervicis

cervical vertebrae 5,6: articular processes

transverse processes

a.v. cervicalis profunda

m. longissimus thoracis

m. iliocostalis thoracis

nn. cervicales VI, VII, VIII, rr. ventrales

oesophagus

a. scapularis dorsalis

rib I

n. thoracis I, r. ventralis

n. phrenicus

a.v. axillaris

costal cartilage, rib I

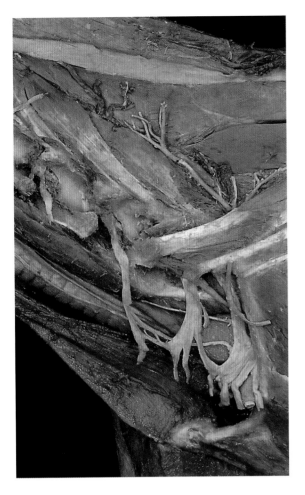

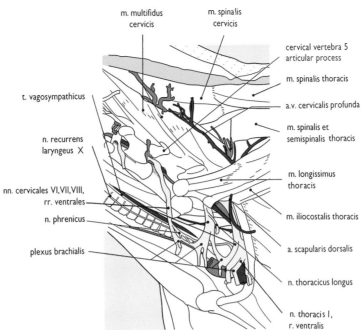

m. multifidus cervicis
m. spinalis cervicis

cervical vertebra 5 articular process

m. spinalis thoracis

t. vagosympathicus

a.v. cervicalis profunda

m. spinalis et semispinalis thoracis

n. recurrens laryngeus X

m. longissimus thoracis

nn. cervicales VI,VII,VIII, rr. ventrales

n. phrenicus

m. iliocostalis thoracis

a. scapularis dorsalis

plexus brachialis

n. thoracicus longus

n. thoracis I, r. ventralis

Fig. 3.24 Deep structures at the thoracic inlet (1). Brachial plexus: left lateral view. The ventral serrate and scalene muscles in the thorax have been removed to uncover nearly the entire length of rib 1. Branches from the costocervical trunk can be seen – the dorsal scapular emerging from around the first rib, and the deep cervical arising from within intercostal space 1.

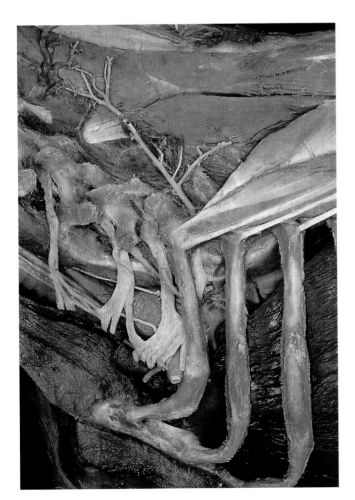

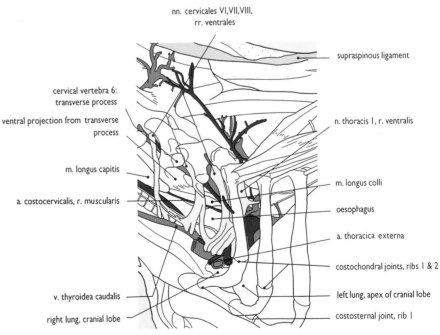

nn. cervicales VI,VII,VIII, rr. ventrales

supraspinous ligament

cervical vertebra 6: transverse process

n. thoracis I, r. ventralis

ventral projection from transverse process

m. longus capitis

m. longus colli

a. costocervicalis, r. muscularis

oesophagus

a. thoracica externa

costochondral joints, ribs I & 2

v. thyroidea caudalis

left lung, apex of cranial lobe

right lung, cranial lobe

costosternal joint, rib I

Fig. 3.25 Deep structures at the thoracic inlet (2). Brachial plexus, vertebral and deep cervical vessels: left lateral view. The rectus thoracis and abdominis muscles have been removed from rib 1, and the intercostal space has been cleared of muscles and fascia, showing nearly all of the first rib in addition to thoracic nerve 1. The remaining component of the cervical longissimus, and the component of the thoracic longissimus inserting on cervical vertebra 7, have been removed, as has the cervical multifidus. Much of cervical vertebrae 6 and 7, the emergence of cervical nerves 7 and 8, and the vertebral vessels entering the neck can now be seen.

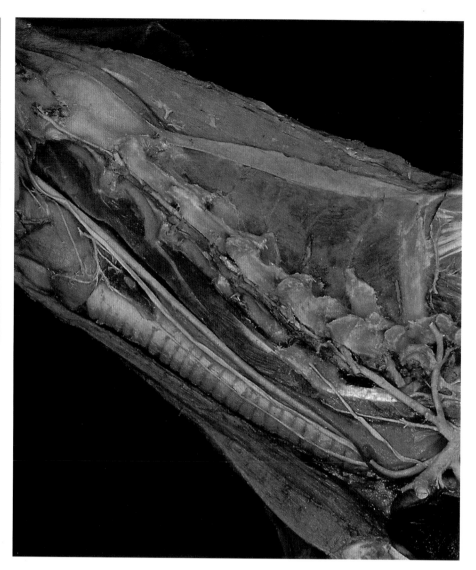

Fig. 3.26 Deep structures (6). Cervical vertebral column and vertebral artery and vein: left lateral view. The remaining multifidus and spinalis muscles of the neck have been removed from the dorsal aspects of the cervical vertebrae, along with the ramifications of the deep cervical vessels. The longus capitis muscle, ventral to the neck vertebrae, has been removed to expose the longus colli muscle. There is almost complete lateral exposure of the neck vertebrae and the entire length of the vertebral artery and vein are displayed.

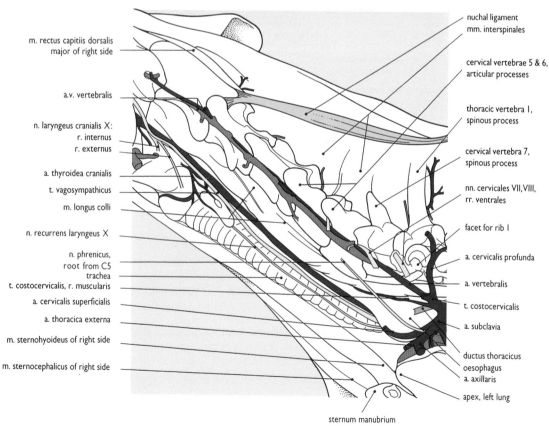

m. rectus capitiis dorsalis major of right side

a.v. vertebralis

n. laryngeus cranialis X:
r. internus
r. externus

a. thyroidea cranialis

t. vagosympathicus

m. longus colli

n. recurrens laryngeus X

n. phrenicus, root from C5
trachea
t. costocervicalis, r. muscularis

a. cervicalis superficialis

a. thoracica externa

m. sternohyoideus of right side

m. sternocephalicus of right side

sternum manubrium

nuchal ligament
mm. interspinales

cervical vertebrae 5 & 6, articular processes

thoracic vertebra I, spinous process

cervical vertebra 7, spinous process

nn. cervicales VII, VIII, rr. ventrales

facet for rib I

a. cervicalis profunda

a. vertebralis

t. costocervicalis

a. subclavia

ductus thoracicus
oesophagus
a. axillaris

apex, left lung

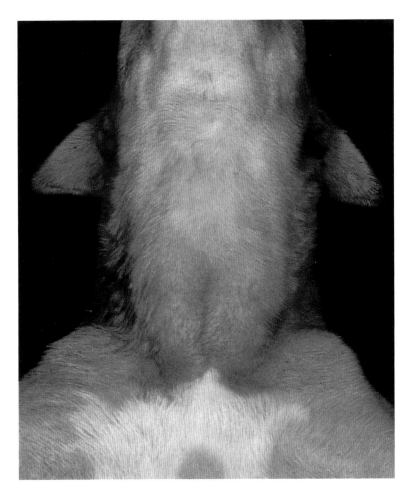

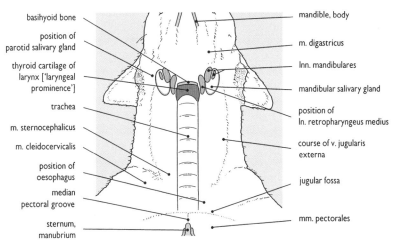

Fig. 3.27 Surface features: ventral view. Practically no bony 'landmarks' are palpable on the underside of the neck, apart from the basihyoid bone cranially, and the sternal manubrium caudally. The cartilages of the larynx and trachea are, however, clearly palpable although no contours are visible.

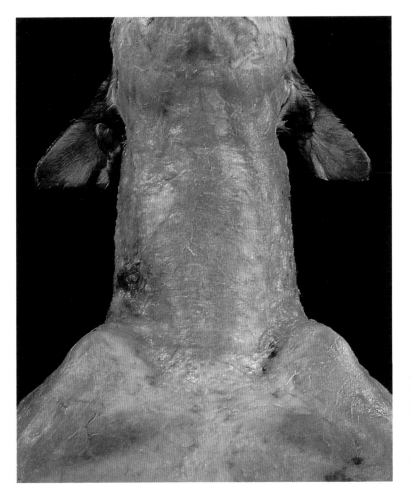

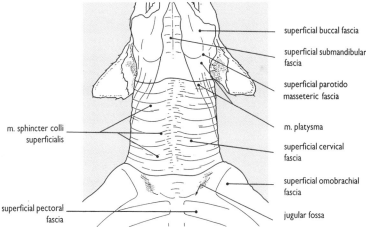

Fig. 3.28 Superficial structures of the intermandibular, subhyoid and ventral cervical regions (1). Superficial fascia: ventral view. The skin has been removed exposing superficial fascia in the form of a loose cylinder around the neck. This is continuous with the superficial fascia of the head at the larynx and parotidomasseteric regions, and with the superficial pectoral and omobrachial fascia in the presternal and shoulder regions. It contains recognizable strands of the sphincter colli superficialis muscle in addition to the platysma muscle.

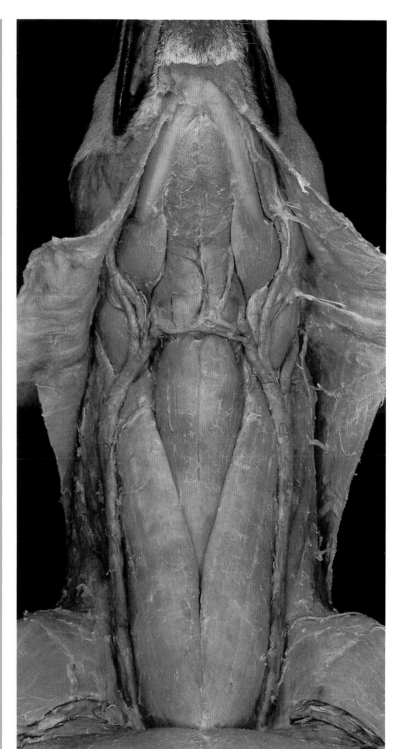

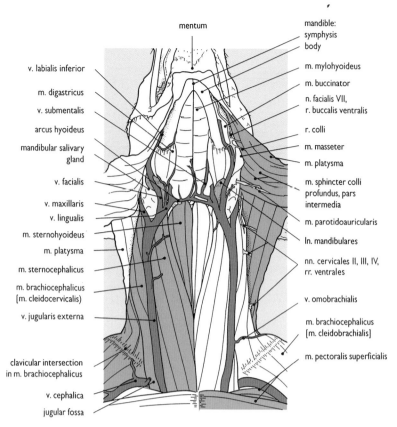

mentum

mandible:
symphysis
body

v. labialis inferior

m. digastricus

v. submentalis

arcus hyoideus

mandibular salivary
gland

v. facialis

v. maxillaris

v. lingualis

m. sternohyoideus

m. platysma

m. sternocephalicus

m. brachiocephalicus
[m. cleidocervicalis]

v. jugularis externa

clavicular intersection
in m. brachiocephalicus

v. cephalica

jugular fossa

m. mylohyoideus

m. buccinator

n. facialis VII,
r. buccalis ventralis

r. colli

m. masseter

m. platysma

m. sphincter colli
profundus, pars
intermedia

m. parotidoauricularis

ln. mandibulares

nn. cervicales II, III, IV,
rr. ventrales

v. omobrachialis

m. brachiocephalicus
[m. cleidobrachialis]

m. pectoralis superficialis

Fig. 3.29 Superficial structures of the intermandibular, subhyoid and ventral cervical regions (2) muscles: cutaneous ventral view. Bilateral removal of the skin and preliminary cleaning of the superficial fascia exposes the muscles and superficial veins on the ventral surface of the neck. The irregular and poorly defined transverse components of the cutaneous muscle of the neck have been removed. These lay in the superficial fascia of the laryngeal and subhyoid region (see Fig. 3.28). In addition, the platysma muscle (see Figs 3.6, 3.7), which extends cranioventrally onto the ventrolateral surface of the subhyoid and intermandibular regions, has been reflected on either side. On its internal surface, strands of the parotidoauricular and intermediate component of the sphincter colli profundus muscles are visible.

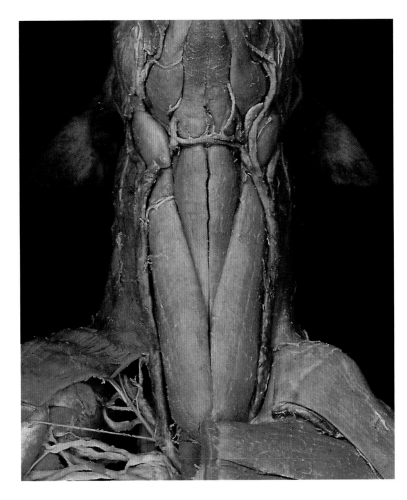

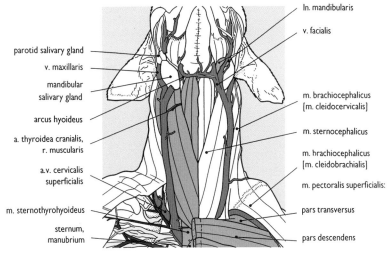

parotid salivary gland
v. maxillaris
mandibular salivary gland
arcus hyoideus
a. thyroidea cranialis, r. muscularis
a.v. cervicalis superficialis
m. sternothyrohyoideus
sternum, manubrium

ln. mandibularis
v. facialis
m. brachiocephalicus [m. cleidocervicalis]
m. sternocephalicus
m. brachiocephalicus [m. cleidobrachialis]
m. pectoralis superficialis:
pars transversus
pars descendens

Fig. 3.30 Superficial structures: ventral view. Part of the facial, lingual and linguofacial veins, together with the mandibular lymph nodes, have been removed from the right side. The mandibular salivary gland is exposed at the junction of the head and neck. In this, and the following three figures, the base of the right side of the neck was disturbed, to some extent, when nerves and vessels to the forelimb were dissected (see Chapter 4).

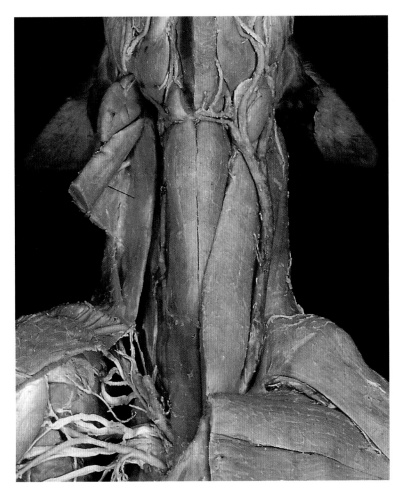

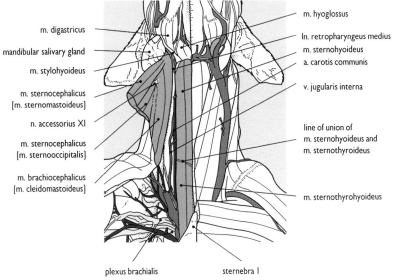

m. digastricus
mandibular salivary gland
m. stylohyoideus
m. sternocephalicus [m. sternomastoideus]
n. accessorius XI
m. sternocephalicus [m. sternooccipitalis]
m. brachiocephalicus [m. cleidomastoideus]
plexus brachialis
sternebra I

m. hyoglossus
ln. retropharyngeus medius
m. sternohyoideus
a. carotis communis
v. jugularis interna
line of union of m. sternohyoideus and m. sternothyroideus
m. sternothyrohyoideus

Fig. 3.31 Sternocephalic muscle and carotid sheath: ventral view. The right sternocephalic muscle has been cut through in the middle of the neck, and its cranial part reflected laterally, displacing the mandibular salivary gland. This exposes the medial retropharyngeal lymph node, the right common carotid artery and the accompanying internal jugular vein. In addition, the ventral branch of the accessory nerve (XI) can be seen emerging through the cleidomastoid muscle.

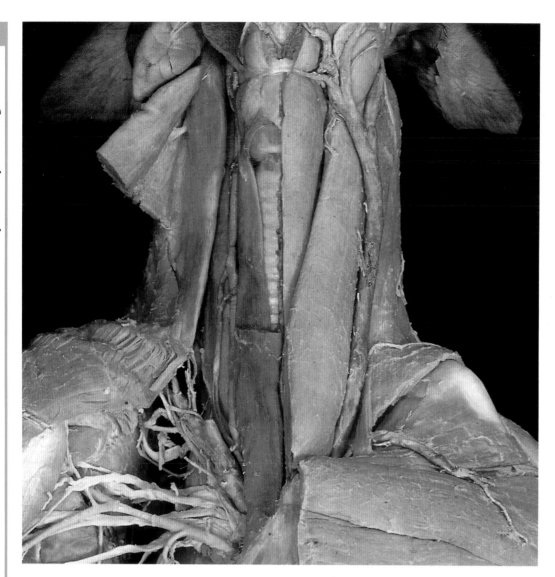

Fig. 3.32 Sternothyrohyoid muscle, larynx and trachea: ventral view. Removal of the cranial half of the right sternohyoid muscle begins exposure of the thyroid, and cricoid cartilages of the larynx, with their associated extrinsic muscles (cricothyroid and thyrohyoid). Despite its removal, the nerve supply from the hypoglossal (XII) has been retained and is visible on the sternothyroid muscle. Removal of the lower half of the sternocephalic muscle exposes that part of the sternohyoid which is fused to the sternothyroid.

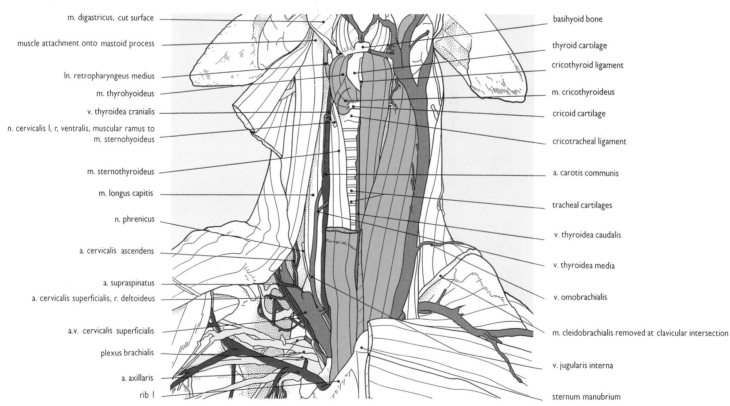

m. digastricus, cut surface

muscle attachment onto mastoid process

ln. retropharyngeus medius

m. thyrohyoideus

v. thyroidea cranialis

n. cervicalis I, r, ventralis, muscular ramus to m. sternohyoideus

m. sternothyroideus

m. longus capitis

n. phrenicus

a. cervicalis ascendens

a. supraspinatus

a. cervicalis superficialis, r. deltoideus

a.v. cervicalis superficialis

plexus brachialis

a. axillaris

rib I

basihyoid bone

thyroid cartilage

cricothyroid ligament

m. cricothyroideus

cricoid cartilage

cricotracheal ligament

a. carotis communis

tracheal cartilages

v. thyroidea caudalis

v. thyroidea media

v. omobrachialis

m. cleidobrachialis removed at clavicular intersection

v. jugularis interna

sternum manubrium

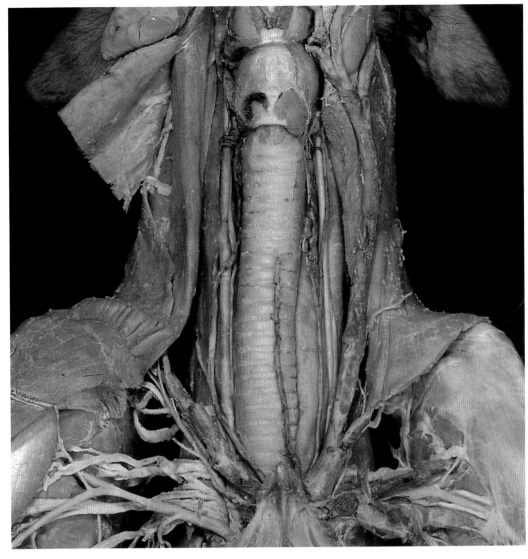

Fig. 3.33 Larynx, trachea, thyroid gland and carotid sheath (1): ventral view. There is complete bilateral removal of the sternohyoid and sternothyroid muscles, along with partial removal of the left sternocephalic muscle. The latter was removed by cutting through the muscle on a line with the lower boundary of the external jugular vein. The entire length of the neck is now 'opened' ventrally, and the trachea and esophagus are exposed. In addition, both lobes of the thyroid gland are visible, although a connecting isthmus was not present across the trachea.

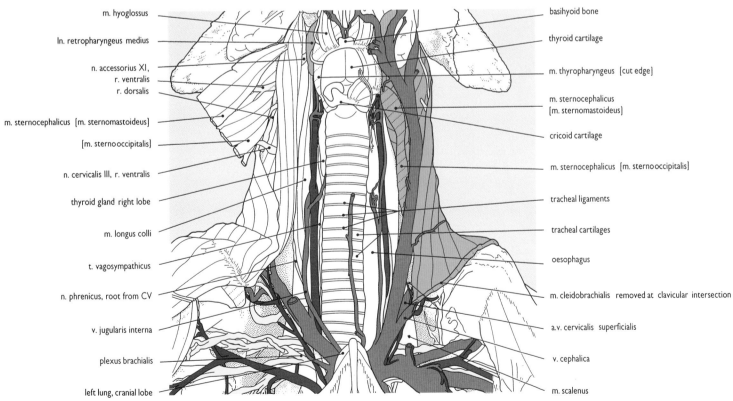

m. hyoglossus

ln. retropharyngeus medius

n. accessorius XI,
r. ventralis
r. dorsalis

m. sternocephalicus [m. sternomastoideus]

[m. sterno occipitalis]

n. cervicalis III, r. ventralis

thyroid gland right lobe

m. longus colli

t. vagosympathicus

n. phrenicus, root from CV

v. jugularis interna

plexus brachialis

left lung, cranial lobe

basihyoid bone

thyroid cartilage

m. thyropharyngeus [cut edge]

m. sternocephalicus
[m. sternomastoideus]

cricoid cartilage

m. sternocephalicus [m. sterno occipitalis]

tracheal ligaments

tracheal cartilages

oesophagus

m. cleidobrachialis removed at clavicular intersection

a.v. cervicalis superficialis

v. cephalica

m. scalenus

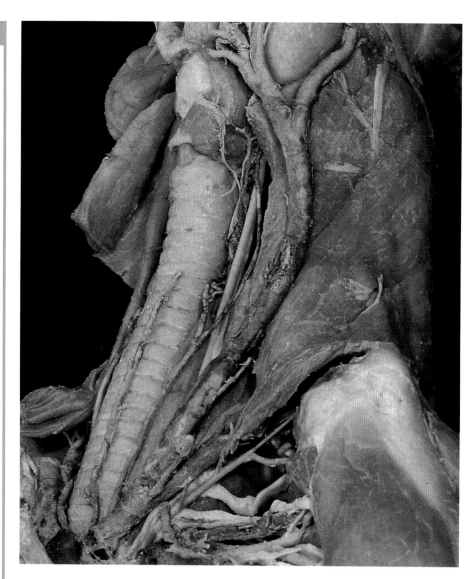

Fig. 3.34 Larynx, trachea, thyroid gland and carotid sheath (2): left ventrolateral view. The cleidobrachial component of the brachiocephalic muscle has been removed by cutting through at the clavicular intersection, thus exposing the branches of the superficial cervical vessels at the base of the neck.

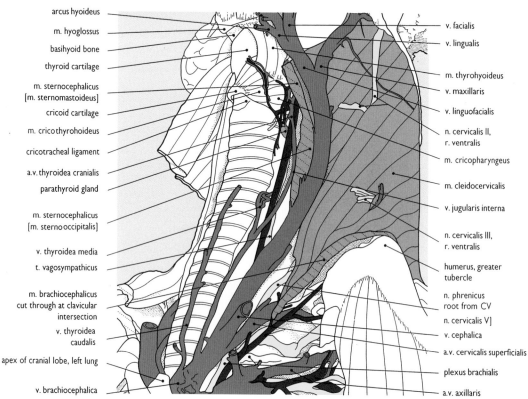

arcus hyoideus

m. hyoglossus

basihyoid bone

thyroid cartilage

m. sternocephalicus
[m. sternomastoideus]

cricoid cartilage

m. cricothyroideus

cricotracheal ligament

a.v. thyroidea cranialis

parathyroid gland

m. sternocephalicus
[m. sternooccipitalis]

v. thyroidea media

t. vagosympathicus

m. brachiocephalicus
cut through at clavicular
intersection

v. thyroidea
caudalis

apex of cranial lobe, left lung

v. brachiocephalica

v. facialis

v. lingualis

m. thyrohyoideus

v. maxillaris

v. linguofacialis

n. cervicalis II,
r. ventralis

m. cricopharyngeus

m. cleidocervicalis

v. jugularis interna

n. cervicalis III,
r. ventralis

humerus, greater
tubercle

n. phrenicus
root from CV

n. cervicalis V]

v. cephalica

a.v. cervicalis superficialis

plexus brachialis

a.v. axillaris

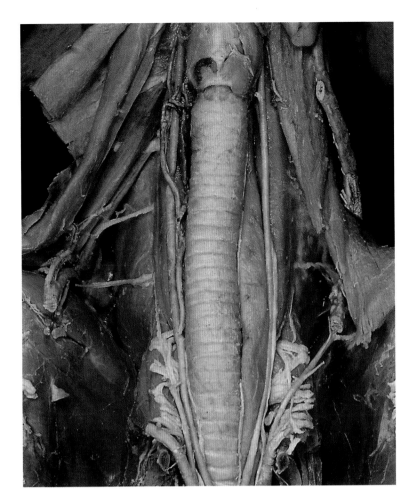

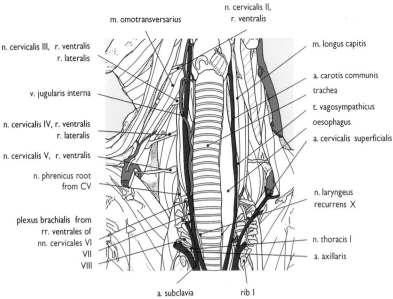

n. cervicalis II,
r. ventralis

m. omotransversarius

n. cervicalis III, r. ventralis
r. lateralis

m. longus capitis

v. jugularis interna

a. carotis communis

trachea

n. cervicalis IV, r. ventralis
r. lateralis

t. vagosympathicus

oesophagus

n. cervicalis V, r. ventralis

a. cervicalis superficialis

n. phrenicus root
from CV

n. laryngeus
recurrens X

plexus brachialis from
rr. ventrales of
nn. cervicales VI
VII
VIII

n. thoracis I

a. axillaris

a. subclavia

rib I

Fig. 3.35 Trachea, esophagus, recurrent nerves and vagosympathetic trunk: ventral view. In the course of thoracic dissection the thoracic inlet was opened and its position is marked by the cut stumps of the first ribs. The veins traversing the inlet have been removed, as have practically all the veins in the neck. The common carotid arteries remain intact on both sides, and the vagosympathetic trunk and recurrent nerve of the left side are both shown in position. The relationship of those structures which run the length of the neck are shown in the series of

transverse sections (Figs 3.36–3.43) and are made at the levels indicated on the accompanying sketch. The first section is viewed from a cranial aspect, whilst the remaining seven sections are viewed from a caudal aspect. The first section (Fig. 3.36) is a direct continuation from the last section through the head (see Chapter 2). The last section (Fig. 3.43) actually passes through the thoracic inlet and is continued by the first section through the thorax (see Chapter 5).

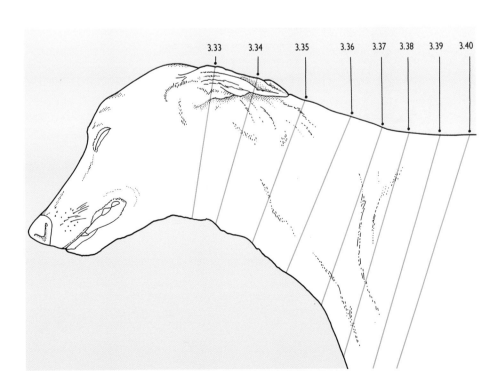

3.33 3.34 3.35 3.36 3.37 3.38 3.39 3.40

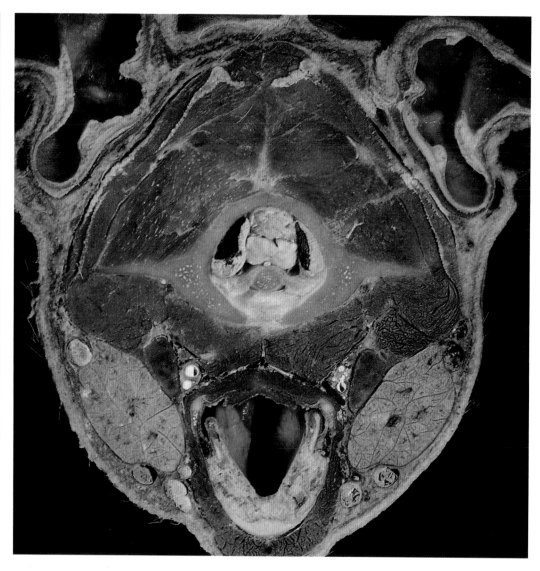

Fig. 3.36 Transverse section (1) through cervical vertebrae 1 (atlas), laryngopharynx, laryngeal vestibule and medial retropharyngeal lymph nodes: cranial view. This section passes through the atlas vertebra (C1) showing its expanded transverse processes (wings) on either side. Within the ventral part of the vertebral canal the dens of the axis vertebra (C2) is visible, held in place by a pronounced transverse atlantal ligament. Also contained in the canal are paired internal vertebral venous plexuses running within the epidural space. Ventral to the atlas wing the medial retropharyngeal lymph node lies lateral to the common carotid artery, the vagosympathetic trunk and the internal jugular vein, and medial to the mandibular salivary gland. This region at the 'border' between head and neck is primarily dealt with in Chapter 2.

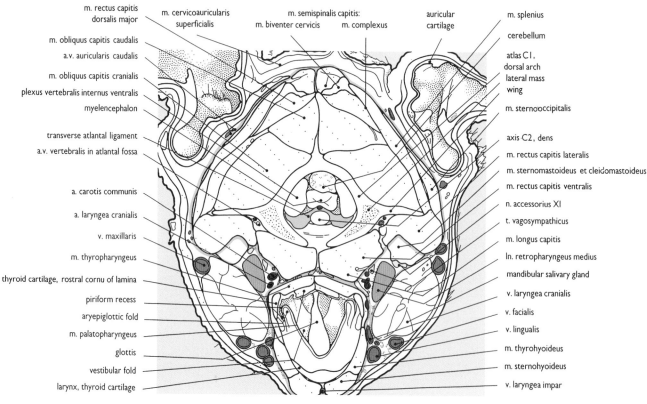

m. rectus capitis dorsalis major
m. obliquus capitis caudalis
a.v. auricularis caudalis
m. obliquus capitis cranialis
plexus vertebralis internus ventralis
myelencephalon
transverse atlantal ligament
a.v. vertebralis in atlantal fossa
a. carotis communis
a. laryngea cranialis
v. maxillaris
m. thyropharyngeus
thyroid cartilage, rostral cornu of lamina
piriform recess
aryepiglottic fold
m. palatopharyngeus
glottis
vestibular fold
larynx, thyroid cartilage

m. cervicoauricularis superficialis

m. semispinalis capitis:
m. biventer cervicis   m. complexus

auricular cartilage

m. splenius
cerebellum
atlas C1,
dorsal arch
lateral mass
wing
m. sternooccipitalis
axis C2, dens
m. rectus capitis lateralis
m. sternomastoideus et cleidomastoideus
m. rectus capitis ventralis
n. accessorius XI
t. vagosympathicus
m. longus capitis
ln. retropharyngeus medius
mandibular salivary gland
v. laryngea cranialis
v. facialis
v. lingualis
m. thyrohyoideus
m. sternohyoideus
v. laryngea impar

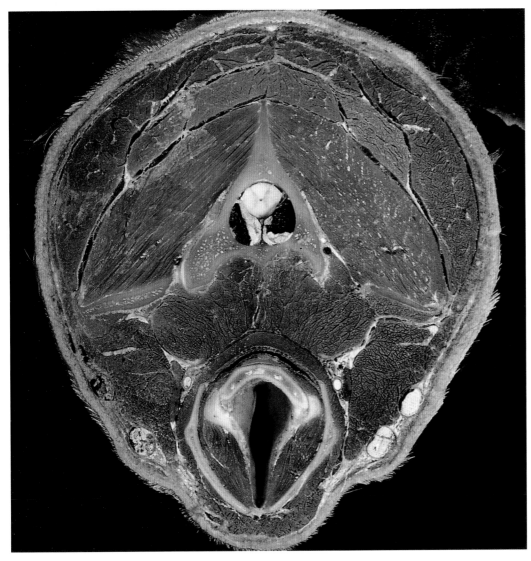

Fig. 3.37 Transverse section (2) through cervical vertebrae 2 (axis) and larynx: caudal view. Identifiable are the four main laryngeal cartilages, as well as the intrinsic muscles associated with the arytenoid cartilages. Further detail of laryngeal anatomy is dealt with in Chapter 2. The laryngopharynx is shown to advantage here, surrounded by the thyropharyngeal muscle, one of the pharyngeal constrictors.

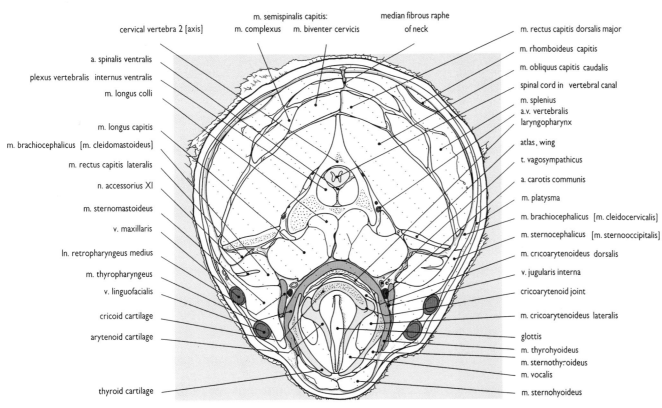

cervical vertebra 2 [axis]
a. spinalis ventralis
plexus vertebralis internus ventralis
m. longus colli
m. longus capitis
m. brachiocephalicus [m. cleidomastoideus]
m. rectus capitis lateralis
n. accessorius XI
m. sternomastoideus
v. maxillaris
ln. retropharyngeus medius
m. thyropharyngeus
v. linguofacialis
cricoid cartilage
arytenoid cartilage
thyroid cartilage

m. semispinalis capitis:
m. complexus   m. biventer cervicis
median fibrous raphe of neck

m. rectus capitis dorsalis major
m. rhomboideus capitis
m. obliquus capitis caudalis
spinal cord in vertebral canal
m. splenius
a.v. vertebralis
laryngopharynx
atlas, wing
t. vagosympathicus
a. carotis communis
m. platysma
m. brachiocephalicus [m. cleidocervicalis]
m. sternocephalicus [m. sternooccipitalis]
m. cricoarytenoideus dorsalis
v. jugularis interna
cricoarytenoid joint
m. cricoarytenoideus lateralis
glottis
m. thyrohyoideus
m. sternothyroideus
m. vocalis
m. sternohyoideus

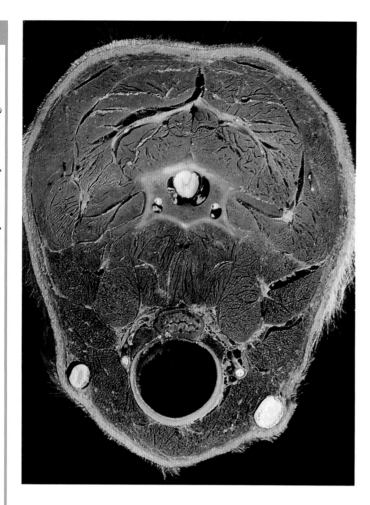

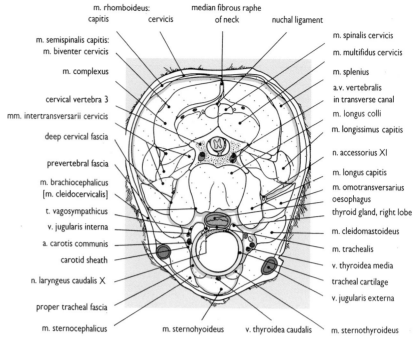

m. rhomboideus:
capitis   cervicis

median fibrous raphe
of neck   nuchal ligament

m. semispinalis capitis:
m. biventer cervicis

m. complexus

cervical vertebra 3

mm. intertransversarii cervicis

deep cervical fascia

prevertebral fascia

m. brachiocephalicus
[m. cleidocervicalis]

t. vagosympathicus

v. jugularis interna

a. carotis communis

carotid sheath

n. laryngeus caudalis X

proper tracheal fascia

m. sternocephalicus

m. spinalis cervicis

m. multifidus cervicis

m. splenius

a.v. vertebralis
in transverse canal

m. longus colli

m. longissimus capitis

n. accessorius XI

m. longus capitis

m. omotransversarius

oesophagus

thyroid gland, right lobe

m. cleidomastoideus

m. trachealis

v. thyroidea media

tracheal cartilage

v. jugularis externa

m. sternohyoideus   v. thyroidea caudalis   m. sternothyroideus

Fig. 3.38 Transverse section (3) through cervical vertebra 3 and the thyroid gland: caudal view. The esophagus is midline and flanked by the lobes of the thyroid gland.

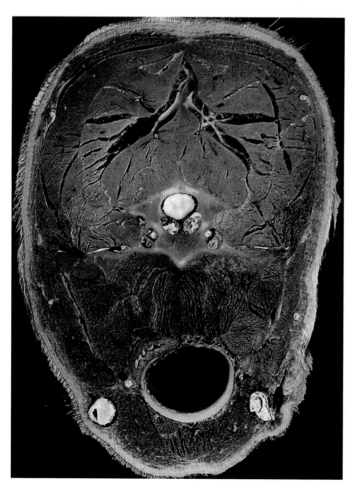

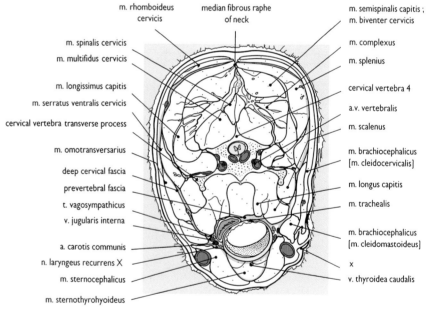

m. rhomboideus
cervicis

median fibrous raphe
of neck

m. semispinalis capitis ;
m. biventer cervicis

m. spinalis cervicis

m. multifidus cervicis

m. longissimus capitis

m. serratus ventralis cervicis

cervical vertebra transverse process

m. omotransversarius

deep cervical fascia

prevertebral fascia

t. vagosympathicus

v. jugularis interna

a. carotis communis

n. laryngeus recurrens X

m. sternocephalicus

m. sternothyrohyoideus

m. complexus

m. splenius

cervical vertebra 4

a.v. vertebralis

m. scalenus

m. brachiocephalicus
[m. cleidocervicalis]

m. longus capitis

m. trachealis

m. brachiocephalicus
[m. cleidomastoideus]

x

v. thyroidea caudalis

Fig. 3.39 Transverse section (4) through cervical vertebra 4: caudal view. The damage indicated at the point labelled 'X' in this section was occasioned by the procedure for cannulating the right common carotid artery for embalming and the subsequent latex injection of the arterial system.

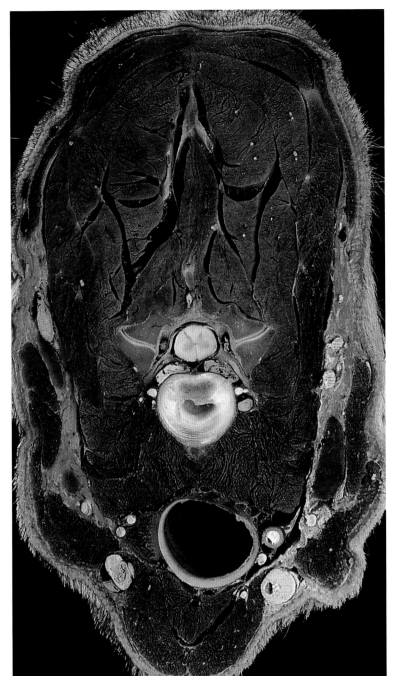

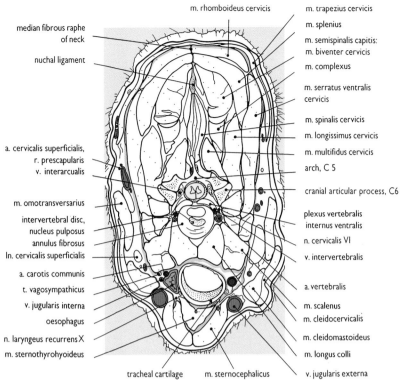

median fibrous raphe of neck

nuchal ligament

a. cervicalis superficialis, r. prescapularis
v. interarcualis

m. omotransversarius

intervertebral disc, nucleus pulposus annulus fibrosus

ln. cervicalis superficialis

a. carotis communis

t. vagosympathicus

v. jugularis interna

oesophagus

n. laryngeus recurrens X

m. sternothyrohyoideus

tracheal cartilage

m. sternocephalicus

m. rhomboideus cervicis

m. trapezius cervicis

m. splenius

m. semispinalis capitis: m. biventer cervicis

m. complexus

m. serratus ventralis cervicis

m. spinalis cervicis

m. longissimus cervicis

m. multifidus cervicis

arch, C 5

cranial articular process, C6

plexus vertebralis internus ventralis

n. cervicalis VI

v. intervertebralis

a. vertebralis

m. scalenus

m. cleidocervicalis

m. cleidomastoideus

m. longus colli

v. jugularis externa

Fig. 3.40 Transverse section (5) through the intervertebral disc, between cervical vertebrae 5 and 6: caudal view. The increased size of the right common carotid artery in this section is due to the pressure in the artery of the plastic cannula used for injection. A completely encircling layer of deep fascia extends down either side from the median fibrous raphe beneath the cleidocervical, omotransverse, cleidomastoid and sternocephalic muscles, to meet in the mid ventral line. A second strong layer passes down on the surface of the splenius beneath the cervical parts of the trapezius, rhomboideus and ventral serrate. The prevertebral fascia, ventral to the longus colli and capitis muscles, joins the lateral layers.

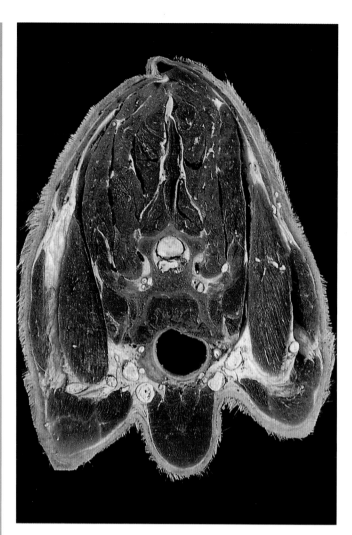

Fig. 3.41 Transverse section (6) through cervical vertebra 6 and the jugular fossa: caudal view. The jugular fossa is displayed in this section towards the base of the neck. It is a deep indentation bordered by the sternocephalic muscle medially, and the brachiocephalic muscle laterally (see Fig. 3.9). The main veins draining the neck and shoulder converge within the fossa i.e. internal and external jugular, caudal thyroid, superficial cervical, and omobrachial.

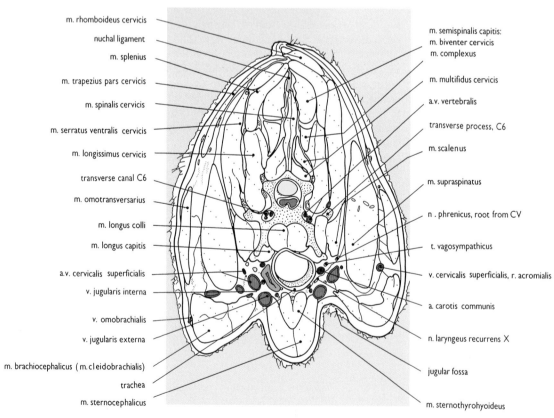

m. rhomboideus cervicis

nuchal ligament

m. splenius

m. trapezius pars cervicis

m. spinalis cervicis

m. serratus ventralis cervicis

m. longissimus cervicis

transverse canal C6

m. omotransversarius

m. longus colli

m. longus capitis

a.v. cervicalis superficialis

v. jugularis interna

v. omobrachialis

v. jugularis externa

m. brachiocephalicus (m. cleidobrachialis)

trachea

m. sternocephalicus

m. semispinalis capitis:
m. biventer cervicis
m. complexus

m. multifidus cervicis

a.v. vertebralis

transverse process, C6

m. scalenus

m. supraspinatus

n . phrenicus, root from CV

t. vagosympathicus

v. cervicalis superficialis, r. acromialis

a. carotis communis

n. laryngeus recurrens X

jugular fossa

m. sternothyrohyoideus

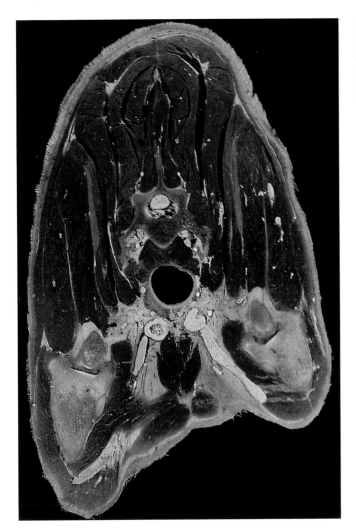

Fig. 3.42 Transverse section (7) through cervical vertebra 7 and the shoulder joint: caudal view. On the left, the pectoral muscle indicates the ventral boundary of the jugular fossa, whilst on the right the limb is somewhat retracted so that the cephalic vein is visible entering the fossa (see Figs 3.29 and 3.30). The vertebral artery and vein can be seen ventral to the transverse processes and body of the vertebrae en route for the transverse canal of C6 (see also Figs 3.24–3.26).

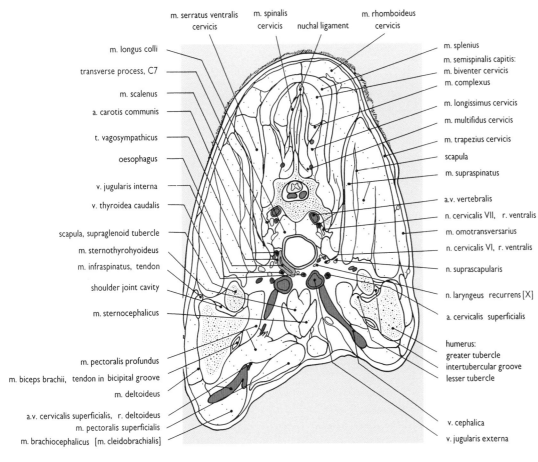

m. serratus ventralis cervicis
m. spinalis cervicis
nuchal ligament
m. rhomboideus cervicis

m. longus colli
transverse process, C7
m. scalenus
a. carotis communis
t. vagosympathicus
oesophagus
v. jugularis interna
v. thyroidea caudalis
scapula, supraglenoid tubercle
m. sternothyrohyoideus
m. infraspinatus, tendon
shoulder joint cavity
m. sternocephalicus
m. pectoralis profundus
m. biceps brachii, tendon in bicipital groove
m. deltoideus
a.v. cervicalis superficialis, r. deltoideus
m. pectoralis superficialis
m. brachiocephalicus [m. cleidobrachialis]

m. splenius
m. semispinalis capitis:
m. biventer cervicis
m. complexus
m. longissimus cervicis
m. multifidus cervicis
m. trapezius cervicis
scapula
m. supraspinatus
a.v. vertebralis
n. cervicalis VII, r. ventralis
m. omotransversarius
n. cervicalis VI, r. ventralis
n. suprascapularis
n. laryngeus recurrens [X]
a. cervicalis superficialis
humerus:
greater tubercle
intertubercular groove
lesser tubercle
v. cephalica
v. jugularis externa

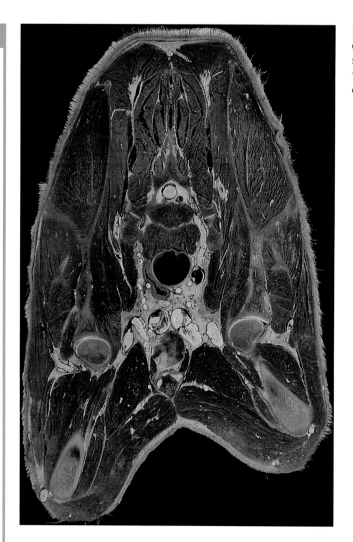

Fig. 3.43 Transverse section (8) through thoracic vertebra 1 and the thoracic inlet: caudal view. This cross-section through the inlet complements those lateral views shown earlier in Figs 3.23–3.25. On either side of the inlet, the scalene muscles extend ventrally from the head of the first rib, and the sternothyrohyoid muscles extend dorsally from the manubrium of the sternum.

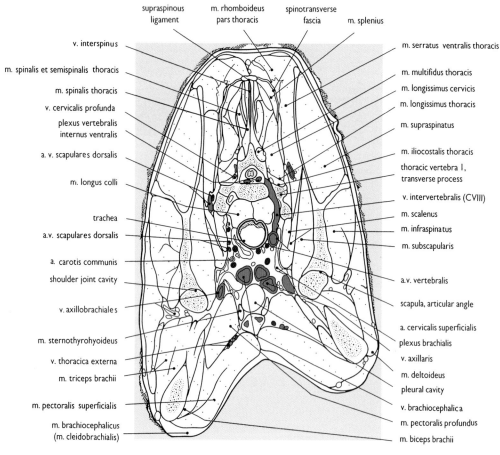

supraspinous ligament
m. rhomboideus pars thoracis
spinotransverse fascia
m. splenius

v. interspinus
m. spinalis et semispinalis thoracis
m. spinalis thoracis
v. cervicalis profunda
plexus vertebralis internus ventralis
a. v. scapulares dorsalis
m. longus colli
trachea
a.v. scapulares dorsalis
a. carotis communis
shoulder joint cavity
v. axillobrachiales
m. sternothyrohyoideus
v. thoracica externa
m. triceps brachii
m. pectoralis superficialis
m. brachiocephalicus (m. cleidobrachialis)

m. serratus ventralis thoracis
m. multifidus thoracis
m. longissimus cervicis
m. longissimus thoracis
m. supraspinatus
m. iliocostalis thoracis
thoracic vertebra I, transverse process
v. intervertebralis (CVIII)
m. scalenus
m. infraspinatus
m. subscapularis
a.v. vertebralis
scapula, articular angle
a. cervicalis superficialis
plexus brachialis
v. axillaris
m. deltoideus
pleural cavity
v. brachiocephalica
m. pectoralis profundus
m. biceps brachii

4. THE FORELIMB

As with the previous two chapters, any part of the limb may be involved in surface trauma with bruising and hemorrhage requiring cleaning, disinfection and debridement. Luckily, most of the important structures are on the medial aspect of the limbs and are therefore protected, in most instances, from such damage.

There is no bony connection of the shoulder to the main vertebral skeleton so the shoulder can be over-abducted from the body leading to trauma to the brachial plexus and damage to axillary vessels. This can occur when inexperienced people lift dogs by the front legs without supporting the weight of the body. In a complete brachial plexus paralysis there is loss of skin sensation over the lateral shoulder region. In radial paralysis, there is loss of skin sensation only over the cranial antebrachium and dorsum of the manus. There is obviously also loss of motor supply to the extensors of the elbow, carpus and digits. Radial paralysis is indicated by dragging of the limb with the dorsum of the manus in contact with the ground. This results in severe dysfunction, as the dog is unable to stabilize the elbow joint and the lower limb. As well as being damaged in the brachial plexus, the radial nerve can also be damaged at the point where it emerges from its passage (in a spiral) down the brachial groove. It can be damaged here in a fracture or when the repair is made. The supraspinatus and infraspinatus muscles may atrophy when there is damage to the suprascapular nerve and increased prominence of the scapular spine is then seen. In working dogs there are conditions involving infraspinatus contracture (with an associated atrophy) possibly secondary to trauma. This results in dogs swinging their legs in a circumferential arc and requires surgical correction by tenotomy. Many bony landmarks are palpable in the forelimb, notably the dorsal border of the scapula, the greater tubercle of the humerus, deltoid tuberosity, olecranon, medial surface of radius and accessory bone of the carpus, spine of scapula, and acromion.

The scapula may be subject to trauma with fracture of the neck or acromion process. The greater tubercle of the humerus and the acromion are palpable and are used to assess the normal position of the shoulder joint. The shoulder joint is often a site of *osteochondritis dissecans* (OCD), inflammatory changes imposed on the underlying condition of osteochondrosis, which is a degenerative condition of cartilage. Fragments of cartilage may separate and cause pain within the joint. They sometimes wedge under the tendon of the subscapular muscle or within the synovial sheath of the biceps. These flaps often originate from the caudal part of the head of the humerus. They may also sit in a large caudal pouch where often they do not cause any pain. Attached pieces of cartilage may also cause lameness. When operating for shoulder OCD, the caudolateral approach tends to be favored. In this a curved incision is made from about the mid-point

of the scapula, over the acromion and extending about one-third of the way down the humerus. The acromial and spinal heads of the deltoid are then retracted cranially and caudally respectively, followed by cranial retraction of the teres minor and internal rotation of the limb.

The body of the humerus is 'S'-shaped and for this reason repair of fractures is difficult as intramedullary pins are difficult to insert. You should always use as big a pin as possible to fill the shaft of the humerus but in this case a smaller pin has to be used so that it will traverse down the curved medullary cavity. Fractures of the body of the humerus tend to be in middle third or distal in position with approximately one-third involving the distal articular surface. This is due to the massive thickness of the bone proximally and the relative thinning distally, i.e. under pressure the fracture is at the weaker points. They also tend to be spiral fractures. Humeral fractures tend to present with a dropped elbow and with the paw resting on its dorsal surface. In young animals the fractures tend to be Salter Harris type but in the older dog the 'Y' fracture of the distal humerus is more common. No structures pass through the supracondylar foramen (covered by connective tissue), whereas in the cat, the brachial artery and median nerve pass through it. The groove immediately medial to the greater tubercle has a great use in that it is used to introduce an intramedullary pin which can be driven distally to effect immobilization of a fracture of the body of the humerus. In Springer spaniels lateral or medial condylar fractures also occur due to failure of ossification in this site.

Essentially there are three sites for intramedullary pinning of the humerus. Proximal fractures are repaired by separating the caudal edge of the M. cleidobrachialis from the cranial edge of the M. triceps (lateral head). A mid-shaft fracture is approached by dividing the caudal edge of the M. cleidobrachialis from the cranial edge of the brachialis muscle. A distal fracture is approached by dissecting between the caudal edge of the M. brachialis and the cranial edge of the M. triceps. This is the point at which the radial nerve is exposed to trauma. Intramedullary pins are rarely used in isolation but are frequently combined with an external fixator or coerciage wires. The pin is generally inserted in a normograde manner starting laterally to the ridge of the greater tuberosity and anchoring it in the medial condyle.

The elbow joint can be a site of several important clinical conditions. The anconeal process of the ulna fits into the olecranon fossa of the humerus and therefore the joint can only dislocate when the joint is in full flexion or when fracture of the humeral epicondyle occurs (repaired by surgery and use of screws). This usually occurs in traumatic accidents. It can also be put back in place with full flexion of the joint. The anconeal process has occasionally a separate centre of ossification from that of the olecranon. In this case, the anconeal process detaches following trauma or fails to unite and is pulled off by M. triceps and may have to be removed surgically. Caudolateral arthrotomy of the elbow is used to remove an anconeal process that is disunited. A curved incision is made over the distal third of the humerus to the proximal third of the radius. The pronator teres and the flexor carpi radialis are then separated to expose the joint capsule.

Medial arthrotomy of the elbow joint is used to treat osteochondritis of the elbow joint but not the underlying osteochondrosis cause, and for removal of a fragmented coronoid process which can also be screwed back into place. This primarily affects large breeds of dogs such as St Bernards. An incision is made over the medial humeral epicondyle.

The styloid process of the ulna fractures easily in the dog. It is important clinically to recognize the sesamoid bones as normal features and not bone chips, and to remember that there is a dorsal sesamoid at the level of the metacarpophalangeal joint. The accessory carpal bone has two centres of ossification and it may therefore be vulnerable to dislocation. It is important to repair these types of fractures as they lead to instability of the carpus which will not resolve without repair. Fracture of the accessory carpal bone is often seen in racing greyhounds. Hyperextension injuries of the carpus are relatively common in medium and large breeds of dog and require carpal arthrodesis.

It is possible for rupture of all the forelimb muscle bellies, especially in working dogs or racing dogs like greyhounds. These heal with a lot of scar tissue. Dogs may also rupture the tendinous support structures. For example, tearing of the flexor retinaculum holding the deep digital flexor in place in the carpal canal. Clinically, remember that all extensors of the carpus and digits arise from the lateral epicondyle of the humerus and all flexors from the medial epicondyle of the humerus.

The other major site of damage in the forelimb may be at the intertubercular site in the humerus where bursitis may occur. The tendon sheath of the M. biceps slides through this groove and is held in place by the transverse ligament of the humerus.

The cephalic vein has considerable importance in clinical practice for collection of blood samples, administration of supportive therapy (intravenous drips) and for intravenous anesthesia and for euthanasia. The cephalic vein is also in close proximity to the medial and lateral branches of the superficial ramus of the radial nerve.

The superficial lymph nodes associated with the front leg are the superficial cervical which takes most of the drainage from the foot, carpus and lateral humeral and shoulder regions and the axillary lymph node which drains the axillary region and part of the lateral chest wall. Neither is normally palpable and the former is by far the most important.

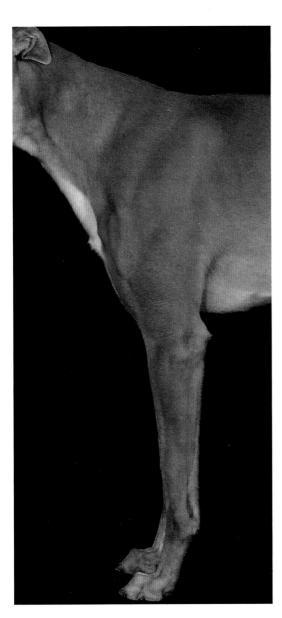

Fig. 4.1 Surface features of the neck and forelimb: left lateral view. The palpable bony prominences of the neck and forelimb are shown. In addition the trachea is clearly palpable on the underside of the neck. 'Soft' structures identifiable include the mandibular lymph nodes at the cranial end of the neck and the superficial cervical nodes in front of the scapula at the caudal end. A pulse may be detected in the common carotid artery in the neck, but also from the brachial/median artery in the cubital fossa on the flexor surface of the elbow joint. The external jugular vein may be raised by pressure in the jugular fossa: the cephalic vein may also be raised in the antebrachium by pressure immediately distal to the elbow joint. Fig. 4.1A at the foot of the page shows the main topographical regions that are recognized for descriptive purposes. The boundaries of regions in the neck are a trifle arbitrary because of the absence of discernible underlying features. The four main topographical regions of the forelimb are based on internal osteological components; the subsidiary topographical regions are related to the underlying joints between segments.

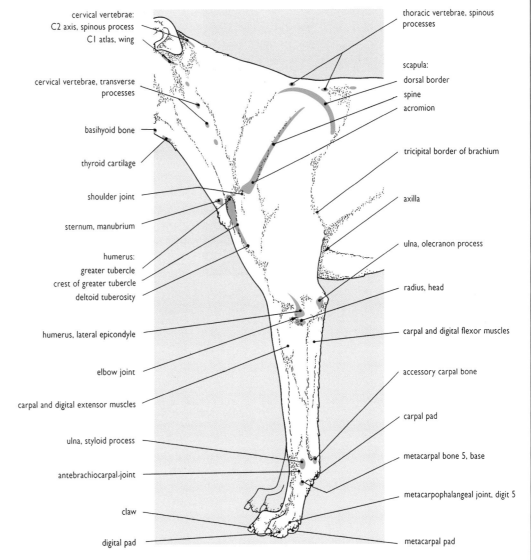

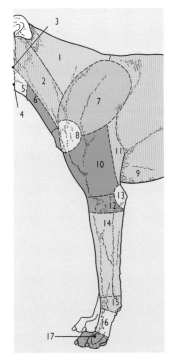

Fig. 4.1A Topographical regions of the neck and forelimb: left lateral view. **1** Dorsal Neck Region. **2** Lateral Neck Region. **3** Parotid Region. **4** Pharyngeal Region. **5** Laryngeal Region. **6** Tracheal Region. **7** Scapular Region. **8** Shoulder Joint Region. **9** Axillary Region. **10** Brachial Region. **11** Tricipital Region. **12** Cubital Region. **13** Olecranon Region. **14** Antebrachial Region. **15** Carpal Region. **16** Metacarpal Region. **17** Phalangeal (Digital) Region.

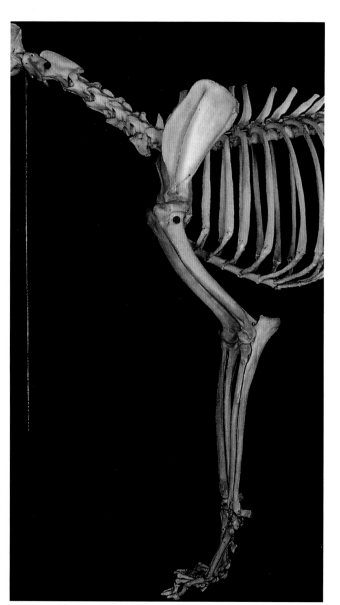

Fig. 4.2 Skeleton of the neck and forelimb: left lateral view. The palpable bony features shown in the surface view are colored green in the accompanying drawing. Additional areas of bone are deeply palpable through overlying musculature. These include the cranial border of the scapula, the humeral shaft proximal to the elbow joint, the distal ends of both radius and ulna approaching the carpus, and much of the carpal, metacarpal and phalangeal bones in the forepaw. Adjacent bones of the vertebral column and ribcage are included in the picture to give the approximate position of the forelimb skeleton in relation to the trunk in the normal standing posture. The position of the olecranon process ('point of the elbow') in relation to the chest is important since it may be used as a reference point for determining the position of thoracic organs. It should be noted that any features of the third to seventh cervical vertebrae are palpable only with difficulty even in thin dogs.

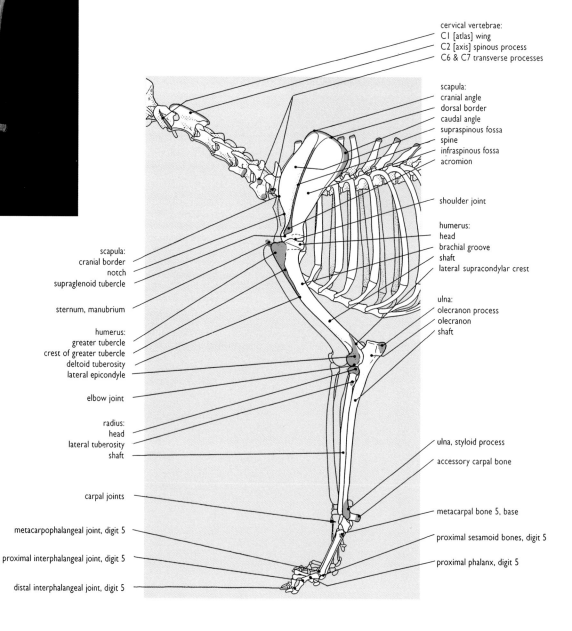

cervical vertebrae:
C1 [atlas] wing
C2 [axis] spinous process
C6 & C7 transverse processes

scapula:
cranial angle
dorsal border
caudal angle
supraspinous fossa
spine
infraspinous fossa
acromion

shoulder joint

humerus:
head
brachial groove
shaft
lateral supracondylar crest

ulna:
olecranon process
olecranon
shaft

ulna, styloid process

accessory carpal bone

metacarpal bone 5, base

proximal sesamoid bones, digit 5

proximal phalanx, digit 5

scapula:
cranial border
notch
supraglenoid tubercle

sternum, manubrium

humerus:
greater tubercle
crest of greater tubercle
deltoid tuberosity
lateral epicondyle

elbow joint

radius:
head
lateral tuberosity
shaft

carpal joints

metacarpophalangeal joint, digit 5

proximal interphalangeal joint, digit 5

distal interphalangeal joint, digit 5

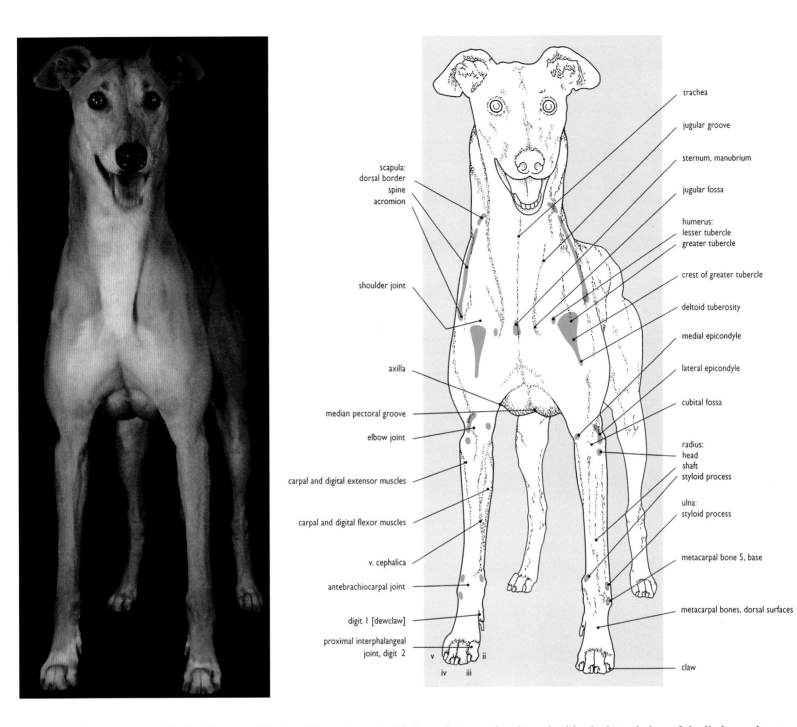

scapula:
dorsal border
spine
acromion

shoulder joint

axilla

median pectoral groove

elbow joint

carpal and digital extensor muscles

carpal and digital flexor muscles

v. cephalica

antebrachiocarpal joint

digit 1 [dewclaw]

proximal interphalangeal
joint, digit 2

trachea

jugular groove

sternum, manubrium

jugular fossa

humerus:
lesser tubercle
greater tubercle

crest of greater tubercle

deltoid tuberosity

medial epicondyle

lateral epicondyle

cubital fossa

radius:
head
shaft
styloid process

ulna:
styloid process

metacarpal bone 5, base

metacarpal bones, dorsal surfaces

claw

v

iv   iii

ii

Fig. 4.3 Surface features of the forelimb: cranial view. The major palpable bony features already noticed in the lateral view of the limb are shown again as reference points and are indicated in the drawing. In addition bony prominences palpable on the medial aspect of the limb are shown. The triangular jugular fossa is a visible depression at the base of the neck lateral to the sternal manubrium. Careful palpation within the fossa may identify the first rib where it borders the thoracic inlet. A second triangular depression, the cubital fossa, is visible and palpable cranial to the elbow joint and within it the median nerve and pulsations in the brachial/median artery may be felt.

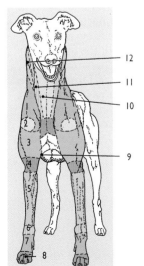

12

11

10

9

Fig. 4.3A Topographical regions of the forelimb: cranial view. **1** Scapular Region. **2** Shoulder Joint Region. **3** Brachial Region. **4** Cubital Region. **5** Antebrachial Region. **6** Carpal Region. **7** Metacarpal Region. **8** Phalangeal (Digital) Region. **9** Axillary Region. **10** Ventral Neck Region. **11** Lateral Neck Region. **12** Dorsal Neck Region.

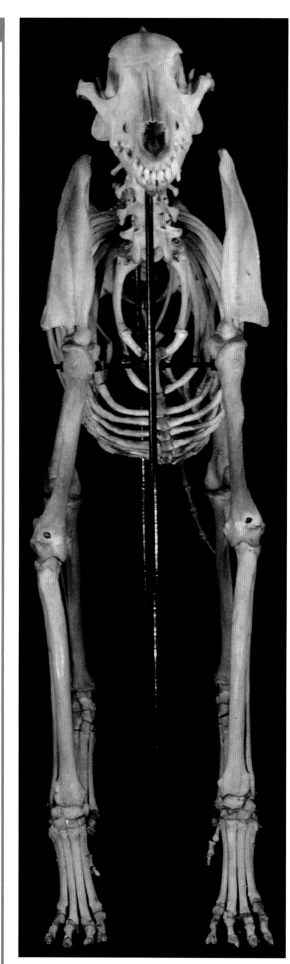

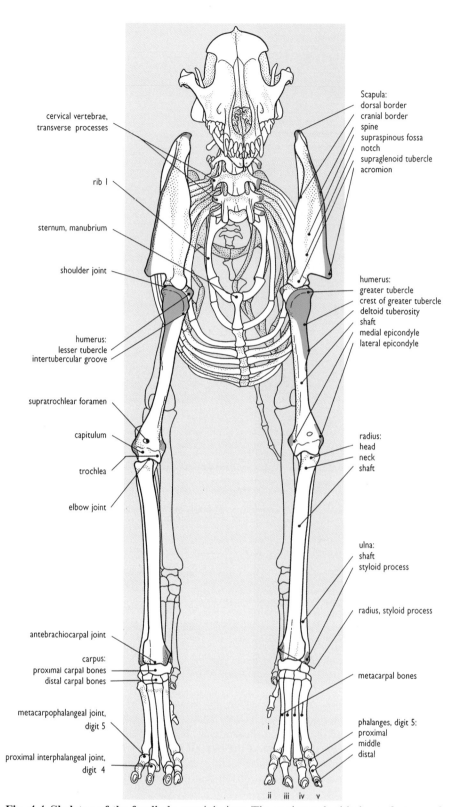

cervical vertebrae,
transverse processes

rib I

sternum, manubrium

shoulder joint

humerus:
lesser tubercle
intertubercular groove

supratrochlear foramen

capitulum

trochlea

elbow joint

antebrachiocarpal joint

carpus:
proximal carpal bones
distal carpal bones

metacarpophalangeal joint,
digit 5

proximal interphalangeal joint,
digit 4

Scapula:
dorsal border
cranial border
spine
supraspinous fossa
notch
supraglenoid tubercle
acromion

humerus:
greater tubercle
crest of greater tubercle
deltoid tuberosity
shaft
medial epicondyle
lateral epicondyle

radius:
head
neck
shaft

ulna:
shaft
styloid process

radius, styloid process

metacarpal bones

phalanges, digit 5:
proximal
middle
distal

i   ii   iii   iv   v

Fig. 4.4 Skeleton of the forelimb: cranial view. The major palpable bony features shown in the surface view are colored in this picture and are illustrated in the accompanying drawing. The complete absence of bony continuity between forelimb and trunk skeleton is now apparent. A clavicle, which in many mammals unites the lower end of the scapula with the manubrial region of the sternum, is only represented in a dog by a tendinous intersection within the brachiocephalic muscle. The entirely muscular 'joint' between the forelimb and trunk is based upon the deeply positioned and therefore impalpable ventral serrate muscle passing from the upper end of the scapula down onto the ribs and cervical vertebrae. This main weight-bearing muscle is assisted by other muscles such as the pectorals, brachiocephalic, latissimus dorsi, trapezius, and rhomboid, a number of which are palpable around the shoulder region and on the chest.

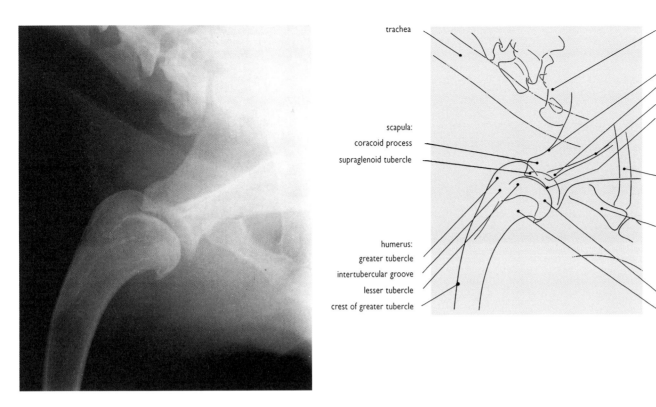

trachea

cervical vertebra 6

scapula:
notch
acromion
spine
glenoid cavity

scapula:
coracoid process
supraglenoid tubercle

rib I

sternum

humerus:
greater tubercle
intertubercular groove
lesser tubercle
crest of greater tubercle

humerus:
head
neck

Fig. 4.5 Radiograph of the shoulder joint: left lateral view. The major osteological features of the shoulder joint are shown in this radiograph. The relatively shallow glenoid fossa in the scapula contrasts with the considerably greater articular surface of the humeral head. However, the depth of the glenoid cavity is increased to some extent by a surrounding lip of fibrocartilage (radiolucent), although the overall articular area is still only about one half the area of the head.

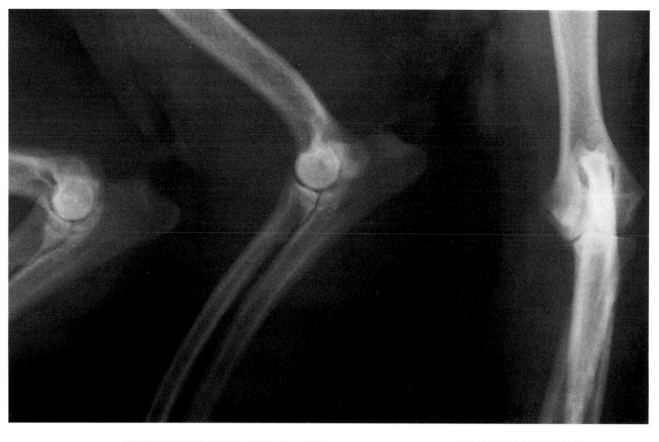

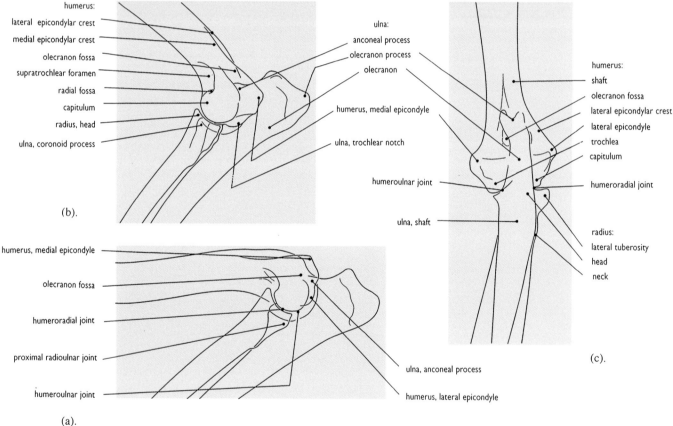

humerus:
lateral epicondylar crest
medial epicondylar crest
olecranon fossa
supratrochlear foramen
radial fossa
capitulum
radius, head
ulna, coronoid process

(b).

ulna:
anconeal process
olecranon process
olecranon

humerus, medial epicondyle

ulna, trochlear notch

humeroulnar joint

ulna, shaft

humerus:
shaft
olecranon fossa
lateral epicondylar crest
lateral epicondyle
trochlea
capitulum

humeroradial joint

radius:
lateral tuberosity
head
neck

(c).

humerus, medial epicondyle

olecranon fossa

humeroradial joint

proximal radioulnar joint

humeroulnar joint

ulna, anconeal process

humerus, lateral epicondyle

(a).

Fig. 4.6 Radiographs of the elbow joint: craniocaudal and lateral views. The major osteological features of the elbow joint are shown. The trochlea of the humeral condyle fits closely into the deep trochlear notch of the ulna providing its very stable hinge-like action. When extended (b) the anconeal process of the olecranon is located within the olecranon fossa stabilizing the joint; when flexed (a) the process is withdrawn and stability is reduced. When a paw is raised and the elbow flexed some measure of rotation occurs at the proximal radioulnar joint, apparent as a limited amount of pronation and supination of the paw. In the craniocaudal view (c) the two main subdivisions of the elbow joint are apparent – the humeroradial joint, a weight-transferring component between forearm and brachium, and the humeroulnar joint, more specifically concerned with movement and stability.

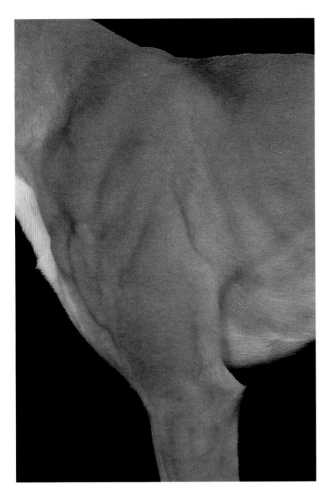

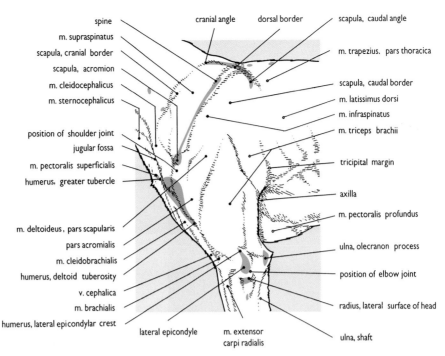

spine
m. supraspinatus
scapula, cranial border
scapula, acromion
m. cleidocephalicus
m. sternocephalicus

position of shoulder joint
jugular fossa
m. pectoralis superficialis
humerus, greater tubercle

m. deltoideus, pars scapularis
pars acromialis
m. cleidobrachialis
humerus, deltoid tuberosity
v. cephalica
m. brachialis
humerus, lateral epicondylar crest

cranial angle   dorsal border   scapula, caudal angle

m. trapezius, pars thoracica
scapula, caudal border
m. latissimus dorsi
m. infraspinatus
m. triceps brachii

tricipital margin

axilla
m. pectoralis profundus

ulna, olecranon process
position of elbow joint

radius, lateral surface of head

ulna, shaft

lateral epicondyle   m. extensor
carpi radialis

Fig. 4.7 Surface features of the shoulder and brachium: left lateral view. Palpable and visible features are indicated.

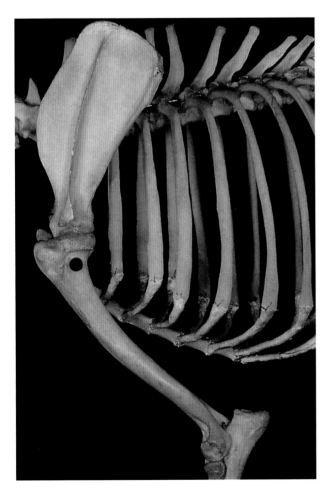

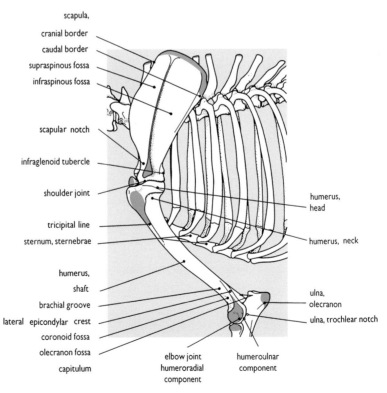

scapula,
cranial border
caudal border
supraspinous fossa
infraspinous fossa

scapular notch

infraglenoid tubercle

shoulder joint

tricipital line
sternum, sternebrae

humerus,
shaft
brachial groove
lateral epicondylar crest
coronoid fossa
olecranon fossa
capitulum

humerus,
head

humerus, neck

ulna,
olecranon
ulna, trochlear notch

elbow joint   humeroulnar
humeroradial   component
component

Fig. 4.8 Skeleton of the shoulder and brachium: left lateral view. The features colored green correspond to the palpable bony features shown in the previous figure (Fig. 4.7).

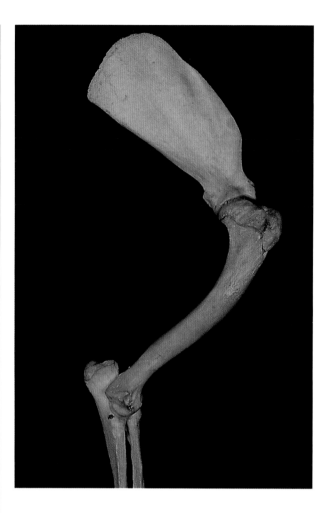

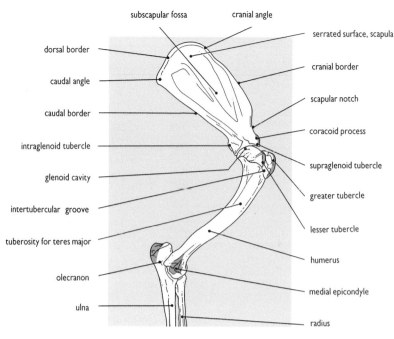

Fig. 4.9 Skeleton of the shoulder and brachium: left medial view. The features colored green are bony features which may be palpable in the live dog.

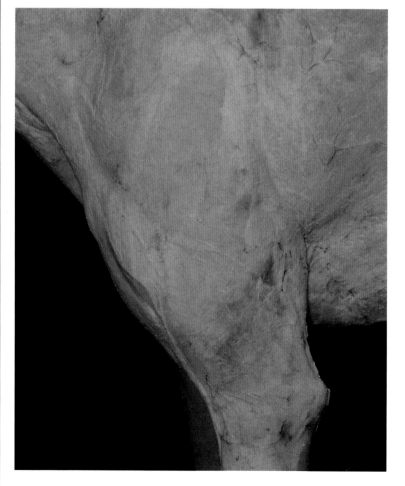

Fig. 4.10 Superficial fascia of the shoulder and brachium: left lateral view. Only the skin has been removed. The superficial fascia of the shoulder and brachium is continuous with the cervical fascia cranially, and with the trunk fascia caudally. This fascia contains a myriad of small blood vessels and nerves. The deep fascia of the lateral shoulder and brachium (fascia omobrachialis lateralis), which is also continuous with that of the neck and trunk, has firm attachments to the spine of the scapula and to the crest of the greater tubercle. Fascia omobrachialis lateralis, together with fascia omobrachialis medialis, are continuous with the fascia antebrachii which covers the muscles of the forearm as a closely applied tube.

Veterinary Anatomy: The Dog and Cat

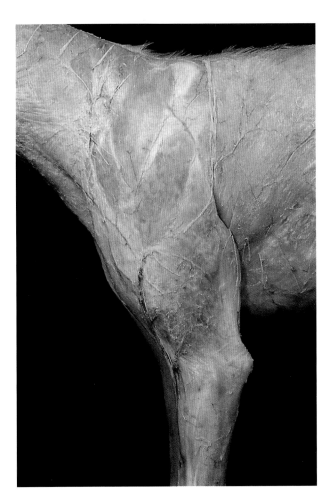

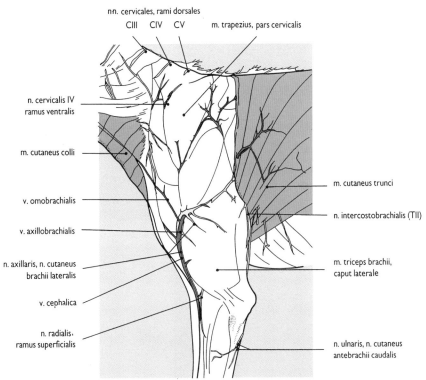

Fig. 4.11 Superficial structures of the shoulder and brachium: left lateral view. Some clearing of superficial fascia has exposed the cutaneous muscles of the neck and trunk, as well as superficial nerves and blood vessels. There is no cutaneous muscle over the forelimb.

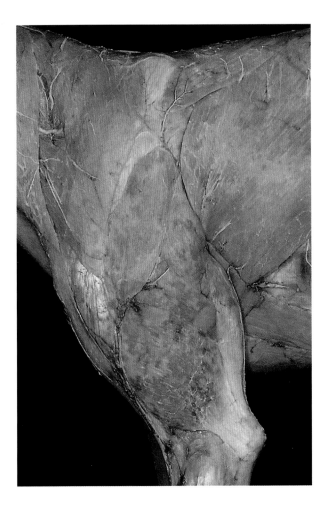

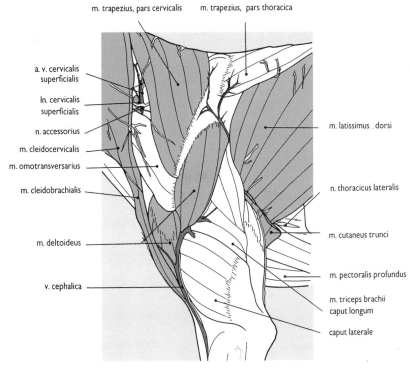

Fig. 4.12 Superficial muscles of the shoulder and brachium: left lateral view. The fascia has been cleared and the cutaneus trunci muscle removed. Many of the extrinsic muscles which attach the forelimb to the trunk (the 'synsarcosis') can be seen.

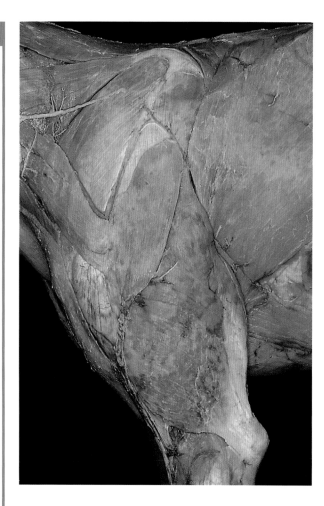

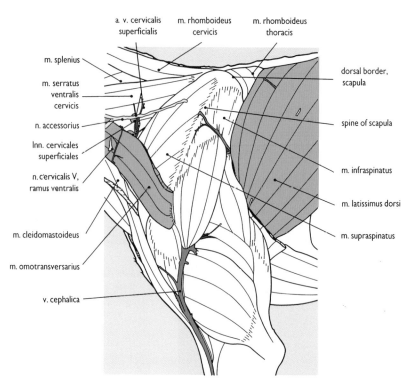

a. v. cervicalis superficialis
m. rhomboideus cervicis
m. rhomboideus thoracis
m. splenius
m. serratus ventralis cervicis
n. accessorius
lnn. cervicales superficiales
n. cervicalis V, ramus ventralis
m. cleidomastoideus
m. omotransversarius
v. cephalica
dorsal border, scapula
spine of scapula
m. infraspinatus
m. latissimus dorsi
m. supraspinatus

Fig. 4.13 Shoulder and brachium after removal of trapezius and cleidocervical muscles: left lateral view. The accessory nerve has been left in position after the removal of the trapezius muscle which it innervates.

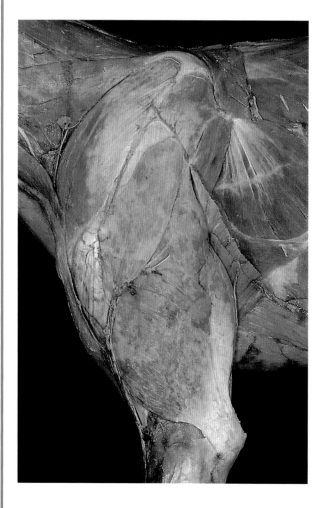

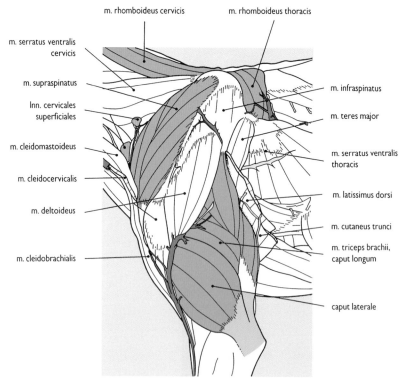

m. rhomboideus cervicis
m. rhomboideus thoracis
m. serratus ventralis cervicis
m. supraspinatus
lnn. cervicales superficiales
m. cleidomastoideus
m. cleidocervicalis
m. deltoideus
m. cleidobrachialis
m. infraspinatus
m. teres major
m. serratus ventralis thoracis
m. latissimus dorsi
m. cutaneus trunci
m. triceps brachii, caput longum
caput laterale

Fig. 4.14 Shoulder and brachium after removal of latissimus dorsi and omotransverse muscles: left lateral view. The superficial cervical lymph nodes are now exposed just cranial to the supraspinatus muscle.

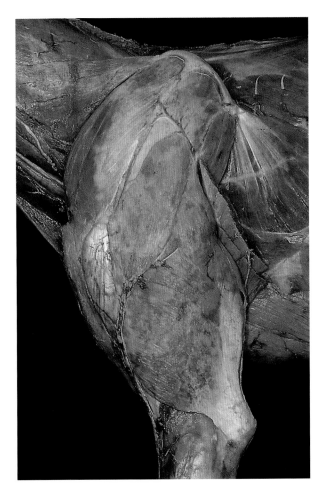

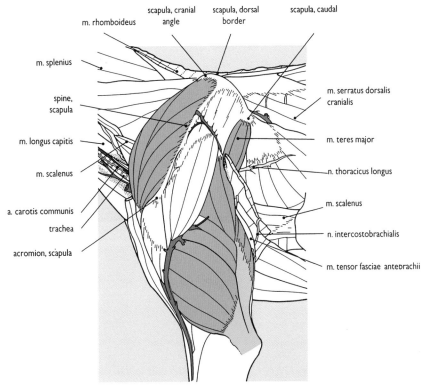

m. rhomboideus

scapula, cranial angle

scapula, dorsal border

scapula, caudal

m. splenius

spine, scapula

m. longus capitis

m. scalenus

a. carotis communis

trachea

acromion, scapula

m. serratus dorsalis cranialis

m. teres major

n. thoracicus longus

m. scalenus

n. intercostobrachialis

m. tensor fasciae antebrachii

Fig. 4.15 Shoulder and brachium after removal of rhomboid and cleidomastoid muscles: left lateral view. The boundary between neck and forelimb is now clearly visible.

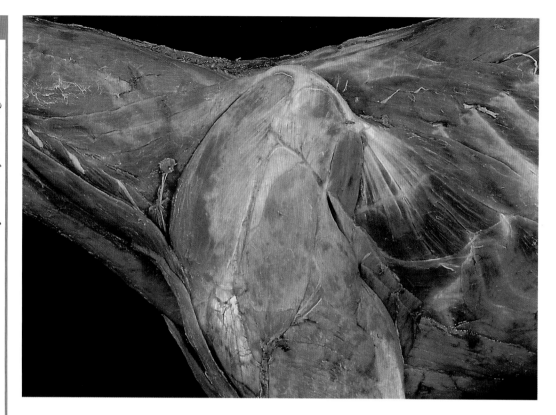

Fig. 4.16 Extent of ventral serrate muscle: left lateral view. This is the same stage of dissection as Fig. 4.14, but the wider view shows the full extent of the fan-shaped ventral serrate muscle. This muscle and the pectoral muscles are the only muscles now attaching the forelimb to the trunk.

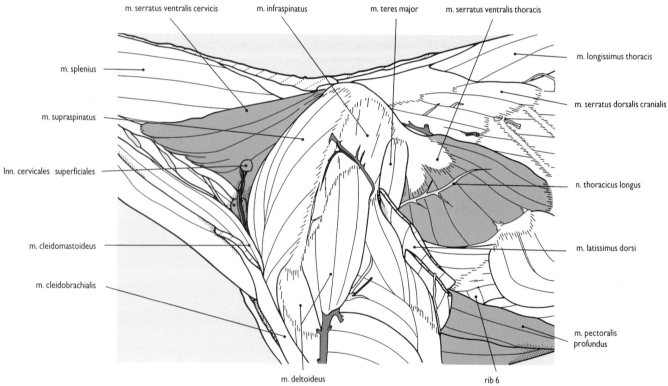

m. serratus ventralis cervicis

m. infraspinatus

m. teres major

m. serratus ventralis thoracis

m. splenius

m. longissimus thoracis

m. supraspinatus

m. serratus dorsalis cranialis

lnn. cervicales superficiales

n. thoracicus longus

m. cleidomastoideus

m. latissimus dorsi

m. cleidobrachialis

m. pectoralis profundus

m. deltoideus

rib 6

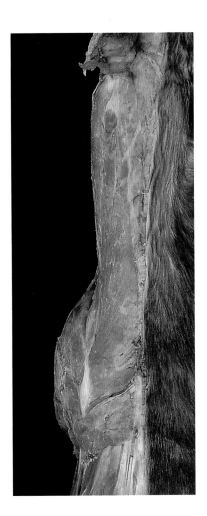

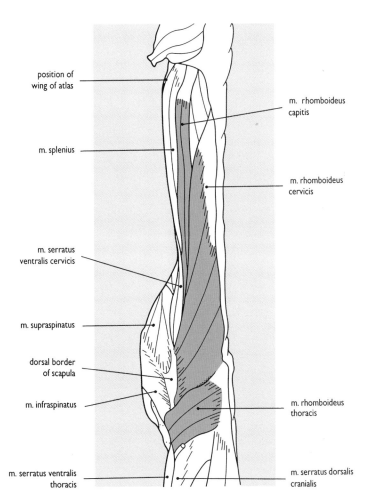

position of
wing of atlas

m. splenius

m. serratus
ventralis cervicis

m. supraspinatus

dorsal border
of scapula

m. infraspinatus

m. serratus ventralis
thoracis

m. rhomboideus
capitis

m. rhomboideus
cervicis

m. rhomboideus
thoracis

m. serratus dorsalis
cranialis

Fig. 4.17 Left rhomboid muscle: dorsal view. The trapezius and latissimus dorsi muscles have been removed. Three parts of the rhomboid muscle can be seen.

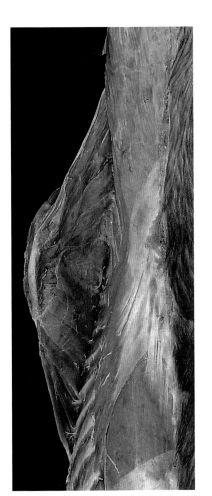

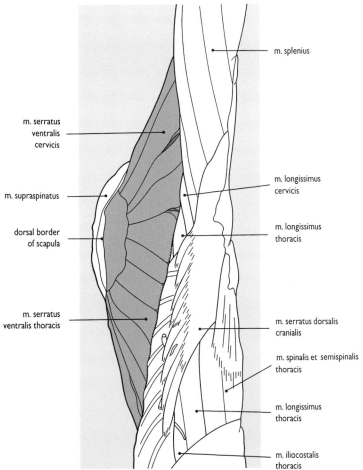

m. serratus
ventralis
cervicis

m. supraspinatus

dorsal border
of scapula

m. serratus
ventralis thoracis

m. splenius

m. longissimus
cervicis

m. longissimus
thoracis

m. serratus dorsalis
cranialis

m. spinalis et semispinalis
thoracis

m. longissimus
thoracis

m. iliocostalis
thoracis

Fig. 4.18 Left ventral serrate muscle after removal of the rhomboid muscle: dorsal view. The medial surface of the ventral serrate muscle has been exposed by abduction of the upper part of the scapula.

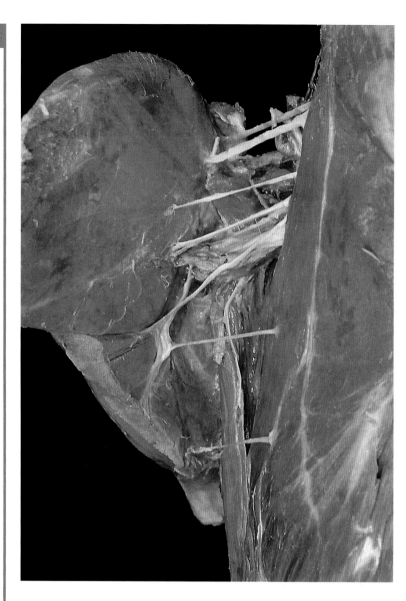

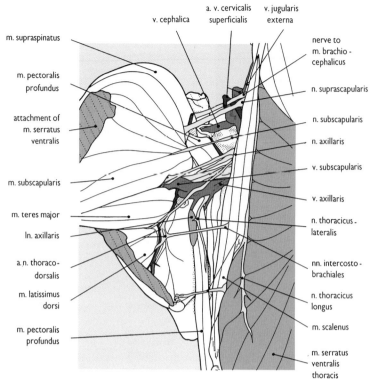

m. supraspinatus

v. cephalica

a. v. cervicalis superficialis

v. jugularis externa

m. pectoralis profundus

nerve to m. brachio-cephalicus

attachment of m. serratus ventralis

n. suprascapularis

n. subscapularis

n. axillaris

m. subscapularis

v. subscapularis

m. teres major

v. axillaris

ln. axillaris

n. thoracicus lateralis

a. n. thoraco-dorsalis

nn. intercosto-brachiales

m. latissimus dorsi

n. thoracicus longus

m. pectoralis profundus

m. scalenus

m. serratus ventralis thoracis

Fig. 4.19 Left axillary structures: dorsal view. The ventral serrate muscle has been separated from the scapula and returned to its position against the trunk. The scapula has been further abducted to expose the axillary structures which have been somewhat stretched.

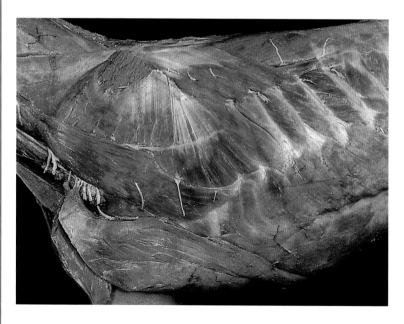

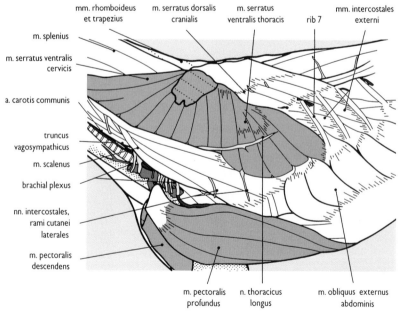

mm. rhomboideus et trapezius

m. serratus dorsalis cranialis

m. serratus ventralis thoracis

mm. intercostales externi

m. splenius

rib 7

m. serratus ventralis cervicis

a. carotis communis

truncus vagosympathicus

m. scalenus

brachial plexus

nn. intercostales, rami cutanei laterales

m. pectoralis descendens

m. pectoralis profundus

n. thoracicus longus

m. obliquus externus abdominis

Fig. 4.20 Pectoral and ventral serrate muscles after removal of the forelimb: left lateral view. The pectoral and ventral serrate muscles were the last muscles of the synsarcosis to be transected.

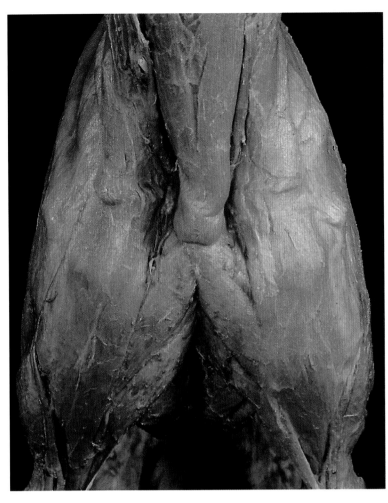

Fig. 4.21 Superficial structures of shoulder and brachium: cranial view. Only the fascia has been removed.

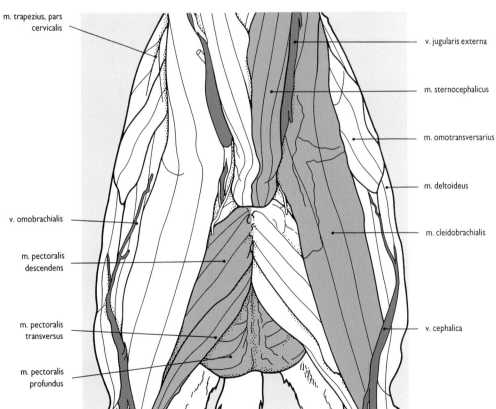

m. trapezius, pars cervicalis

v. omobrachialis

m. pectoralis descendens

m. pectoralis transversus

m. pectoralis profundus

v. jugularis externa

m. sternocephalicus

m. omotransversarius

m. deltoideus

m. cleidobrachialis

v. cephalica

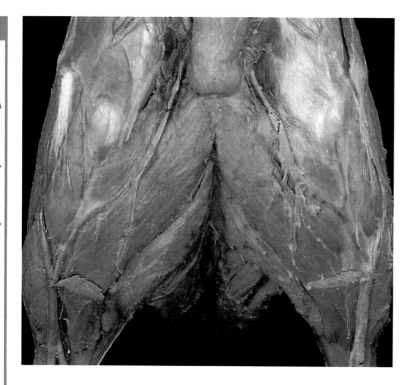

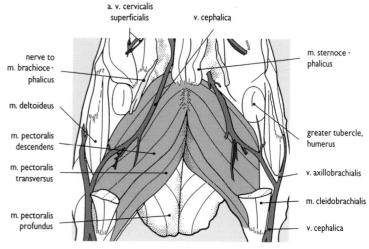

Fig. 4.22 Shoulder and brachium after removal of the brachiocephalic muscle: cranial view. The 'point of the shoulder' and course of the cephalic vein are now exposed.

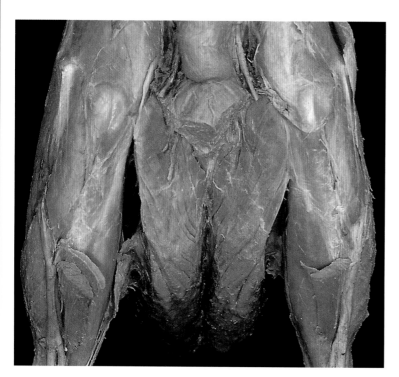

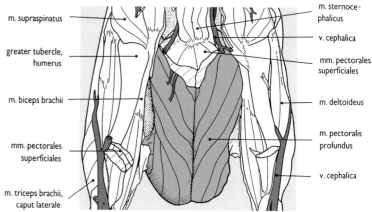

Fig. 4.23 Shoulder and brachium after removal of the superficial pectoral muscles: cranial view. The deep pectoral muscle is now exposed.

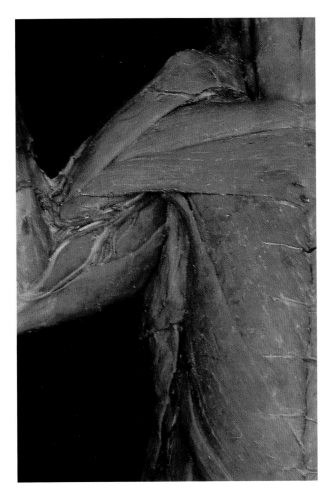

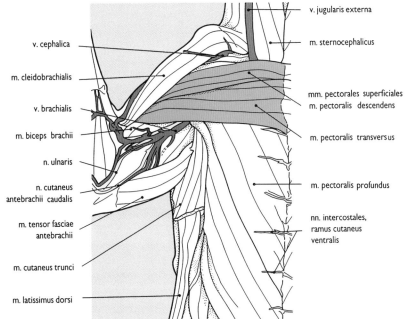

v. jugularis externa

v. cephalica

m. cleidobrachialis

v. brachialis

m. biceps brachii

n. ulnaris

n. cutaneus
antebrachii caudalis

m. tensor fasciae
antebrachii

m. cutaneus trunci

m. latissimus dorsi

m. sternocephalicus

mm. pectorales superficiales
m. pectoralis descendens

m. pectoralis transversus

m. pectoralis profundus

nn. intercostales,
ramus cutaneus
ventralis

Fig. 4.24 Right pectoral muscles: ventral view. Only the fascia and cutaneous muscles have been removed.

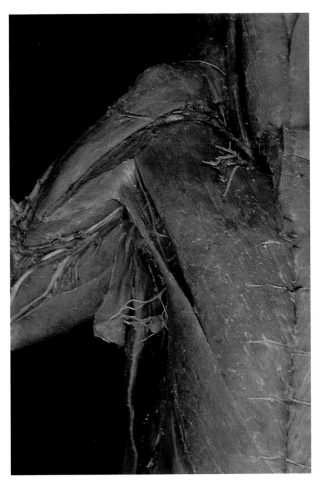

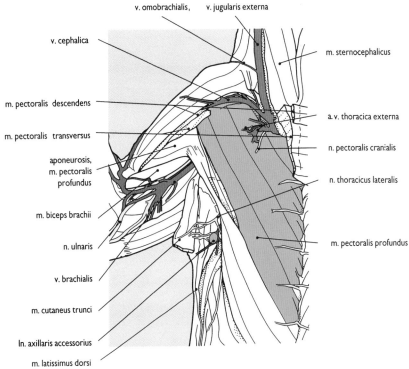

v. omobrachialis,   v. jugularis externa

v. cephalica

m. pectoralis descendens

m. pectoralis transversus

aponeurosis,
m. pectoralis
profundus

m. biceps brachii

n. ulnaris

v. brachialis

m. cutaneus trunci

ln. axillaris accessorius

m. latissimus dorsi

m. sternocephalicus

a. v. thoracica externa

n. pectoralis cranialis

n. thoracicus lateralis

m. pectoralis profundus

Fig. 4.25 Right deep pectoral muscle after removal of superficial pectoral muscles: ventral view. The latissimus dorsi muscle has been partly reflected to expose the accessory axillary lymph node and the lateral thoracic nerve supplying the cutaneus trunci muscle. The blood vessels and nerves supplying the superficial pectoral muscles can be seen in their cranial position.

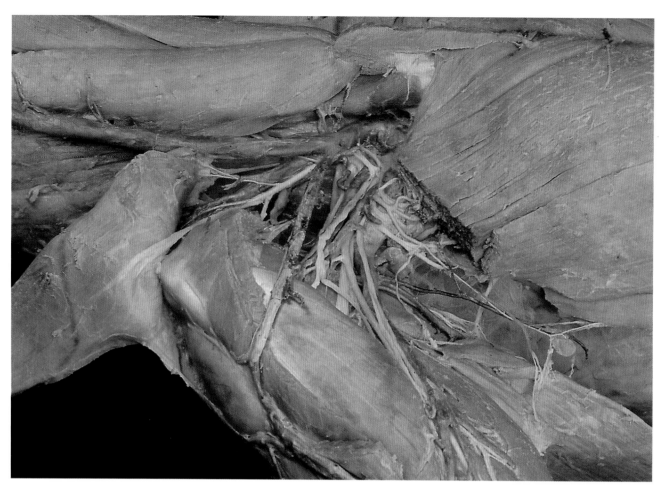

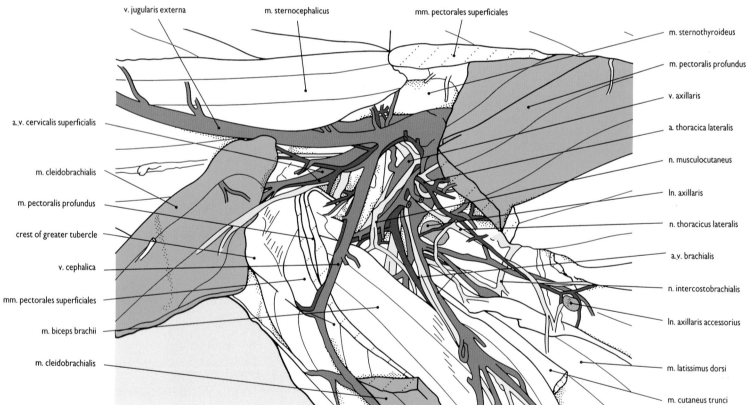

v. jugularis externa   m. sternocephalicus   mm. pectorales superficiales

m. sternothyroideus

m. pectoralis profundus

v. axillaris

a.v. cervicalis superficialis

a. thoracica lateralis

n. musculocutaneus

m. cleidobrachialis

ln. axillaris

m. pectoralis profundus

n. thoracicus lateralis

crest of greater tubercle

a.v. brachialis

v. cephalica

n. intercostobrachialis

mm. pectorales superficiales

ln. axillaris accessorius

m. biceps brachii

m. cleidobrachialis

m. latissimus dorsi

m. cutaneus trunci

Fig. 4.26 Right axillary structures: ventral view. Part of the deep pectoral muscle has been removed and the cleidobrachial muscle has been transected and reflected. Note that for Figures 4.26–4.30 the dissection photographs have been turned through 90° compared to Figures 4.24 & 4.25; i.e. the head is to the left in these figures.

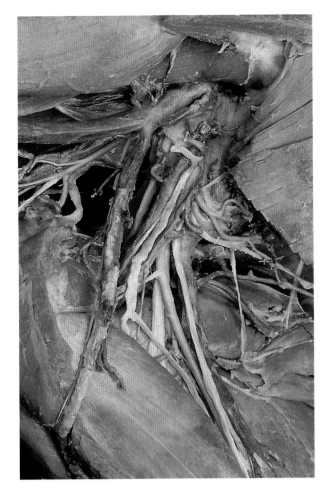

Fig. 4.27 Right axillary structures: ventral view. This is a closer view of part of the dissection shown in the previous figure (Fig. 4.26). Many of the nerves of the brachial plexus can be identified.

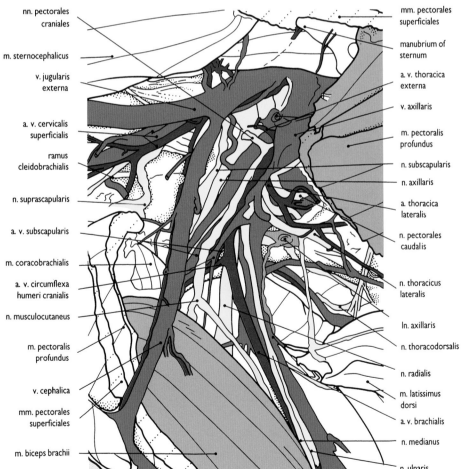

nn. pectorales craniales

m. sternocephalicus

v. jugularis externa

a. v. cervicalis superficialis

ramus cleidobrachialis

n. suprascapularis

a. v. subscapularis

m. coracobrachialis

a. v. circumflexa humeri cranialis

n. musculocutaneus

m. pectoralis profundus

v. cephalica

mm. pectorales superficiales

m. biceps brachii

mm. pectorales superficiales

manubrium of sternum

a. v. thoracica externa

v. axillaris

m. pectoralis profundus

n. subscapularis

n. axillaris

a. thoracica lateralis

n. pectorales caudalis

n. thoracicus lateralis

ln. axillaris

n. thoracodorsalis

n. radialis

m. latissimus dorsi

a. v. brachialis

n. medianus

n. ulnaris

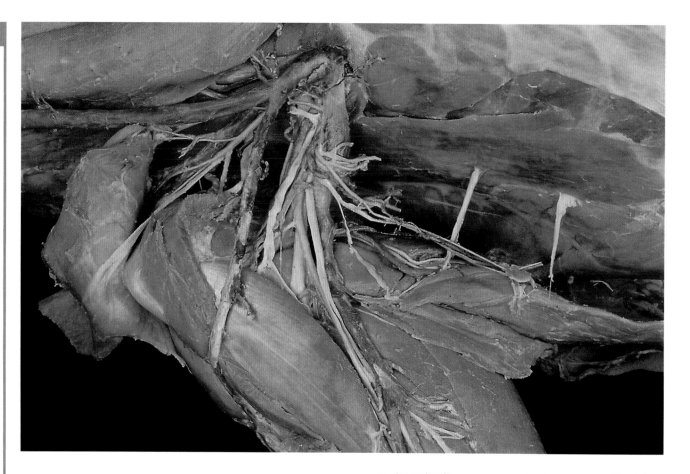

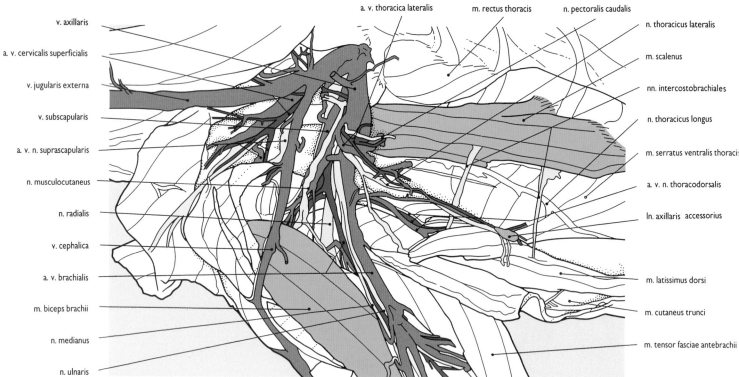

v. axillaris

a. v. cervicalis superficialis

v. jugularis externa

v. subscapularis

a. v. n. suprascapularis

n. musculocutaneus

n. radialis

v. cephalica

a. v. brachialis

m. biceps brachii

n. medianus

n. ulnaris

a. v. thoracica lateralis

m. rectus thoracis

n. pectoralis caudalis

n. thoracicus lateralis

m. scalenus

nn. intercostobrachiales

n. thoracicus longus

m. serratus ventralis thoracis

a. v. n. thoracodorsalis

ln. axillaris accessorius

m. latissimus dorsi

m. cutaneus trunci

m. tensor fasciae antebrachii

Fig. 4.28 Right axillary structures after removal of the deep pectoral muscle: ventral view.

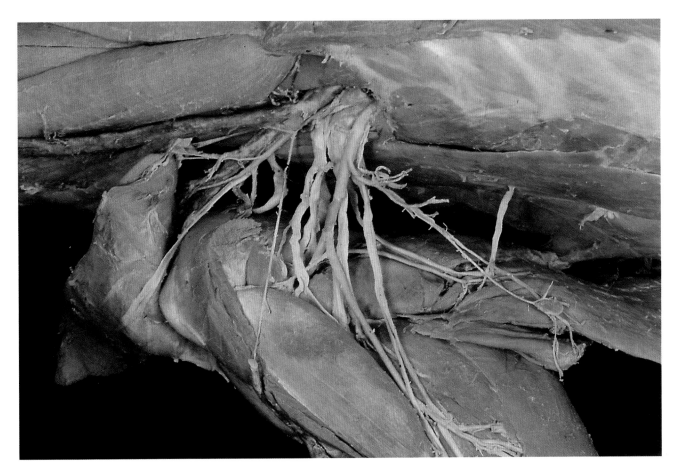

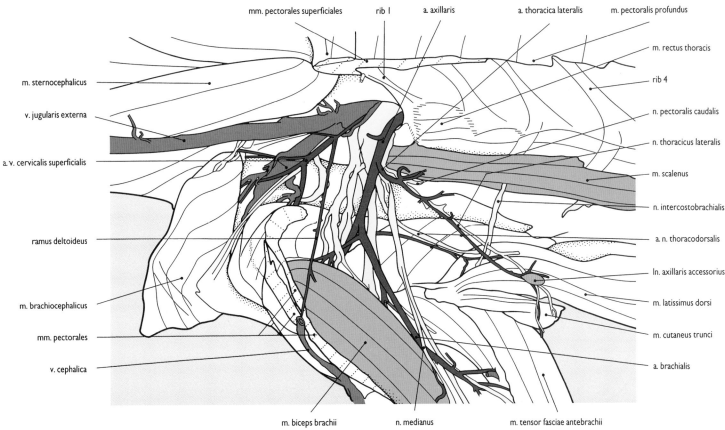

mm. pectorales superficiales   rib I   a. axillaris   a. thoracica lateralis   m. pectoralis profundus

m. rectus thoracis

m. sternocephalicus

rib 4

v. jugularis externa

n. pectoralis caudalis

a. v. cervicalis superficialis

n. thoracicus lateralis

m. scalenus

n. intercostobrachialis

ramus deltoideus

a. n. thoracodorsalis

ln. axillaris accessorius

m. brachiocephalicus

m. latissimus dorsi

mm. pectorales

m. cutaneus trunci

v. cephalica

a. brachialis

m. biceps brachii   n. medianus   m. tensor fasciae antebrachii

Fig. 4.29 Right axillary structures after removal of veins: ventral view. Arteries and nerves of the brachial plexus are now more clearly visible after the removal of the axillary vein and its branches, and part of the cephalic vein.

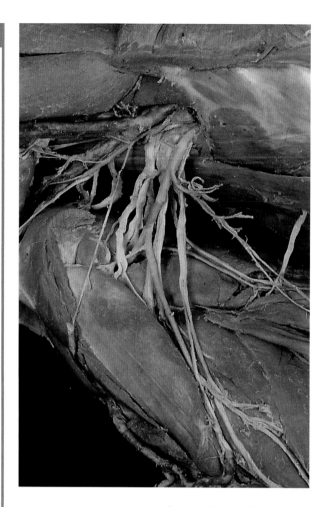

Fig. 4.30 Right axillary structures after removal of veins: ventral view. This is a closer view of part of the dissection shown in the previous figure (Fig. 4.29).

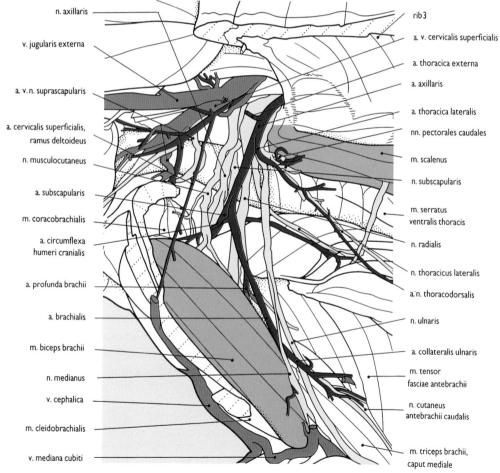

n. axillaris

v. jugularis externa

a. v. n. suprascapularis

a. cervicalis superficialis, ramus deltoideus

n. musculocutaneus

a. subscapularis

m. coracobrachialis

a. circumflexa humeri cranialis

a. profunda brachii

a. brachialis

m. biceps brachii

n. medianus

v. cephalica

m. cleidobrachialis

v. mediana cubiti

rib 3

a. v. cervicalis superficialis

a. thoracica externa

a. axillaris

a. thoracica lateralis

nn. pectorales caudales

m. scalenus

n. subscapularis

m. serratus ventralis thoracis

n. radialis

n. thoracicus lateralis

a. n. thoracodorsalis

n. ulnaris

a. collateralis ulnaris

m. tensor fasciae antebrachii

n. cutaneus antebrachii caudalis

m. triceps brachii, caput mediale

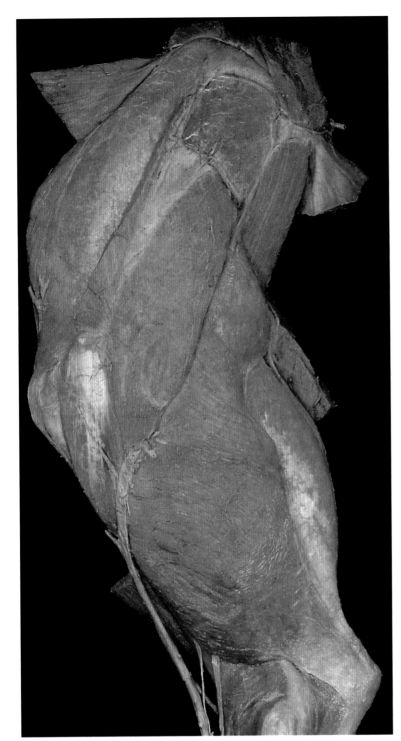

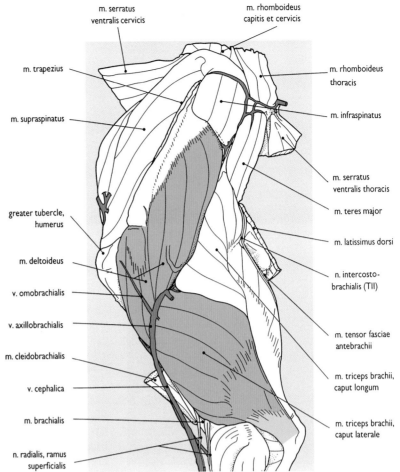

m. serratus
ventralis cervicis

m. rhomboideus
capitis et cervicis

m. trapezius

m. rhomboideus
thoracis

m. supraspinatus

m. infraspinatus

m. serratus
ventralis thoracis

m. teres major

greater tubercle,
humerus

m. latissimus dorsi

m. deltoideus

n. intercosto-
brachialis (TII)

v. omobrachialis

v. axillobrachialis

m. cleidobrachialis

m. tensor fasciae
antebrachii

v. cephalica

m. triceps brachii,
caput longum

m. brachialis

m. triceps brachii,
caput laterale

n. radialis, ramus
superficialis

Fig. 4.31 Shoulder and brachium of the separated forelimb: left lateral view. Many of the muscles which have been transected in order to separate the forelimb from the trunk may be seen (includes ventral serrate, trapezius, rhomboid, latissimus dorsi and cleidobrachialis muscles).

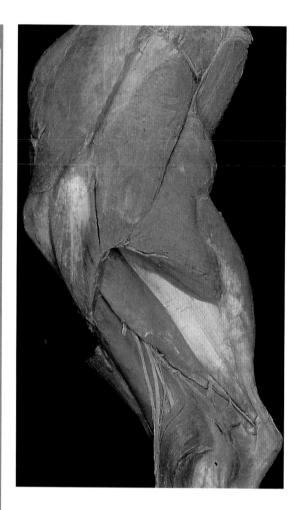

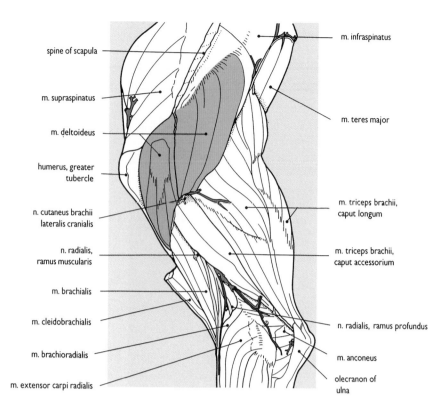

spine of scapula

m. infraspinatus

m. supraspinatus

m. deltoideus

m. teres major

humerus, greater tubercle

n. cutaneus brachii lateralis cranialis

m. triceps brachii, caput longum

n. radialis, ramus muscularis

m. triceps brachii, caput accessorium

m. brachialis

m. cleidobrachialis

n. radialis, ramus profundus

m. brachioradialis

m. anconeus

m. extensor carpi radialis

olecranon of ulna

Fig. 4.32 Shoulder and brachium after removal of the lateral head of the triceps brachii muscle: left lateral view. The transected branch of the radial nerve supplying the lateral head of the triceps brachii muscle can be seen. Latissimus dorsi and ventral serrate muscles have also been removed.

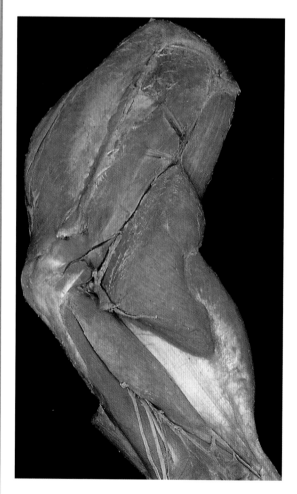

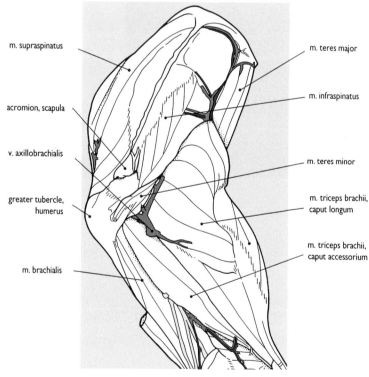

m. supraspinatus

m. teres major

acromion, scapula

m. infraspinatus

v. axillobrachialis

m. teres minor

greater tubercle, humerus

m. triceps brachii, caput longum

m. triceps brachii, caput accessorium

m. brachialis

Fig. 4.33 Shoulder and brachium after removal of the deltoid muscle: left lateral view. The infraspinatus and teres minor muscles are now exposed. The rhomboid muscles have also been removed.

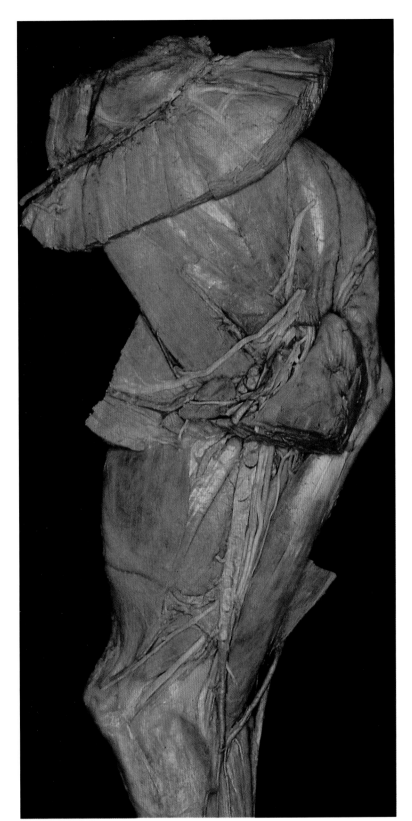

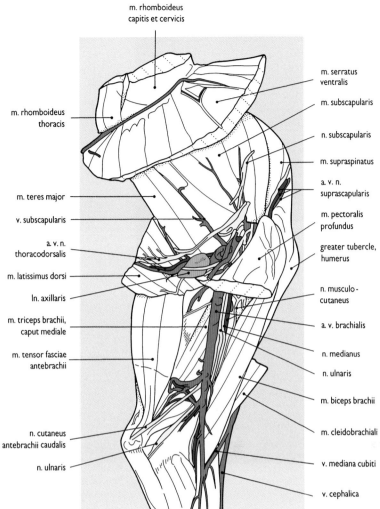

m. rhomboideus
capitis et cervicis

m. rhomboideus
thoracis

m. teres major

v. subscapularis

a. v. n.
thoracodorsalis

m. latissimus dorsi

ln. axillaris

m. triceps brachii,
caput mediale

m. tensor fasciae
antebrachii

n. cutaneus
antebrachii caudalis

n. ulnaris

m. serratus
ventralis

m. subscapularis

n. subscapularis

m. supraspinatus

a. v. n.
suprascapularis

m. pectoralis
profundus

greater tubercle,
humerus

n. musculo-
cutaneus

a. v. brachialis

n. medianus

n. ulnaris

m. biceps brachii

m. cleidobrachiali

v. mediana cubiti

v. cephalica

Fig. 4.34 Left shoulder and brachium: medial view. Many of the muscles
which have been transected, in order to separate the forelimb from the
trunk, may be seen (includes rhomboid, ventral serrate, latissimus dorsi,
cleidobrachialis and deep pectoral muscles).

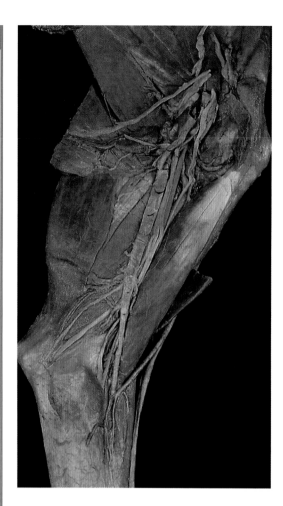

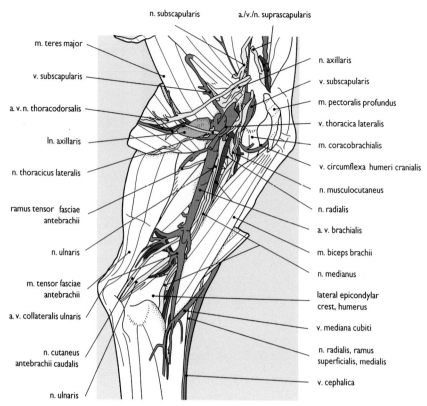

n. subscapularis   a./v./n. suprascapularis

m. teres major

v. subscapularis

a. v. n. thoracodorsalis

ln. axillaris

n. thoracicus lateralis

ramus tensor fasciae antebrachii

n. ulnaris

m. tensor fasciae antebrachii

a. v. collateralis ulnaris

n. cutaneus antebrachii caudalis

n. ulnaris

n. axillaris

v. subscapularis

m. pectoralis profundus

v. thoracica lateralis

m. coracobrachialis

v. circumflexa humeri cranialis

n. musculocutaneus

n. radialis

a. v. brachialis

m. biceps brachii

n. medianus

lateral epicondylar crest, humerus

v. mediana cubiti

n. radialis, ramus superficialis, medialis

v. cephalica

Fig. 4.35 Left shoulder and brachium: medial view. More of the deep pectoral muscle has been removed.

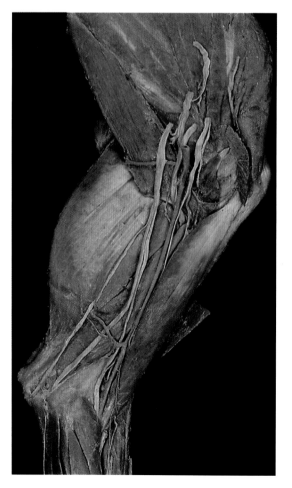

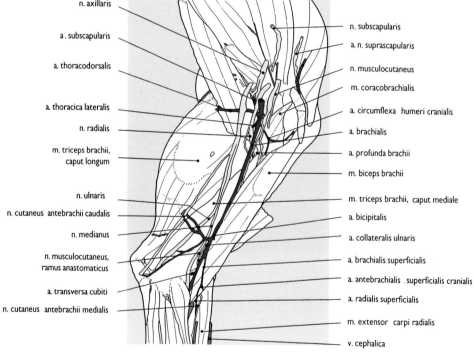

n. axillaris

a. subscapularis

a. thoracodorsalis

a. thoracica lateralis

n. radialis

m. triceps brachii, caput longum

n. ulnaris

n. cutaneus antebrachii caudalis

n. medianus

n. musculocutaneus, ramus anastomaticus

a. transversa cubiti

n. cutaneus antebrachii medialis

n. subscapularis

a. n. suprascapularis

n. musculocutaneus

m. coracobrachialis

a. circumflexa humeri cranialis

a. brachialis

a. profunda brachii

m. biceps brachii

m. triceps brachii, caput mediale

a. bicipitalis

a. collateralis ulnaris

a. brachialis superficialis

a. antebrachialis . superficialis cranialis

a. radialis superficialis

m. extensor carpi radialis

v. cephalica

Fig. 4.36 Left shoulder and brachium after removal of veins: medial view. Veins have been removed to expose more clearly the arteries and nerves of the medial shoulder and brachium.

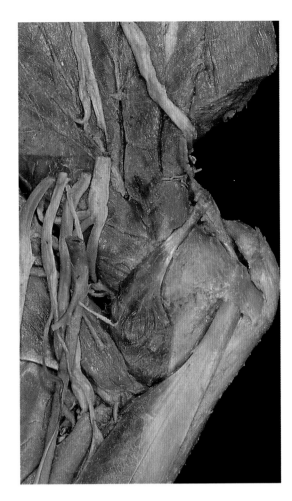

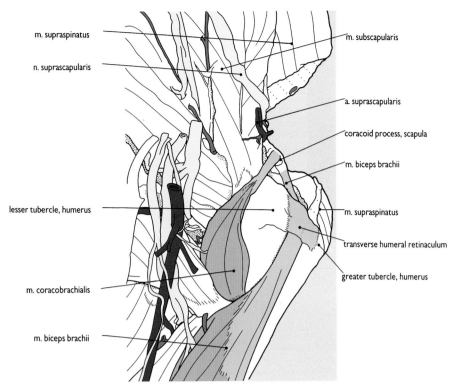

m. supraspinatus

n. suprascapularis

m. subscapularis

a. suprascapularis

coracoid process, scapula

m. biceps brachii

lesser tubercle, humerus

m. supraspinatus

transverse humeral retinaculum

greater tubercle, humerus

m. coracobrachialis

m. biceps brachii

Fig. 4.37 Left shoulder: medial view. Part of the supraspinatus muscle has been removed to expose the origins of the coracobrachialis and biceps brachii muscles.

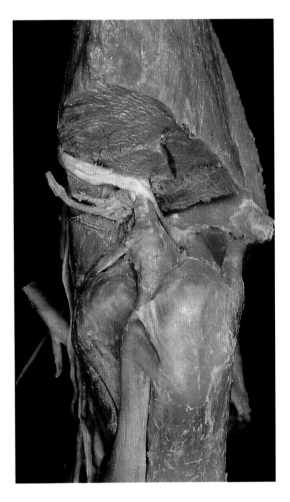

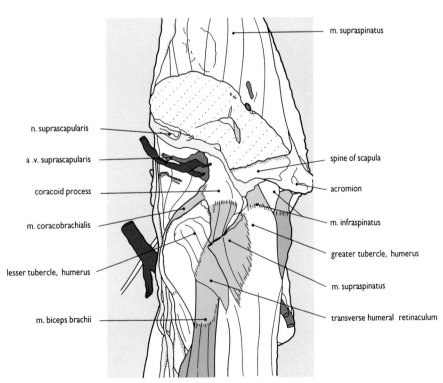

m. supraspinatus

n. suprascapularis

a .v. suprascapularis

spine of scapula

coracoid process

acromion

m. coracobrachialis

m. infraspinatus

greater tubercle, humerus

lesser tubercle, humerus

m. supraspinatus

m. biceps brachii

transverse humeral retinaculum

Fig. 4.38 Left shoulder: cranial view. Part of the supraspinatus muscle has been removed. The origin of the coracobrachialis and biceps brachii muscles on the coracoid process can be seen. Notice also the course of the suprascapular nerve around the neck of the scapula, and of the branch to the infraspinatus muscle around the distal border of the spine of the scapula.

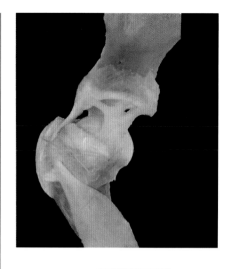

Fig. 4.39 Left shoulder joint: medial view.

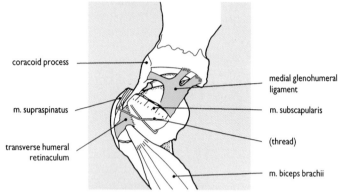

coracoid process

medial glenohumeral ligament

m. supraspinatus

m. subscapularis

transverse humeral retinaculum

(thread)

m. biceps brachii

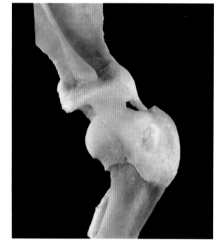

Fig. 4.40 Left shoulder joint: lateral view. Both the lateral and medial glenohumeral ligaments are weak. The joint is largely stabilized by muscles functioning as active collateral ligaments.

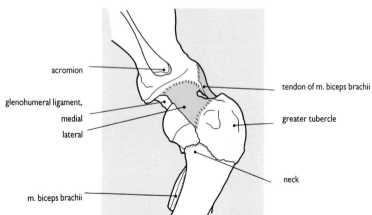

acromion

glenohumeral ligament,

medial

lateral

m. biceps brachii

tendon of m. biceps brachii

greater tubercle

neck

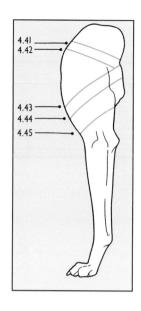

4.41
4.42

4.43
4.44
4.45

Figs 4.41–4.45 Transverse sections through the left scapular and brachial regions at the levels indicated in the above drawing: view of proximal surface of sections.

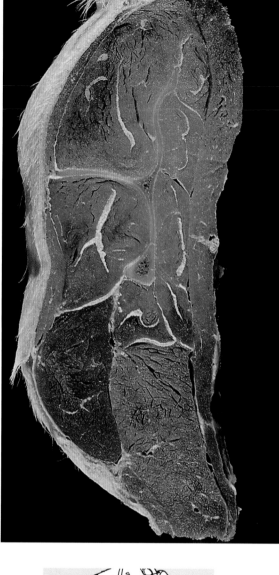

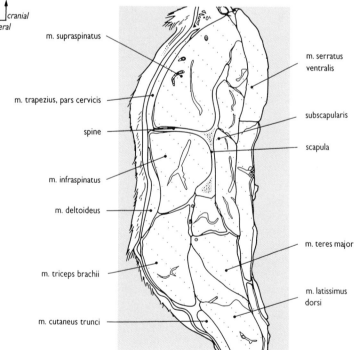

cranial
lateral

m. supraspinatus

m. trapezius, pars cervicis

spine

m. infraspinatus

m. deltoideus

m. triceps brachii

m. cutaneus trunci

m. serratus ventralis

subscapularis

scapula

m. teres major

m. latissimus dorsi

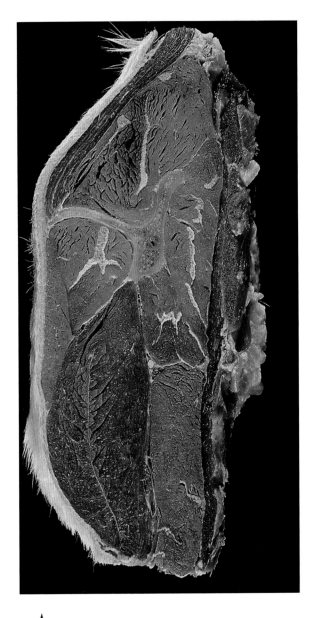

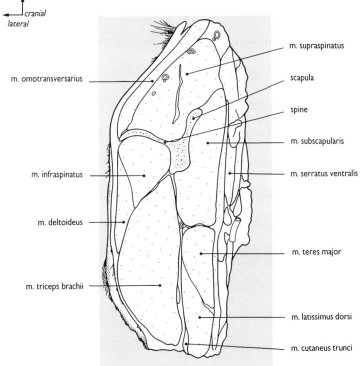

↑ cranial
← lateral

m. omotransversarius

m. infraspinatus

m. deltoideus

m. triceps brachii

m. supraspinatus

scapula

spine

m. subscapularis

m. serratus ventralis

m. teres major

m. latissimus dorsi

m. cutaneus trunci

Fig. 4.42

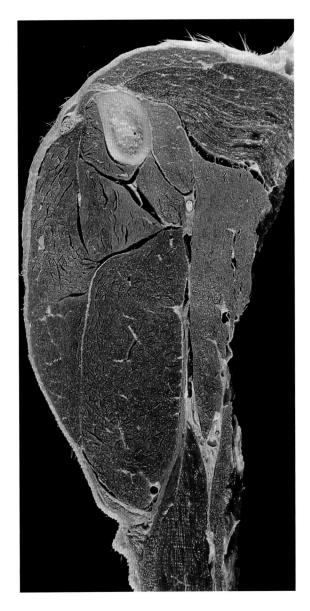

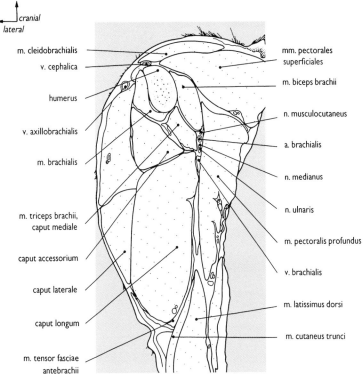

↑ cranial
← lateral

m. cleidobrachialis

v. cephalica

humerus

v. axillobrachialis

m. brachialis

m. triceps brachii,
caput mediale

caput accessorium

caput laterale

caput longum

m. tensor fasciae
antebrachii

mm. pectorales
superficiales

m. biceps brachii

n. musculocutaneus

a. brachialis

n. medianus

n. ulnaris

m. pectoralis profundus

v. brachialis

m. latissimus dorsi

m. cutaneus trunci

Fig. 4.43

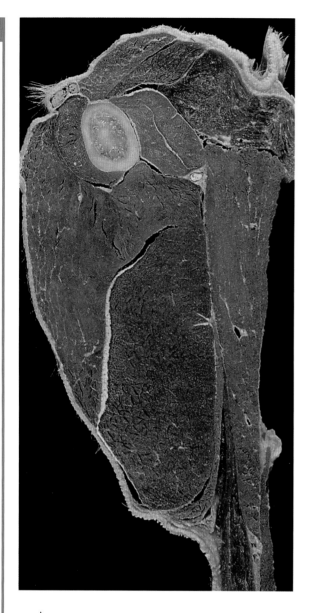

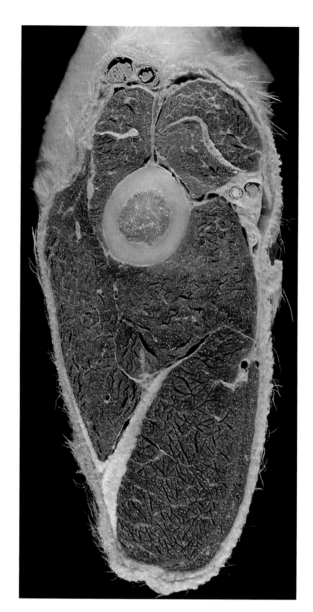

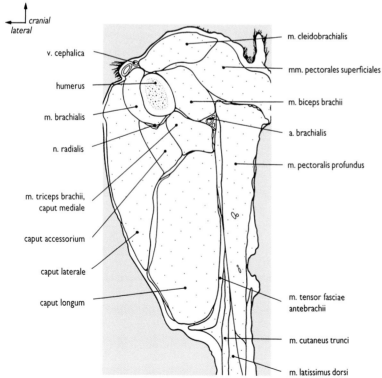

cranial
lateral

v. cephalica

humerus

m. brachialis

n. radialis

m. triceps brachii,
caput mediale

caput accessorium

caput laterale

caput longum

m. cleidobrachialis

mm. pectorales superficiales

m. biceps brachii

a. brachialis

m. pectoralis profundus

m. tensor fasciae
antebrachii

m. cutaneus trunci

m. latissimus dorsi

Fig. 4.44

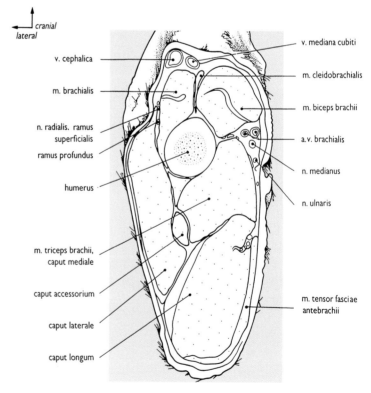

cranial
lateral

v. cephalica

m. brachialis

n. radialis, ramus
superficialis

ramus profundus

humerus

m. triceps brachii,
caput mediale

caput accessorium

caput laterale

caput longum

v. mediana cubiti

m. cleidobrachialis

m. biceps brachii

a.v. brachialis

n. medianus

n. ulnaris

m. tensor fasciae
antebrachii

Fig. 4.45

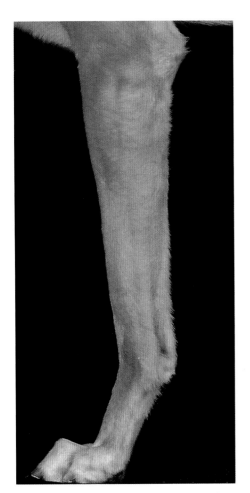

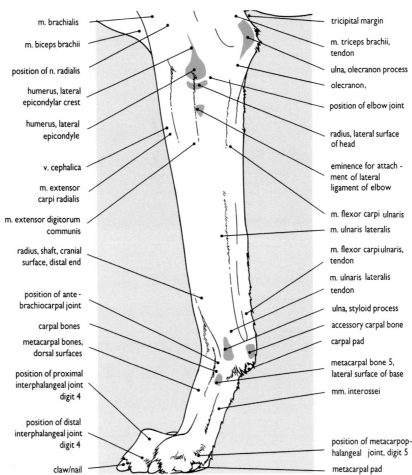

m. brachialis
m. biceps brachii
position of n. radialis
humerus, lateral epicondylar crest
humerus, lateral epicondyle
v. cephalica
m. extensor carpi radialis
m. extensor digitorum communis
radius, shaft, cranial surface, distal end
position of ante-brachiocarpal joint
carpal bones
metacarpal bones, dorsal surfaces
position of proximal interphalangeal joint digit 4
position of distal interphalangeal joint digit 4
claw/nail

tricipital margin
m. triceps brachii, tendon
ulna, olecranon process
olecranon,
position of elbow joint
radius, lateral surface of head
eminence for attachment of lateral ligament of elbow
m. flexor carpi ulnaris
m. ulnaris lateralis
m. flexor carpi ulnaris, tendon
m. ulnaris lateralis tendon
ulna, styloid process
accessory carpal bone
carpal pad
metacarpal bone 5, lateral surface of base
mm. interossei
position of metacarpophalangeal joint, digit 5
metacarpal pad

Fig. 4.46 Surface features of the antebrachium and manus: left lateral view. Palpable and visible features are indicated.

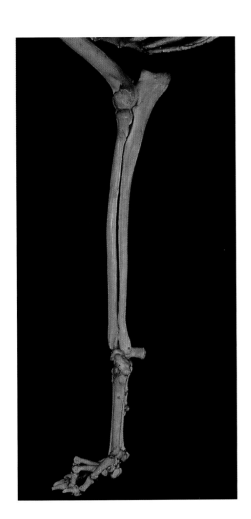

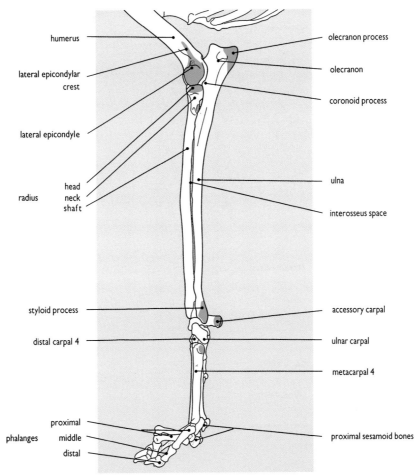

humerus
lateral epicondylar crest
lateral epicondyle
radius — head / neck / shaft
styloid process
distal carpal 4
phalanges — proximal / middle / distal

olecranon process
olecranon
coronoid process
ulna
interosseus space
accessory carpal
ulnar carpal
metacarpal 4
proximal sesamoid bones

Fig. 4.47 Skeleton of the antebrachium and manus: left lateral view. The features colored green correspond to the palpable bony features shown in the previous figure (Fig. 4.46).

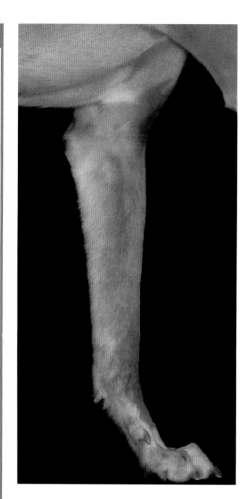

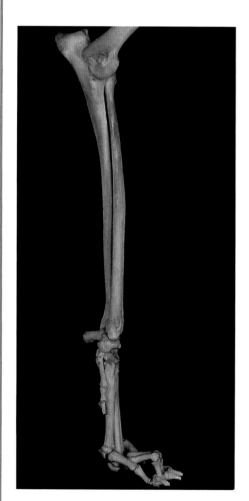

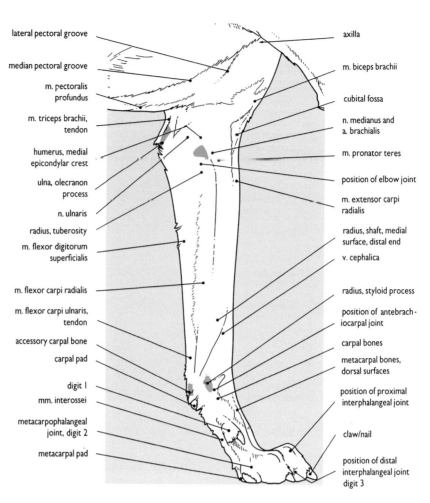

lateral pectoral groove
median pectoral groove
m. pectoralis profundus
m. triceps brachii, tendon
humerus, medial epicondylar crest
ulna, olecranon process
n. ulnaris
radius, tuberosity
m. flexor digitorum superficialis
m. flexor carpi radialis
m. flexor carpi ulnaris, tendon
accessory carpal bone
carpal pad
digit 1
mm. interossei
metacarpophalangeal joint, digit 2
metacarpal pad

axilla
m. biceps brachii
cubital fossa
n. medianus and a. brachialis
m. pronator teres
position of elbow joint
m. extensor carpi radialis
radius, shaft, medial surface, distal end
v. cephalica
radius, styloid process
position of antebrachiocarpal joint
carpal bones
metacarpal bones, dorsal surfaces
position of proximal interphalangeal joint
claw/nail
position of distal interphalangeal joint digit 3

Fig. 4.48 Surface features of the antebrachium and manus: left medial view. Palpable and visible features are indicated.

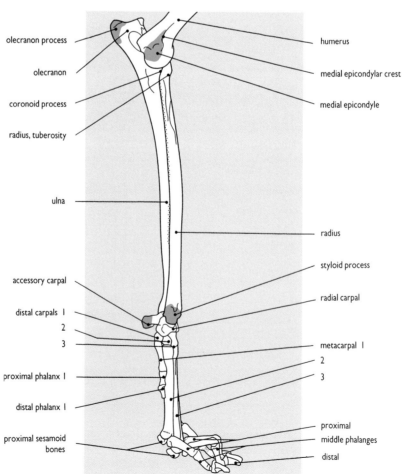

olecranon process
olecranon
coronoid process
radius, tuberosity
ulna
accessory carpal
distal carpals 1
2
3
proximal phalanx 1
distal phalanx 1
proximal sesamoid bones

humerus
medial epicondylar crest
medial epicondyle
radius
styloid process
radial carpal
metacarpal 1
2
3
proximal
middle phalanges
distal

Fig. 4.49 Skeleton of the antebrachium and manus: left medial view. The features colored green correspond to the palpable bony features shown in the previous figure (Fig. 4.48).

Fig. 4.50 Superficial fascia of the antebrachium and manus: left lateral view. The superficial fascia of the antebrachium is thinner and less movable than the more proximal superficial fascia. It contains many cutaneous vessels and nerves. The deep fascia of the antebrachium is closely applied to the muscles (although less so over flexor muscles) and sends septa between the muscles to the radius and ulna. The antebrachial fascia is thickest medially. At the carpus the antebrachial fascia becomes the fascia of the manus. This fascia forms a sheath around all tendons, and is attached to all pads and projecting bones.

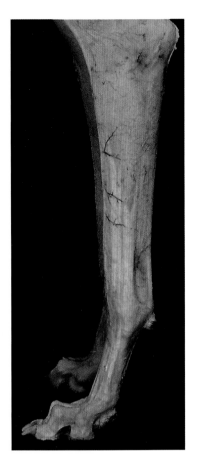

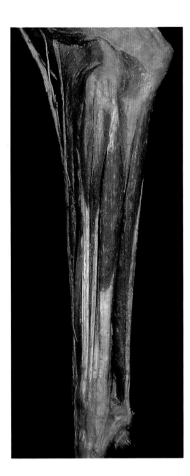

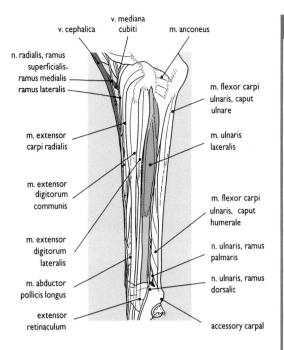

Fig. 4.51 Antebrachium: left lateral view. Only the fascia has been removed, although the extensor retinaculum remains in place.

v. mediana cubiti

v. cephalica

m. anconeus

n. radialis, ramus superficialis, ramus medialis, ramus lateralis

m. flexor carpi ulnaris, caput ulnare

m. extensor carpi radialis

m. ulnaris lateralis

m. extensor digitorum communis

m. flexor carpi ulnaris, caput humerale

m. extensor digitorum lateralis

n. ulnaris, ramus palmaris

m. abductor pollicis longus

n. ulnaris, ramus dorsalis

extensor retinaculum

accessory carpal

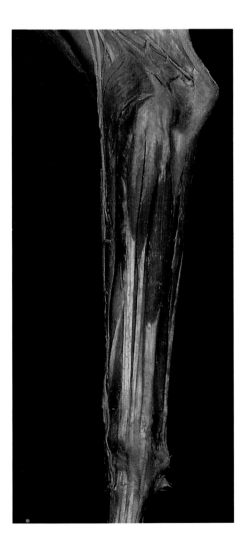

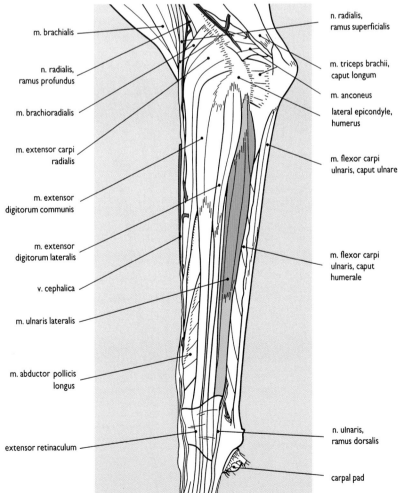

Fig. 4.52 Antebrachium: left lateral view. The cephalic vein has been removed proximally.

m. brachialis

n. radialis, ramus superficialis

n. radialis, ramus profundus

m. triceps brachii, caput longum

m. brachioradialis

m. anconeus

m. extensor carpi radialis

lateral epicondyle, humerus

m. flexor carpi ulnaris, caput ulnare

m. extensor digitorum communis

m. extensor digitorum lateralis

v. cephalica

m. flexor carpi ulnaris, caput humerale

m. ulnaris lateralis

m. abductor pollicis longus

n. ulnaris, ramus dorsalis

extensor retinaculum

carpal pad

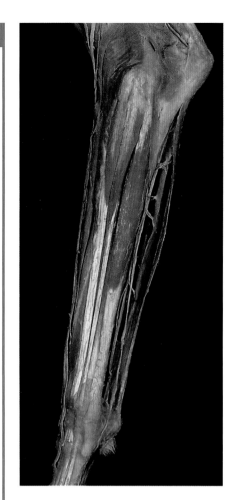
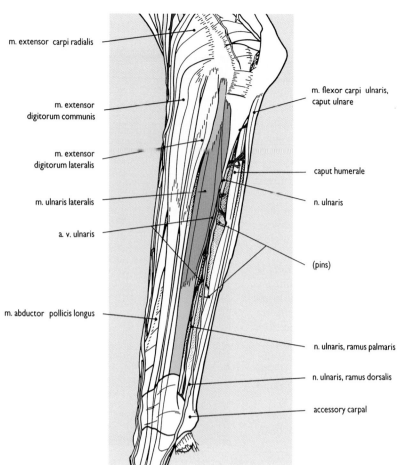

m. extensor carpi radialis

m. extensor
digitorum communis

m. extensor
digitorum lateralis

m. ulnaris lateralis

a. v. ulnaris

m. abductor pollicis longus

m. flexor carpi ulnaris,
caput ulnare

caput humerale

n. ulnaris

(pins)

n. ulnaris, ramus palmaris

n. ulnaris, ramus dorsalis

accessory carpal

Fig. 4.53 Antebrachium showing ulnar nerve: left lateral view. The ulnar carpal flexor has been separated from the lateral ulnar muscle in order to expose the ulnar nerve.

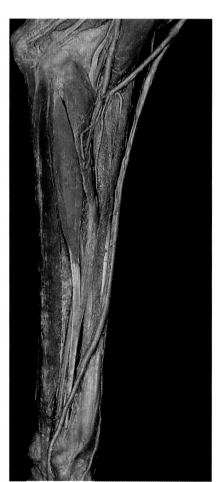
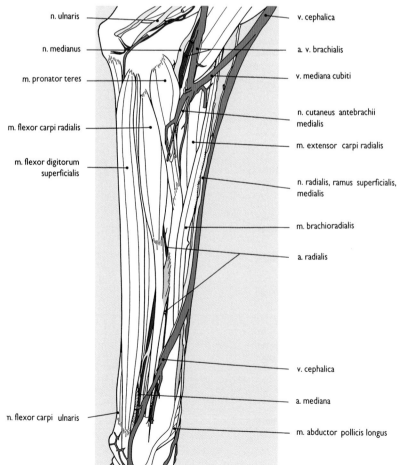

n. ulnaris

n. medianus

m. pronator teres

m. flexor carpi radialis

m. flexor digitorum
superficialis

n. flexor carpi ulnaris

v. cephalica

a. v. brachialis

v. mediana cubiti

n. cutaneus antebrachii
medialis

m. extensor carpi radialis

n. radialis, ramus superficialis,
medialis

m. brachioradialis

a. radialis

v. cephalica

a. mediana

m. abductor pollicis longus

Fig. 4.54 Antebrachium: left medial view. Only the fascia has been removed.

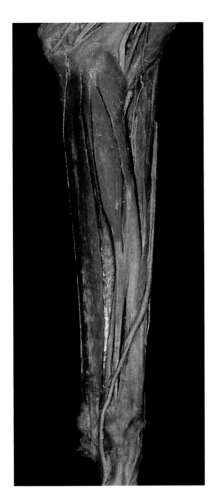

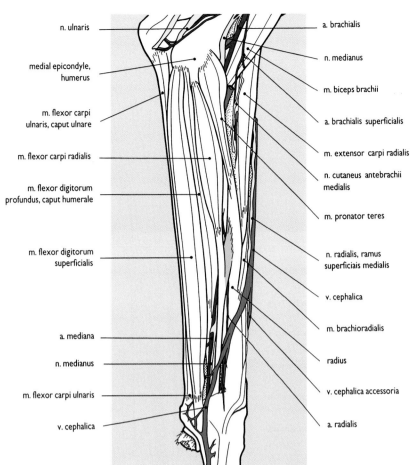

n. ulnaris

medial epicondyle, humerus

m. flexor carpi ulnaris, caput ulnare

m. flexor carpi radialis

m. flexor digitorum profundus, caput humerale

m. flexor digitorum superficialis

a. mediana

n. medianus

m. flexor carpi ulnaris

v. cephalica

a. brachialis

n. medianus

m. biceps brachii

a. brachialis superficialis

m. extensor carpi radialis

n. cutaneus antebrachii medialis

m. pronator teres

n. radialis, ramus superficiais medialis

v. cephalica

m. brachioradialis

radius

v. cephalica accessoria

a. radialis

Fig. 4.55 Antebrachium after removal of superficial veins: left medial view. The proximal cephalic, median and median cubital veins have been removed.

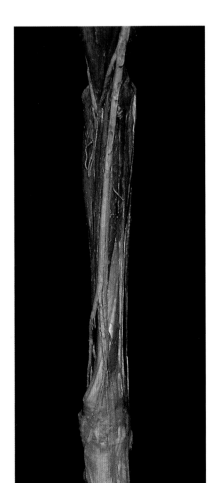

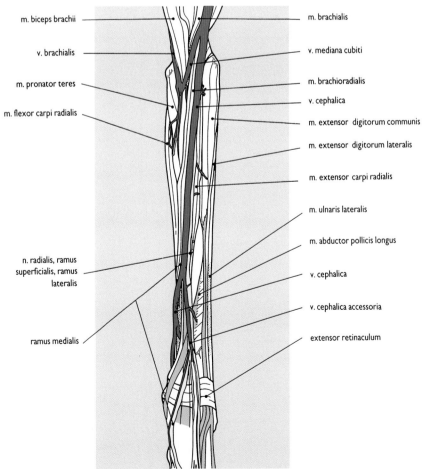

m. biceps brachii

v. brachialis

m. pronator teres

m. flexor carpi radialis

n. radialis, ramus superficialis, ramus lateralis

ramus medialis

m. brachialis

v. mediana cubiti

m. brachioradialis

v. cephalica

m. extensor digitorum communis

m. extensor digitorum lateralis

m. extensor carpi radialis

m. ulnaris lateralis

m. abductor pollicis longus

v. cephalica

v. cephalica accessoria

extensor retinaculum

Fig. 4.56 Left antebrachium: cranial view. Only the fascia has been removed.

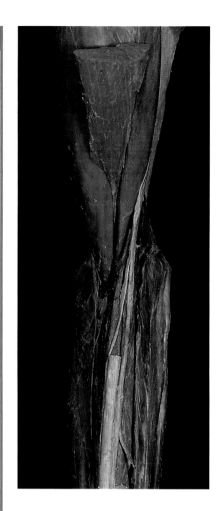

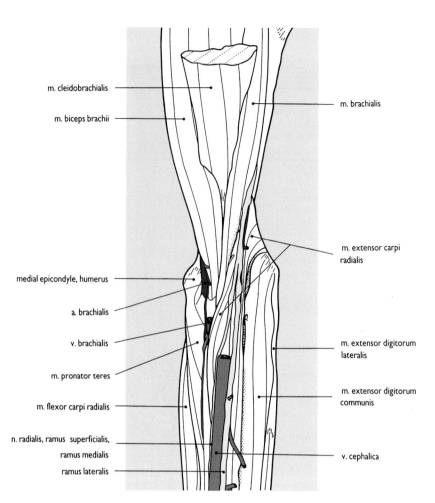

m. cleidobrachialis

m. biceps brachii

m. brachialis

m. extensor carpi radialis

medial epicondyle, humerus

a. brachialis

v. brachialis

m. pronator teres

m. flexor carpi radialis

n. radialis, ramus superficialis, ramus medialis

ramus lateralis

m. extensor digitorum lateralis

m. extensor digitorum communis

v. cephalica

Fig. 4.57 Left elbow after removal of veins: cranial view. The course of the lateral and medial branches of the superficial radial nerve can be clearly seen.

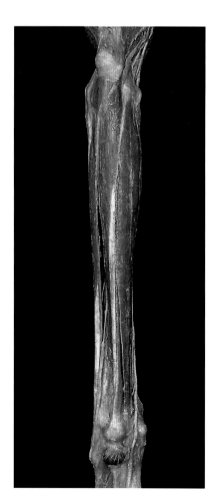

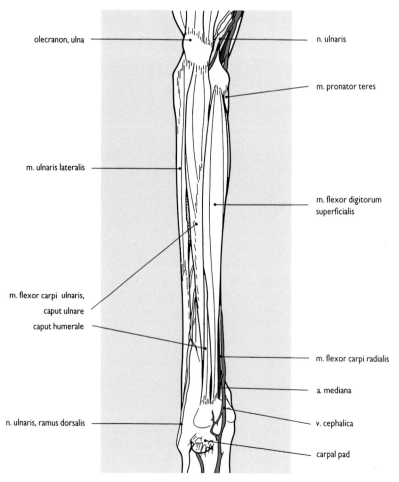

olecranon, ulna

n. ulnaris

m. pronator teres

m. ulnaris lateralis

m. flexor digitorum superficialis

m. flexor carpi ulnaris, caput ulnare

caput humerale

m. flexor carpi radialis

a. mediana

v. cephalica

n. ulnaris, ramus dorsalis

carpal pad

Fig. 4.58 Left antebrachium: caudal view. Only the fascia has been removed.

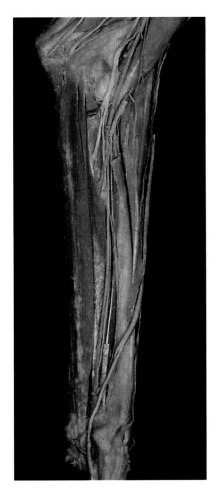

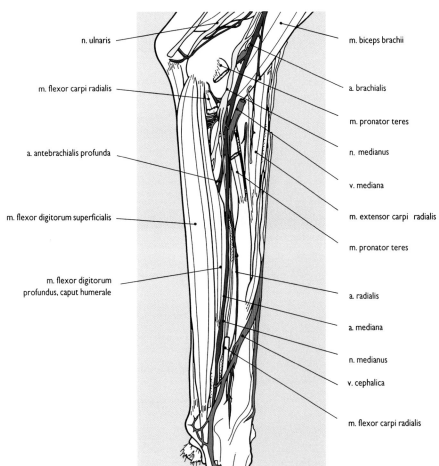

n. ulnaris

m. flexor carpi radialis

a. antebrachialis profunda

m. flexor digitorum superficialis

m. flexor digitorum profundus, caput humerale

m. biceps brachii

a. brachialis

m. pronator teres

n. medianus

v. mediana

m. extensor carpi radialis

m. pronator teres

a. radialis

a. mediana

n. medianus

v. cephalica

m. flexor carpi radialis

Fig. 4.59 Antebrachium after removal of pronator teres and radial carpal flexor muscles: left medial views. The passage of the median vessels and nerve deep to the pronator teres muscle can be seen.

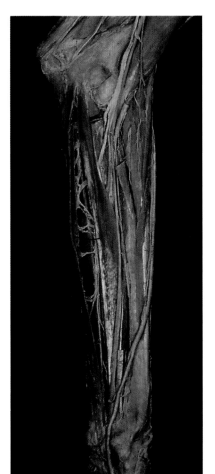

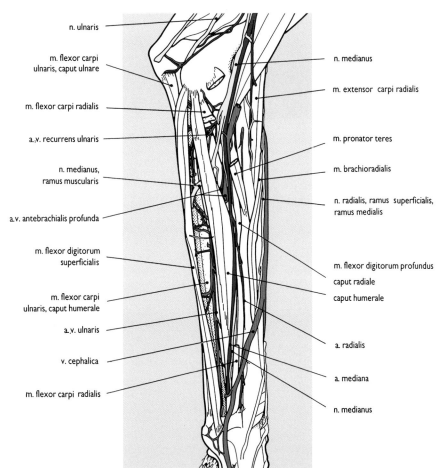

n. ulnaris

m. flexor carpi ulnaris, caput ulnare

m. flexor carpi radialis

a.,v. recurrens ulnaris

n. medianus, ramus muscularis

a.v. antebrachialis profunda

m. flexor digitorum superficialis

m. flexor carpi ulnaris, caput humerale

a.,v. ulnaris

v. cephalica

m. flexor carpi radialis

n. medianus

m. extensor carpi radialis

m. pronator teres

m. brachioradialis

n. radialis, ramus superficialis, ramus medialis

m. flexor digitorum profundus
caput radiale
caput humerale

a. radialis

a. mediana

n. medianus

Fig. 4.60 Antebrachium showing ulnar vessels: left medial view. The superficial and deep digital flexor muscles have been separated in order to expose the ulnar vessels (which anastomose with the deep antebrachial vessels).

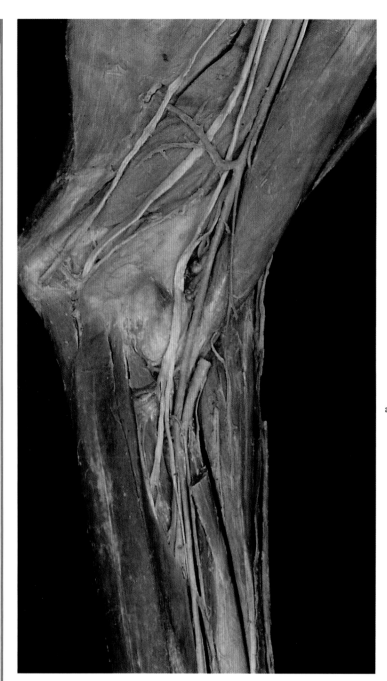

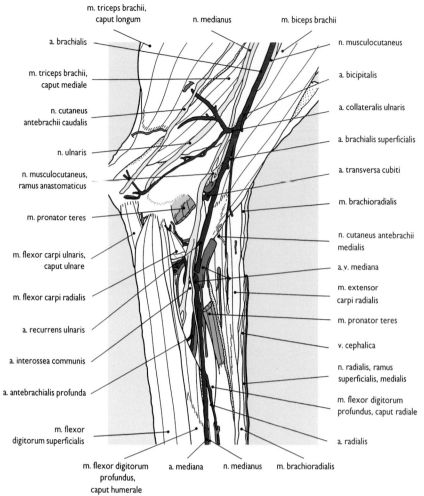

m. triceps brachii, caput longum

n. medianus

m. biceps brachii

a. brachialis

n. musculocutaneus

m. triceps brachii, caput mediale

a. bicipitalis

n. cutaneus antebrachii caudalis

a. collateralis ulnaris

a. brachialis superficialis

n. ulnaris

a. transversa cubiti

n. musculocutaneus, ramus anastomaticus

m. brachioradialis

m. pronator teres

n. cutaneus antebrachii medialis

m. flexor carpi ulnaris, caput ulnare

a. v. mediana

m. extensor carpi radialis

m. flexor carpi radialis

m. pronator teres

a. recurrens ulnaris

v. cephalica

a. interossea communis

n. radialis, ramus superficialis, medialis

a. antebrachialis profunda

m. flexor digitorum profundus, caput radiale

m. flexor digitorum superficialis

a. radialis

m. flexor digitorum profundus, caput humerale

a. mediana

n. medianus

m. brachioradialis

Fig. 4.61 Elbow after removal of pronator teres and radial carpal flexor muscles: left medial view. This is a closer view of part of the dissection shown in the previous figure (Fig. 4.60). The connection between the musculocutaneous and median nerves just above the elbow can be seen, as well as all the major branches of the brachial and median arteries in this region. Most of the median and cephalic veins have been removed.

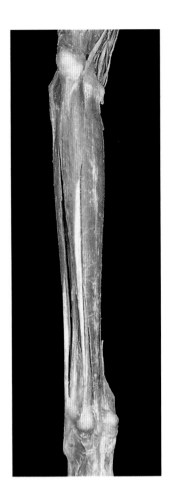

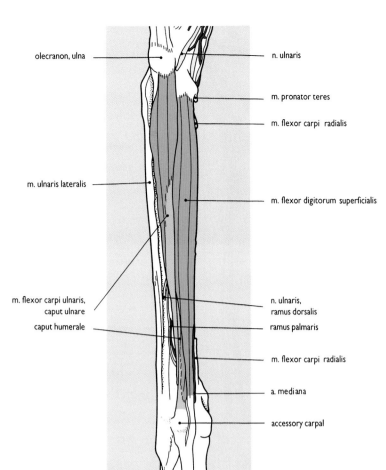

olecranon, ulna

m. pronator teres

m. flexor carpi radialis

m. ulnaris lateralis

m. flexor digitorum superficialis

n. ulnaris

n. ulnaris,
ramus dorsalis

ramus palmaris

m. flexor carpi ulnaris,
caput ulnare

caput humerale

m. flexor carpi radialis

a. mediana

accessory carpal

Fig. 4.62 Left antebrachium after removal of cephalic vein: caudal view. The pronator teres and radial carpal flexor muscles have also been removed, as well as the carpal pad and the dorsal branch of the ulnar nerve.

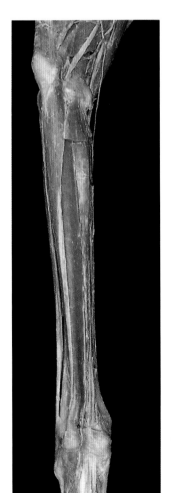

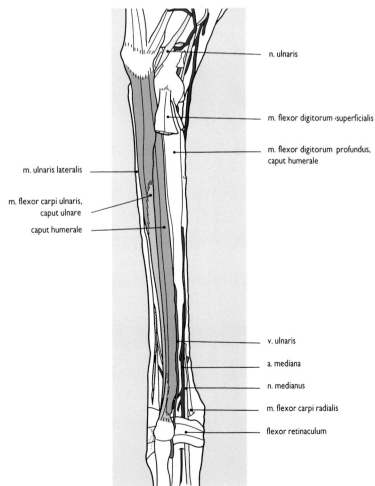

n. ulnaris

m. flexor digitorum superficialis

m. flexor digitorum profundus,
caput humerale

m. ulnaris lateralis

m. flexor carpi ulnaris,
caput ulnare

caput humerale

v. ulnaris

a. mediana

n. medianus

m. flexor carpi radialis

flexor retinaculum

Fig. 4.63 Left antebrachium after removal of the superficial digital flexor muscle: caudal view. Notice the flexor retinaculum is deep to the superficial digital flexor muscle.

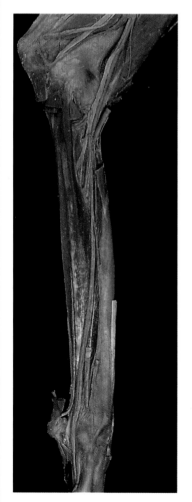

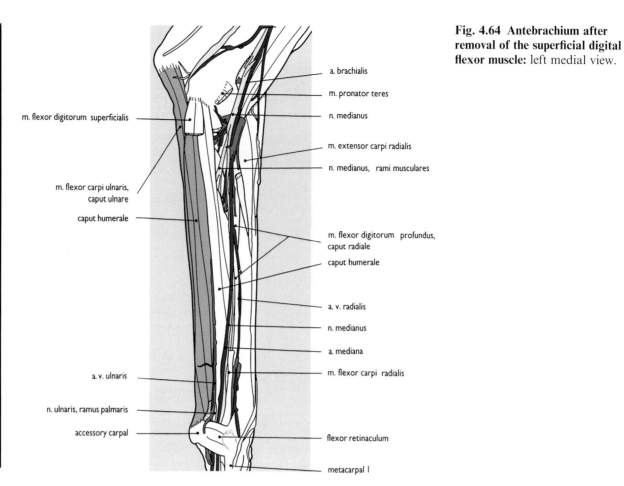

m. flexor digitorum superficialis

m. flexor carpi ulnaris, caput ulnare

caput humerale

a. v. ulnaris

n. ulnaris, ramus palmaris

accessory carpal

a. brachialis

m. pronator teres

n. medianus

m. extensor carpi radialis

n. medianus, rami musculares

m. flexor digitorum profundus, caput radiale

caput humerale

a. v. radialis

n. medianus

a. mediana

m. flexor carpi radialis

flexor retinaculum

metacarpal I

Fig. 4.64 Antebrachium after removal of the superficial digital flexor muscle: left medial view.

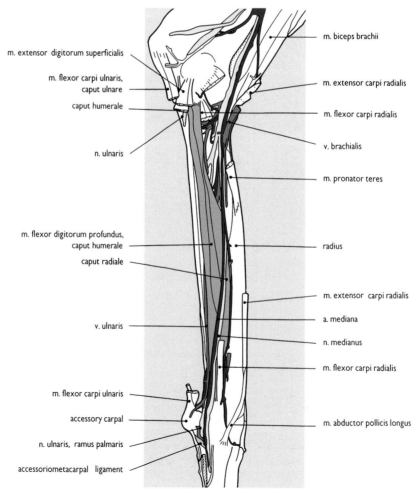

m. extensor digitorum superficialis

m. flexor carpi ulnaris, caput ulnare

caput humerale

n. ulnaris

m. flexor digitorum profundus, caput humerale

caput radiale

v. ulnaris

m. flexor carpi ulnaris

accessory carpal

n. ulnaris, ramus palmaris

accessoriometacarpal ligament

m. biceps brachii

m. extensor carpi radialis

m. flexor carpi radialis

v. brachialis

m. pronator teres

radius

m. extensor carpi radialis

a. mediana

n. medianus

m. flexor carpi radialis

m. abductor pollicis longus

Fig. 4.65 Antebrachium after removal of the ulnar carpal flexor muscle: left medial view. The flexor retinaculum has also been removed, as well as the radial carpal extensor muscle.

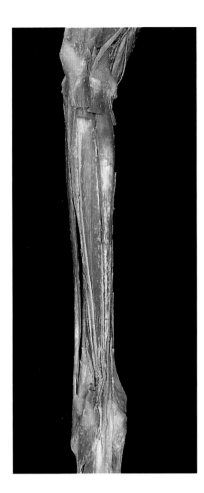

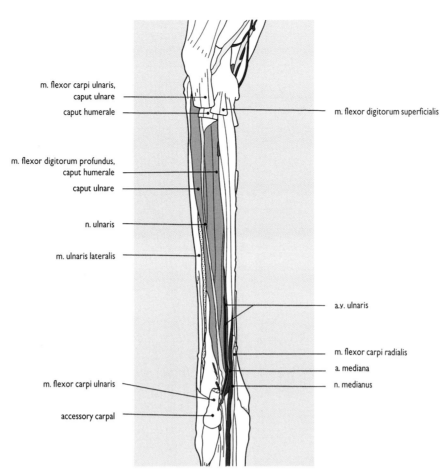

m. flexor carpi ulnaris, caput ulnare
caput humerale

m. flexor digitorum profundus, caput humerale
caput ulnare

n. ulnaris

m. ulnaris lateralis

m. flexor digitorum superficialis

a.v. ulnaris

m. flexor carpi radialis
a. mediana
n. medianus

m. flexor carpi ulnaris

accessory carpal

Fig. 4.66 Left antebrachium after removal of the ulnar carpal flexor muscle: caudal view. Removal of the flexor retinaculum exposes the median artery and nerve, and ulnar nerve, as they pass through the carpal canal.

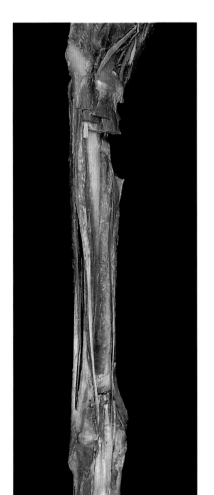

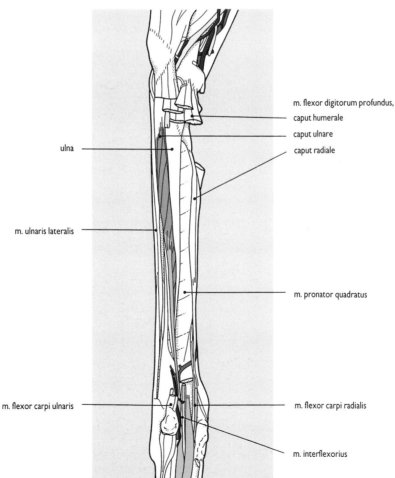

ulna

m. ulnaris lateralis

m. flexor carpi ulnaris

m. flexor digitorum profundus, caput humerale
caput ulnare
caput radiale

m. pronator quadratus

m. flexor carpi radialis

m. interflexorius

Fig. 4.67 Left antebrachium after removal of the humeral head of the deep digital flexor muscle: caudal view. The radial and ulnar heads of the deep digital flexor muscle are clearly visible, as is the pronator quadratus muscle between the radius and ulna.

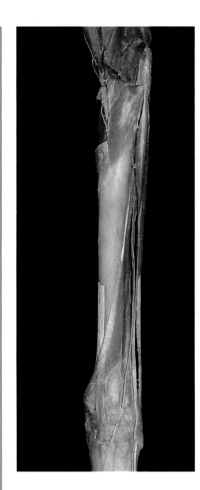

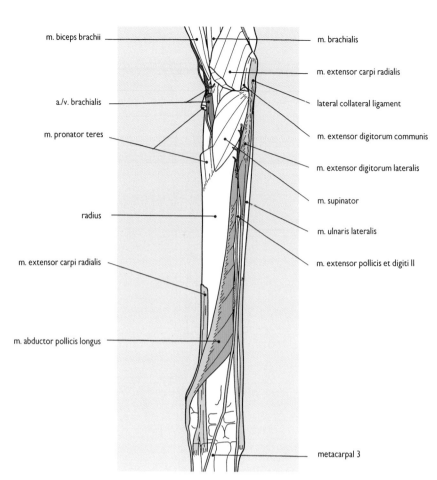

m. biceps brachii

m. brachialis

a./v. brachialis

m. extensor carpi radialis

m. pronator teres

lateral collateral ligament

m. extensor digitorum communis

m. extensor digitorum lateralis

radius

m. supinator

m. ulnaris lateralis

m. extensor carpi radialis

m. extensor pollicis et digiti II

m. abductor pollicis longus

metacarpal 3

Fig. 4.68 Left antebrachium after removal of the radial carpal extensor muscle: cranial view.

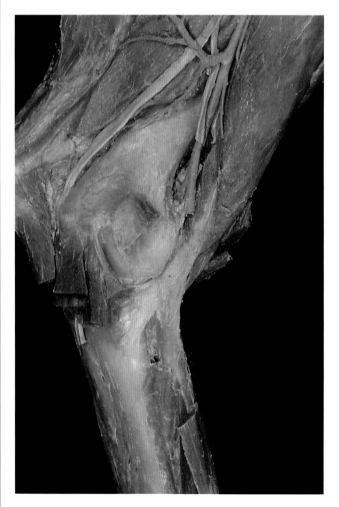

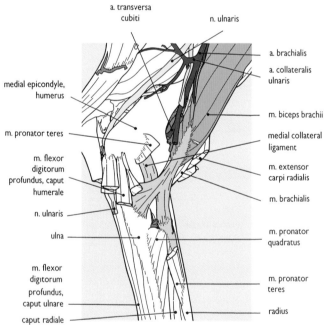

a. transversa cubiti

n. ulnaris

a. brachialis

a. collateralis ulnaris

medial epicondyle, humerus

m. biceps brachii

m. pronator teres

medial collateral ligament

m. flexor digitorum profundus, caput humerale

m. extensor carpi radialis

m. brachialis

n. ulnaris

m. pronator quadratus

ulna

m. flexor digitorum profundus, caput ulnare

m. pronator teres

caput radiale

radius

Fig. 4.69 Deep structures of the elbow region: left medial view. The dual insertion of the biceps brachii muscle on the radius and ulna can be seen in addition to the medial collateral ligament.

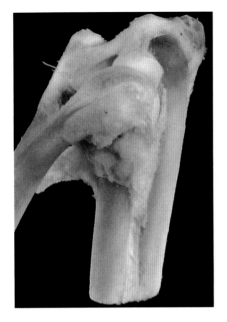

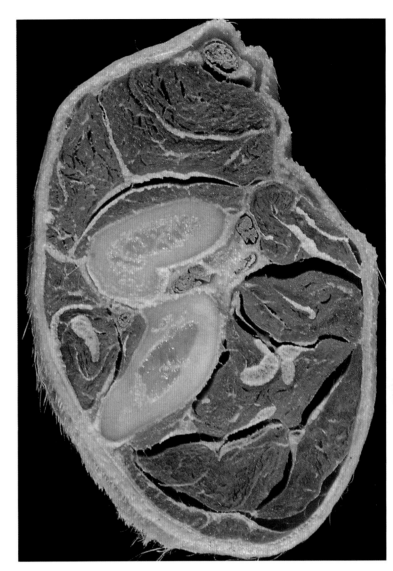

Fig. 4.70 Left elbow joint: lateral view. The olecranon ligament helps to dampen overflexion.

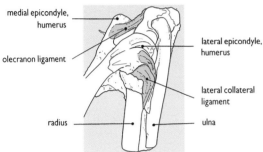

medial epicondyle, humerus

olecranon ligament

lateral epicondyle, humerus

lateral collateral ligament

radius

ulna

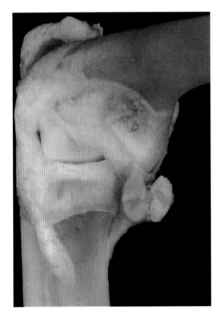

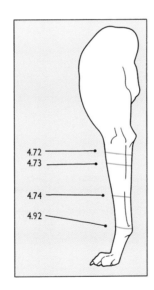

4.72
4.73

4.74

4.92

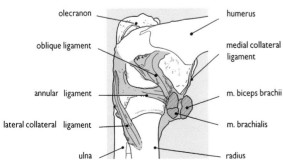

olecranon

oblique ligament

annular ligament

lateral collateral ligament

ulna

humerus

medial collateral ligament

m. biceps brachii

m. brachialis

radius

Fig. 4.71 Right elbow joint: cranial view. The annular ligament surrounds the head of the radius and the oblique ligament helps to dampen overextension.

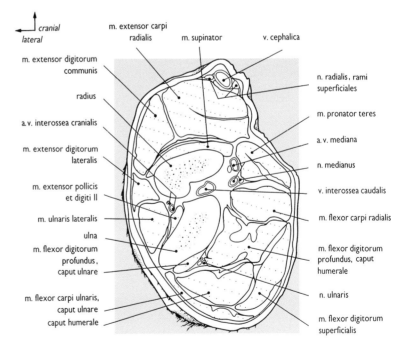

cranial
lateral

m. extensor carpi radialis

m. extensor digitorum communis

radius

a. v. interossea cranialis

m. extensor digitorum lateralis

m. extensor pollicis et digiti II

m. ulnaris lateralis

ulna

m. flexor digitorum profundus, caput ulnare

m. flexor carpi ulnaris, caput ulnare

caput humerale

m. supinator

v. cephalica

n. radialis, rami superficiales

m. pronator teres

a. v. mediana

n. medianus

v. interossea caudalis

m. flexor carpi radialis

m. flexor digitorum profundus, caput humerale

n. ulnaris

m. flexor digitorum superficialis

Figs. 4.72–4.74 Transverse sections through the left antebrachium at the levels indicated in the accompanying drawing: view of proximal surface of sections.

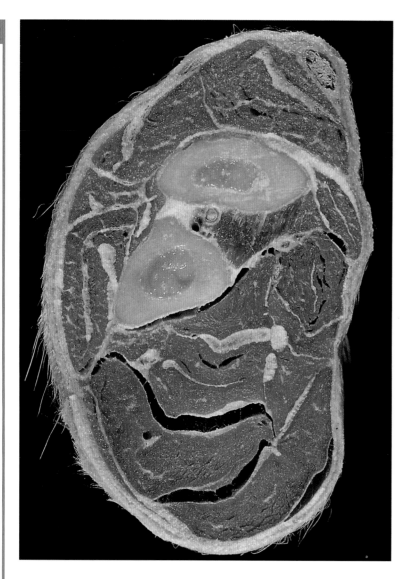

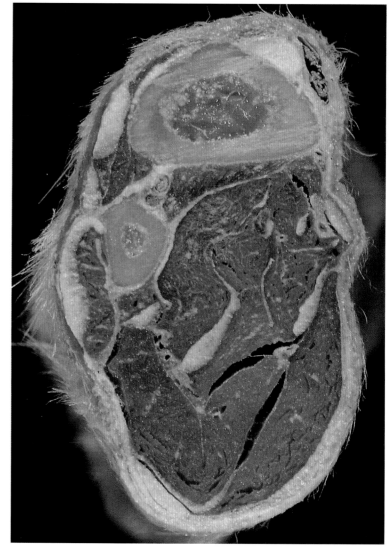

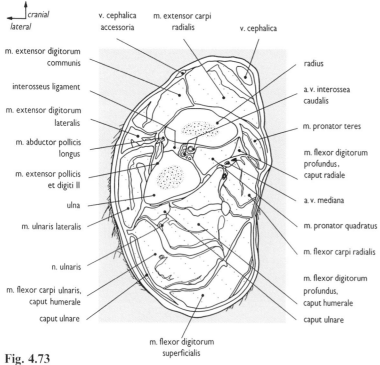

cranial
lateral

v. cephalica
accessoria

m. extensor carpi
radialis

v. cephalica

m. extensor digitorum
communis

interosseus ligament

m. extensor digitorum
lateralis

m. abductor pollicis
longus

m. extensor pollicis
et digiti II

ulna

m. ulnaris lateralis

n. ulnaris

m. flexor carpi ulnaris,
caput humerale

caput ulnare

radius

a. v. interossea
caudalis

m. pronator teres

m. flexor digitorum
profundus,
caput radiale

a. v. mediana

m. pronator quadratus

m. flexor carpi radialis

m. flexor digitorum
profundus,
caput humerale

caput ulnare

m. flexor digitorum
superficialis

Fig. 4.73

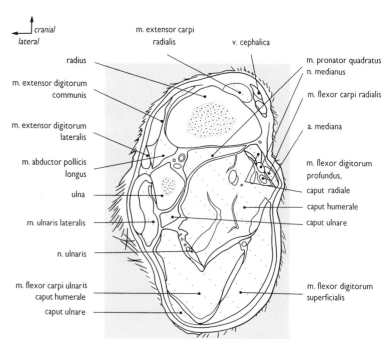

cranial
lateral

m. extensor carpi
radialis

v. cephalica

radius

m. extensor digitorum
communis

m. extensor digitorum
lateralis

m. abductor pollicis
longus

ulna

m. ulnaris lateralis

n. ulnaris

m. flexor carpi ulnaris
caput humerale

caput ulnare

m. pronator quadratus
n. medianus

m. flexor carpi radialis

a. mediana

m. flexor digitorum
profundus,
caput radiale

caput humerale

caput ulnare

m. flexor digitorum
superficialis

Fig. 4.74

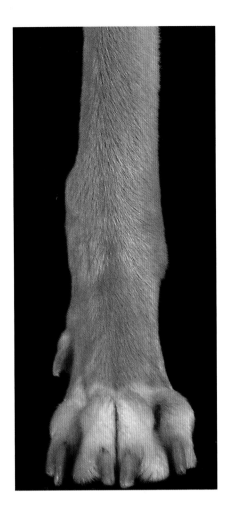

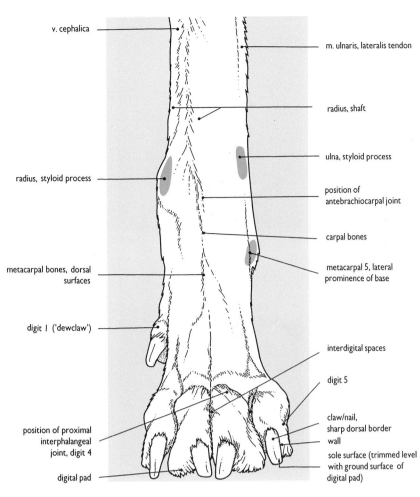

Fig. 4.75 Surface features of the left carpus and manus: dorsal view. Palpable and visible features are indicated.

v. cephalica

m. ulnaris, lateralis tendon

radius, shaft

ulna, styloid process

radius, styloid process

position of antebrachiocarpal joint

carpal bones

metacarpal 5, lateral prominence of base

metacarpal bones, dorsal surfaces

digit I ('dewclaw')

interdigital spaces

digit 5

claw/nail, sharp dorsal border

wall

sole surface (trimmed level with ground surface of digital pad)

position of proximal interphalangeal joint, digit 4

digital pad

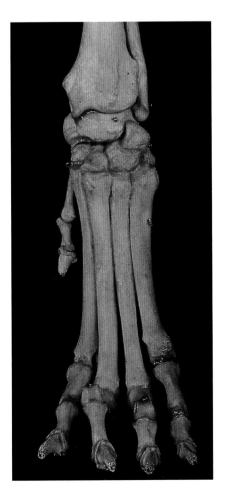

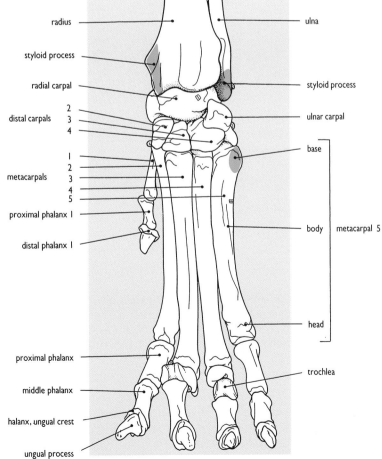

Fig. 4.76 Skeleton of the left carpus and manus: dorsal view. The features colored green correspond to the palpable bony features shown in the previous figure (Fig. 4.75).

radius

ulna

styloid process

styloid process

radial carpal

distal carpals 2 3 4

ulnar carpal

base

metacarpals 1 2 3 4 5

proximal phalanx I

body | metacarpal 5

distal phalanx I

head

proximal phalanx

middle phalanx

trochlea

halanx, ungual crest

ungual process

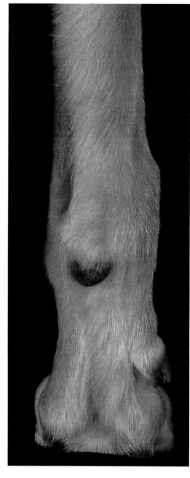

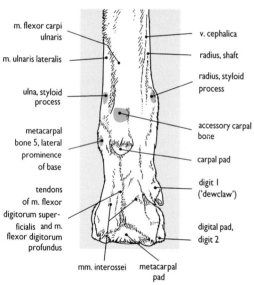

m. flexor carpi ulnaris

m. ulnaris lateralis

ulna, styloid process

metacarpal bone 5, lateral prominence of base

tendons of m. flexor digitorum superficialis and m. flexor digitorum profundus

mm. interossei   metacarpal pad

v. cephalica

radius, shaft

radius, styloid process

accessory carpal bone

carpal pad

digit I ('dewclaw')

digital pad, digit 2

Fig. 4.77 Surface features of the left carpus and manus: palmar view. Palpable and visible features are indicated.

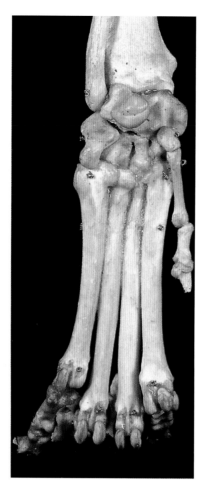

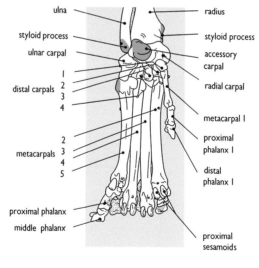

ulna

styloid process

ulnar carpal

distal carpals
1
2
3
4

metacarpals
2
3
4
5

proximal phalanx

middle phalanx

radius

styloid process

accessory carpal

radial carpal

metacarpal I

proximal phalanx I

distal phalanx I

proximal sesamoids

Fig. 4.78 Skeleton of the left carpus and manus: palmar view. The features colored green correspond to the palpable bony features shown in the previous figure (Fig. 4.77).

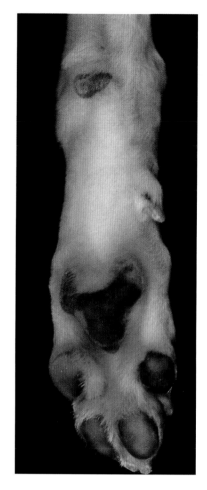

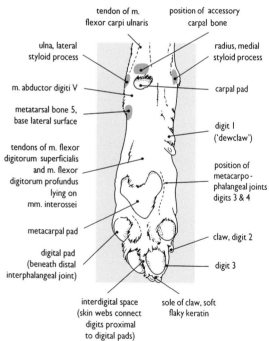

tendon of m. flexor carpi ulnaris

position of accessory carpal bone

ulna, lateral styloid process

m. abductor digiti V

metatarsal bone 5, base lateral surface

tendons of m. flexor digitorum superficialis and m. flexor digitorum profundus lying on mm. interossei

metacarpal pad

digital pad (beneath distal interphalangeal joint)

interdigital space (skin webs connect digits proximal to digital pads)

radius, medial styloid process

carpal pad

digit I ('dewclaw')

position of metacarpo-phalangeal joints digits 3 & 4

claw, digit 2

digit 3

sole of claw, soft flaky keratin

Fig. 4.79 Surface features of the left carpus and manus (manus off the ground): palmar view. Palpable and visible features are indicated.

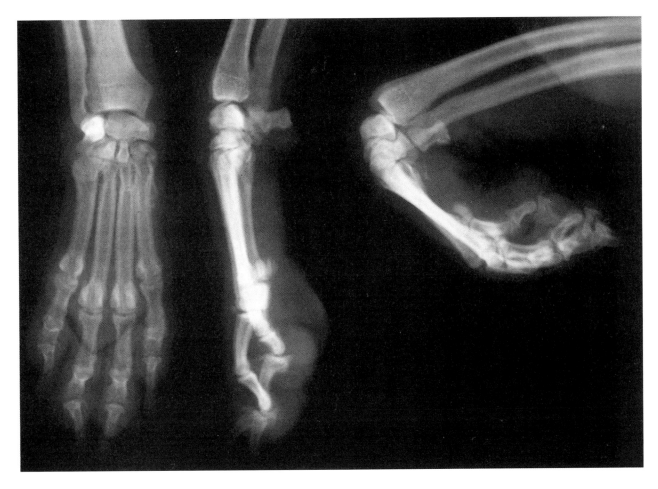

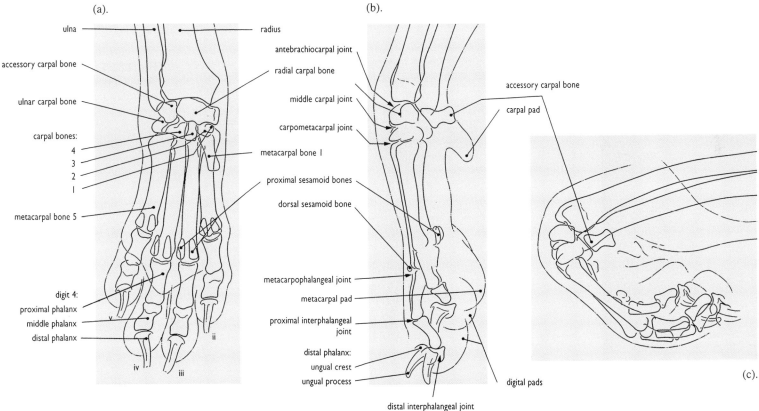

(a).

(b).

ulna

radius

accessory carpal bone

antebrachiocarpal joint

radial carpal bone

ulnar carpal bone

middle carpal joint

accessory carpal bone

carpal pad

carpal bones:

carpometacarpal joint

4

metacarpal bone I

3

2

I

proximal sesamoid bones

metacarpal bone 5

dorsal sesamoid bone

metacarpophalangeal joint

metacarpal pad

digit 4:

proximal phalanx

proximal interphalangeal

middle phalanx

joint

distal phalanx

distal phalanx:

ungual crest

ungual process

digital pads

(c).

distal interphalangeal joint

Fig. 4.80 Radiographs of the carpus and forepaw: dorsopalmar and lateral views. The major osteological features of the manus are shown, most comprehensively in the dorsopalmar view (a). It is only the prominent accessory carpal bone that is somewhat obscured, being superimposed on the image of the ulnar carpal bone. A dorsopalmar view also shows sesamoid bone distribution, especially the pair behind each metacarpophalangeal joint. The lateral view (b) gives a clearer picture of the disposition of carpal and forepaw joints and (c) shows the 'levels' at which movement occurs in the carpus. Most takes place at the antebrachiocarpal joint, less at the middle carpal joint and not to any noticeable extent at the carpometacarpal joints. The relationship of the metacarpal and digital pads to the underlying joints is also clearly demonstrated, as are the dorsal sesamoid bones of the metacarpophalangeal joints. In normal standing these joints are overextended and body weight is transferred to the metacarpal pads underlying them. When the paw is raised there is considerable flexion at these joints.

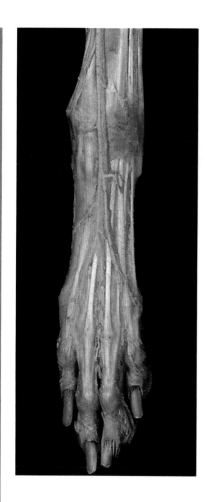

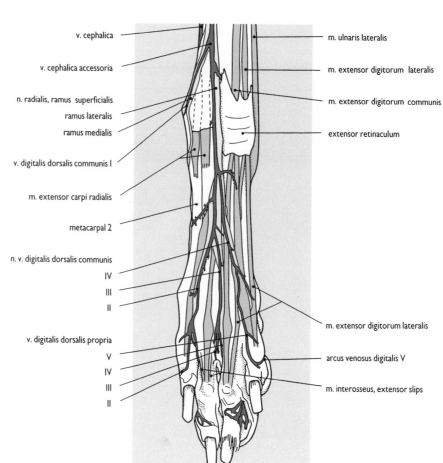

v. cephalica

v. cephalica accessoria

n. radialis, ramus superficialis

ramus lateralis

ramus medialis

v. digitalis dorsalis communis I

m. extensor carpi radialis

metacarpal 2

n. v. digitalis dorsalis communis

IV

III

II

v. digitalis dorsalis propria

V

IV

III

II

m. ulnaris lateralis

m. extensor digitorum lateralis

m. extensor digitorum communis

extensor retinaculum

m. extensor digitorum lateralis

arcus venosus digitalis V

m. interosseus, extensor slips

Fig. 4.81 Left manus: dorsal view. Only the fascia has been removed, although the extensor retinaculum remains in place. The manus used in this dissection, and in the next figure, was fixed with the foot off the ground (the digits are therefore not overextended at the mctacarpophalangcal joints).

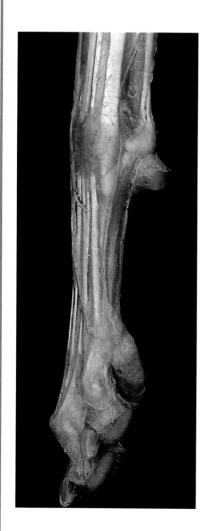

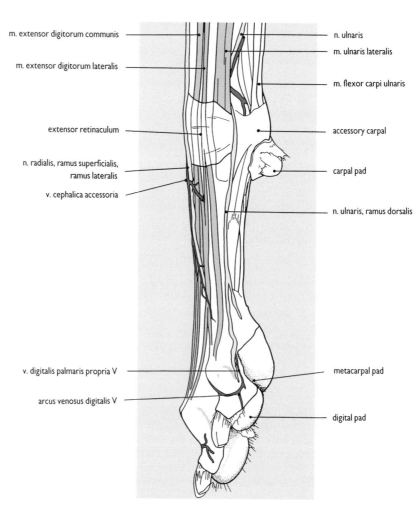

m. extensor digitorum communis

m. extensor digitorum lateralis

extensor retinaculum

n. radialis, ramus superficialis, ramus lateralis

v. cephalica accessoria

v. digitalis palmaris propria V

arcus venosus digitalis V

n. ulnaris

m. ulnaris lateralis

m. flexor carpi ulnaris

accessory carpal

carpal pad

n. ulnaris, ramus dorsalis

metacarpal pad

digital pad

Fig. 4.82 Left manus: lateral view. Only the fascia has been removed.

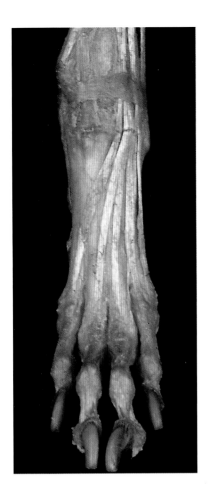

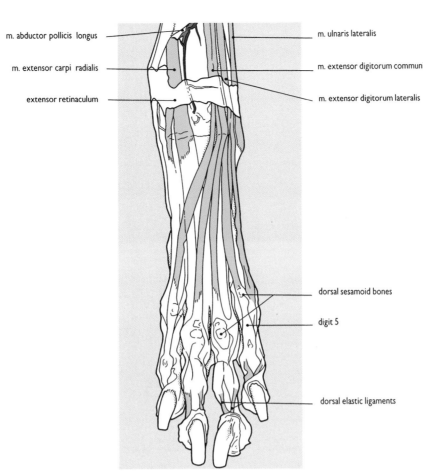

m. abductor pollicis longus

m. extensor carpi radialis

extensor retinaculum

m. ulnaris lateralis

m. extensor digitorum communis

m. extensor digitorum lateralis

dorsal sesamoid bones

digit 5

dorsal elastic ligaments

Fig. 4.83 Left manus after removal of the accessory cephalic vein and superficial radial nerves: dorsal view.

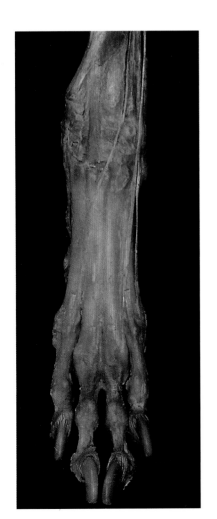

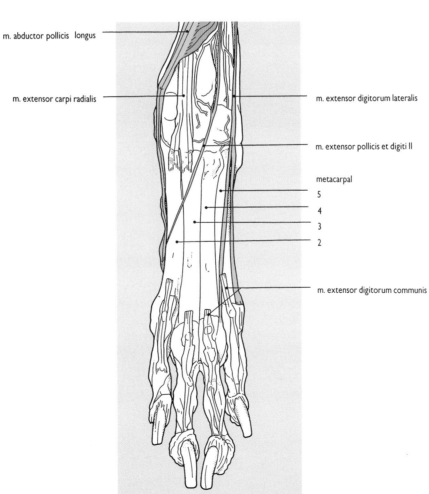

m. abductor pollicis longus

m. extensor carpi radialis

m. extensor digitorum lateralis

m. extensor pollicis et digiti II

metacarpal

5

4

3

2

m. extensor digitorum communis

Fig. 4.84 Left manus after removal of the common digital extensor tendons: dorsal view. The lateral digital extensor muscle would more commonly insert on digit 3, as well as digits 4 and 5.

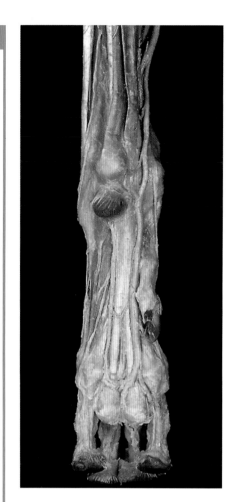

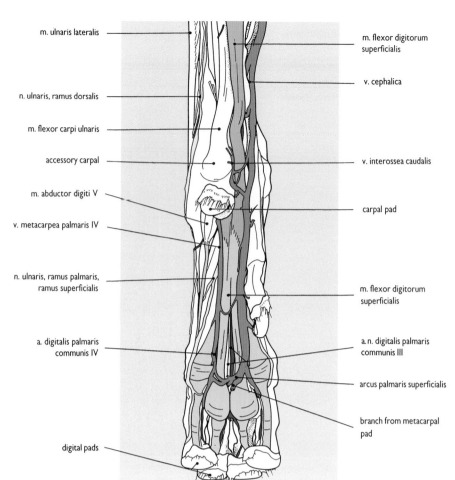

m. ulnaris lateralis

m. flexor digitorum superficialis

n. ulnaris, ramus dorsalis

v. cephalica

m. flexor carpi ulnaris

accessory carpal

v. interossea caudalis

m. abductor digiti V

carpal pad

v. metacarpea palmaris IV

n. ulnaris, ramus palmaris, ramus superficialis

m. flexor digitorum superficialis

a. digitalis palmaris communis IV

a.n. digitalis palmaris communis III

arcus palmaris superficialis

branch from metacarpal pad

digital pads

Fig. 4.85 Left manus: palmar view. Only the fascia and the metacarpal pad have been removed.

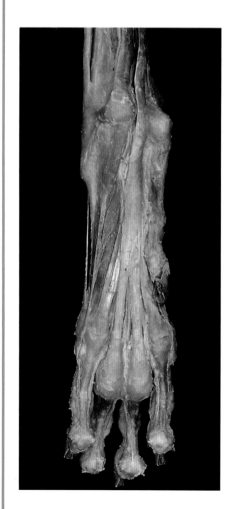

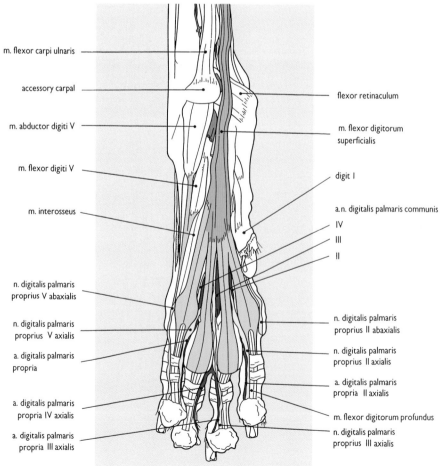

m. flexor carpi ulnaris

accessory carpal

flexor retinaculum

m. abductor digiti V

m. flexor digitorum superficialis

m. flexor digiti V

digit I

m. interosseus

a.n. digitalis palmaris communis

IV

III

II

n. digitalis palmaris proprius V abaxialis

n. digitalis palmaris proprius II abaxialis

n. digitalis palmaris proprius V axialis

n. digitalis palmaris proprius II axialis

a. digitalis palmaris propria

a. digitalis palmaris propria II axialis

m. flexor digitorum profundus

a. digitalis palmaris propria IV axialis

n. digitalis palmaris proprius III axialis

a. digitalis palmaris propria III axialis

Fig. 4.86 Left manus after the removal of the cephalic vein: palmar view.

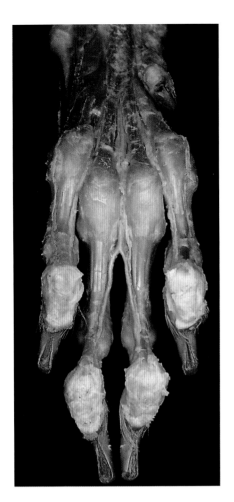

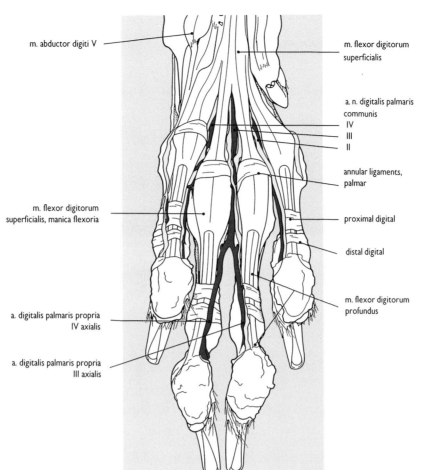

m. abductor digiti V

m. flexor digitorum superficialis

a. n. digitalis palmaris communis
IV
III
II

annular ligaments, palmar

m. flexor digitorum superficialis, manica flexoria

proximal digital

distal digital

m. flexor digitorum profundus

a. digitalis palmaris propria IV axialis

a. digitalis palmaris propria III axialis

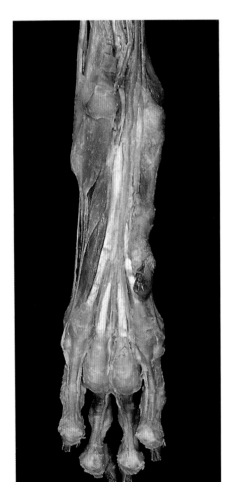

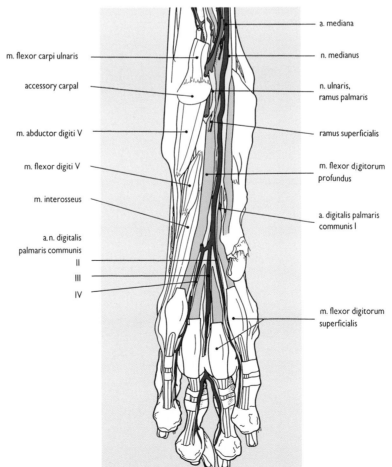

Fig. 4.88 Left manus after removal of superficial digital flexor tendons: palmar view. The flexor retinaculum deep to the superficial digital flexor has also been removed.

m. flexor carpi ulnaris

accessory carpal

m. abductor digiti V

m. flexor digiti V

m. interosseus

a. n. digitalis palmaris communis
II
III
IV

a. mediana

n. medianus

n. ulnaris, ramus palmaris

ramus superficialis

m. flexor digitorum profundus

a. digitalis palmaris communis I

m. flexor digitorum superficialis

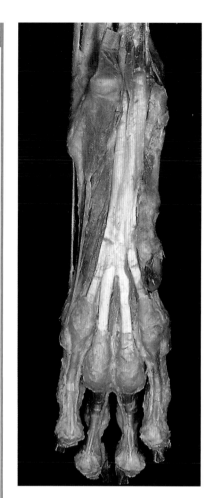

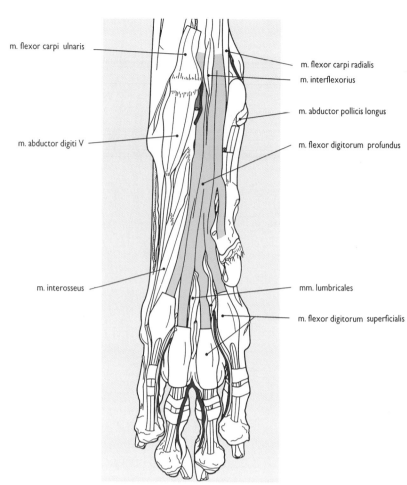

m. flexor carpi ulnaris

m. abductor digiti V

m. interosseus

m. flexor carpi radialis

m. interflexorius

m. abductor pollicis longus

m. flexor digitorum profundus

mm. lumbricales

m. flexor digitorum superficialis

Fig. 4.89 Left manus after the removal of the median artery and nerve: palmar view.

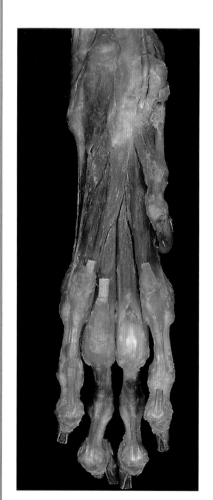

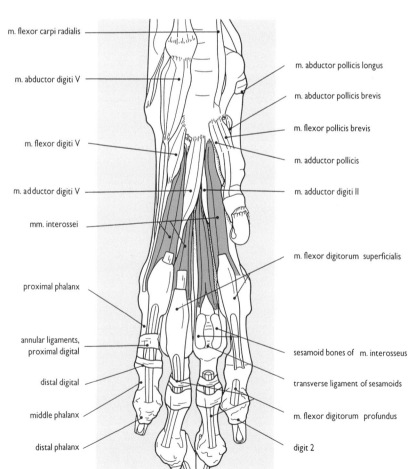

m. flexor carpi radialis

m. abductor digiti V

m. flexor digiti V

m. adductor digiti V

mm. interossei

proximal phalanx

annular ligaments, proximal digital

distal digital

middle phalanx

distal phalanx

m. abductor pollicis longus

m. abductor pollicis brevis

m. flexor pollicis brevis

m. adductor pollicis

m. adductor digiti II

m. flexor digitorum superficialis

sesamoid bones of m. interosseus

transverse ligament of sesamoids

m. flexor digitorum profundus

digit 2

Fig. 4.90 Left manus after removal of the deep digital flexor tendons: palmar view.

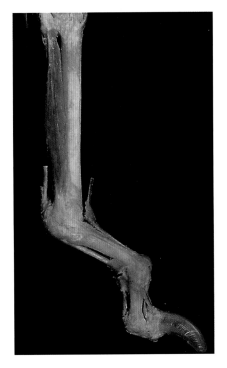

Fig. 4.91 Separated 4th digit: medial view.

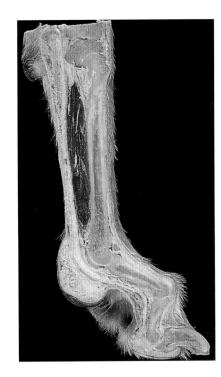

Fig. 4.93 Longitudinal section through the 3rd metacarpus and digit. Transverse sections of the metapodium and digits are illustrated in Chapter 7.

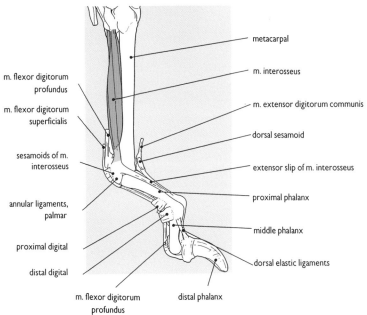

m. flexor digitorum profundus
m. flexor digitorum superficialis
sesamoids of m. interosseus
annular ligaments, palmar
proximal digital
distal digital
m. flexor digitorum profundus

metacarpal
m. interosseus
m. extensor digitorum communis
dorsal sesamoid
extensor slip of m. interosseus
proximal phalanx
middle phalanx
dorsal elastic ligaments
distal phalanx

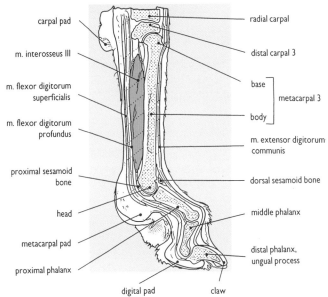

carpal pad
m. interosseus III
m. flexor digitorum superficialis
m. flexor digitorum profundus
proximal sesamoid bone
head
metacarpal pad
proximal phalanx
digital pad
claw

radial carpal
distal carpal 3
base
metacarpal 3
body
m. extensor digitorum communis
dorsal sesamoid bone
middle phalanx
distal phalanx, ungual process

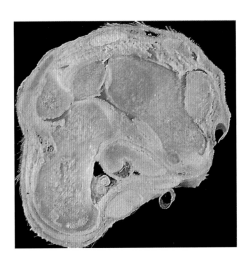

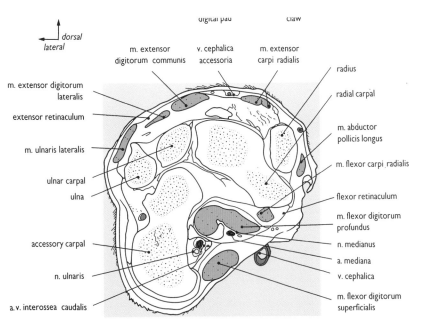

dorsal *lateral*

m. extensor digitorum communis
v. cephalica accessoria
m. extensor carpi radialis
m. extensor digitorum lateralis
extensor retinaculum
m. ulnaris lateralis
ulnar carpal
ulna
accessory carpal
n. ulnaris
a. v. interossea caudalis

radius
radial carpal
m. abductor pollicis longus
m. flexor carpi radialis
flexor retinaculum
m. flexor digitorum profundus
n. medianus
a. mediana
v. cephalica
m. flexor digitorum superficialis

Fig. 4.92 Transverse section through the left carpus: view of proximal surface of section.

5. THE THORAX

Clinically, the thorax is important because of the wealth of problems that may affect the heart, lungs and trachea, esophagus and diaphragm. The regions are presternal, sternal, cardiac and costal regions.

The thorax can be examined by palpation (which is limited), auscultation and percussion. In the dog, the forelimbs can be brought forward.

The heart is situated in the 3rd to 5th intercostal spaces and occasionally as far caudally as the 7th. The cardiac notch in the lung acts as a valuable window to examine the heart more effectively, by auscultation and echocardiography. Here, there is direct access to the heart without any overlying lung tissue. It is more pronounced on the right side. Horizontally, the heart is situated at the level of the middle of the first rib and this forms the dorsal boundary. There is wide variation in the shape and size of the heart due to the tremendous variation between breeds of dog. In deep-chested dogs it is tall, narrow and upright; in barrel-chested dogs, almost globular. In the standing dog, the heart lies at the olecranon at 5th rib – therefore need to draw leg before. It occupies usually 2.5 to 3.5 intercostal spaces and the height of the heart is about two-thirds of the length of the thoracic cavity. In width, it occupies two-thirds of the width of the thoracic cavity with the apex tilted to the left of the midline. The vertebral heart score is the most useful assessment of cardiac size and is normally 10.5–12.5. The apex beat of the heart is found on the left and right in the 4th to 5th intercostal space near the mitral valve. The left atrioventricular valve (mitral) is heard best on the left in the 5th intercostal space at the costochondral junction, the aortic valves in the 4th intercostal space on the left at the level of the shoulder, and the pulmonary valves best in the 3rd intercostal space on the left above costochondral junction. On the right side, the right atrioventricular valves (tricuspid) are best heard in the 4th intercostal space at the level of the costochondral junction. The costomediastinal recess occupies the 4th to 6th intercostal spaces on the left and on the right as well.

Left-sided enlargement of the heart is important in the dog. In this you can see elevation of the trachea, the caudal border of the heart straightens. There is tensing of the left atrium and loss of the caudal heart waist. In right-sided enlargement, there is also elevation of the trachea, increased sternal contact, rounding of the cranial border, loss of cranial waist and dorsal displacement of the cranial vessels of the heart. Cardiomyopathy in the form of enlarged heart can be seen in myocardial disease, myocarditis and associated with the presence of *Angiostrongylus* the canine heartworm. It is particularly common in large breeds such as Dobermans.

A whole variety of heart problems both congenital and acquired can be found in dogs and are beyond this short introduction. Suffice to say that patent *ductus arteriosus* and persistent right aortic arch can be treated surgically. Mention of thoracotomy will be made later but for this, surgical openings are made in the left 4th or 5th intercostal space, and during repair care must be taken to protect the recurrent laryngeal nerve and thoracic duct. A patent ductus leads to a left-to-right shunt with the left ventricle continuously overloaded leading to dyspnoea (difficulty breathing), shortness of breadth and other problems with the only treatment surgical closure. Interestingly, it may produce signs of esophageal stricture because the esophagus is partially obstructed by the ductus and eventually this may lead to an extensive esophageal diverticulum, left-sided atrial and ventricular enlargement and subsequent failure.

The majority of esophageal strictures are probably associated with persistent 4th right aortic arches.

At the base of the heart, the aorta is on the left side of the esophagus so access is best from the right. In the caudal mediastinal space, the esophagus lies to the left, and the aorta is now dorsal so the right surgical approach to the esophagus is from the left. In all cases, care is needed to avoid the vagal nerves.

Esophageal surgery will also require a transthoracic esophagotomy. The blockage is found by use of a stomach tube and then you can make an entry at the appropriate intercostal space for thoracotomy. In most instances these days esophageal foreign bodies are found using flexible gastroscopes with the majority of removals via rigid endoscopes.

The thoracotomy can be used for all intrathoracic surgery. You have to cut mm latissimus dorsi, so be careful with the thoraco-dorsal nerve. It can be done in several ways. The lateral intercostal is usually used and gives good exposure and a good repair. Approximately one-third of the half of the thorax can be viewed from your incision. The incisions are made equidistant from the vertebrae to avoid the vessels and nerves. There is nowadays perceived to be no higher incidence of postoperative complications with median sternotomy than intercostal methods. In median sternotomy the manubrium or the xiphoid is left intact to aid stabilization of the ribcage when it is closed. Occasionally, transcostal is performed and the last method involves midline trans-sternal incision and this may be used for repair of the ruptured diaphragm where entrapment or adhesion of abdominal viscera within the thorax is anticipated. It is possible to remove a rib completely and then approach through the rib cage. Cranial thoracotomy requires incision through the M. scalenus and caudal thoracotomy through the external abdominal oblique and serratus ventralis muscles. Hiatus hernia of the esophagus is also repaired through a left thoracotomy or through a midline celiotomy (laparotomy). Pulmonary lobectomy for removal of a lung is usually for neoplasia, pneumothorax or emphysema, torsion of a lobe lung or foreign body infection can be carried out at the 5th intercostal space on either the left or right side or via a median sternotomy. For thoracolumbar disc protrusion, incision can be made over the intercostal muscle which is then transected and further incisions can be made to the spine.

Thorascopic techniques are now increasingly used to examine the thoracic contents with minimal postoperative problems.

Thoracentesis or puncturing of the chest is carried out to empty fluid (transudate, exudate, blood, pus or chyle) or air from the chest when a pneumothorax has occurred. The key is to make sure that the skin wound does not overlay the puncturing through the intercostal region. If it does, there is danger of creating a pneumothorax.

Dyspnoea or difficult breathing is a major clinical entity and is investigated in several ways. The respiratory pattern is studied, the mucous membrane color is noted and auscultation and percussion of the chest carried out. Radiography, thoracentesis, fluoroscopy and other techniques can be used to aid diagnosis including bronchoalveolar lavage where sterile fluid is introduced into the lungs and collected for analysis. Ultrasound scanning techniques are useful for cardiac pathology but with Doppler techniques it can be very useful. A cough is a similar entity and may originate in the larynx, pharynx or trachea or main bronchi, and is investigated by a similar range of techniques.

Thoracic respiratory sounds may originate from the bronchi, pulmonary parenchyma or the pleura. Auscultation of these sounds may indicate pathological processes.

In practice, the cranial border of the lung is the caudal border of the long head of the triceps. The dorsal border is a line from the coxal tuberosity lateral to the iliocostalis line and the caudal border is to the 11th intercostal space from the olecranon.

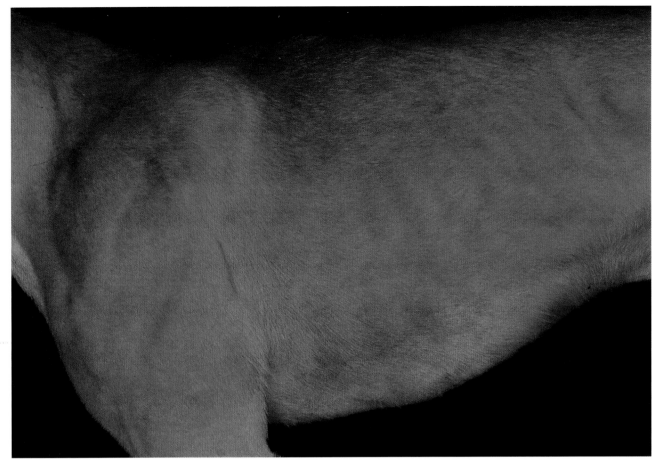

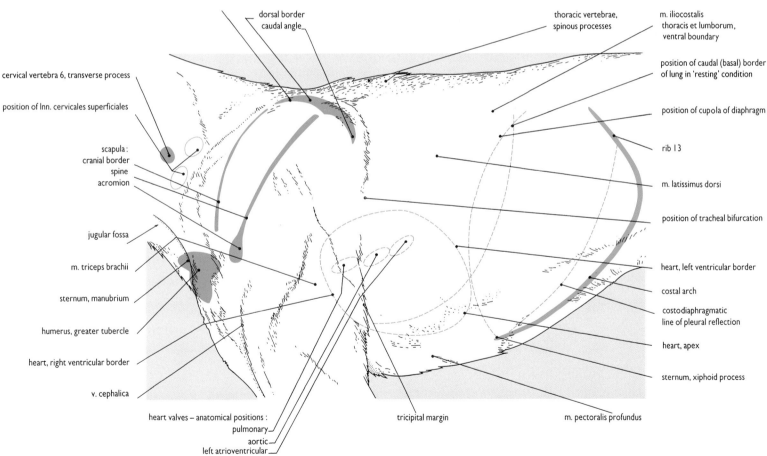

cervical vertebra 6, transverse process

position of lnn. cervicales superficiales

scapula :
cranial border
spine
acromion

jugular fossa

m. triceps brachii

sternum, manubrium

humerus, greater tubercle

heart, right ventricular border

v. cephalica

heart valves – anatomical positions :
pulmonary
aortic
left atrioventricular

dorsal border
caudal angle

thoracic vertebrae,
spinous processes

m. iliocostalis
thoracis et lumborum,
ventral boundary

position of caudal (basal) border
of lung in 'resting' condition

position of cupola of diaphragm

rib 13

m. latissimus dorsi

position of tracheal bifurcation

heart, left ventricular border

costal arch

costodiaphragmatic
line of pleural reflection

heart, apex

sternum, xiphoid process

tricipital margin

m. pectoralis profundus

Fig. 5.1 Surface features of the shoulder and thorax: left lateral view. The palpable bony 'landmarks' and those muscles whose contours are clearly recognizable on palpation are indicated. In the normal standing posture the scapula and its associated muscles cover ribs 1 to 4 completely. The broken green lines indicate the position of structures as they are seen in subsequent dissections. It is extremely important to appreciate that these are not the normal positions in the live animal (see Fig. 1.3). In the live animal, the heart is more cranially placed and the cupola of the diaphragm may extend as far cranially as rib 6.

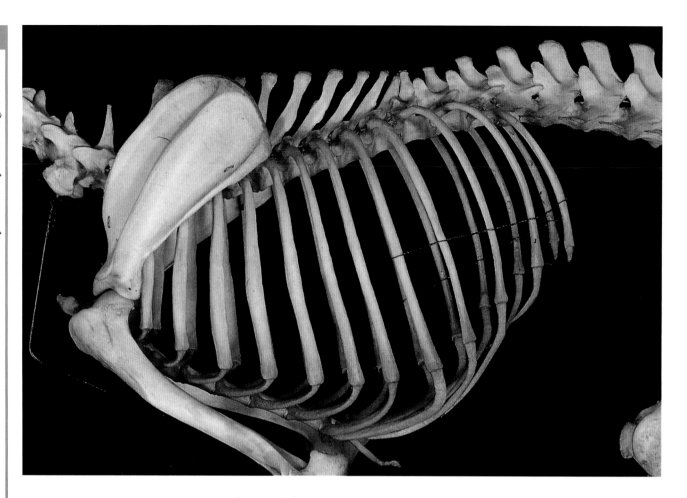

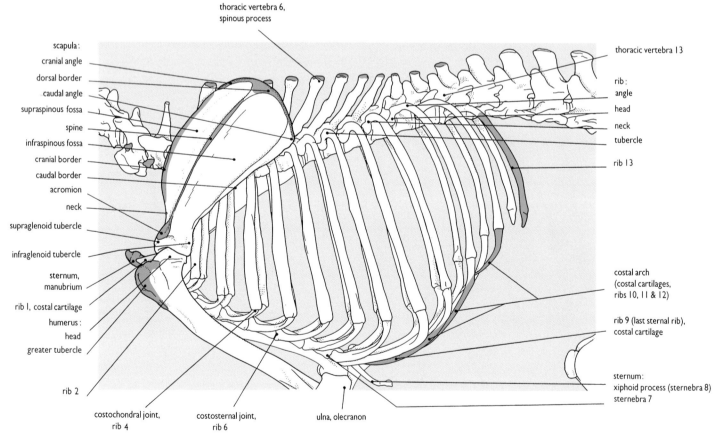

thoracic vertebra 6,
spinous process

scapula :
cranial angle
dorsal border
caudal angle
supraspinous fossa
spine
infraspinous fossa
cranial border
caudal border
acromion
neck
supraglenoid tubercle
infraglenoid tubercle
sternum,
manubrium
rib I, costal cartilage
humerus :
head
greater tubercle
rib 2

thoracic vertebra 13

rib :
angle
head
neck
tubercle

rib 13

costal arch
(costal cartilages,
ribs 10, 11 & 12)

rib 9 (last sternal rib),
costal cartilage

sternum:
xiphoid process (sternebra 8)
sternebra 7

costochondral joint,
rib 4

costosternal joint,
rib 6

ulna, olecranon

Fig. 5.2 Skeleton of the shoulder and thorax: left lateral view. Palpable bony features shown in the surface view are colored green for reference. In addition, the more caudal ribs and the entire length of the sternum within the median pectoral groove are palpable. Passing caudally from the small cranial thoracic aperture (thoracic inlet) between the first pair of ribs, the sternum and vertebral column diverge, and the ribs lengthen (up to rib 9) and increase in their outward curvature.

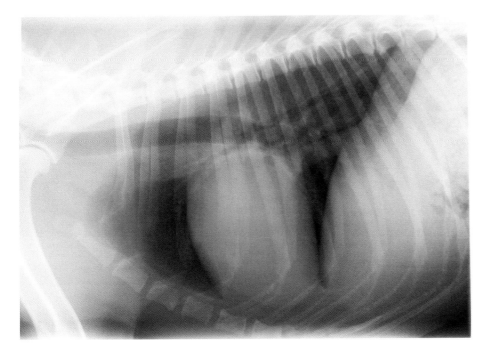

Fig. 5.3 Radiograph of the thorax: lateral view. Air within its lumen highlights the trachea. The heart is clearly visible. The lungs can be seen by virtue of their air content. The majority of other structures are soft tissue and mediastinal and so cannot be clearly distinguished from one another. The position, shape and relationship of structures may alter quite markedly according to breed type, body condition and stage of respiration.

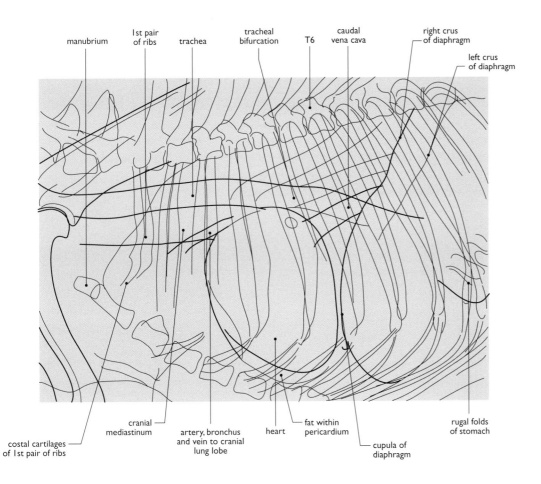

manubrium   1st pair of ribs   trachea   tracheal bifurcation   T6   caudal vena cava   right crus of diaphragm   left crus of diaphragm

costal cartilages of 1st pair of ribs   cranial mediastinum   artery, bronchus and vein to cranial lung lobe   heart   fat within pericardium   cupula of diaphragm   rugal folds of stomach

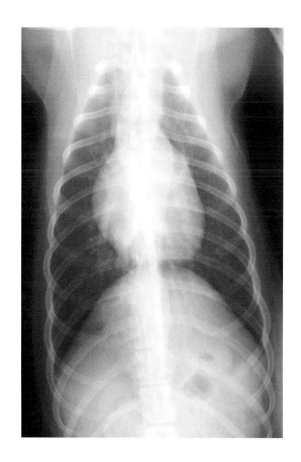

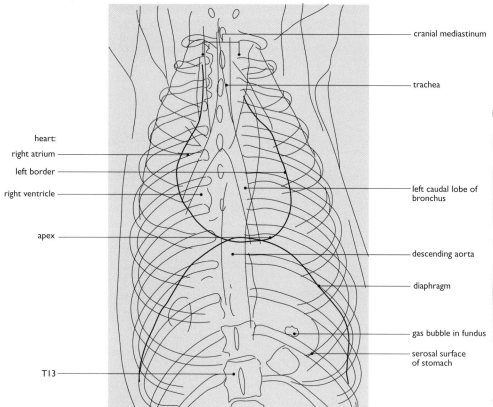

cranial mediastinum

trachea

heart:
right atrium

left border

right ventricle

left caudal lobe of bronchus

apex

descending aorta

diaphragm

gas bubble in fundus

serosal surface of stomach

T13

Fig. 5.4 Radiograph of the thorax: dorsoventral view. Only the lungs and the heart can be easily appreciated in this view as other structures are mediastinal and thus superimposed on the spine and sternum.

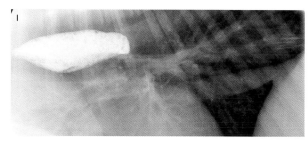

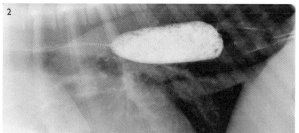

bolus of barium and food passing down oesophagus to enter stomach at the cardia showing longitudinal folds

aorta

heartbase

caudal vena cava

l crus of diaphragm

r crus of diaphragm

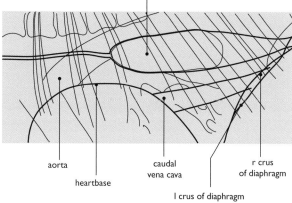

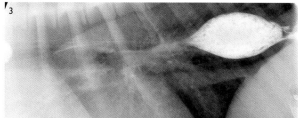

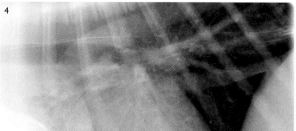

Fig. 5.5 Radiograph of the thorax: lateral view, immediately after oral administration of barium mixed with dog food. (1), (2) & (3) A bolus of food mixed with contrast medium can be seen within the esophagus. The longitudinal mucosal folds can be seen in the distal esophagus. (4) Streaks of barium remaining within the esophagus highlight its path and the mucosal folds.

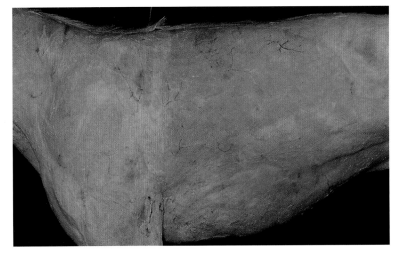

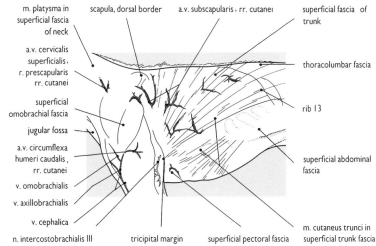

m. platysma in superficial fascia of neck

scapula, dorsal border

a.v. subscapularis, rr. cutanei

superficial fascia of trunk

a.v. cervicalis superficialis, r. prescapularis rr. cutanei

thoracolumbar fascia

superficial omobrachial fascia

rib 13

jugular fossa

a.v. circumflexa humeri caudalis, rr. cutanei

superficial abdominal fascia

v. omobrachialis

v. axillobrachialis

v. cephalica

m. cutaneus trunci in superficial trunk fascia

n. intercostobrachialis III

tricipital margin

superficial pectoral fascia

Fig. 5.6 Superficial fascia of the shoulder thorax: left lateral view. The superficial fascia is not attached to the skeleton and may be variably infiltrated with fat. The cutaneous muscle of the trunk is visible embedded in the fascial layer.

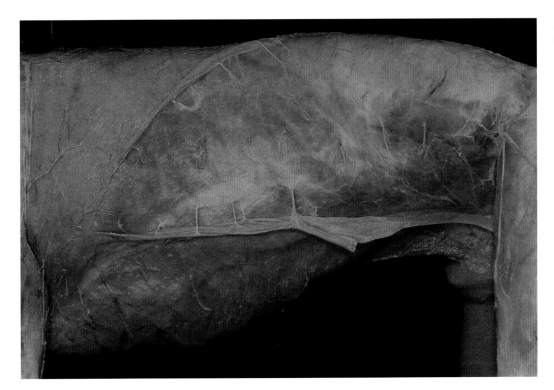

Fig. 5.7 Cutaneous muscle of the trunk and cutaneous nerves of the thorax: left lateral view. Limited cleaning of superficial fascia has exposed the cutaneous muscle. It has been cut into and reflected ventrally, revealing two series of lateral cutaneous nerves, with their accompanying small cutaneous blood vessels which originate from the intercostal vessels.

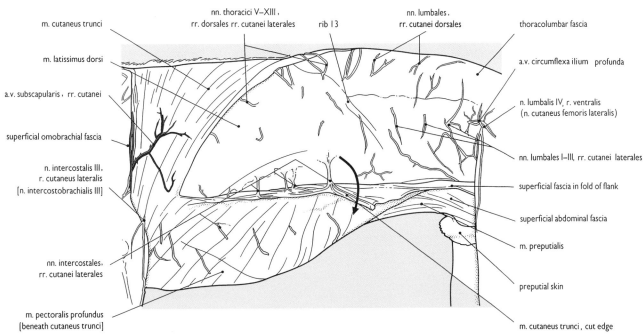

m. cutaneus trunci

nn. thoracici V–XIII, rr. dorsales rr. cutanei laterales

rib 13

nn. lumbales, rr. cutanei dorsales

thoracolumbar fascia

m. latissimus dorsi

a.v. circumflexa ilium profunda

a.v. subscapularis, rr. cutanei

n. lumbalis IV, r. ventralis (n. cutaneus femoris lateralis)

superficial omobrachial fascia

n. intercostalis III, r. cutaneus lateralis [n. intercostobrachialis III]

nn. lumbales I–III, rr. cutanei laterales

superficial fascia in fold of flank

superficial abdominal fascia

m. preputialis

nn. intercostales, rr. cutanei laterales

preputial skin

m. pectoralis profundus [beneath cutaneus trunci]

m. cutaneus trunci, cut edge

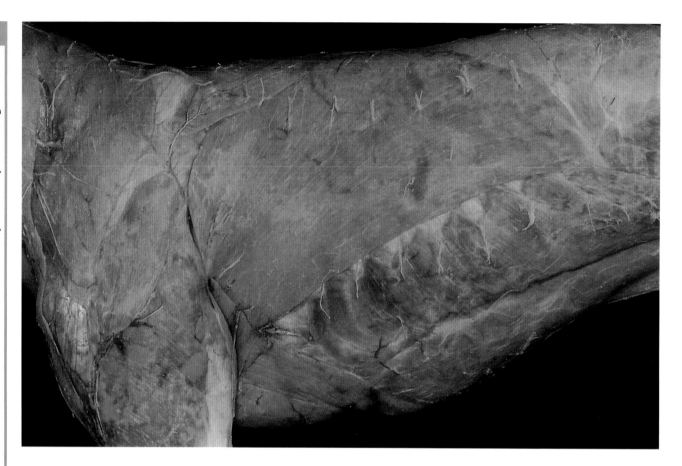

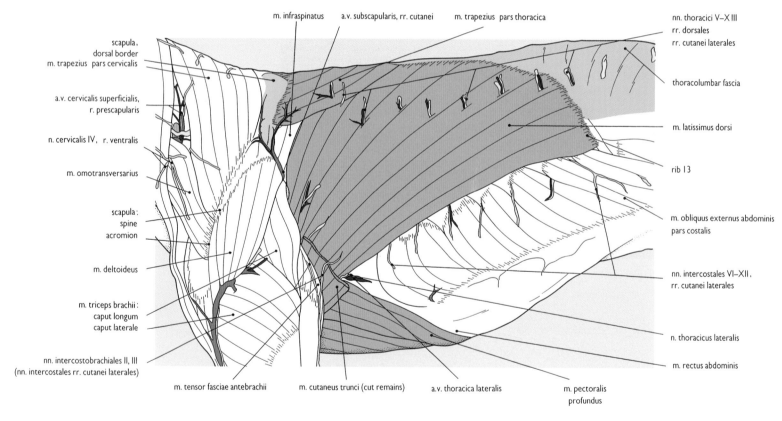

scapula,
dorsal border
m. trapezius pars cervicalis

a.v. cervicalis superficialis,
r. prescapularis

n. cervicalis IV, r. ventralis

m. omotransversarius

scapula :
spine
acromion

m. deltoideus

m. triceps brachii :
caput longum
caput laterale

nn. intercostobrachiales II, III
(nn. intercostales rr. cutanei laterales)

m. tensor fasciae antebrachii

m. infraspinatus

a.v. subscapularis, rr. cutanei

m. trapezius pars thoracica

m. cutaneus trunci (cut remains)

a.v. thoracica lateralis

m. pectoralis
profundus

nn. thoracici V–XIII
rr. dorsales
rr. cutanei laterales

thoracolumbar fascia

m. latissimus dorsi

rib 13

m. obliquus externus abdominis
pars costalis

nn. intercostales VI–XII,
rr. cutanei laterales

n. thoracicus lateralis

m. rectus abdominis

Fig. 5.8 Superficial structures of the shoulder and thorax (1) cutaneous nerves: left lateral view. The remaining superficial fascia and most of the cutaneous muscle have been cleaned. The lateral thoracic vessels and nerve emerge from between the diverging pectoral and latissimus dorsi muscles which extend from the axilla caudally onto the chest.

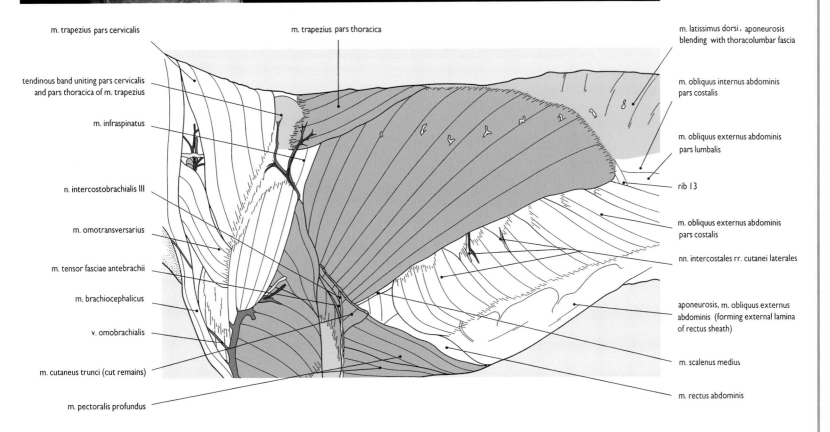

m. trapezius pars cervicalis

m. trapezius pars thoracica

m. latissimus dorsi, aponeurosis blending with thoracolumbar fascia

tendinous band uniting pars cervicalis and pars thoracica of m. trapezius

m. obliquus internus abdominis pars costalis

m. infraspinatus

m. obliquus externus abdominis pars lumbalis

n. intercostobrachialis III

rib 13

m. omotransversarius

m. obliquus externus abdominis pars costalis

m. tensor fasciae antebrachii

nn. intercostales rr. cutanei laterales

m. brachiocephalicus

aponeurosis, m. obliquus externus abdominis (forming external lamina of rectus sheath)

v. omobrachialis

m. cutaneus trunci (cut remains)

m. scalenus medius

m. pectoralis profundus

m. rectus abdominis

Fig. 5.9 Superficial structures of the shoulder and thorax (2) extrinsic forelimb muscles: left lateral view. Extrinsic muscles of the forelimb are exposed after removal of the superficial fascia and trimming of lateral cutaneous nerves. The basis of the caudal boundary of the upper arm, the tricipital margin, is clearly displayed. Deep thoracic fascia passes internal to the latissimus dorsi and pectoral muscles and medial to the upper arm, and forms the medial lining layer of the axilla (see Figs 3.43 and 5.82).

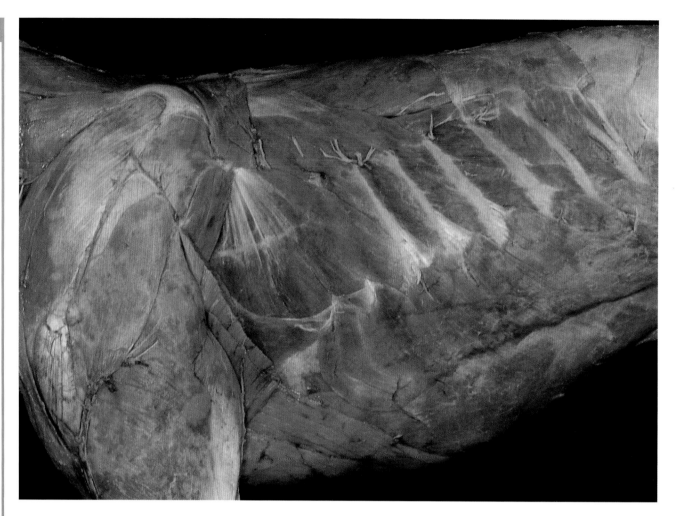

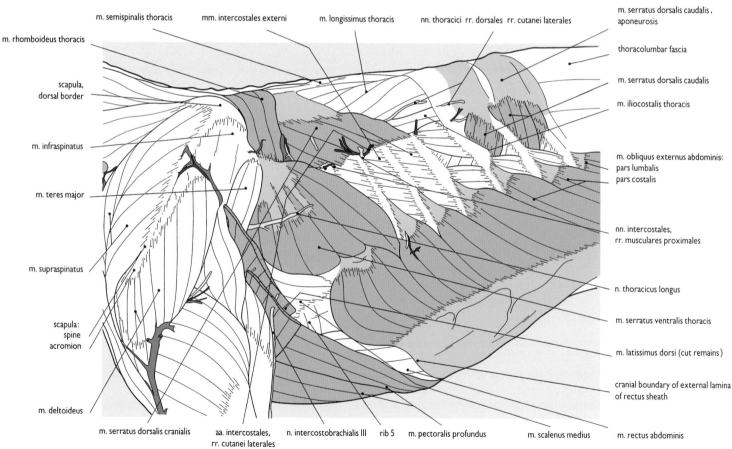

m. semispinalis thoracis   mm. intercostales externi   m. longissimus thoracis   nn. thoracici rr. dorsales rr. cutanei laterales   m. serratus dorsalis caudalis, aponeurosis

m. rhomboideus thoracis

thoracolumbar fascia

scapula, dorsal border

m. serratus dorsalis caudalis

m. iliocostalis thoracis

m. infraspinatus

m. obliquus externus abdominis: pars lumbalis pars costalis

m. teres major

nn. intercostales, rr. musculares proximales

m. supraspinatus

n. thoracicus longus

scapula: spine acromion

m. serratus ventralis thoracis

m. latissimus dorsi (cut remains)

cranial boundary of external lamina of rectus sheath

m. deltoideus

m. serratus dorsalis cranialis   aa. intercostales, rr. cutanei laterales   n. intercostobrachialis III   rib 5   m. pectoralis profundus   m. scalenus medius   m. rectus abdominis

Fig. 5.10 Thoracic wall (1) after removal of the latissimus dorsi muscle: left lateral view. The latissimus dorsi and trapezius muscles have been removed to begin exposure of the thoracic wall, displaying the entire thoracic origin of the external abdominal oblique muscle from rib 13 cranially to rib 6; the caudal attachments of the thoracic ventral serrate muscle from ribs 5 to 8; the thoracic rhomboid at the dorsal end of the scapula related to its caudal angle and vertebral border. Part of the deep thoracolumbar fascia covering the epaxial musculature has been removed in order to demarcate those areas of the fascia which also act as aponeurotic attachments for the cranial and caudal dorsal serrate muscles.

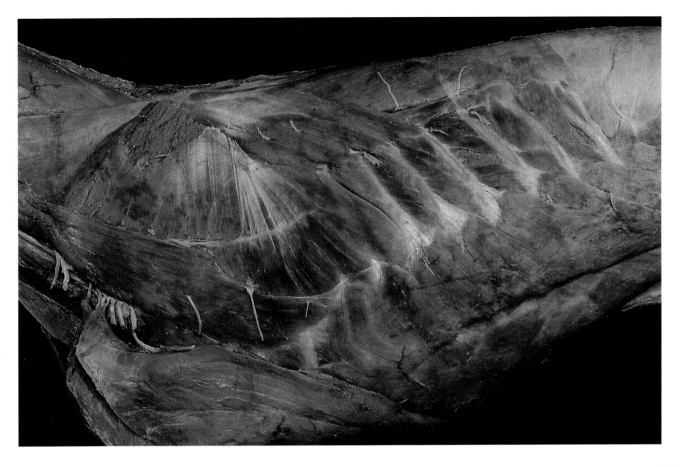

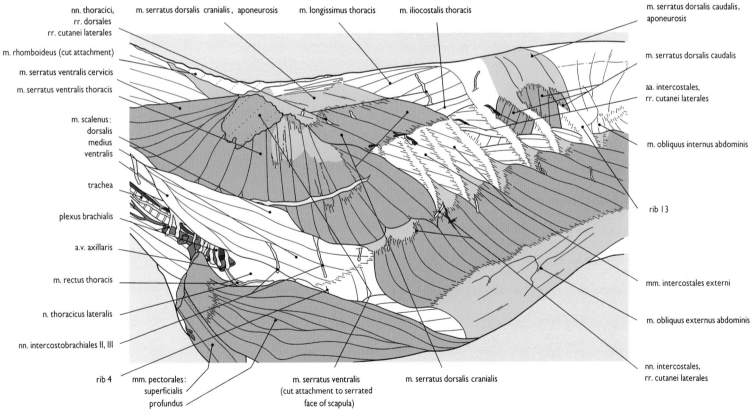

nn. thoracici,
rr. dorsales
rr. cutanei laterales

m. rhomboideus (cut attachment)

m. serratus ventralis cervicis

m. serratus ventralis thoracis

m. scalenus :
dorsalis
medius
ventralis

trachea

plexus brachialis

a.v. axillaris

m. rectus thoracis

n. thoracicus lateralis

nn. intercostobrachiales II, III

rib 4

mm. pectorales :
superficialis
profundus

m. serratus dorsalis cranialis , aponeurosis

m. longissimus thoracis

m. iliocostalis thoracis

m. serratus ventralis
(cut attachment to serrated
face of scapula)

m. serratus dorsalis cranialis

m. serratus dorsalis caudalis,
aponeurosis

m. serratus dorsalis caudalis

aa. intercostales,
rr. cutanei laterales

m. obliquus internus abdominis

rib 13

mm. intercostales externi

m. obliquus externus abdominis

nn. intercostales,
rr. cutanei laterales

Fig. 5.11 Thoracic wall (2) after removal of the forelimb: left lateral view. The forelimb was removed by severing the rhomboid muscle at its attachment to the supraspinous and nuchal ligament, and the mid dorsal tendinous raphe of the neck; cutting the ventral serrate muscle from its attachment onto the serrated face of the scapula; freeing the superficial and deep pectoral muscles from their humeral attachments and severing axillary vessels and nerves arising from the brachial plexus.

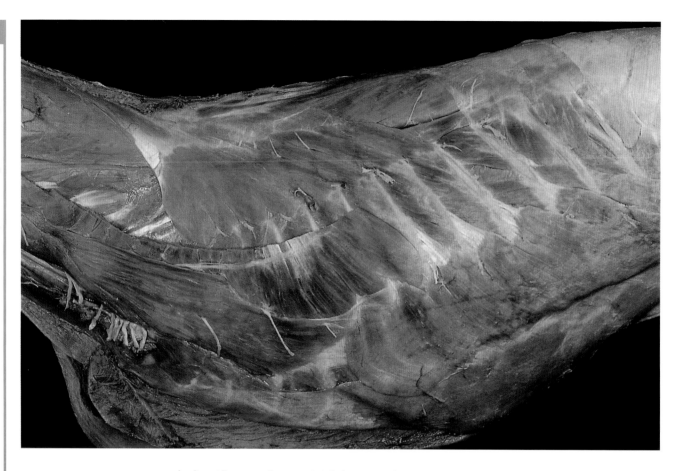

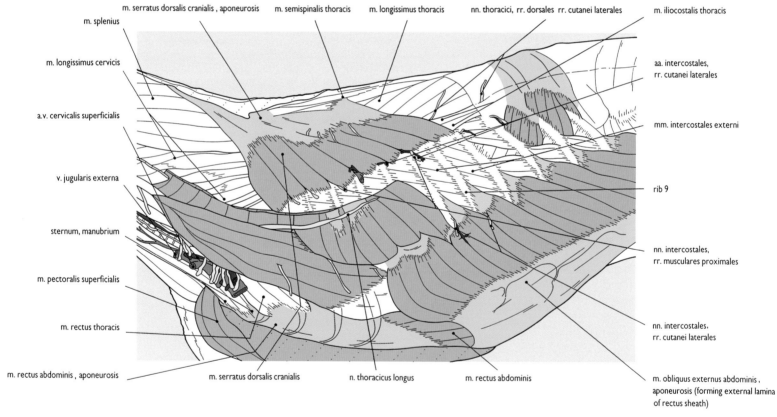

m. splenius

m. longissimus cervicis

a.v. cervicalis superficialis

v. jugularis externa

sternum, manubrium

m. pectoralis superficialis

m. rectus thoracis

m. rectus abdominis , aponeurosis

m. serratus dorsalis cranialis , aponeurosis

m. semispinalis thoracis

m. longissimus thoracis

nn. thoracici, rr. dorsales rr. cutanei laterales

m. iliocostalis thoracis

aa. intercostales, rr. cutanei laterales

mm. intercostales externi

rib 9

nn. intercostales, rr. musculares proximales

nn. intercostales, rr. cutanei laterales

m. obliquus externus abdominis , aponeurosis (forming external lamina of rectus sheath)

m. serratus dorsalis cranialis

n. thoracicus longus

m. rectus abdominis

Fig. 5.12 Thoracic wall (3) dorsal serrate and scalene muscles: left lateral view. The ventral serrate muscle has been removed (bar its ventral rib attachment) exposing the cranial dorsal serrate muscle. Left pectoral musculature has been removed exposing the medial surface of the right pectoral muscles abutting onto the left pectoral muscles ventral to the sternum; the small rectus thoracis muscle; the aponeurosis of origin of the rectus abdominis muscle; and the manubrium of the sternum.

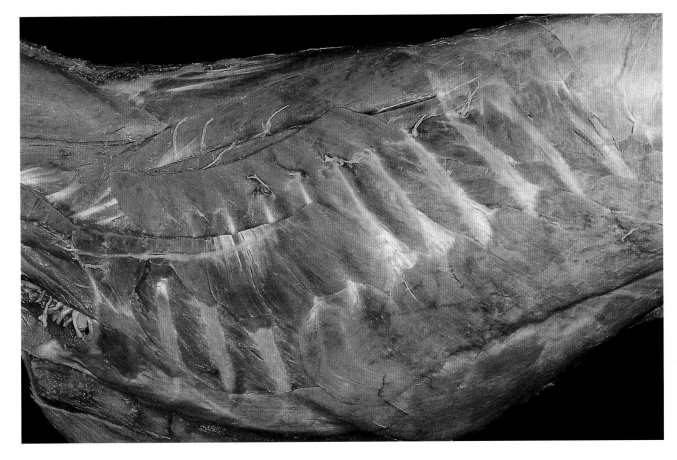

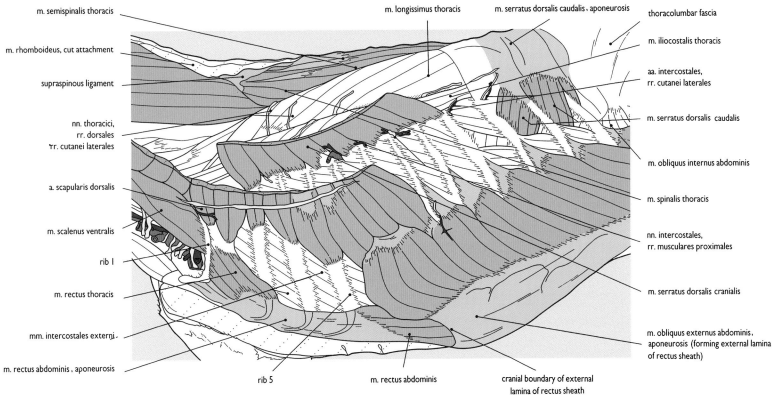

m. semispinalis thoracis

m. rhomboideus, cut attachment

supraspinous ligament

nn. thoracici,
rr. dorsales
rr. cutanei laterales

a. scapularis dorsalis

m. scalenus ventralis

rib I

m. rectus thoracis

mm. intercostales externi

m. rectus abdominis , aponeurosis

rib 5

m. rectus abdominis

m. longissimus thoracis

m. serratus dorsalis caudalis , aponeurosis

thoracolumbar fascia

m. iliocostalis thoracis

aa. intercostales,
rr. cutanei laterales

m. serratus dorsalis caudalis

m. obliquus internus abdominis

m. spinalis thoracis

nn. intercostales,
rr. musculares proximales

m. serratus dorsalis cranialis

m. obliquus externus abdominis,
aponeurosis (forming external lamina
of rectus sheath)

cranial boundary of external
lamina of rectus sheath

Fig. 5.13 Thoracic wall (4) external abdominal oblique muscle: left lateral view. The thoracolumbar fascia has been removed exposing the origin of the splenius muscle (see also Chapter 3), the supraspinous ligament and the spinalis and semispinalis thoracis muscles. Component parts of the scalenus muscle (dorsal and middle) which extended caudally onto ribs 2–6 have been removed leaving only the rib 1 attachment. This has exposed rib 1, parts of ribs 2–5 and the external intercostal muscles in the intervening intercostal spaces.

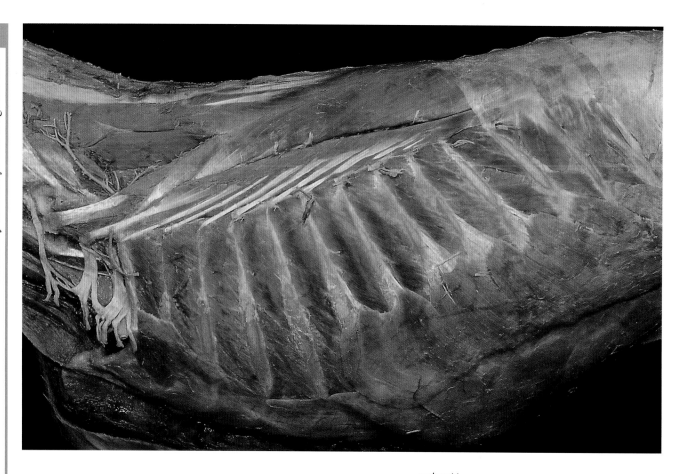

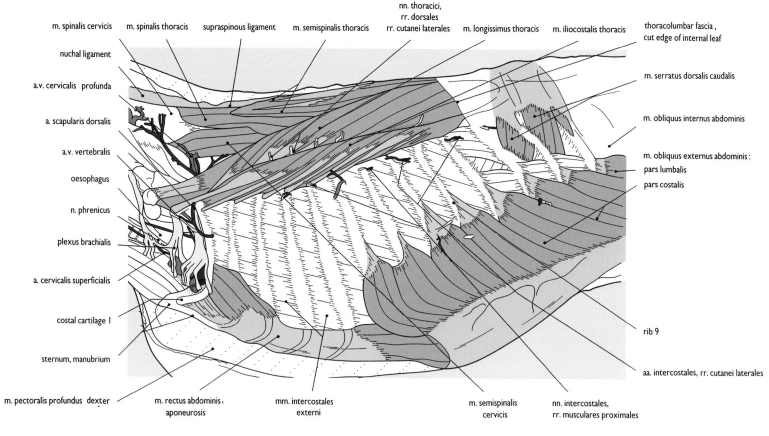

m. spinalis cervicis   m. spinalis thoracis   supraspinous ligament   m. semispinalis thoracis   nn. thoracici, rr. dorsales rr. cutanei laterales   m. longissimus thoracis   m. iliocostalis thoracis   thoracolumbar fascia , cut edge of internal leaf

nuchal ligament   m. serratus dorsalis caudalis

a.v. cervicalis profunda   m. obliquus internus abdominis

a. scapularis dorsalis   m. obliquus externus abdominis : pars lumbalis

a.v. vertebralis   pars costalis

oesophagus

n. phrenicus

plexus brachialis

a. cervicalis superficialis

costal cartilage I   rib 9

sternum, manubrium   aa. intercostales, rr. cutanei laterales

m. pectoralis profundus dexter   m. rectus abdominis , aponeurosis   mm. intercostales externi   m. semispinalis cervicis   nn. intercostales, rr. musculares proximales

Fig. 5.14 Thoracic wall (5) longissimus and iliocostalis thoracis muscles: left lateral view. The rest of the ventral serrate and cranial dorsal serrate muscles and the component of the scalene muscle which attached to rib 1 have been removed. The overall extent of the ribcage is now becoming apparent with all 13 ribs at least partly exposed. Splenius and semispinalis capitis muscles have been removed from the neck (see Chapter 3) with much of the longissimus cervicis muscle. This has exposed the spinalis thoracis and semispinalis thoracis muscles, the longissimus thoracis extending cranially to cervical vertebra 6, and the iliocostalis thoracis muscle extending cranially onto cervical vertebra 7.

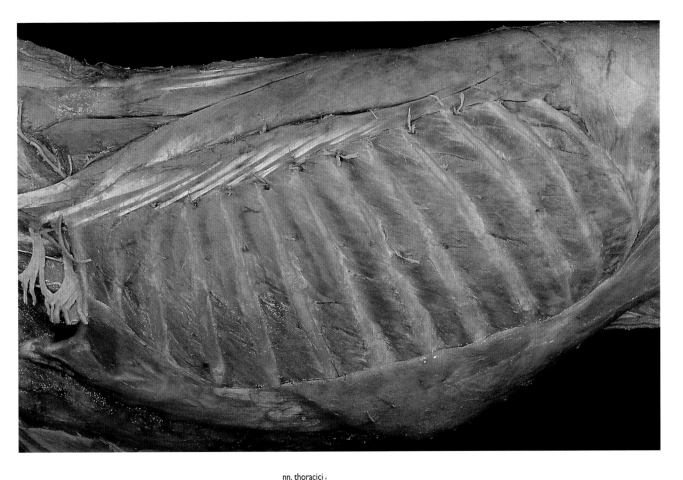

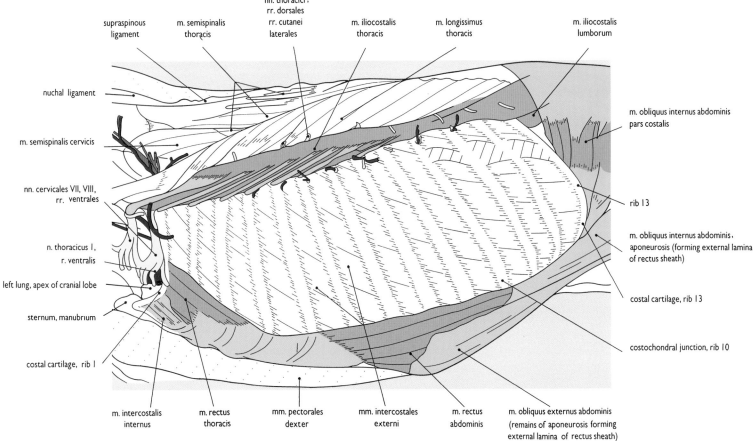

supraspinous ligament

m. semispinalis thoracis

nn. thoracici , rr. dorsales rr. cutanei laterales

m. iliocostalis thoracis

m. longissimus thoracis

m. iliocostalis lumborum

nuchal ligament

m. semispinalis cervicis

nn. cervicales VII, VIII, rr. ventrales

n. thoracicus I, r. ventralis

left lung, apex of cranial lobe

sternum, manubrium

costal cartilage, rib I

m. obliquus internus abdominis pars costalis

rib 13

m. obliquus internus abdominis, aponeurosis (forming external lamina of rectus sheath)

costal cartilage, rib 13

costochondral junction, rib 10

m. intercostalis internus

m. rectus thoracis

mm. pectorales dexter

mm. intercostales externi

m. rectus abdominis

m. obliquus externus abdominis (remains of aponeurosis forming external lamina of rectus sheath)

Fig. 5.15 Thoracic wall (6) rectus abdominis muscle and rectus sheath: left lateral view. The rib attachments of the external abdominal oblique muscle have been removed leaving that part of the ventral aponeurosis which contributes to the external lamina of the rectus sheath closely adherent to the rectus muscle surface. Caudally the contribution of the internal abdominal oblique aponeurosis to the rectus sheath remains intact. The rectus abdominis muscle is now exposed along the length of the thorax.

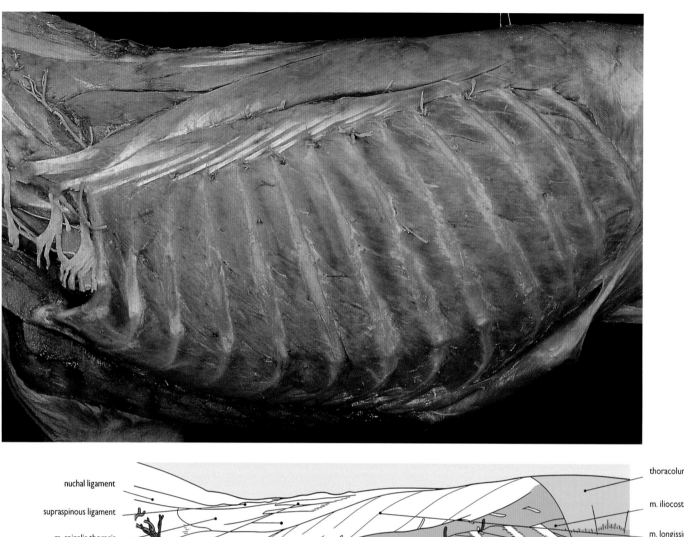

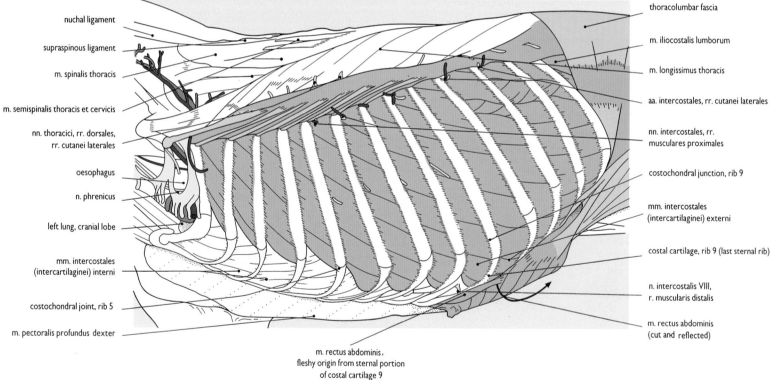

nuchal ligament

supraspinous ligament

m. spinalis thoracis

m. semispinalis thoracis et cervicis

nn. thoracici, rr. dorsales,
rr. cutanei laterales

oesophagus

n. phrenicus

left lung, cranial lobe

mm. intercostales
(intercartilaginei) interni

costochondral joint, rib 5

m. pectoralis profundus dexter

thoracolumbar fascia

m. iliocostalis lumborum

m. longissimus thoracis

aa. intercostales, rr. cutanei laterales

nn. intercostales, rr.
musculares proximales

costochondral junction, rib 9

mm. intercostales
(intercartilaginei) externi

costal cartilage, rib 9 (last sternal rib)

n. intercostalis VIII,
r. muscularis distalis

m. rectus abdominis
(cut and reflected)

m. rectus abdominis,
fleshy origin from sternal portion
of costal cartilage 9

Fig. 5.16 Ribcage (1) external intercostal muscles: left lateral view. The rectus thoracis muscle has been removed and the rectus abdominis muscle is reflected caudally, although a fleshy attachment of the rectus abdominis muscle to the sternal portion of costal cartilage 9 prevents total reflection. Practically the entire ribcage is now exposed with the external intercostal muscles occupying much of the intercostal spaces.

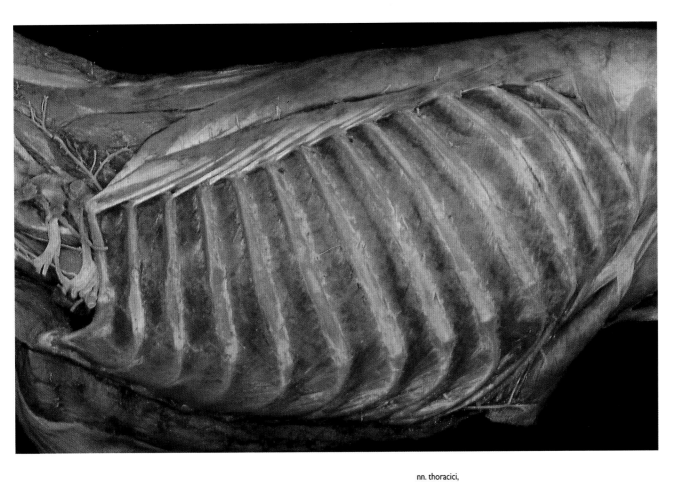

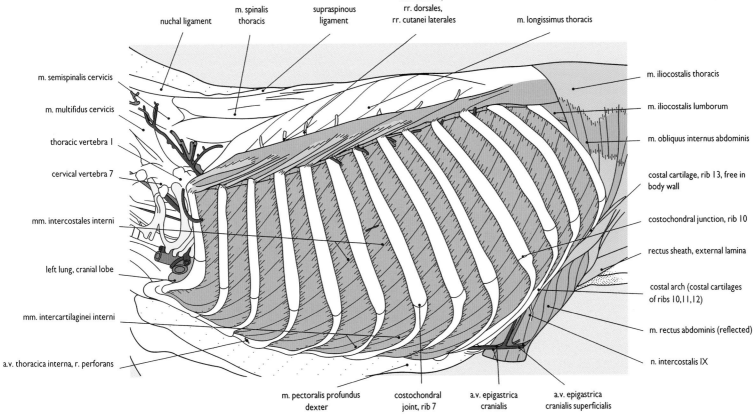

nn. thoracici,
rr. dorsales,
rr. cutanei laterales

nuchal ligament

m. spinalis
thoracis

supraspinous
ligament

m. longissimus thoracis

m. semispinalis cervicis

m. multifidus cervicis

thoracic vertebra 1

cervical vertebra 7

mm. intercostales interni

left lung, cranial lobe

mm. intercartilaginei interni

a.v. thoracica interna, r. perforans

m. iliocostalis thoracis

m. iliocostalis lumborum

m. obliquus internus abdominis

costal cartilage, rib 13, free in
body wall

costochondral junction, rib 10

rectus sheath, external lamina

costal arch (costal cartilages
of ribs 10,11,12)

m. rectus abdominis (reflected)

n. intercostalis IX

m. pectoralis profundus
dexter

costochondral
joint, rib 7

a.v. epigastrica
cranialis

a.v. epigastrica
cranialis superficialis

Fig. 5.17 Ribcage (2) internal intercostal muscles: left lateral view. The rectus abdominis muscle is fully reflected following the severance of its fleshy attachment (see Fig. 5.16). Exposed by this procedure are the costal arch, the continuation of the rectus sheath and the cranial epigastric vessels. The external intercostal muscles have also been removed from all of the intercostal and caudal interchondral spaces exposing the internal intercostal muscles.

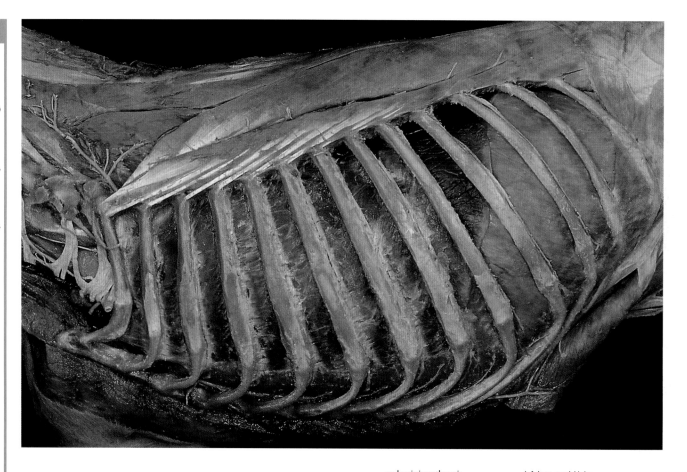

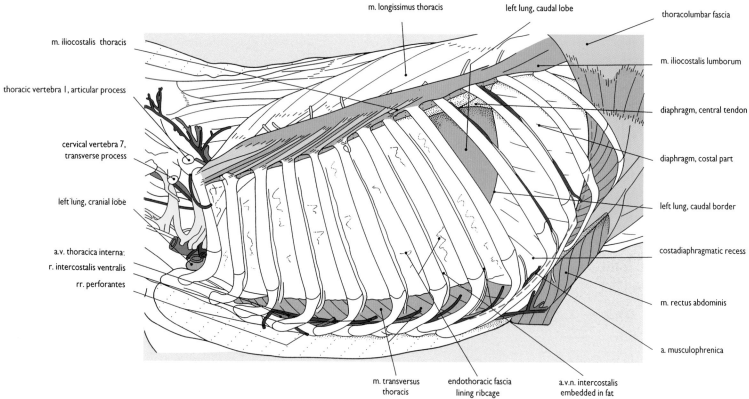

m. longissimus thoracis

left lung, caudal lobe

thoracolumbar fascia

m. iliocostalis thoracis

thoracic vertebra 1, articular process

cervical vertebra 7, transverse process

left lung, cranial lobe

a.v. thoracica interna:
r. intercostalis ventralis
rr. perforantes

m. iliocostalis lumborum

diaphragm, central tendon

diaphragm, costal part

left lung, caudal border

costadiaphragmatic recess

m. rectus abdominis

a. musculophrenica

m. transversus thoracis

endothoracic fascia lining ribcage

a.v.n. intercostalis embedded in fat

Fig. 5.18 Ribcage (3) transverse thoracic muscle and endothoracic fascia: left lateral view. The internal intercostal muscles and their interchondral components have been removed, bar those small portions in interchondral spaces 11 & 12 lying caudal to the costodiaphragmatic line of pleural reflection. In the last four intercostal spaces the endothoracic fascia has also been removed. In those intercostal spaces in which the fascia is intact, an intercostal artery, vein and nerve 'triad' lies embedded in fat against the caudal border of a rib.

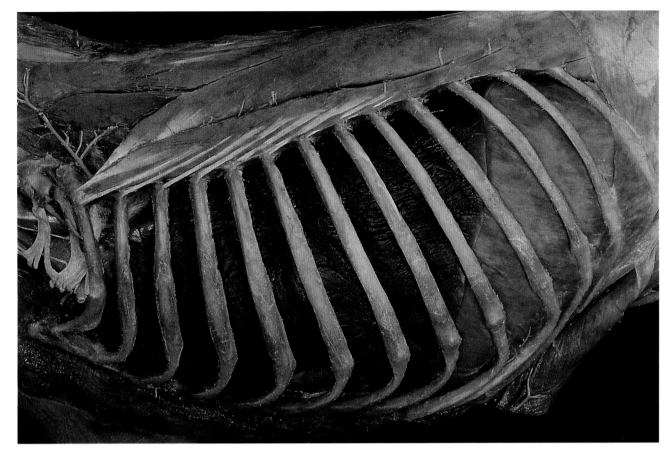

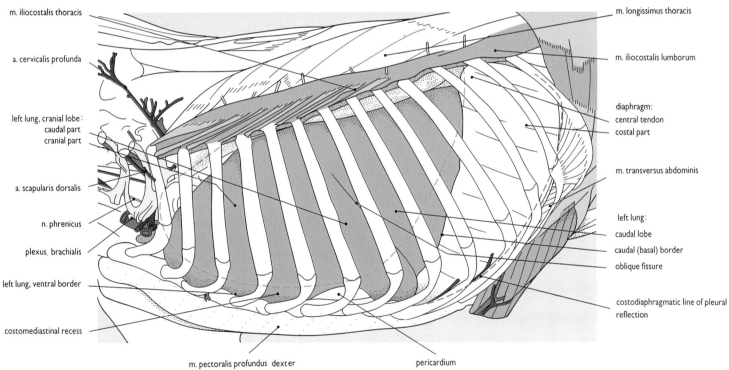

m. iliocostalis thoracis

a. cervicalis profunda

left lung, cranial lobe :
caudal part
cranial part

a. scapularis dorsalis

n. phrenicus

plexus, brachialis

left lung, ventral border

costomediastinal recess

m. pectoralis profundus dexter

pericardium

m. longissimus thoracis

m. iliocostalis lumborum

diaphragm:
central tendon
costal part

m. transversus abdominis

left lung:
caudal lobe
caudal (basal) border
oblique fissure

costodiaphragmatic line of pleural
reflection

Fig. 5.19 Ribcage (4) topography of the thorax: left lateral view. Intercostal spaces were cleared by removing the endothoracic fascia, transverse thoracic muscle, internal thoracic vessels, and intercostal arteries, veins and nerves. The ribs are outlined and the costal surface of the left lung is viewed through the intercostal spaces. An accurate representation of the position and extent of the lungs is sometimes difficult to obtain in embalmed material. The broken green line indicates the approximate contour of the caudal and ventral borders of the lung in a 'resting' position.

213

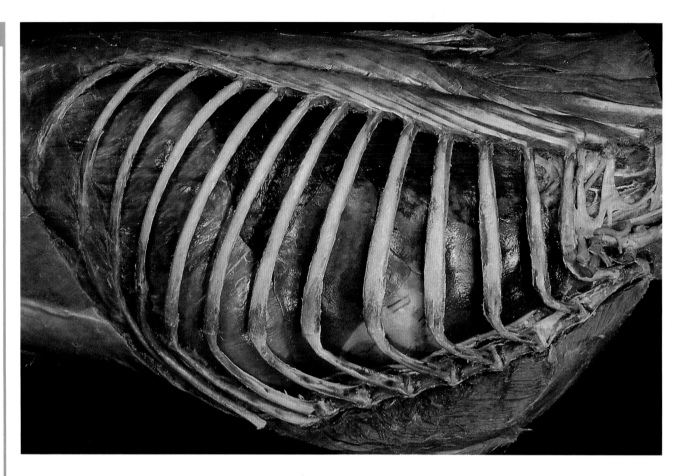

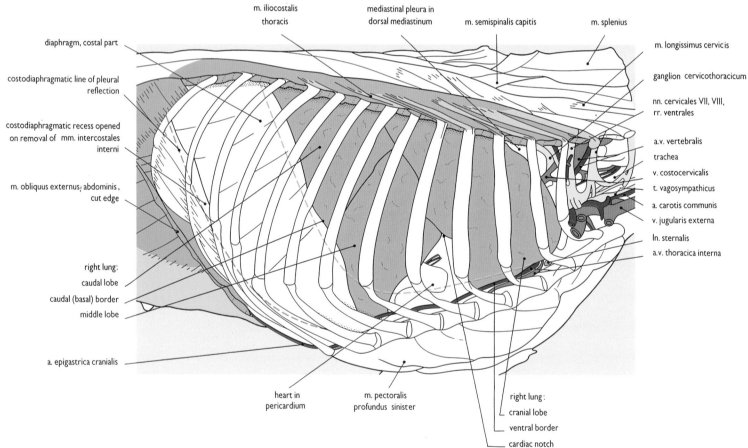

m. iliocostalis thoracis

mediastinal pleura in dorsal mediastinum

m. semispinalis capitis

m. splenius

diaphragm, costal part

costodiaphragmatic line of pleural reflection

costodiaphragmatic recess opened on removal of mm. intercostales interni

m. obliquus externus, abdominis, cut edge

right lung:
caudal lobe
caudal (basal) border
middle lobe

a. epigastrica cranialis

m. longissimus cervicis

ganglion cervicothoracicum

nn. cervicales VII, VIII, rr. ventrales

a.v. vertebralis
trachea
v. costocervicalis
t. vagosympathicus
a. carotis communis
v. jugularis externa
ln. sternalis
a.v. thoracica interna

heart in pericardium

m. pectoralis profundus sinister

right lung:
cranial lobe
ventral border
cardiac notch

Fig. 5.20 Ribcage (5) topography of the thorax: right lateral view. The lung has been preserved in a fairly normal 'resting' condition, its outer contour conforming quite closely to the proposed borders – the broken green line on the drawing. This line passes cranioventrally from the upper end of the penultimate intercostal space at the lateral border of the iliocostalis muscle and parallels the costodiaphragmatic line of pleural reflection (broken blue line) down to the costochondral junction of rib 6 where it continues cranially parallel with the sternum.

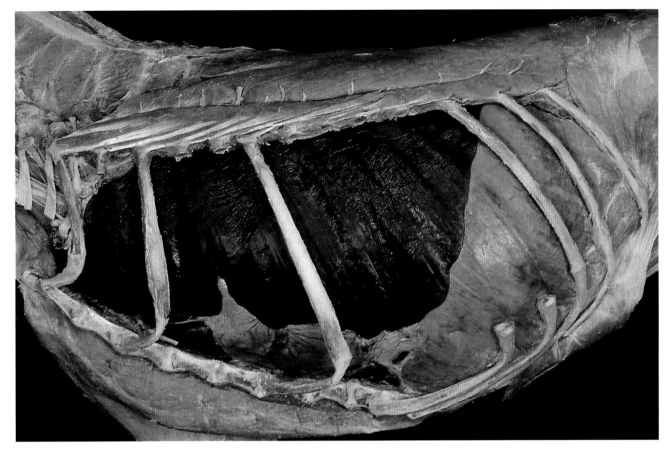

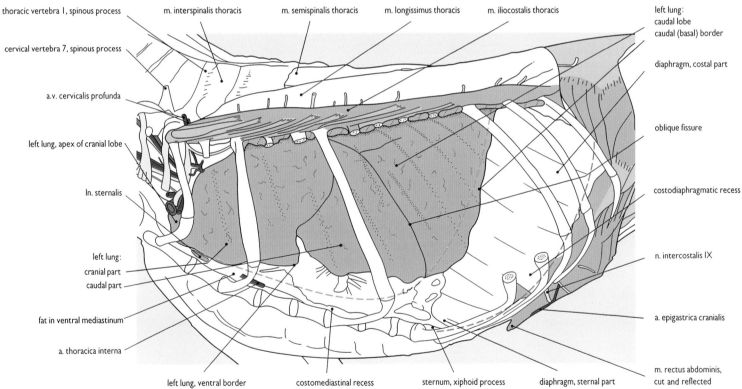

thoracic vertebra 1, spinous process	m. interspinalis thoracis	m. semispinalis thoracis	m. longissimus thoracis	m. iliocostalis thoracis

left lung:
caudal lobe
caudal (basal) border

cervical vertebra 7, spinous process

diaphragm, costal part

a.v. cervicalis profunda

oblique fissure

left lung, apex of cranial lobe

ln. sternalis

costodiaphragmatic recess

left lung:
cranial part
caudal part

n. intercostalis IX

fat in ventral mediastinum

a. epigastrica cranialis

a. thoracica interna

m. rectus abdominis,
cut and reflected

left lung, ventral border   costomediastinal recess   sternum, xiphoid process   diaphragm, sternal part

Fig. 5.21 Thoracic viscera in situ: left lateral view. Ribs 1, 3 and 6 are left in place to show the costal relationships of the viscera. The lungs in this specimen had hardened on fixation rather than becoming 'waterlogged' (unlike Fig. 5.19), presenting a more 'normal' outer contour. The costodiaphragmatic line of pleural reflection is indicated on this, and accompanying drawings by the broken blue line. It follows the attachment of the diaphragm to the ribcage from the midpoint of rib 13, through the distal part of rib 12 and the costochondral junction of rib 11 and follows the costal cartilages of ribs 10 and 9.

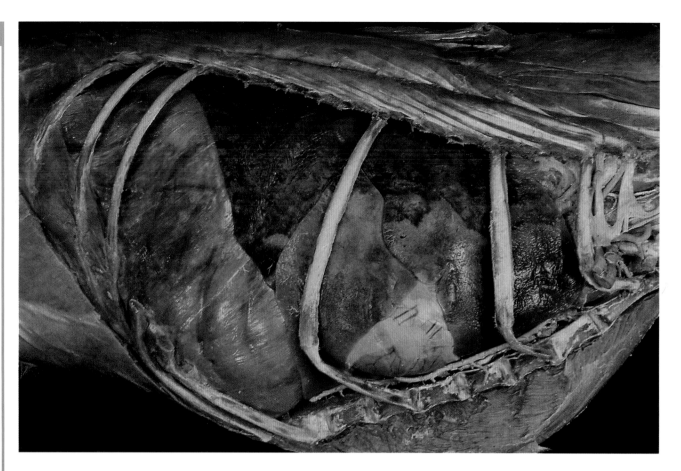

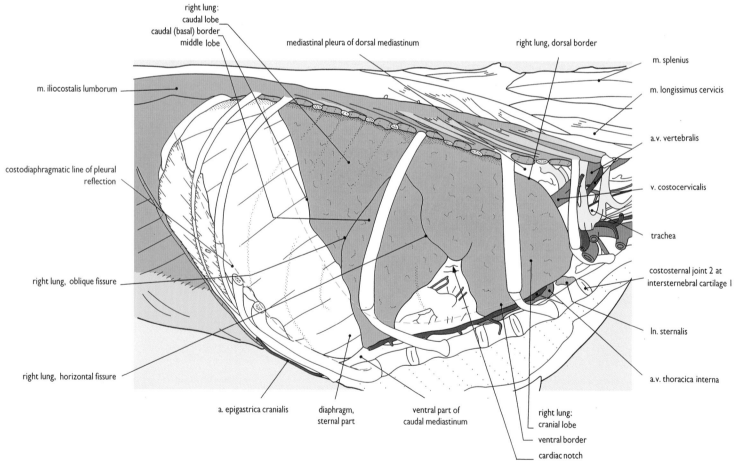

right lung:
caudal lobe
caudal (basal) border
middle lobe

mediastinal pleura of dorsal mediastinum

right lung, dorsal border

m. splenius

m. iliocostalis lumborum

m. longissimus cervicis

a.v. vertebralis

costodiaphragmatic line of pleural
reflection

v. costocervicalis

trachea

right lung, oblique fissure

costosternal joint 2 at
intersternebral cartilage I

ln. sternalis

right lung, horizontal fissure

a.v. thoracica interna

a. epigastrica cranialis

diaphragm,
sternal part

ventral part of
caudal mediastinum

right lung:
cranial lobe

ventral border

cardiac notch

Fig. 5.22 Thoracic viscera in situ: right lateral view. Removal of ribs 4 and 5 has exposed the cardiac notch in the ventral border of the lung between cranial and middle lobes. Through the notch the fat-infiltrated pericardium is exposed on the surface of the heart. The cranial extent of the pleural cavity does not show at all well in any of the dissections – it is represented on either side by a pleural pocket at the thoracic inlet medial to rib 1.

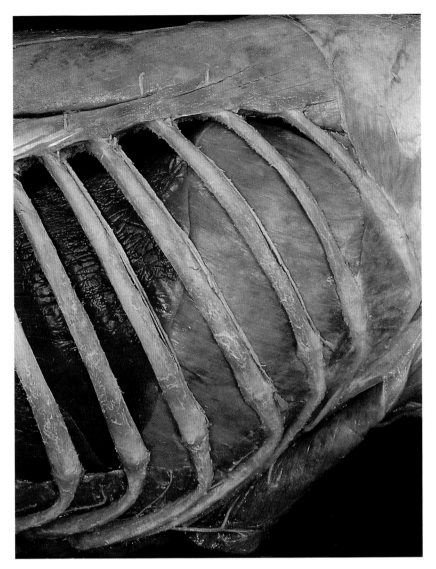

Fig. 5.23 Caudal ribs, costal arch, intercostal arteries and nerves: left lateral view. This is an enlarged view of the caudal end of Fig. 5.18. Intercostal arteries and nerves in intercostal spaces 9, 10 and 11 are displayed after removal of the endothoracic fascia. Continuations of intercostal nerves in spaces 10 and 11 penetrate between interdigitating fibers of the diaphragm and transverse abdominal muscle dorsal to the costal arch. Some internal intercostal muscles remain between the ribs caudal to the costodiaphragmatic line of pleura reflection.

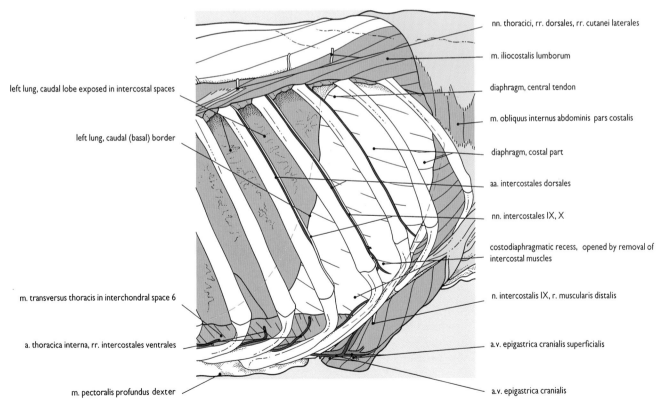

nn. thoracici, rr. dorsales, rr. cutanei laterales

m. iliocostalis lumborum

left lung, caudal lobe exposed in intercostal spaces

diaphragm, central tendon

m. obliquus internus abdominis pars costalis

left lung, caudal (basal) border

diaphragm, costal part

aa. intercostales dorsales

nn. intercostales IX, X

costodiaphragmatic recess, opened by removal of intercostal muscles

m. transversus thoracis in interchondral space 6

n. intercostalis IX, r. muscularis distalis

a. thoracica interna, rr. intercostales ventrales

a.v. epigastrica cranialis superficialis

m. pectoralis profundus dexter

a.v. epigastrica cranialis

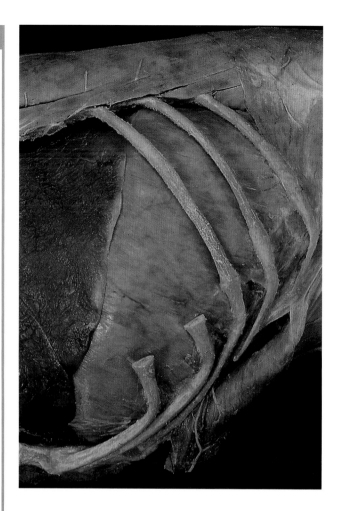

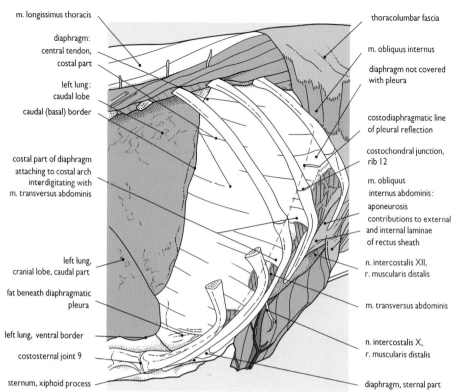

m. longissimus thoracis

diaphragm:
central tendon,
costal part

left lung:
caudal lobe

caudal (basal) border

costal part of diaphragm
attaching to costal arch
interdigitating with
m. transversus abdominis

left lung,
cranial lobe, caudal part

fat beneath diaphragmatic
pleura

left lung, ventral border

costosternal joint 9

sternum, xiphoid process

thoracolumbar fascia

m. obliquus internus

diaphragm not covered
with pleura

costodiaphragmatic line
of pleural reflection

costochondral junction,
rib 12

m. obliquus
internus abdominis:
aponeurosis
contributions to external
and internal laminae
of rectus sheath

n. intercostalis XII,
r. muscularis distalis

m. transversus abdominis

n. intercostalis X,
r. muscularis distalis

diaphragm, sternal part

Fig. 5.24 Caudal ribs, costal arch and diaphragm: left lateral view. The remaining components of the internal intercostal muscles caudal to the costodiaphragmatic line of pleural reflection have been removed from interchondral spaces 11 and 12, exposing the costal arch and overall attachment of the costal part of the diaphragm.

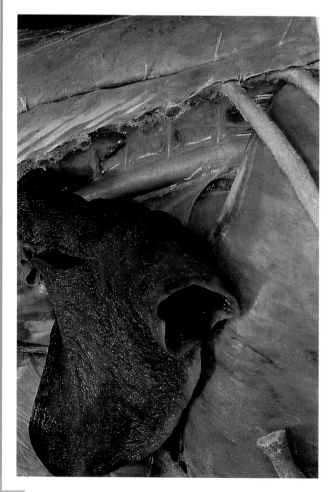

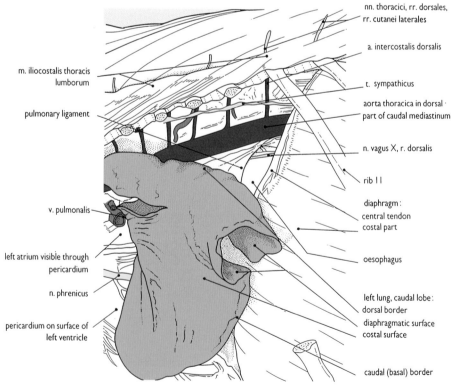

m. iliocostalis thoracis
lumborum

pulmonary ligament

v. pulmonalis

left atrium visible through
pericardium

n. phrenicus

pericardium on surface of
left ventricle

nn. thoracici, rr. dorsales,
rr. cutanei laterales

a. intercostalis dorsalis

t. sympathicus

aorta thoracica in dorsal
part of caudal mediastinum

n. vagus X, r. dorsalis

rib 11

diaphragm:
central tendon
costal part

oesophagus

left lung, caudal lobe:
dorsal border
diaphragmatic surface
costal surface

caudal (basal) border

Fig. 5.25 Pulmonary ligament and caudal lobe of the left lung: left lateral view. The caudal lobe has been pulled ventrally as far as possible without rupturing the pulmonary ligament.

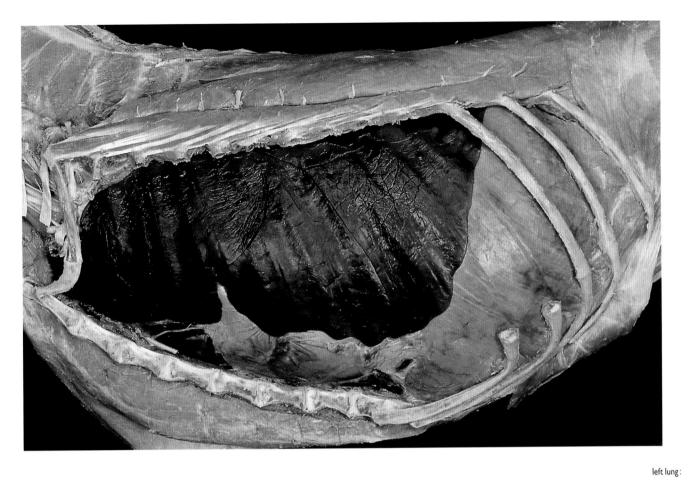

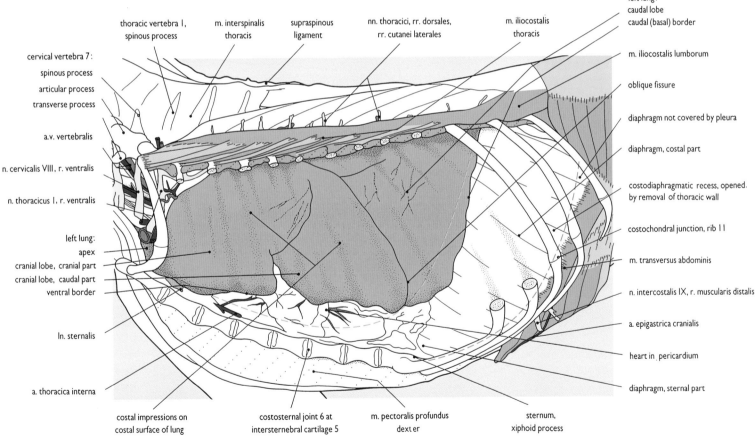

cervical vertebra 7 :

spinous process

articular process

transverse process

a.v. vertebralis

n. cervicalis VIII, r. ventralis

n. thoracicus I, r. ventralis

left lung:
apex
cranial lobe, cranial part
cranial lobe, caudal part
ventral border

ln. sternalis

a. thoracica interna

thoracic vertebra I,
spinous process

m. interspinalis
thoracis

supraspinous
ligament

nn. thoracici, rr. dorsales,
rr. cutanei laterales

m. iliocostalis
thoracis

left lung :
caudal lobe
caudal (basal) border

m. iliocostalis lumborum

oblique fissure

diaphragm not covered by pleura

diaphragm, costal part

costodiaphragmatic recess, opened
by removal of thoracic wall

costochondral junction, rib II

m. transversus abdominis

n. intercostalis IX, r. muscularis distalis

a. epigastrica cranialis

heart in pericardium

diaphragm, sternal part

costal impressions on
costal surface of lung

costosternal joint 6 at
intersternebral cartilage 5

m. pectoralis profundus
dexter

sternum,
xiphoid process

Fig. 5.26 Left lung after removal of the ribs: left lateral view. Ribs 2 to 10 have been removed exposing the costal surface of the lung. The rib impressions remain visible on the surface of the lung (hardened on preservation). The lung subdivision into cranial and caudal lobes is now seen with an incomplete subdivision of the large cranial lobe into cranial and caudal parts. The apex of the cranial lobe is shown projecting through the thoracic inlet into the base of the neck ventral to the axillary vessels (see also Figs 5.32 and 5.35). Cranial to rib 3, the dorsal border is visible passing cranioventrally to the apex of the lung.

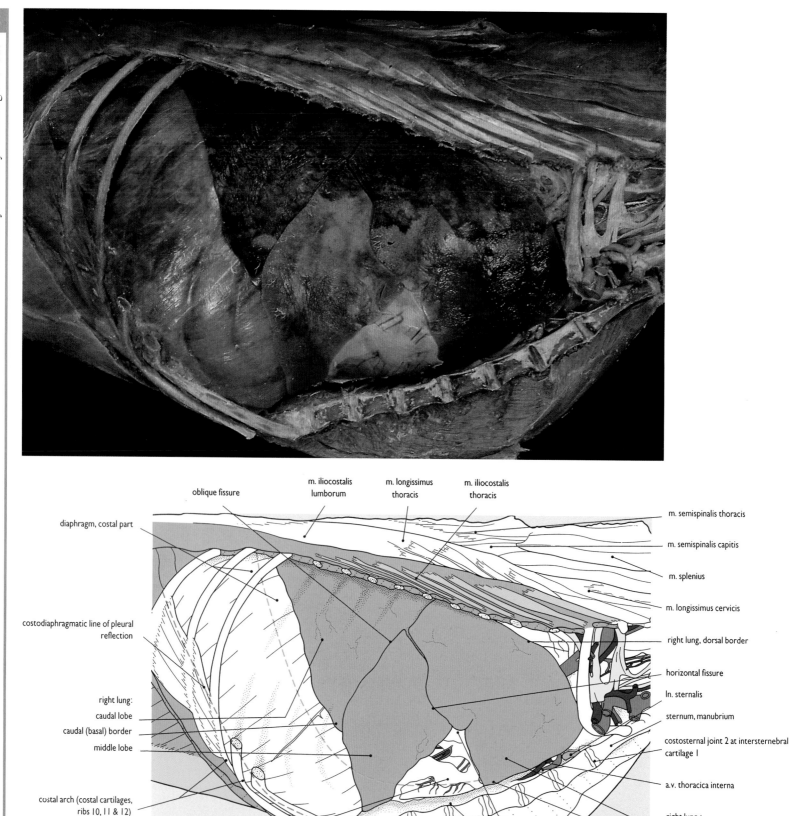

oblique fissure

m. iliocostalis lumborum

m. longissimus thoracis

m. iliocostalis thoracis

diaphragm, costal part

costodiaphragmatic line of pleural reflection

right lung:
caudal lobe
caudal (basal) border
middle lobe

costal arch (costal cartilages, ribs 10, 11 & 12)

heart in pericardium

diaphragm, sternal part

m. pectoralis profundus sinister

m. transversus thoracis sinister (visible, after disruption of ventral mediastinum)

m. semispinalis thoracis

m. semispinalis capitis

m. splenius

m. longissimus cervicis

right lung, dorsal border

horizontal fissure

ln. sternalis

sternum, manubrium

costosternal joint 2 at intersternebral cartilage 1

a.v. thoracica interna

right lung :
cranial lobe
ventral border
cardiac notch

Fig. 5.27 Right lung after removal of the ribs: right lateral view. The subdivision of the lung into three visible lobes is apparent in this right side view. The fourth, accessory, lobe will only be seen if these lobes are removed (see Fig. 5.29) or if viewed from the left side, since it lies to the left of the caudal vena cava in the mediastinal recess of the right pleural cavity (see Figs 5.31 and 5.86).

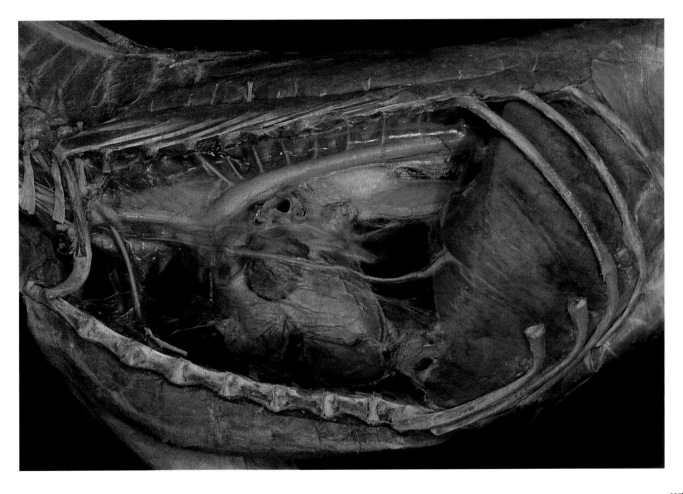

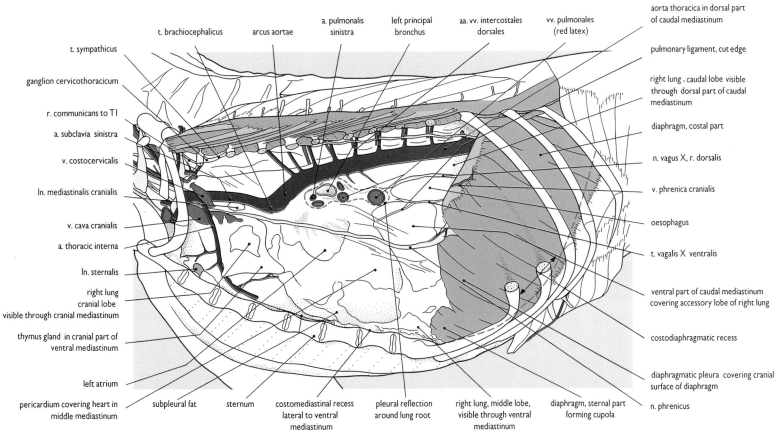

aorta thoracica in dorsal part of caudal mediastinum

pulmonary ligament, cut edge

right lung . caudal lobe visible through dorsal part of caudal mediastinum

diaphragm, costal part

n. vagus X, r. dorsalis

v. phrenica cranialis

oesophagus

t. vagalis X ventralis

ventral part of caudal mediastinum covering accessory lobe of right lung

costodiaphragmatic recess

diaphragmatic pleura covering cranial surface of diaphragm

n. phrenicus

t. sympathicus

ganglion cervicothoracicum

r. communicans to T1

a. subclavia sinistra

v. costocervicalis

ln. mediastinalis cranialis

v. cava cranialis

a. thoracic interna

ln. sternalis

right lung cranial lobe visible through cranial mediastinum

thymus gland in cranial part of ventral mediastinum

left atrium

pericardium covering heart in middle mediastinum

t. brachiocephalicus

arcus aortae

a. pulmonalis sinistra

left principal bronchus

aa. vv. intercostales dorsales

vv. pulmonales (red latex)

subpleural fat

sternum

costomediastinal recess lateral to ventral mediastinum

pleural reflection around lung root

right lung, middle lobe, visible through ventral mediastinum

diaphragm, sternal part forming cupola

Fig. 5.28 Mediastinum after removal of the left lung: left lateral view. The lung has been removed at its hilus and the root of the lung is exposed. The mediastinum dividing left from right pleural cavities can be seen. It is covered by a layer of mediastinal pleura that, together with some underlying fat deposits, obscures many details of the mediastinal 'contents'. The disposition of the mediastinum in the thorax is complicated by two factors – the caudal vena cava in its fold of mediastinum (plica vena cava) and the accessory lobe of the right lung 'pushing' the mediastinum away from its midline position.

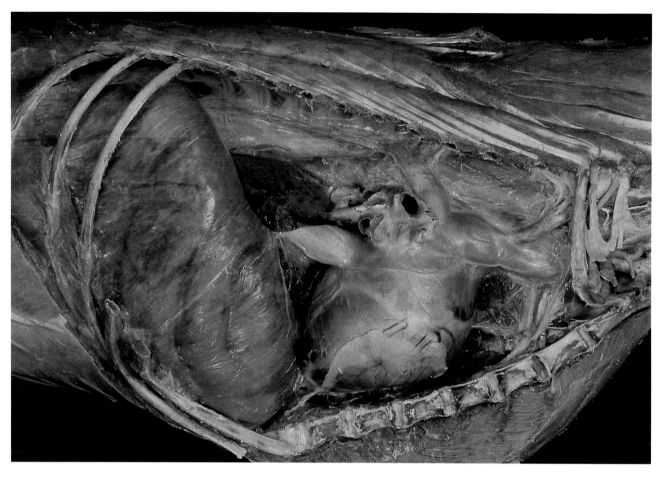

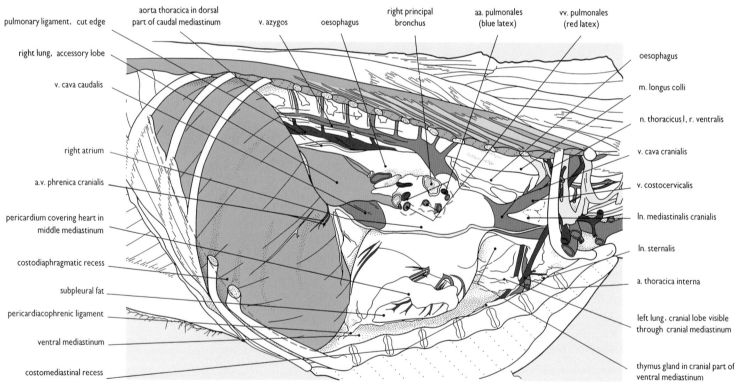

pulmonary ligament, cut edge

aorta thoracica in dorsal part of caudal mediastinum

v. azygos

oesophagus

right principal bronchus

aa. pulmonales (blue latex)

vv. pulmonales (red latex)

right lung, accessory lobe

v. cava caudalis

right atrium

a.v. phrenica cranialis

pericardium covering heart in middle mediastinum

costodiaphragmatic recess

subpleural fat

pericardiacophrenic ligament

ventral mediastinum

costomediastinal recess

oesophagus

m. longus colli

n. thoracicus I, r. ventralis

v. cava cranialis

v. costocervicalis

ln. mediastinalis cranialis

ln. sternalis

a. thoracica interna

left lung, cranial lobe visible through cranial mediastinum

thymus gland in cranial part of ventral mediastinum

Fig. 5.29 Mediastinum after removal of the cranial, middle and caudal lobes of the right lung: right lateral view. The cranial, middle and caudal lobes of the lung have been removed, the accessory lobe remaining in position, slightly obscuring the root of the lung (see also Figs 5.86 & 5.92). Note the extreme thinness and fragility of the ventral mediastinum where it meets the sternum ventrally.

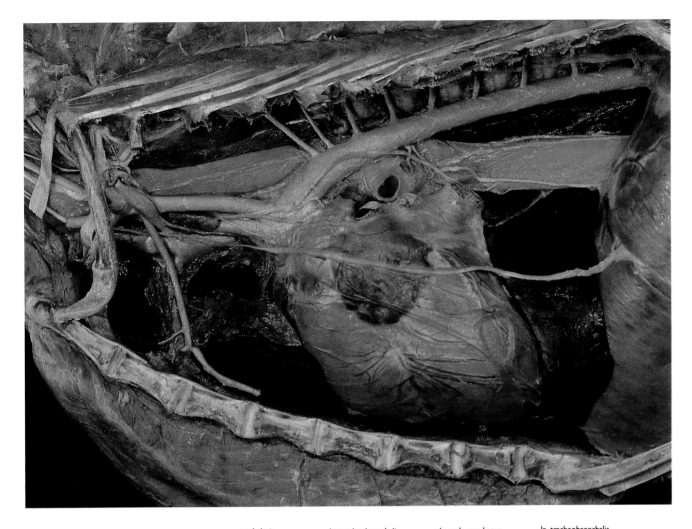

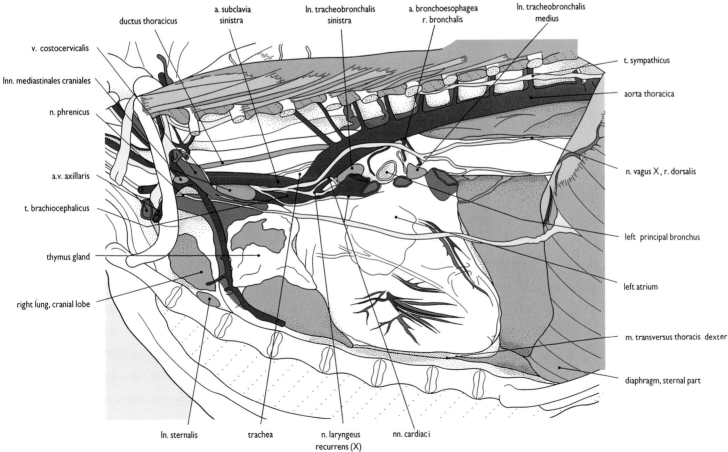

ductus thoracicus · a. subclavia sinistra · ln. tracheobronchalis sinistra · a. bronchoesophagea r. bronchalis · ln. tracheobronchalis medius

v. costocervicalis

lnn. mediastinales craniales

n. phrenicus

a.v. axillaris

t. brachiocephalicus

thymus gland

right lung, cranial lobe

t. sympathicus

aorta thoracica

n. vagus X , r. dorsalis

left principal bronchus

left atrium

m. transversus thoracis dexter

diaphragm, sternal part

ln. sternalis · trachea · n. laryngeus recurrens (X) · nn. cardiaci

Fig. 5.30 Vessels and nerves of the mediastinum: left lateral view. The mediastinal pleura and underlying deposits of fat have been removed. The thin mediastinum, consisting of a connective tissue sheet sandwiched by pleural layers, has been removed, opening the right pleural cavity. The cranial, caudal and accessory lobes of the right lung are exposed. Dissection around the lung root and base of the heart exposes the tracheobronchial lymph nodes, the course of the vagus nerve (X) and its recurrent and cardiac branches, and vagal branching on the esophagus. The pericardium remains intact along with the phrenic nerve.

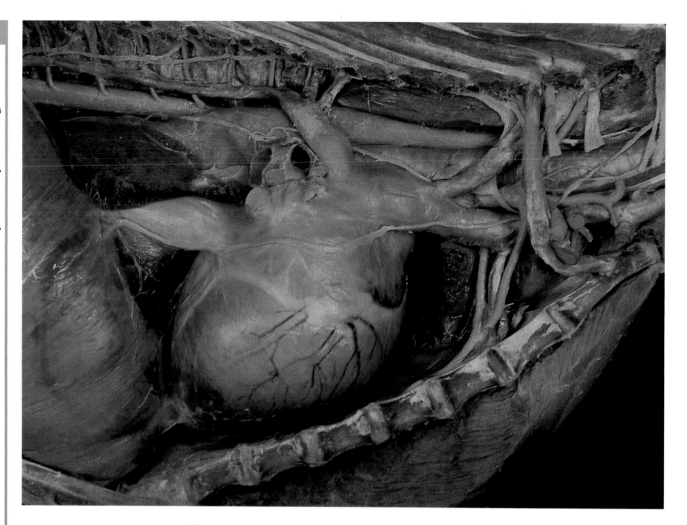

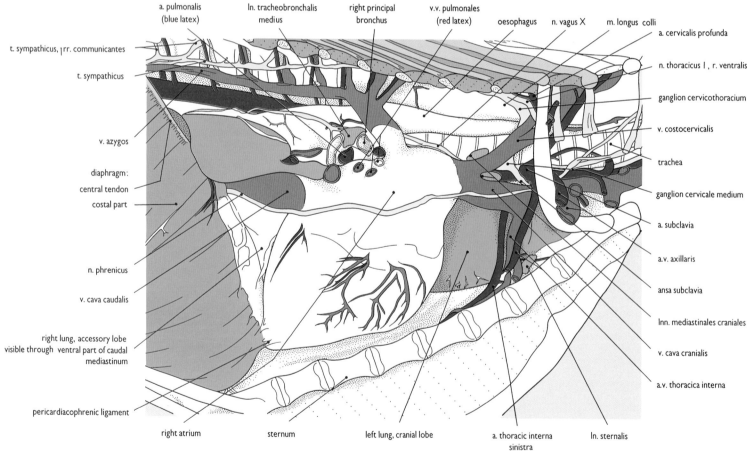

a. pulmonalis (blue latex)

ln. tracheobronchalis medius

right principal bronchus

v.v. pulmonales (red latex)

oesophagus

n. vagus X

m. longus colli

t. sympathicus, ₁rr. communicantes

t. sympathicus

v. azygos

diaphragm:
central tendon
costal part

n. phrenicus

v. cava caudalis

right lung, accessory lobe
visible through ventral part of caudal
mediastinum

pericardiacophrenic ligament

a. cervicalis profunda

n. thoracicus I , r. ventralis

ganglion cervicothoracium

v. costocervicalis

trachea

ganglion cervicale medium

a. subclavia

a.v. axillaris

ansa subclavia

lnn. mediastinales craniales

v. cava cranialis

a.v. thoracica interna

right atrium

sternum

left lung, cranial lobe

a. thoracic interna sinistra

ln. sternalis

Fig. 5.31 Vessels and nerves of the mediastinum: right lateral view. Removal of mediastinal pleura and subpleural fat has exposed the mediastinal 'contents' but the mediastinum, where it forms an additional fold (plica) for the caudal vena cava and phrenic nerve, is still intact. The ventral part of the accessory lobe is visible and the middle tracheobronchial lymph node is exposed.

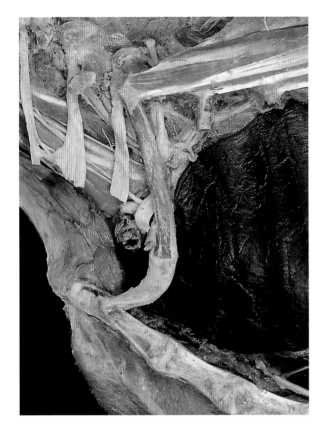

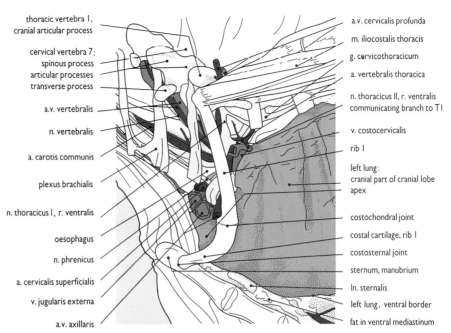

thoracic vertebra I, cranial articular process

cervical vertebra 7:
spinous process
articular processes
transverse process

a.v. vertebralis

n. vertebralis

a. carotis communis

plexus brachialis

n. thoracicus I, r. ventralis

oesophagus

n. phrenicus

a. cervicalis superficialis

v. jugularis externa

a.v. axillaris

a.v. cervicalis profunda

m. iliocostalis thoracis

g. cervicothoracicum

a. vertebralis thoracica

n. thoracicus II, r. ventralis communicating branch to T I

v. costocervicalis

rib I

left lung:
cranial part of cranial lobe
apex

costochondral joint

costal cartilage, rib I

costosternal joint

sternum, manubrium

ln. sternalis

left lung, ventral border

fat in ventral mediastinum

Fig. 5.32 Thoracic inlet and apex of the left lung: left lateral view. This is an enlarged view of the cranial end of the dissection in Fig. 5.26. Note the apex of the left lung projecting through the lower part of the thoracic inlet below the axillary vessels. (See Chapter 3 for relationship of thoracic inlet to structures in the neck – the thoracic inlet in section is shown in Fig. 3.43.) Several structures which were *not* covered by mediastinal pleura are exposed in the dorsal end of intercostal space 1.

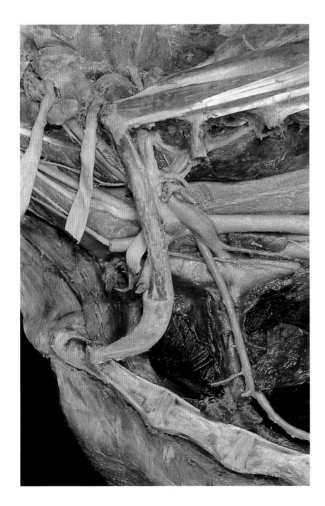

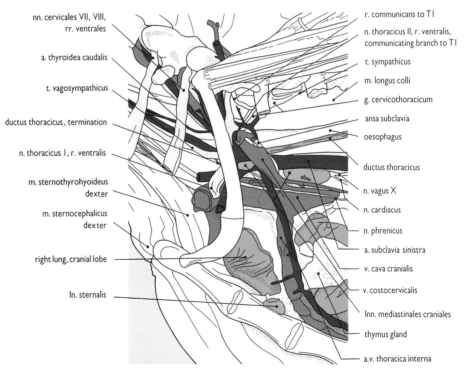

nn. cervicales VII, VIII, rr. ventrales

a. thyroidea caudalis

t. vagosympathicus

ductus thoracicus, termination

n. thoracicus I, r. ventralis

m. sternothyrohyoideus dexter

m. sternocephalicus dexter

right lung, cranial lobe

ln. sternalis

r. communicans to T I

n. thoracicus II, r. ventralis, communicating branch to T I

t. sympathicus

m. longus colli

g. cervicothoracicum

ansa subclavia

oesophagus

ductus thoracicus

n. vagus X

n. cardiacus

n. phrenicus

a. subclavia sinistra

v. cava cranialis

v. costocervicalis

lnn. mediastinales craniales

thymus gland

a.v. thoracica interna

Fig. 5.33 Thoracic inlet after removal of the left lung: left lateral view. This is an enlarged view of the cranial end of the dissection in Fig. 5.30. Removal of the lung exposes the blood vessels and nerves passing through the thoracic inlet and shows cranial mediastinal lymph nodes and the thoracic duct. The esophagus is slightly dilated at the base of the neck as it passes through the thoracic inlet. The termination of the thoracic duct is just visible and it contains a small quantity of blue latex which entered it from the external jugular vein.

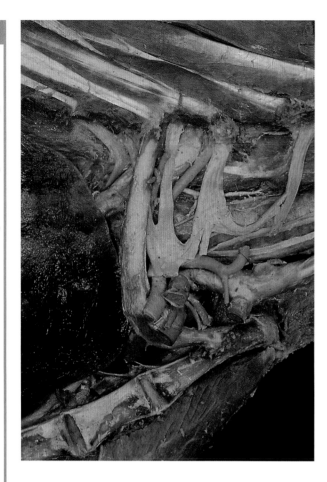

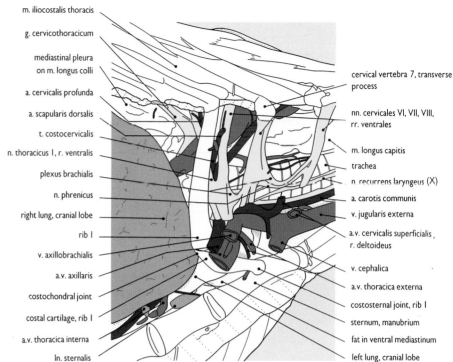

m. iliocostalis thoracis
g. cervicothoracicum
mediastinal pleura
on m. longus colli
a. cervicalis profunda
a. scapularis dorsalis
t. costocervicalis
n. thoracicus I, r. ventralis
plexus brachialis
n. phrenicus
right lung, cranial lobe
rib I
v. axillobrachialis
a.v. axillaris
costochondral joint
costal cartilage, rib I
a.v. thoracica interna
ln. sternalis

cervical vertebra 7, transverse process
nn. cervicales VI, VII, VIII, rr. ventrales
m. longus capitis
trachea
n. recurrens laryngeus (X)
a. carotis communis
v. jugularis externa
a.v. cervicalis superficialis, r. deltoideus
v. cephalica
a.v. thoracica externa
costosternal joint, rib I
sternum, manubrium
fat in ventral mediastinum
left lung, cranial lobe

Fig. 5.34 Thoracic inlet and apex of the right lung: right lateral view. This is an enlarged view of the cranial end of the dissection in Fig. 5.27. The apex of the right lung does not extend for any distance through the thoracic inlet – compare with left lung in Fig. 5.32. The entry of the cephalic vein into the external jugular vein, and the axillobrachial vein union with the axillary vein are clearly displayed.

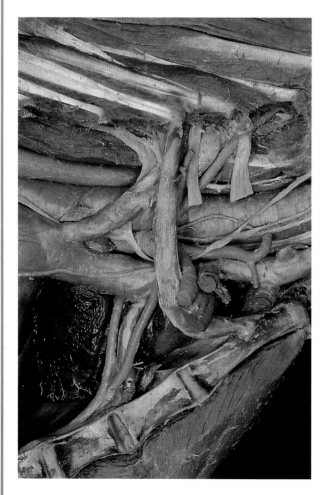

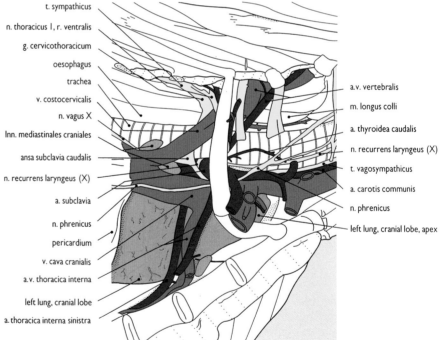

t. sympathicus
n. thoracicus I, r. ventralis
g. cervicothoracicum
oesophagus
trachea
v. costocervicalis
n. vagus X
lnn. mediastinales craniales
ansa subclavia caudalis
n. recurrens laryngeus (X)
a. subclavia
n. phrenicus
pericardium
v. cava cranialis
a.v. thoracica interna
left lung, cranial lobe
a. thoracica interna sinistra

a.v. vertebralis
m. longus colli
a. thyroidea caudalis
n. recurrens laryngeus (X)
t. vagosympathicus
a. carotis communis
n. phrenicus
left lung, cranial lobe, apex

Fig. 5.35 Thoracic inlet after removal of the right lung: right lateral view. This is an enlarged view of the cranial end of the dissection in Fig. 5.31. Lung removal has exposed blood vessels and nerves passing through the thoracic inlet. Note particularly the costocervical vein flanked at its entry into the cranial vena cava by two cranial mediastinal lymph nodes. The partial removal of the brachial plexus reveals the recurrent laryngeal nerve, the phrenic nerve and the vagosympathetic trunk en route through the inlet.

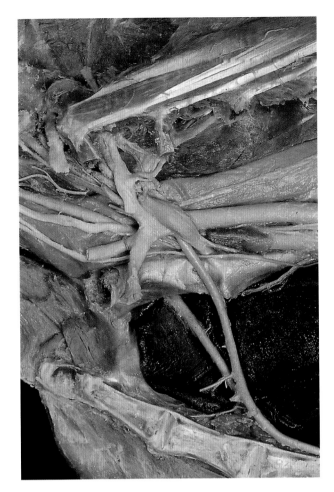

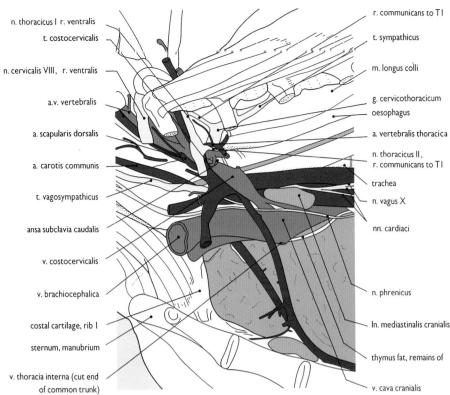

n. thoracicus I r. ventralis

t. costocervicalis

n. cervicalis VIII, r. ventralis

a.v. vertebralis

a. scapularis dorsalis

a. carotis communis

t. vagosympathicus

ansa subclavia caudalis

v. costocervicalis

v. brachiocephalica

costal cartilage, rib I

sternum, manubrium

v. thoracia interna (cut end of common trunk)

r. communicans to T I

t. sympathicus

m. longus colli

g. cervicothoracicum

oesophagus

a. vertebralis thoracica

n. thoracicus II, r. communicans to T I

trachea

n. vagus X

nn. cardiaci

n. phrenicus

ln. mediastinalis cranialis

thymus fat, remains of

v. cava cranialis

Fig. 5.36 Vessels and nerves of the cranial mediastinum: left lateral view (1). Rib 1 has been removed. Exposure of structures medial to it is completed by the removal of the ventral rami of those spinal nerves forming the brachial plexus. Remnants of the thymus gland and mediastinal pleura have been removed from the cranial mediastinum.

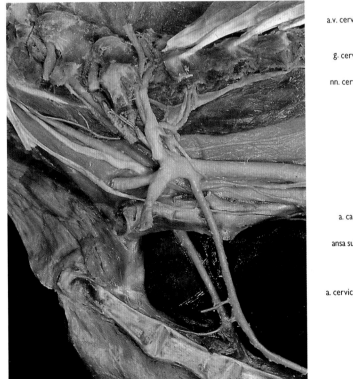

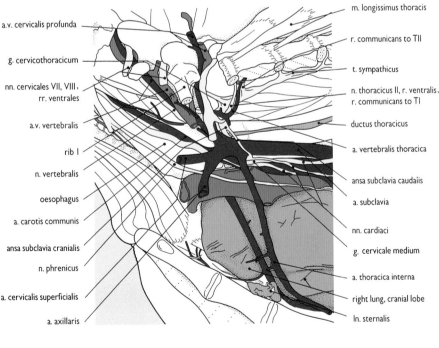

a.v. cervicalis profunda

g. cervicothoracicum

nn. cervicales VII, VIII, rr. ventrales

a.v. vertebralis

rib I

n. vertebralis

oesophagus

a. carotis communis

ansa subclavia cranialis

n. phrenicus

a. cervicalis superficialis

a. axillaris

m. longissimus thoracis

r. communicans to T II

t. sympathicus

n. thoracicus II, r. ventralis, r. communicans to T I

ductus thoracicus

a. vertebralis thoracica

ansa subclavia caudalis

a. subclavia

nn. cardiaci

g. cervicale medium

a. thoracica interna

right lung, cranial lobe

ln. sternalis

Fig. 5.37 Vessels and nerves of the cranial mediastinum: left lateral view (2). The ansa subclavia and middle cervical sympathetic ganglion have been exposed after removal of the costocervical vein and cranial mediastinal lymph nodes. The iliocostalis thoracis muscle and most of the cranial longissimus thoracis muscle components onto the upper end of rib 1 have been removed. Exposed by these removals are the deep cervical vessels, the emergence of thoracic spinal nerve 1, the remaining branches of the left subclavian artery and the sympathetic chain extending caudally from the cervicothoracic ganglion.

5

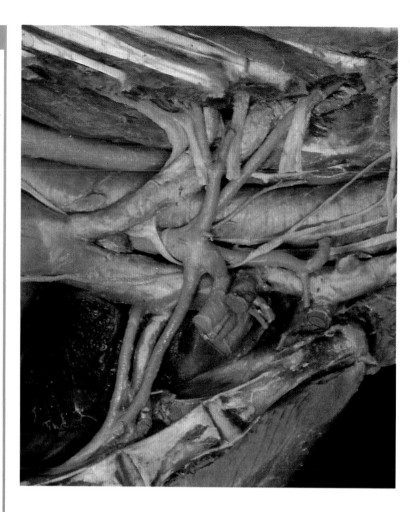

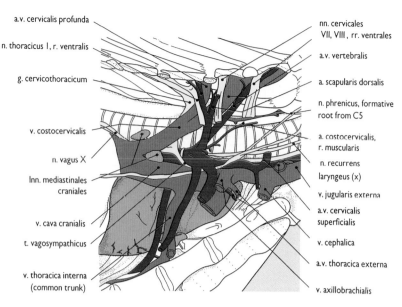

a.v. cervicalis profunda

n. thoracicus I, r. ventralis

g. cervicothoracicum

v. costocervicalis

n. vagus X

lnn. mediastinales craniales

v. cava cranialis

t. vagosympathicus

v. thoracica interna (common trunk)

nn. cervicales VII, VIII, rr. ventrales

a.v. vertebralis

a. scapularis dorsalis

n. phrenicus, formative root from C5

a. costocervicalis, r. muscularis

n. recurrens laryngeus (x)

v. jugularis externa

a.v. cervicalis superficialis

v. cephalica

a.v. thoracica externa

v. axillobrachialis

Fig. 5.38 Vessels and nerves of the cranial mediastinum: right lateral view (1). Removal of rib 1 exposes the initial branching of the subclavian artery and the passage of the phrenic nerve. The recurrent laryngeal nerve (vagus X) is clearly displayed running cranially on the trachea.

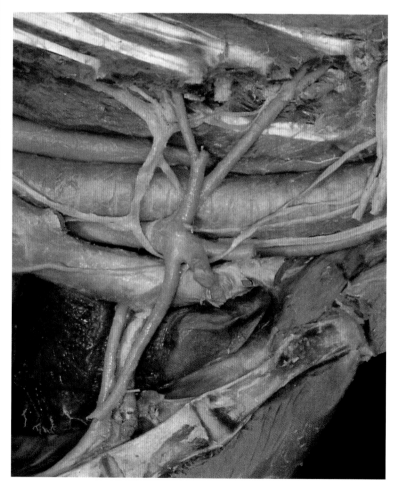

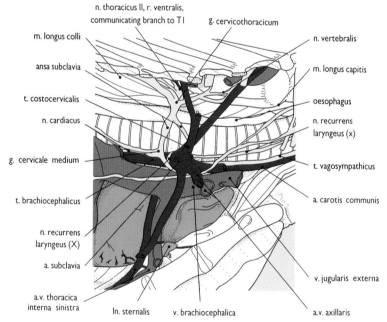

n. thoracicus II, r. ventralis, communicating branch to TI

m. longus colli

ansa subclavia

t. costocervicalis

n. cardiacus

g. cervicale medium

t. brachiocephalicus

n. recurrens laryngeus (X)

a. subclavia

a.v. thoracica interna sinistra

g. cervicothoracicum

n. vertebralis

m. longus capitis

oesophagus

n. recurrens laryngeus (x)

t. vagosympathicus

a. carotis communis

v. jugularis externa

v. brachiocephalica

lnn. sternalis

a.v. axillaris

Fig. 5.39 Vessels and nerves of the cranial mediastinum: right lateral view (2). The ansa subclavia, the origin of the recurrent laryngeal nerve and the formation of the vertebral nerve from combined rami communicates from the cervicothoracic ganglion, are all clearly displayed following removal of the costocervical vein and cranial mediastinal lymph nodes, and further trimming of ventral rami of the spinal nerves. This view clearly shows the cranial extent of the apex of the left lung.

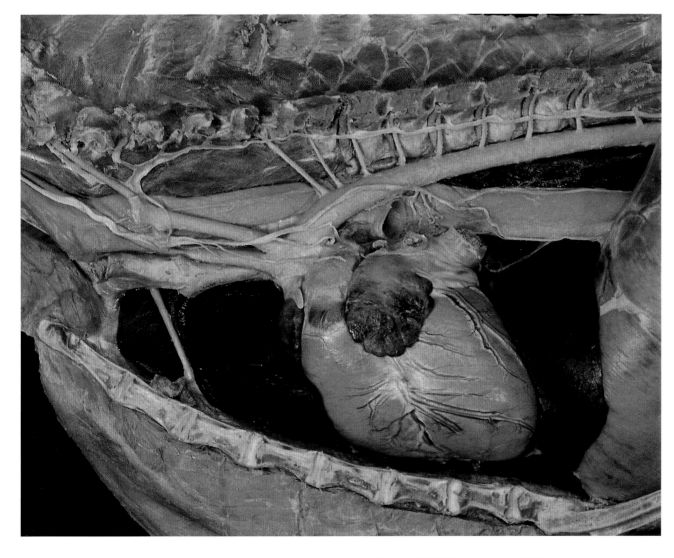

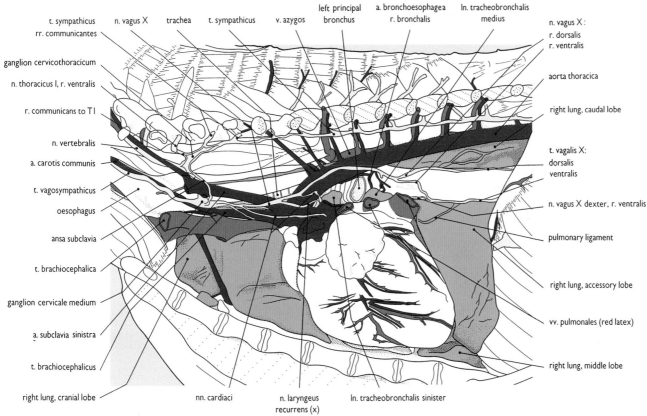

t. sympathicus
rr. communicantes

ganglion cervicothoracicum

n. thoracicus I, r. ventralis

r. communicans to T I

n. vertebralis

a. carotis communis

t. vagosympathicus

oesophagus

ansa subclavia

t. brachiocephalica

ganglion cervicale medium

a. subclavia sinistra

t. brachiocephalicus

right lung, cranial lobe

n. vagus X   trachea   t. sympathicus   v. azygos

left principal
bronchus

a. bronchoesophagea
r. bronchalis

ln. tracheobronchalis
medius

nn. cardiaci

n. laryngeus
recurrens (x)

ln. tracheobronchalis sinister

n. vagus X :
r. dorsalis
r. ventralis

aorta thoracica

right lung, caudal lobe

t. vagalis X:
dorsalis
ventralis

n. vagus X dexter, r. ventralis

pulmonary ligament

right lung, accessory lobe

vv. pulmonales (red latex)

right lung, middle lobe

Fig. 5.40 Autonomic nerves of the thorax: left lateral view. The middle cervical and cervicothoracic ganglia, joined by an ansa subclavia, have been exposed by removal of the subclavian artery (bar its vertebral branch). Removal of the iliocostalis and longissimus thoracis muscles and the upper ends of the ribs exposes the thoracic sympathetic chain with rami communicates. Division of the vagus into dorsal and ventral branches on the esophagus caudal to the heart, and union of the ventral branch with that of right side to give the ventral vagal trunk are shown. Union of the dorsal vagal branches occurs close to the diaphragm. The recurrent laryngeal nerve is visible at its origin from the vagus, curving medially around the ligamentum arteriosum.

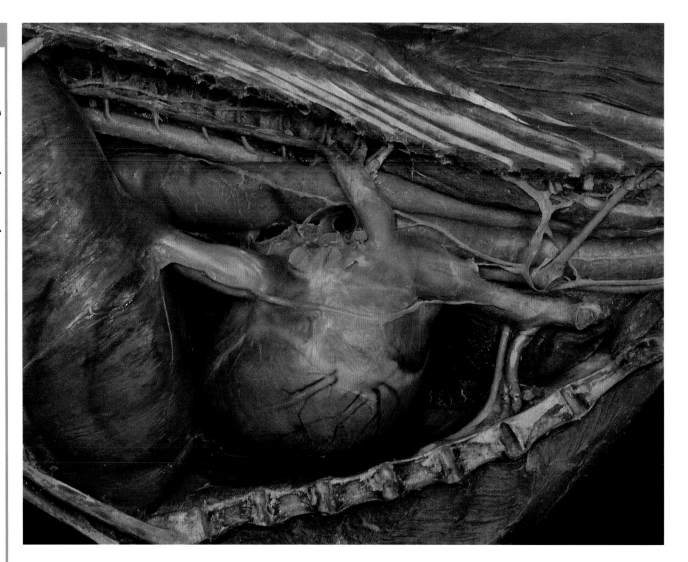

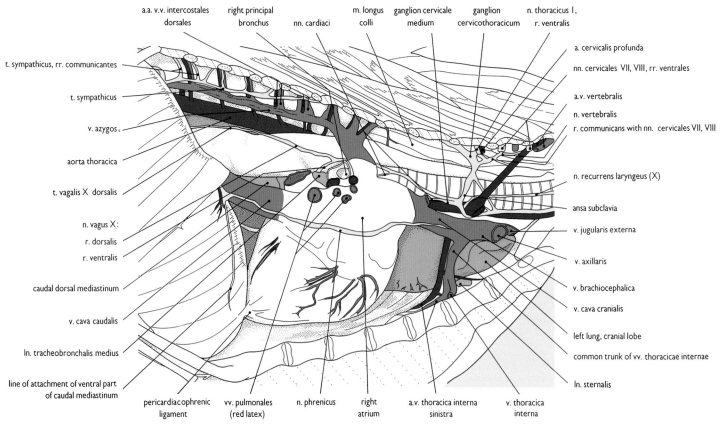

a.a. v.v. intercostales dorsales | right principal bronchus | nn. cardiaci | m. longus colli | ganglion cervicale medium | ganglion cervicothoracicum | n. thoracicus I, r. ventralis

t. sympathicus, rr. communicantes

t. sympathicus

v. azygos

aorta thoracica

t. vagalis X dorsalis

n. vagus X:
r. dorsalis
r. ventralis

caudal dorsal mediastinum

v. cava caudalis

ln. tracheobronchalis medius

line of attachment of ventral part of caudal mediastinum

pericardiacophrenic ligament | vv. pulmonales (red latex) | n. phrenicus | right atrium | a.v. thoracica interna sinistra | v. thoracica interna

a. cervicalis profunda

nn. cervicales VII, VIII, rr. ventrales

a.v. vertebralis

n. vertebralis

r. communicans with nn. cervicales VII, VIII

n. recurrens laryngeus (X)

ansa subclavia

v. jugularis externa

v. axillaris

v. brachiocephalica

v. cava cranialis

left lung, cranial lobe

common trunk of vv. thoracicae internae

ln. sternalis

Fig. 5.41 Autonomic nerves of the thorax: right lateral view. Removal of the subclavian artery (bar its vertebral branch) has exposed the middle cervical and cervicothoracic ganglia and their linking ansa. The right recurrent laryngeal nerve is also exposed at this point as it passes dorsally and cranially around the subclavian artery. Cardiac nerves arise from the vagus nerve (X); its division into dorsal and ventral branches is visible on the esophagus caudal to the heart. The esophagus and caudal vena cava are exposed further after removal of the accessory lobe of the right lung.

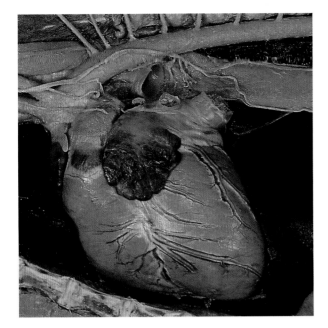
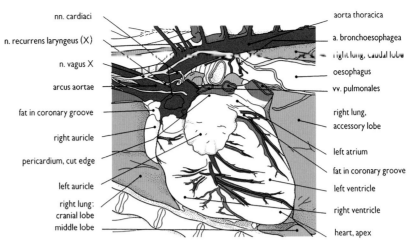

nn. cardiaci
n. recurrens laryngeus (X)
n. vagus X
arcus aortae
fat in coronary groove
right auricle
pericardium, cut edge
left auricle
right lung:
cranial lobe
middle lobe

aorta thoracica
a. bronchoesophagea
right lung, caudal lobe
oesophagus
vv. pulmonales
right lung,
accessory lobe
left atrium
fat in coronary groove
left ventricle
right ventricle
heart, apex

Fig. 5.42 Heart (1) surface after pericardial removal: left lateral view. The pericardium has been removed from the left side of the heart by cutting through at its attachment onto the base of the heart. This has exposed the epicardium applied to the auricular surface of the heart. Both auricles are visible.

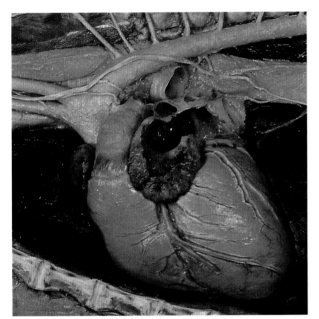
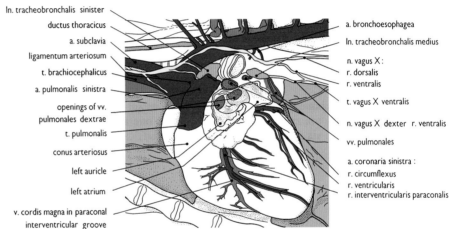

ln. tracheobronchalis sinister
ductus thoracicus
a. subclavia
ligamentum arteriosum
t. brachiocephalicus
a. pulmonalis sinistra
openings of vv. pulmonales dextrae
t. pulmonalis
conus arteriosus
left auricle
left atrium
v. cordis magna in paraconal interventricular groove

a. bronchoesophagea
ln. tracheobronchalis medius
n. vagus X :
r. dorsalis
r. ventralis
t. vagus X ventralis
n. vagus X dexter r. ventralis
vv. pulmonales
a. coronaria sinistra :
r. circumflexus
r. ventricularis
r. interventricularis paraconalis

Fig. 5.43 Heart (2) coronary vessels and interior of the left atrium: left lateral view. The epicardium has been removed along with subepicardial fat exposing the left coronary artery branches and the great cardiac vein. Part of the lateral wall of the left atrium has also been cut away displaying the entry of left and right pulmonary veins.

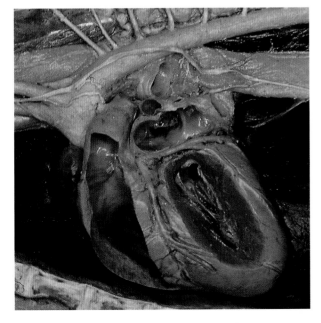
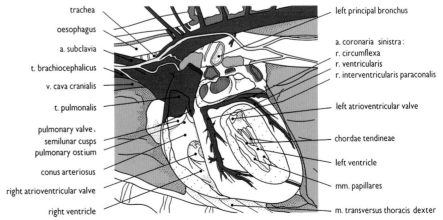

trachea
oesophagus
a. subclavia
t. brachiocephalicus
v. cava cranialis
t. pulmonalis
pulmonary valve, semilunar cusps
pulmonary ostium
conus arteriosus
right atrioventricular valve
right ventricle

left principal bronchus
a. coronaria sinistra :
r. circumflexa
r. ventricularis
r. interventricularis paraconalis
left atrioventricular valve
chordae tendineae
left ventricle
mm. papillares
m. transversus thoracis dexter

Fig. 5.44 Heart (3) left coronary artery and interior of the ventricles: left lateral view. Both ventricles have been opened. In the right, atrioventricular and pulmonary ostia are visible with their constituent valves. In the left, the atrioventricular valve is visible but the aortic ostium and valve are still hidden by the interventricular septum.

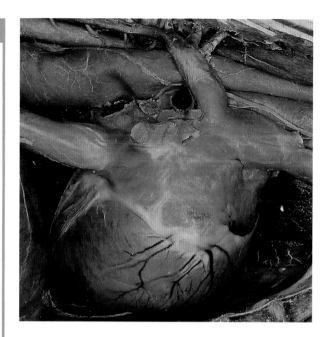
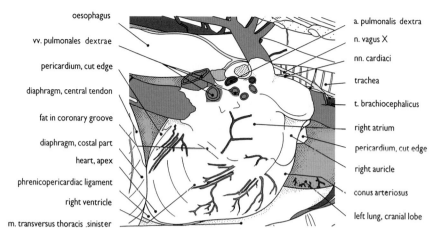

oesophagus
vv. pulmonales dextrae
pericardium, cut edge
diaphragm, central tendon
fat in coronary groove
diaphragm, costal part
heart, apex
phrenicopericardiac ligament
right ventricle
m. transversus thoracis .sinister

a. pulmonalis dextra
n. vagus X
nn. cardiaci
trachea
t. brachiocephalicus
right atrium
pericardium, cut edge
right auricle
conus arteriosus
left lung, cranial lobe

Fig. 5.45 Heart (4) surface after pericardial removal: right lateral view. The pericardium has been removed from the atrial surface of the heart by cutting through its attachment around the heart's base. The limits of atrial myocardium are clearly apparent on the venae cavae and azygos vein where they enter the heart.

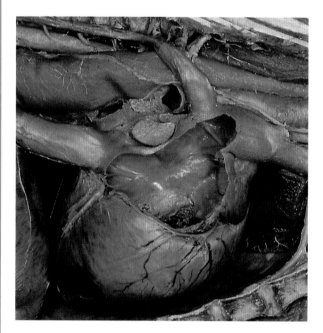
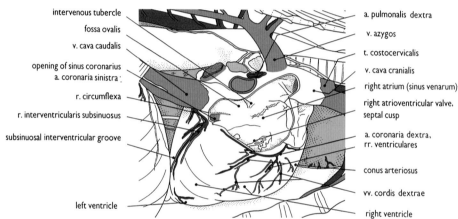

intervenous tubercle
fossa ovalis
v. cava caudalis
opening of sinus coronarius
a. coronaria sinistra
r. circumflexa
r. interventricularis subsinuosus
subsinuosal interventricular groove
left ventricle

a. pulmonalis dextra
v. azygos
t. costocervicalis
v. cava cranialis
right atrium (sinus venarum)
right atrioventricular valve, septal cusp
a. coronaria dextra, rr. ventriculares
conus arteriosus
vv. cordis dextrae
right ventricle

Fig. 5.46 Heart (5) coronary vessels and interior of the right atrium: right lateral view. The epicardium has been stripped from coronary and interventricular grooves and its underlying fat dissected, displaying the right coronary artery and the interventricular branch of the left coronary artery.

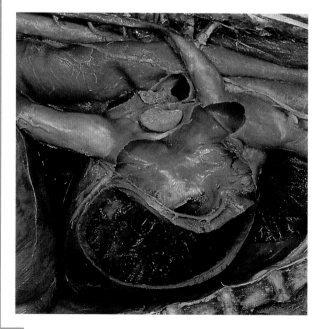
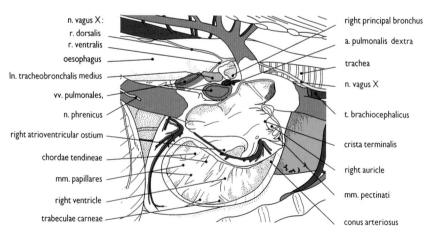

n. vagus X:
r. dorsalis
r. ventralis
oesophagus
ln. tracheobronchalis medius
vv. pulmonales,
n. phrenicus
right atrioventricular ostium
chordae tendineae
mm. papillares
right ventricle
trabeculae carneae

right principal bronchus
a. pulmonalis dextra
trachea
n. vagus X
t. brachiocephalicus
crista terminalis
right auricle
mm. pectinati
conus arteriosus

Fig. 5.47 Heart (6) coronary arteries and interior of the right ventricle: right lateral view. The right ventricle has been opened. The right atrioventricular valve is displayed with its chordae tendineae and papillary muscles, although the valve cusps are not clear (see Fig. 5.56).

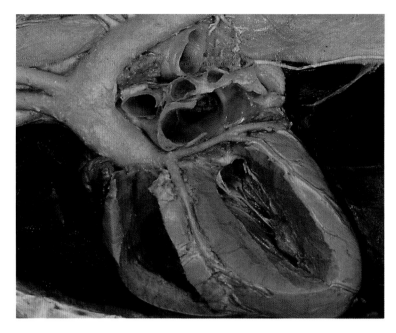

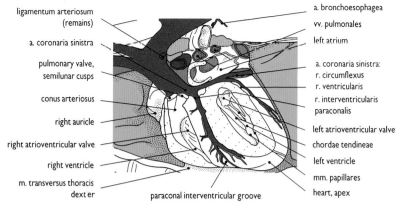

ligamentum arteriosum (remains)
a. coronaria sinistra
pulmonary valve, semilunar cusps
conus arteriosus
right auricle
right atrioventricular valve
right ventricle
m. transversus thoracis dexter
paraconal interventricular groove

a. bronchoesophagea
vv. pulmonales
left atrium
a. coronaria sinistra:
r. circumflexus
r. ventricularis
r. interventricularis paraconalis
left atrioventricular valve
chordae tendineae
left ventricle
mm. papillares
heart, apex

Fig. 5.48 Heart (7) left coronary artery and aortic arch after removal of the pulmonary trunk: left lateral view. The pulmonary trunk has been removed exposing the base of the aorta (the ascending component) on its emergence from the left ventricle.

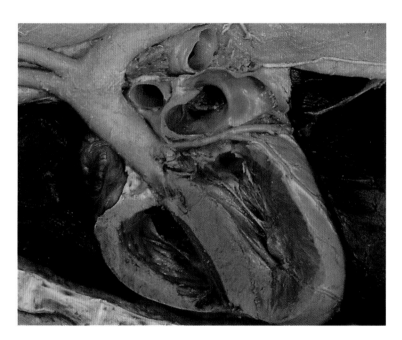

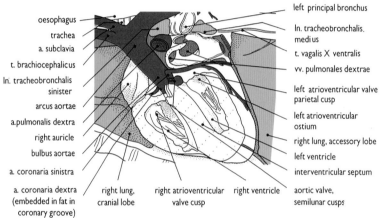

oesophagus
trachea
a. subclavia
t. brachiocephalicus
ln. tracheobronchalis sinister
arcus aortae
a. pulmonalis dextra
right auricle
bulbus aortae
a. coronaria sinistra
a. coronaria dextra (embedded in fat in coronary groove)
right lung, cranial lobe
right atrioventricular valve cusp
right ventricle

left principal bronchus
ln. tracheobronchalis. medius
t. vagalis X ventralis
vv. pulmonales dextrae
left atrioventricular valve parietal cusp
left atrioventricular ostium
right lung, accessory lobe
left ventricle
interventricular septum
aortic valve, semilunar cusps

Fig. 5.49 Heart (8) aortic valve: left lateral view. The paraconal interventricular branch of the left coronary artery has been removed with some of the interventricular septum and some of the muscle at the base of the left ventricle. The left atrioventricular valve is exposed in addition to the left semilunar cusp of the aortic valve.

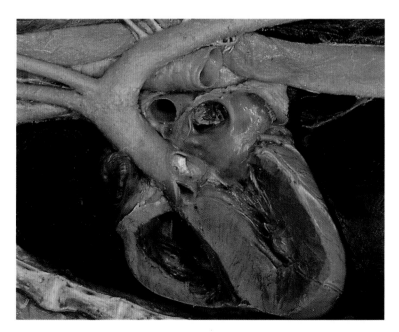

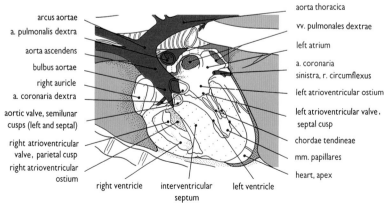

arcus aortae
a. pulmonalis dextra
aorta ascendens
bulbus aortae
right auricle
a. coronaria dextra
aortic valve, semilunar cusps (left and septal)
right atrioventricular valve, parietal cusp
right atrioventricular ostium
right ventricle
interventricular septum
left ventricle

aorta thoracica
vv. pulmonales dextrae
left atrium
a. coronaria sinistra, r. circumflexus
left atrioventricular ostium
left atrioventricular valve, septal cusp
chordae tendineae
mm. papillares
heart, apex

Fig. 5.50 Heart (9) left atrioventricular valve and aortic valve: left lateral view. The circumflex branch of the left coronary artery has been removed to allow the base of the left ventricle to be excised completely, thereby opening the left atrioventricular ostium. The left atrioventricular valve with its septal cusp and chordae tendineae is displayed.

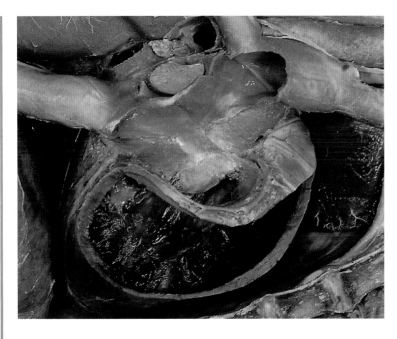

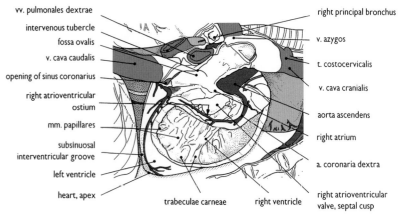

vv. pulmonales dextrae
intervenous tubercle
fossa ovalis
v. cava caudalis
opening of sinus coronarius
right atrioventricular ostium
mm. papillares
subsinuosal interventricular groove
left ventricle
heart, apex

right principal bronchus
v. azygos
t. costocervicalis
v. cava cranialis
aorta ascendens
right atrium
a. coronaria dextra
right atrioventricular valve, septal cusp

trabeculae carneae   right ventricle

Fig. 5.51 Heart (10) right coronary artery: right lateral view. The remainder of the right auricle has been removed leaving only the sinus venarum of the right atrium. The base of the aorta and the origin from it of the right coronary artery are displayed.

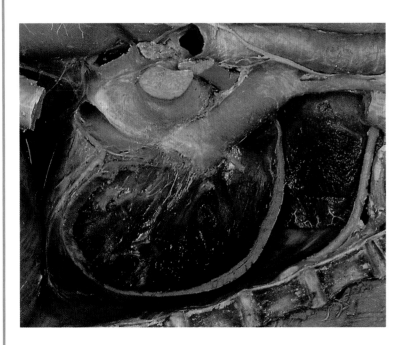

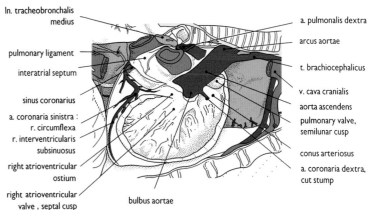

ln. tracheobronchalis medius
pulmonary ligament
interatrial septum
sinus coronarius
a. coronaria sinistra : r. circumflexa
r. interventricularis subsinuosus
right atrioventricular ostium
right atrioventricular valve , septal cusp

a. pulmonalis dextra
arcus aortae
t. brachiocephalicus
v. cava cranialis
aorta ascendens
pulmonary valve, semilunar cusp
conus arteriosus
a. coronaria dextra, cut stump

bulbus aortae

Fig. 5.52 Heart (11) right atrioventricular valve and pulmonary valve: right lateral view. The sinus venarum of the right atrium and the cranial and caudal venae cavae have been removed, exposing the entire ascending aorta. Removal of the circumflex branch of the right coronary artery has allowed the base of the right ventricle to be excised, opening both right atrioventricular ostium and pulmonary ostium and displaying their valves.

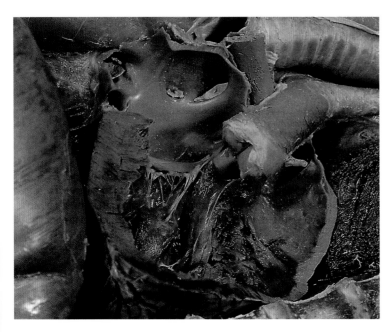

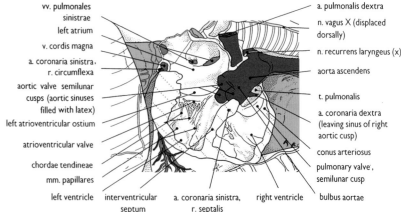

vv. pulmonales sinistrae
left atrium
v. cordis magna
a. coronaria sinistra, r. circumflexa
aortic valve semilunar cusps (aortic sinuses filled with latex)
left atrioventricular ostium
atrioventricular valve
chordae tendineae
mm. papillares
left ventricle   interventricular septum

a. pulmonalis dextra
n. vagus X (displaced dorsally)
n. recurrens laryngeus (x)
aorta ascendens
t. pulmonalis
a. coronaria dextra (leaving sinus of right aortic cusp)
conus arteriosus
pulmonary valve , semilunar cusp
a. coronaria sinistra, r. septalis   right ventricle   bulbus aortae

Fig. 5.53 Heart (12) left atrioventricular valve, aortic valve and pulmonary valve: right caudolateral view. The interventricular septum is partially removed, opening the left ventricle. The remains of the right atrium and interatrial septum have also been removed, opening the left atrium. The left atrioventricular ostium, one of the valve cusps, its chordae tendineae and the three cusps of the aortic valve are clearly displayed.

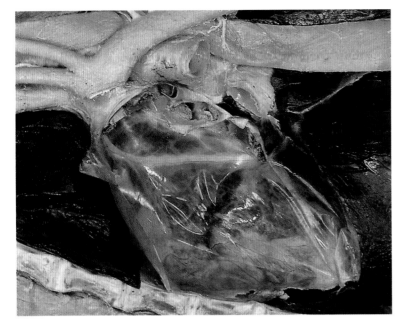

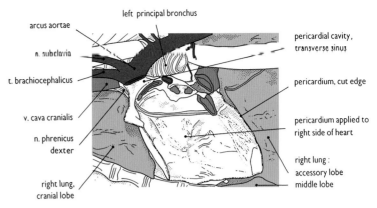

left principal bronchus

arcus aortae

n. subclavia

t. brachiocephalicus

v. cava cranialis

n. phrenicus dexter

right lung, cranial lobe

pericardial cavity, transverse sinus

pericardium, cut edge

pericardium applied to right side of heart

right lung : accessory lobe middle lobe

Fig. 5.54 Pericardium after removal of the heart: medial view of right side. The remainder of the heart has been removed by cutting through the aortic arch, cranial and caudal venae cavae and right pulmonary veins. These cuts were made as close to the heart as possible leaving the pericardium in place against the medial surface of the right lung.

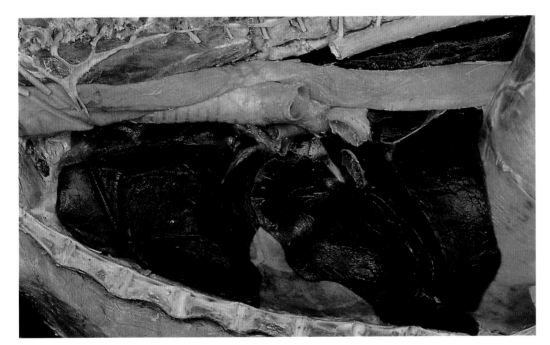

Fig. 5.55 Right lung in situ after removal of the heart and great vessels: medial view. The medial face of the right lung has been cleared of viscera (bar the trachea and esophagus). Note those structures entering into the 'root' of the lung and the impressions made in the lung by such structures as the heart and internal thoracic vessels. (Compare with Fig. 5.27.) The accessory lobe of the right lung is now clearly displayed. The caudal vena cava is just visible at the cranial boundary.

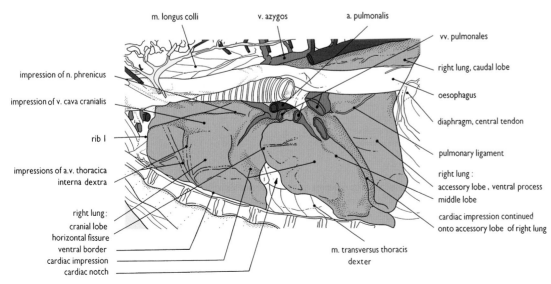

m. longus colli

v. azygos

a. pulmonalis

vv. pulmonales

impression of n. phrenicus

right lung, caudal lobe

impression of v. cava cranialis

oesophagus

rib I

diaphragm, central tendon

impressions of a.v. thoracica interna dextra

pulmonary ligament

right lung : cranial lobe horizontal fissure ventral border cardiac impression cardiac notch

right lung : accessory lobe , ventral process middle lobe

cardiac impression continued onto accessory lobe of right lung

m. transversus thoracis dexter

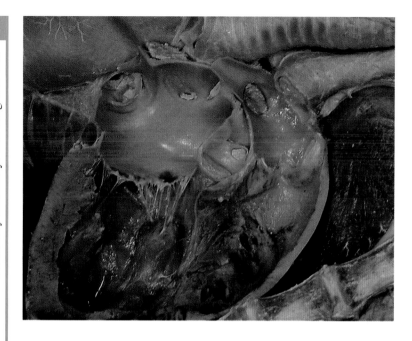
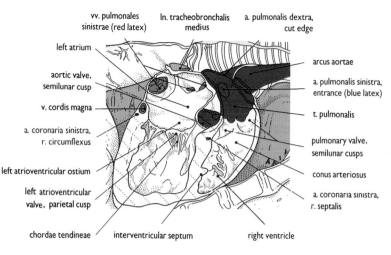

Fig. 5.56 Heart (13) left atrioventricular valve, aortic valve and pulmonary valve: right lateral view. The base of the aorta, aortic valve and ascending component have been removed, completing the exposure of the pulmonary valve and conus arteriosus. Opening of the pulmonary trunk exposes the origin of the left pulmonary artery. At the base of the aorta the opening leading into the left coronary artery is displayed in the aortic sinus of the left semilunar cusp of the valve.

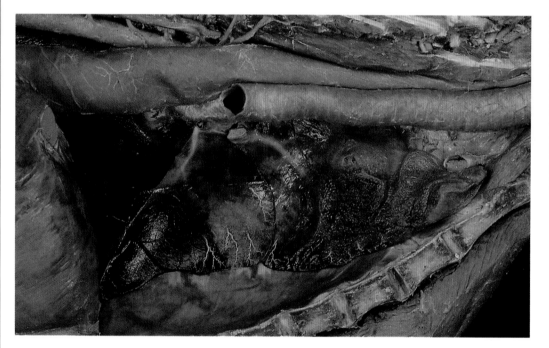

Fig. 5.57 Left lung in situ after removal of the heart and great vessels: medial view. The medial face of the left lung has been cleared of viscera (bar the trachea and esophagus). Those structures comprising the 'root' of the lung are evident, as are impressions in the lung made by the heart and internal thoracic vessels. (Compare with Fig. 5.28.) The acute, projecting apex of the cranial lobe of the lung is sharply contrasted with the deep and bluntly rounded apex of the right (see Fig. 5.55).

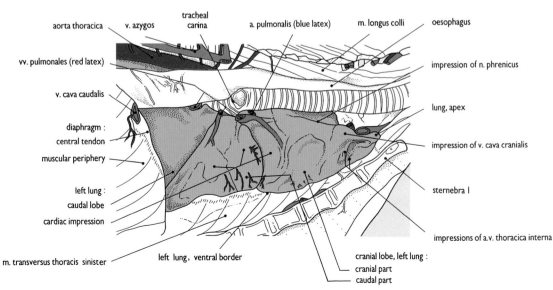

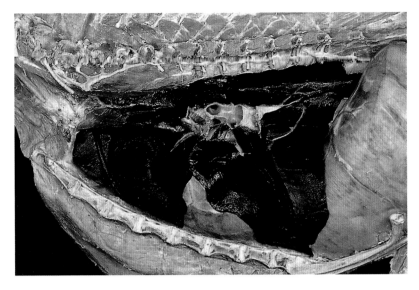

Fig. 5.58 Right lung in situ after removal of the mediastinum and its contents: medial view. The remaining mediastinal structures, the trachea, esophagus and aorta, have been removed and the right lung is left in position in the chest. This medial view of the lung hardened in situ shows the surface indentations which indicate the relationship to mediastinal structures no longer present. The root of the lung (those structures which pass between the mediastinum and hilus of the lung) is completely displayed with principal bronchus positioned most dorsally in the root and the pulmonary veins most ventrally.

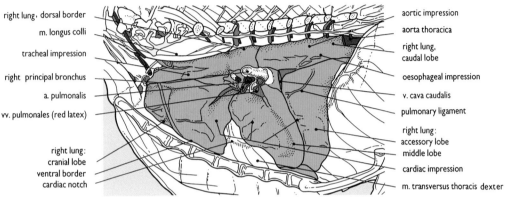

right lung, dorsal border
m. longus colli
tracheal impression
right principal bronchus
a. pulmonalis
vv. pulmonales (red latex)
right lung: cranial lobe
ventral border
cardiac notch

aortic impression
aorta thoracica
right lung, caudal lobe
oesophageal impression
v. cava caudalis
pulmonary ligament
right lung: accessory lobe
middle lobe
cardiac impression
m. transversus thoracis dexter

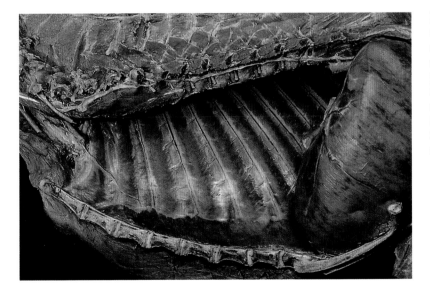

Fig. 5.59 Ribcage (6) transverse thoracic muscle and endothoracic fascia of the right side: medial view. The right lung has been removed, clearing the entire thoracic cavity of viscera. The medial surface of the right thoracic wall is displayed covered by a glistening layer of parietal pleura underlain by endothoracic fascia. Through the pleura and fascia the internal intercostal muscles are visible filling each intercostal space. The transverse thoracic muscle is evident in the thoracic floor from rib 3 caudally. Close against the caudal borders of the ribs lie intercostal vessels and nerves embedded in a small amount of fat (cf. Figs 5.18 and 5.23).

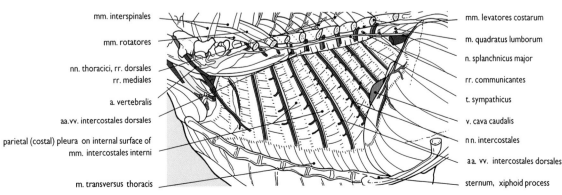

mm. interspinales
mm. rotatores
nn. thoracici, rr. dorsales
rr. mediales
a. vertebralis
aa.vv. intercostales dorsales
parietal (costal) pleura on internal surface of mm. intercostales interni
m. transversus thoracis

mm. levatores costarum
m. quadratus lumborum
n. splanchnicus major
rr. communicantes
t. sympathicus
v. cava caudalis
nn. intercostales
aa. vv. intercostales dorsales
sternum, xiphoid process

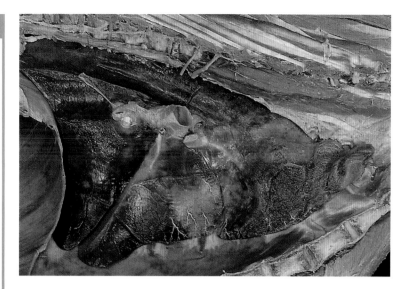

Fig. 5.60 Left lung in situ after removal of the mediastinum and its contents: medial view. The remaining mediastinal structures have been removed and the medial surface of the left lung is viewed in position. In comparison with the equivalent view of the right lung (Fig. 5.58) the pointed apex of the left lung is contrasted with the blunt rounded apex of the right. In addition the pronounced cardiac notch in the ventral border of the right lung has no equivalent in the left.

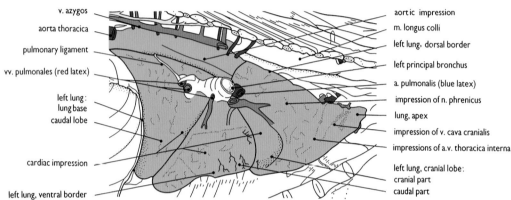

v. azygos

aorta thoracica

pulmonary ligament

vv. pulmonales (red latex)

left lung:
lung base
caudal lobe

cardiac impression

left lung, ventral border

aortic impression

m. longus colli

left lung, dorsal border

left principal bronchus

a. pulmonalis (blue latex)

impression of n. phrenicus

lung, apex

impression of v. cava cranialis

impressions of a.v. thoracica interna

left lung, cranial lobe:
cranial part
caudal part

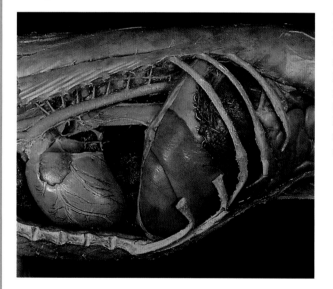

Fig. 5.61 Accessory lobe of the right lung and the liver after removal of the diaphragm: left lateral view. In this dissection the left lung and the left half of the diaphragm have been removed whilst leaving the caudal ribs and costal arch intact. The position of the costodiaphragmatic line of pleural reflection is shown in the drawing by the broken blue line. This is an indication of the effective caudal extent of the pleural cavity. The close relationship of abdominal contents with the caudal and accessory lobes of the right lung and the heart is clearly demonstrated (cf. Fig. 5.92). NB In this specimen a persistent left cranial vena cava was present. It has been removed but its course around the left coronary groove is still apparent and the point at which it emptied into an enlarged coronary sinus is clearly demonstrated.

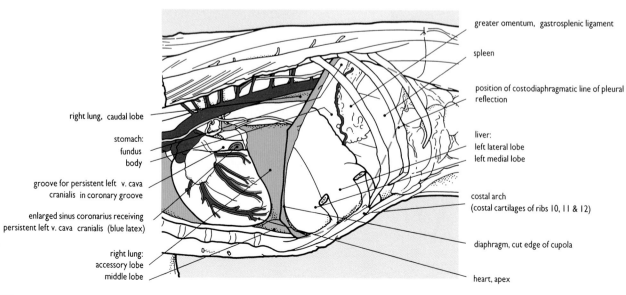

greater omentum, gastrosplenic ligament

spleen

position of costodiaphragmatic line of pleural reflection

right lung, caudal lobe

stomach:
fundus
body

groove for persistent left v. cava cranialis in coronary groove

enlarged sinus coronarius receiving persistent left v. cava cranialis (blue latex)

right lung:
accessory lobe
middle lobe

liver:
left lateral lobe
left medial lobe

costal arch
(costal cartilages of ribs 10, 11 & 12)

diaphragm, cut edge of cupola

heart, apex

The Thorax

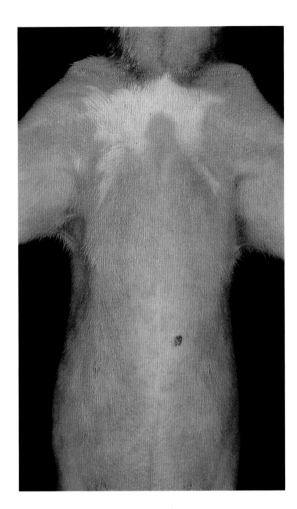

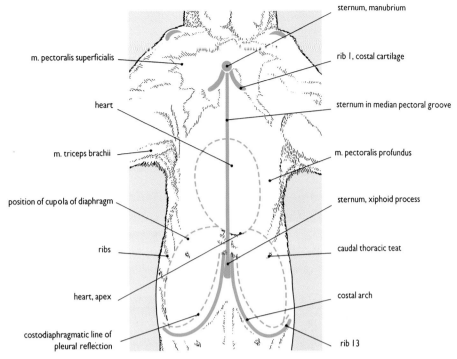

sternum, manubrium

m. pectoralis superficialis

rib I, costal cartilage

heart

sternum in median pectoral groove

m. triceps brachii

m. pectoralis profundus

position of cupola of diaphragm

sternum, xiphoid process

ribs

caudal thoracic teat

heart, apex

costal arch

costodiaphragmatic line of pleural reflection

rib 13

Fig. 5.62 Surface features of the thorax and upper fore-leg: ventral view. The palpable bony 'landmarks' of the thorax and upper fore-leg are shown here. In addition a number of muscles which are palpable are indicated.

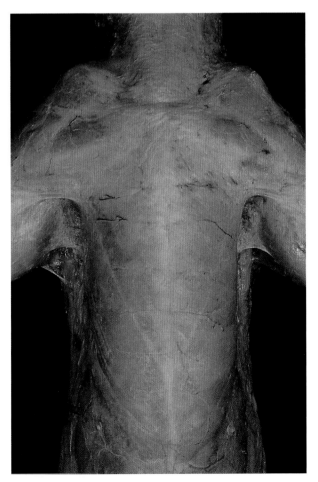

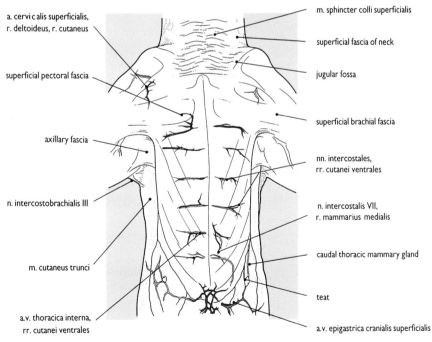

a. cervicalis superficialis, r. deltoideus, r. cutaneus

m. sphincter colli superficialis

superficial pectoral fascia

superficial fascia of neck

jugular fossa

axillary fascia

superficial brachial fascia

n. intercostobrachialis III

nn. intercostales, rr. cutanei ventrales

n. intercostalis VII, r. mammarius medialis

caudal thoracic mammary gland

m. cutaneus trunci

teat

a.v. thoracica interna, rr. cutanei ventrales

a.v. epigastrica cranialis superficialis

Fig. 5.63 Superficial structures of the thorax and upper fore-leg (1) superficial fascia and cutaneous nerves: ventral view. The skin has been removed to expose superficial fascia forming a complete investment of the trunk as external trunk fascia. It is continuous cranially with superficial fascia of the neck and caudally extends back over the abdomen where it contains the mammary glands and cutaneous muscle of the trunk (see Fig. 5.7).

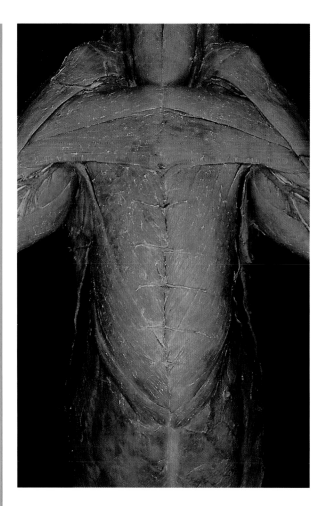

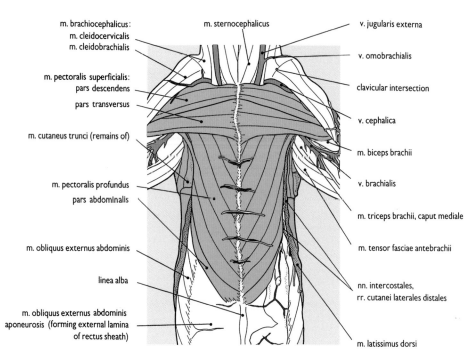

m. brachiocephalicus:
m. cleidocervicalis
m. cleidobrachialis

m. sternocephalicus

v. jugularis externa

v. omobrachialis

clavicular intersection

m. pectoralis superficialis:
pars descendens
pars transversus

v. cephalica

m. cutaneus trunci (remains of)

m. biceps brachii

v. brachialis

m. pectoralis profundus
pars abdominalis

m. triceps brachii, caput mediale

m. tensor fasciae antebrachii

m. obliquus externus abdominis

linea alba

nn. intercostales,
rr. cutanei laterales distales

m. obliquus externus abdominis
aponeurosis (forming external lamina
of rectus sheath)

m. latissimus dorsi

Fig. 5.64 Superficial structures of the thorax and upper fore-leg (2) pectoral and cleidobrachial muscles: ventral view. The superficial thoracic musculature is exposed after removing superficial fascia and cutaneous muscle. A small component of cutaneous muscle is left in place where it blends with pectoral musculature in the axillary region. Adipose tissue present in superficial fascia in such places as the jugular fossa and axilla has also been removed, as has the right caudal thoracic mammary gland.

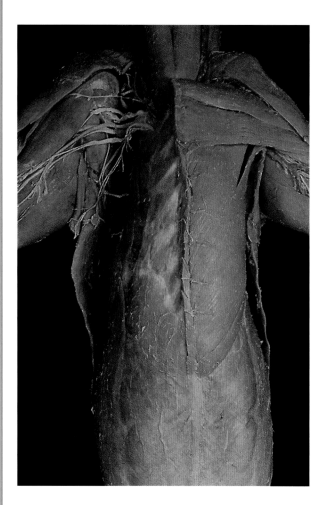

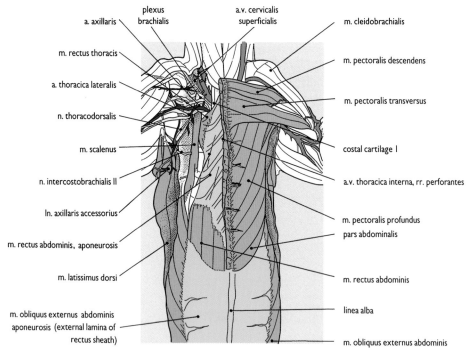

a. axillaris

plexus
brachialis

a.v. cervicalis
superficialis

m. cleidobrachialis

m. rectus thoracis

m. pectoralis descendens

a. thoracica lateralis

m. pectoralis transversus

n. thoracodorsalis

m. scalenus

costal cartilage I

n. intercostobrachialis II

a.v. thoracica interna, rr. perforantes

ln. axillaris accessorius

m. rectus abdominis, aponeurosis

m. pectoralis profundus
pars abdominalis

m. latissimus dorsi

m. rectus abdominis

m. obliquus externus abdominis
aponeurosis (external lamina of
rectus sheath)

linea alba

m. obliquus externus abdominis

Fig. 5.65 Thoracic wall, axilla and pectoral muscles: ventral view (1). Pectoral musculature has been removed from the right side opening out the axilla and exposing nerves and blood vessels to and from the fore-leg and neck. This procedure has allowed some additional limb abduction, thereby displacing the latissimus dorsi muscle laterally and 'straightening' nerves and blood vessels across the axilla. The costal cartilages of ribs 1–5 and interchondral components of the internal intercostal muscles are visible through the aponeurosis of the rectus abdominis muscle.

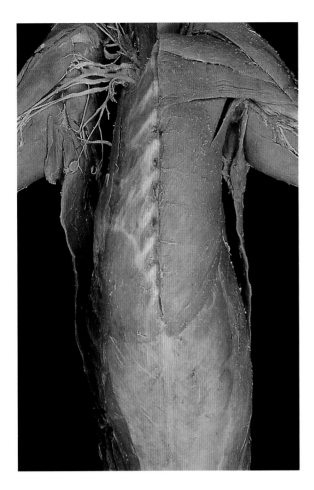

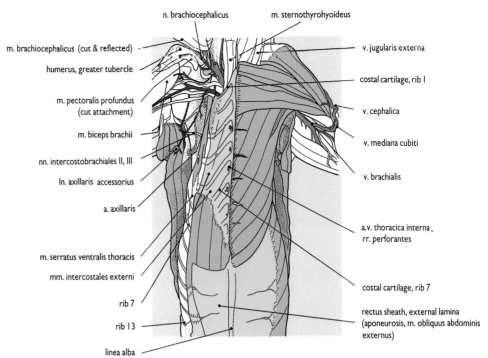

n. brachiocephalicus   m. sternothyrohyoideus

m. brachiocephalicus (cut & reflected)   v. jugularis externa

humerus, greater tubercle   costal cartilage, rib I

m. pectoralis profundus (cut attachment)   v. cephalica

m. biceps brachii   v. mediana cubiti

nn. intercostobrachiales II, III   v. brachialis

ln. axillaris accessorius

a. axillaris

a.v. thoracica interna, rr. perforantes

m. serratus ventralis thoracis

mm. intercostales externi   costal cartilage, rib 7

rib 7   rectus sheath, external lamina (aponeurosis, m. obliquus abdominis externus)

rib 13

linea alba

Fig. 5.66 Thoracic wall, axilla and pectoral muscles: ventral view (2). The more caudal ribs (7–13) have been partially exposed on removal of the external abdominal oblique muscle from its costal origins. Part of the aponeurosis of the muscle is preserved where it contributes to the external lamina of the rectus sheath. The rectus abdominis muscle is outlined on the right side of the thorax, from rib 1 to the abdominal wall.

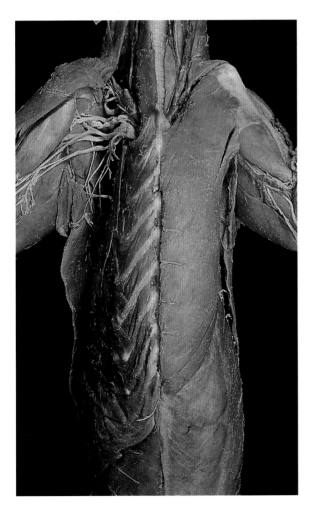

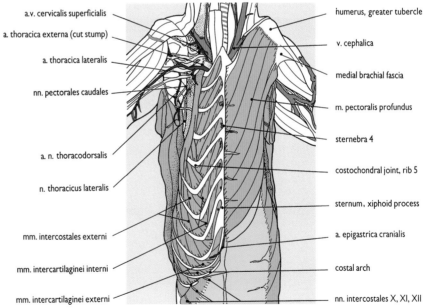

a.v. cervicalis superficialis   humerus, greater tubercle

a. thoracica externa (cut stump)   v. cephalica

a. thoracica lateralis   medial brachial fascia

nn. pectorales caudales   m. pectoralis profundus

sternebra 4

a. n. thoracodorsalis   costochondral joint, rib 5

n. thoracicus lateralis   sternum, xiphoid process

mm. intercostales externi   a. epigastrica cranialis

mm. intercartilaginei interni   costal arch

mm. intercartilaginei externi   nn. intercostales X, XI, XII

Fig. 5.67 Thoracic wall, axilla and pectoral muscles: ventral view (3). Superficial pectoral and cleidobrachial muscles have been removed from the left side, exposing the deep pectoral muscle. Note its extensive attachment in the arm to the humerus and deep brachial fascia. The vessels leading into the neck cranial to rib 1 are also exposed following removal of the sternocephalic and sternothyrohyoid muscles. On the right the rectus thoracis and rectus abdominis muscles have been removed, exposing the entire ribcage back to and including the costal arch.

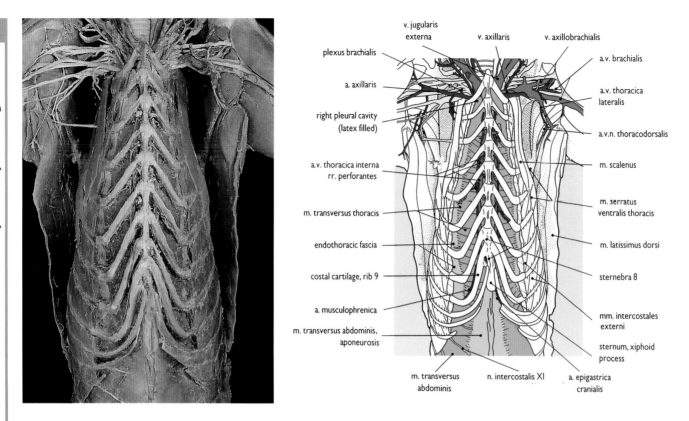

Fig. 5.68 Ribcage, transverse thoracic muscle and internal thoracic vessels: ventral view. Pectoral musculature has been cleared from the left side and intercartilaginous parts of the internal intercostal muscles have been removed from interchondral spaces on both sides back to rib 10. Transverse thoracic muscles and internal thoracic vessels flanking the sternum are exposed caudally from space 2. In interchondral spaces 1 and 2 endothoracic fascia has been removed exposing the cranial extent of the pleural cavities.

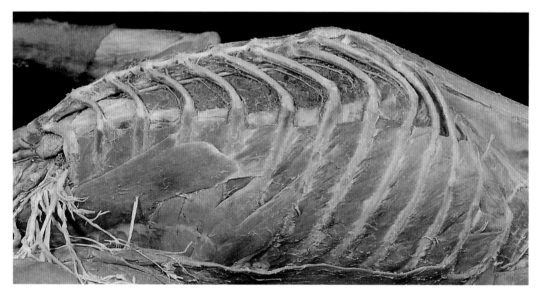

Fig. 5.69 Ribcage, transverse thoracic muscle and internal thoracic vessels: right lateral view. A lateral view of the preceding dissection shows perforating and ventral intercostal branches from the internal thoracic vessels in several of the interchondral spaces. Lateral to the lateral border of the transverse thoracic muscle the endothoracic fascia is thickened and especially prominent.

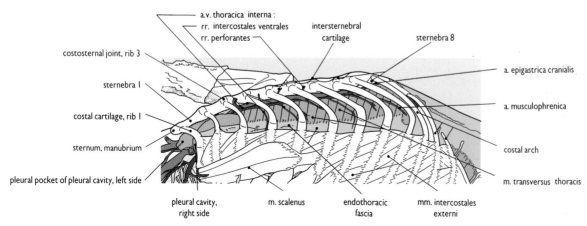

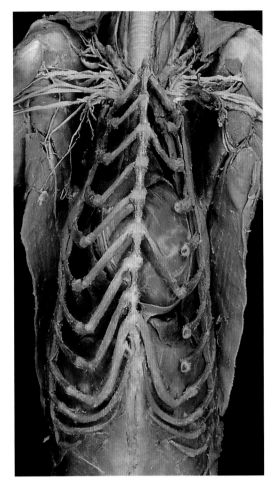

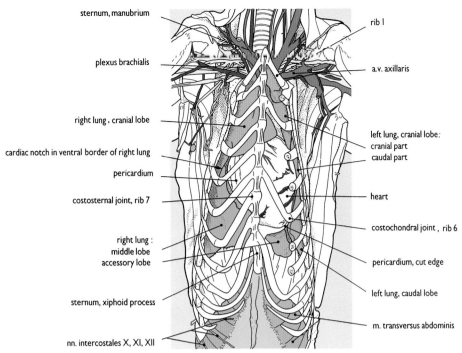

sternum, manubrium
plexus brachialis
right lung , cranial lobe
cardiac notch in ventral border of right lung
pericardium
costosternal joint, rib 7
right lung :
middle lobe
accessory lobe
sternum, xiphoid process
nn. intercostales X, XI, XII

rib I
a.v. axillaris
left lung, cranial lobe:
cranial part
caudal part
heart
costochondral joint , rib 6
pericardium, cut edge
left lung, caudal lobe
m. transversus abdominis

Fig. 5.70 Thoracic viscera *in situ*: ventral view. The transverse thoracic muscles and internal thoracic vessels have been removed, exposing pleural cavities filled with colored latex. This was removed 'piecemeal' through gaps in the ribcage after removal of several costal cartilages on the left side. A large area of pericardium on the left side has been removed, opening the pericardial cavity and exposing the heart.

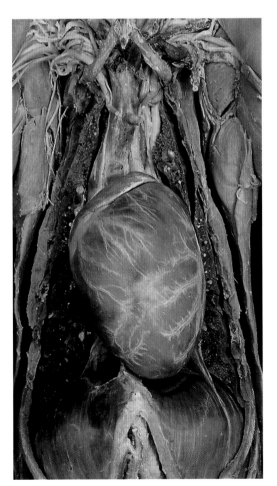

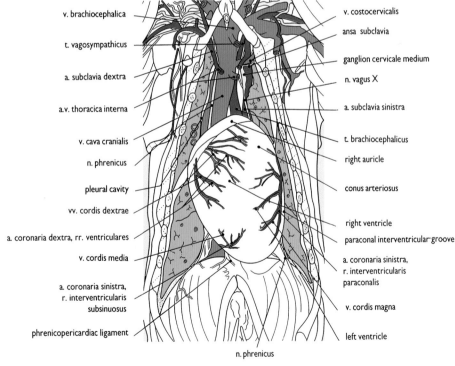

v. brachiocephalica
t. vagosympathicus
a. subclavia dextra
a.v. thoracica interna
v. cava cranialis
n. phrenicus
pleural cavity
vv. cordis dextrae
a. coronaria dextra, rr. ventriculares
v. cordis media
a. coronaria sinistra,
r. interventricularis
subsinuosus
phrenicopericardiac ligament
n. phrenicus

v. costocervicalis
ansa subclavia
ganglion cervicale medium
n. vagus X
a. subclavia sinistra
t. brachiocephalicus
right auricle
conus arteriosus
right ventricle
paraconal interventricular groove
a. coronaria sinistra,
r. interventricularis
paraconalis
v. cordis magna
left ventricle

Fig. 5.71 Thoracic viscera *in situ* after removal of the sternum and costal cartilages: ventral view. Ribs 2 to 8 have been cut back and removed with the sternum. Intercostal muscles were cut back to the same level, as were the lungs. The remains of the pericardium have been removed from the right side of the heart. The right phrenic nerve has been left intact on the vena cava, but the left phrenic nerve was removed to expose the vagus nerve (X) and the subclavian artery on the left side cranial to the heart.

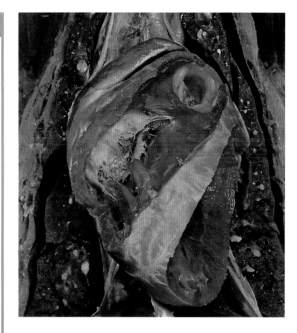

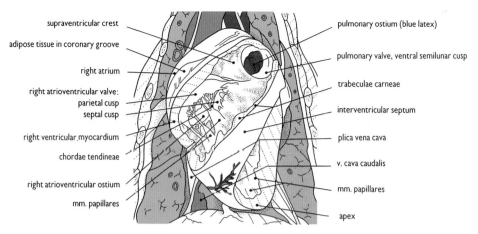

supraventricular crest
adipose tissue in coronary groove
right atrium
right atrioventricular valve:
parietal cusp
septal cusp
right ventricular myocardium
chordae tendineae
right atrioventricular ostium
mm. papillares

pulmonary ostium (blue latex)
pulmonary valve, ventral semilunar cusp
trabeculae carneae
interventricular septum
plica vena cava
v. cava caudalis
mm. papillares
apex

Fig. 5.72 Heart (1) interior of ventricles: ventral view. Both ventricles have been opened and the mass of blue latex which filled the right ventricle was removed 'piecemeal'. The relative positions and thickness of the walls are demonstrated. Note the pulmonary and right atrioventricular valves in the right ventricle, in particular the cusps and chordae tendineae of the latter. A clearer appreciation of the relative position of heart valves is shown below and in Figs 5.53 and 5.56.

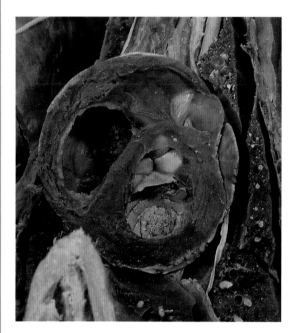

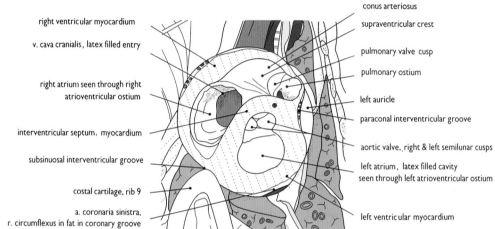

right ventricular myocardium
v. cava cranialis, latex filled entry
right atrium seen through right atrioventricular ostium
interventricular septum, myocardium
subsinuosal interventricular groove
costal cartilage, rib 9
a. coronaria sinistra,
r. circumflexus in fat in coronary groove

conus arteriosus
supraventricular crest
pulmonary valve cusp
pulmonary ostium
left auricle
paraconal interventricular groove
aortic valve, right & left semilunar cusps
left atrium, latex filled cavity
seen through left atrioventricular ostium
left ventricular myocardium

Fig. 5.73 Heart (2) base after ventricular removal: left caudoventral view. Almost all of the ventricular muscle has been removed along with the cusps of the atrioventricular valves to give a view into the 'base' of the heart. The relative positions of the four valve ostia are shown, as are the relative shapes of the ventricles. Much of the blue latex that filled the right atrium has been removed but the left atrium is still filled.

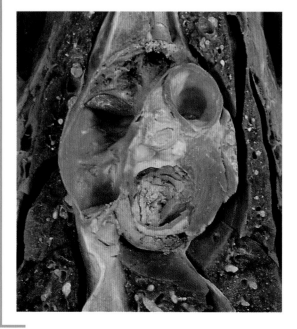

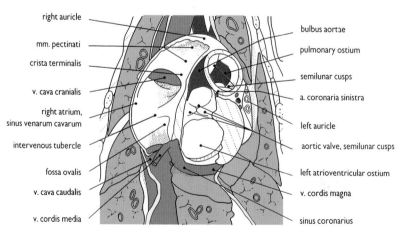

right auricle
mm. pectinati
crista terminalis
v. cava cranialis
right atrium, sinus venarum cavarum
intervenous tubercle
fossa ovalis
v. cava caudalis
v. cordis media

bulbus aortae
pulmonary ostium
semilunar cusps
a. coronaria sinistra
left auricle
aortic valve, semilunar cusps
left atrioventricular ostium
v. cordis magna
sinus coronarius

Fig. 5.74 Heart (3) interior of atria, aortic valve and pulmonary valve: ventral view. The remainder of the ventricular muscle has been removed with some of the right atrial wall to give a clear view into the interior of the sinus venarum of the right atrium and the right auricle. The position of the intervenous tubercle in relation to the openings of the venae cavae is clearly demonstrated (see also Fig. 5.47).

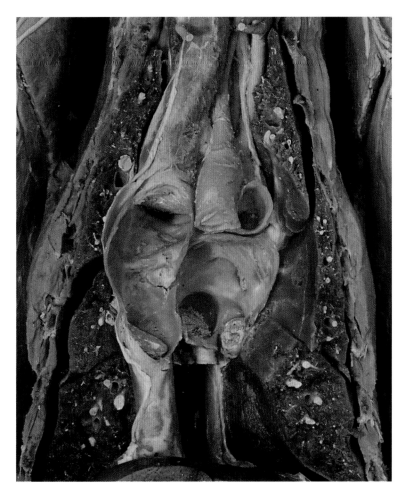

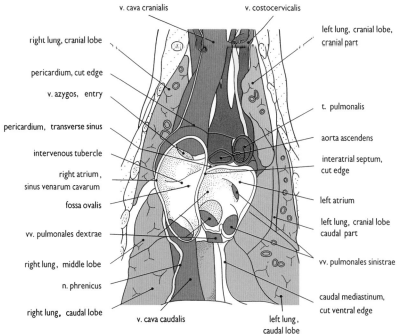

Fig. 5.75 Heart (4) atria and great vessels: ventral view. Left and right auricles have been removed along with the origins of the aorta and pulmonary trunk. All that remains of the right atrium is the roof of the sinus venarum with the entering venae cavae. Several pulmonary veins enter the left atrium which is bounded cranially by the aortic arch encircling the pulmonary trunk. The pericardial attachment to the great vessels is shown by a distinct line crossing the cranial vena cava and the arch of the aorta. The transverse sinus of the pericardial cavity is seen between the great vessels and the left atrium.

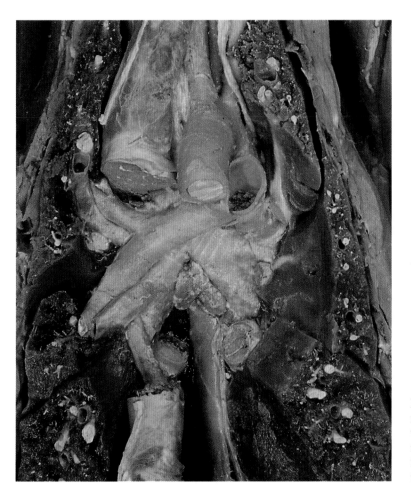

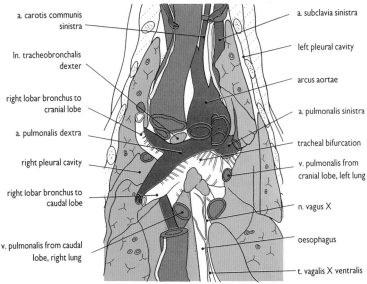

Fig. 5.76 Pulmonary vessels and roots of the lungs: ventral view. The remains of the atria have been removed: the right by cutting through the venae cavae; the left by severing the pulmonary veins. Exposed are the roots of the lungs. Right and left pulmonary arteries originate from the pulmonary trunk; the prominent right crosses dorsal to the base of the heart caudal to the aortic arch.

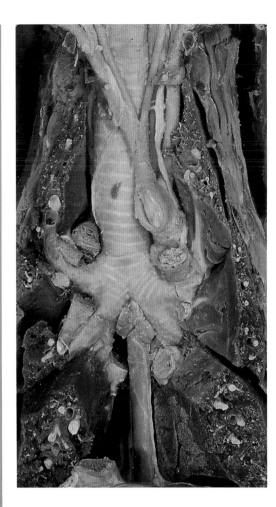

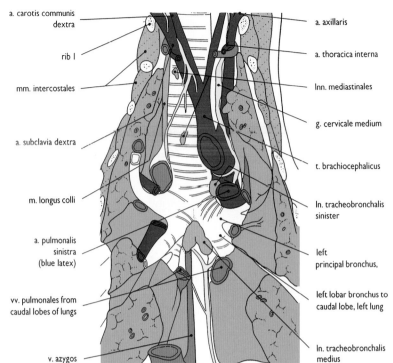

a. carotis communis dextra

rib I

mm. intercostales

a. subclavia dextra

m. longus colli

a. pulmonalis sinistra (blue latex)

vv. pulmonales from caudal lobes of lungs

v. azygos

a. axillaris

a. thoracica interna

lnn. mediastinales

g. cervicale medium

t. brachiocephalicus

ln. tracheobronchalis sinister

left principal bronchus,

left lobar bronchus to caudal lobe, left lung

ln. tracheobronchalis medius

Fig. 5.77 Tracheal bifurcation and tracheobronchial lymph nodes: ventral view. The venae cavae, right pulmonary artery and ascending part of the aortic arch have been removed. Note the trachea, its bifurcation and the initial branching of the principal bronchi into lobar branches. The left and right vagus nerves in the cranial part of the mediastinum disappear dorsal to the lung roots. The union of ventral vagal branches forms a ventral trunk on the esophagus, caudal to the middle tracheobronchial lymph node. The left tracheobronchial lymph node is visible between the trachea and the pulmonary trunk.

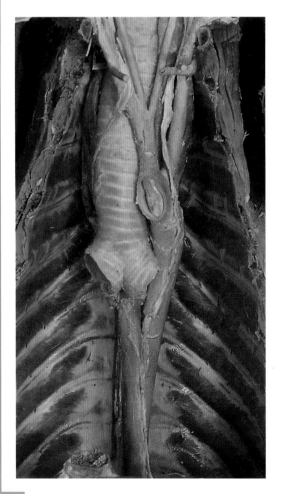

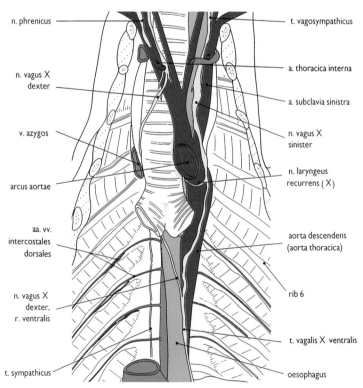

n. phrenicus

n. vagus X dexter

v. azygos

arcus aortae

aa. vv. intercostales dorsales

n. vagus X dexter, r. ventralis

t. sympathicus

t. vagosympathicus

a. thoracica interna

a. subclavia sinistra

n. vagus X sinister

n. laryngeus recurrens (X)

aorta descendens (aorta thoracica)

rib 6

t. vagalis X ventralis

oesophagus

Fig. 5.78 Viscera of the dorsal mediastinum: ventral view. The principal bronchi have been cut, allowing the remains of the lungs to be removed. All that is left are those structures which occupied the dorsal parts of the mediastinum. The esophagus, with its associated ventral vagal trunk, the descending aorta and azygos vein all converge on the midline caudal to the tracheal bifurcation.

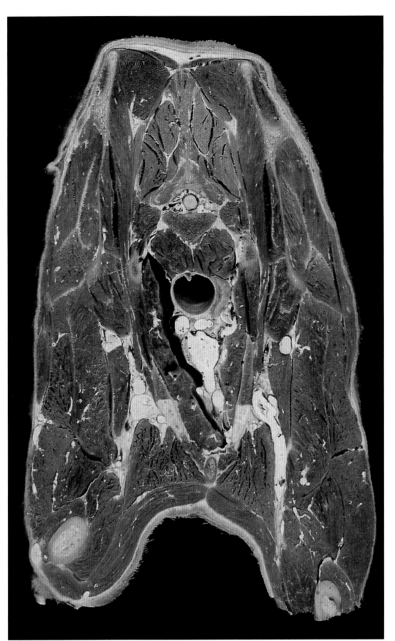

Fig. 5.79 Transverse section (1) through thoracic vertebra 2 and the cranial mediastinum: cranial view. This transverse section and the following eight sections are all viewed from the cranial aspect. The accompanying sketch of the thorax shows the approximate levels at which the sections were taken. The series is a direct continuation of the sections illustrated in the neck chapter (Figs 3.36–3.43), the last one of which passed through thoracic vertebra 1 at the thoracic inlet. The dorsal and ventral boundaries of the axilla are indicated by the points labelled 1 and 2.

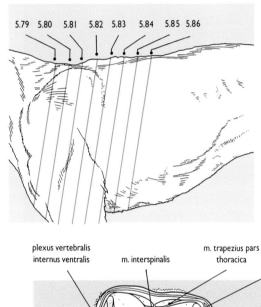

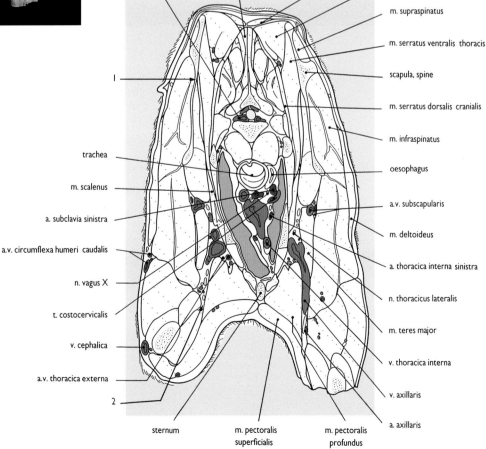

plexus vertebralis internus ventralis

m. interspinalis

m. trapezius pars thoracica

m. rhomboideus thoracis

m. supraspinatus

m. serratus ventralis thoracis

scapula, spine

m. serratus dorsalis cranialis

m. infraspinatus

trachea

oesophagus

m. scalenus

a. subclavia sinistra

a.v. subscapularis

m. deltoideus

a.v. circumflexa humeri caudalis

a. thoracica interna sinistra

n. vagus X

n. thoracicus lateralis

t. costocervicalis

m. teres major

v. cephalica

v. thoracica interna

a.v. thoracica externa

v. axillaris

2

a. axillaris

sternum

m. pectoralis superficialis

m. pectoralis profundus

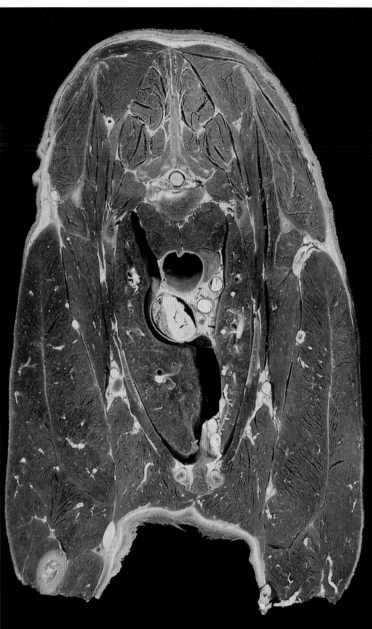

Fig. 5.80 Transverse section (2) through thoracic vertebra 4 and the cranial mediastinum: cranial view. These first two sections through the cranial (precardial) mediastinum show the cranial lobes of both lungs on either side of a mediastinal partition which is more or less a midline structure. Visible mediastinal structures include: trachea and esophagus, cranial vena cava, brachiocephalic trunk and left subclavian artery. The dorsal and ventral boundaries of the axilla are indicated by the points labelled 1 and 2.

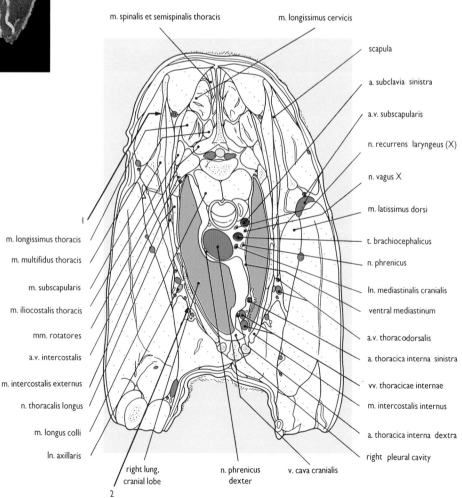

m. spinalis et semispinalis thoracis

m. longissimus cervicis

scapula

a. subclavia sinistra

a.v. subscapularis

n. recurrens laryngeus (X)

n. vagus X

m. latissimus dorsi

t. brachiocephalicus

n. phrenicus

ln. mediastinalis cranialis

ventral mediastinum

a.v. thoracodorsalis

a. thoracica interna sinistra

vv. thoracicae internae

m. intercostalis internus

a. thoracica interna dextra

right pleural cavity

m. longissimus thoracis

m. multifidus thoracis

m. subscapularis

m. iliocostalis thoracis

mm. rotatores

a.v. intercostalis

m. intercostalis externus

n. thoracalis longus

m. longus colli

ln. axillaris

right lung, cranial lobe

n. phrenicus dexter

v. cava cranialis

2

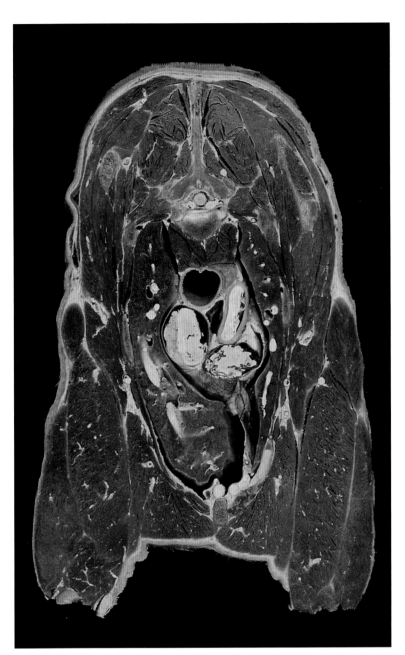

Fig. 5.81 Transverse section (3) through thoracic vertebra 5 and the aortic arch: cranial view. The ventral mediastinum is displaced onto the left side by the considerably larger cranial lobe of the right lung. The internal thoracic vessels have reached the floor of the thorax but at this level, costal cartilage 2, the transverse thoracic muscle is not yet present (see Figs 5.61 and 5.69). Ribs 2, 3 and 4 appear on the left side.

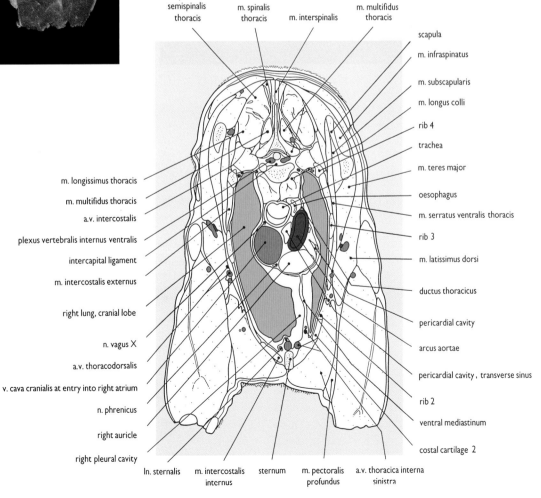

m. spinalis et semispinalis thoracis
m. spinalis thoracis
m. interspinalis
m. multifidus thoracis
scapula
m. infraspinatus
m. subscapularis
m. longus colli
rib 4
trachea
m. teres major
oesophagus
m. serratus ventralis thoracis
rib 3
m. latissimus dorsi
ductus thoracicus
pericardial cavity
arcus aortae
pericardial cavity, transverse sinus
rib 2
ventral mediastinum
costal cartilage 2

m. longissimus thoracis
m. multifidus thoracis
a.v. intercostalis
plexus vertebralis internus ventralis
intercapital ligament
m. intercostalis externus
right lung, cranial lobe
n. vagus X
a.v. thoracodorsalis
v. cava cranialis at entry into right atrium
n. phrenicus
right auricle
right pleural cavity

ln. sternalis
m. intercostalis internus
sternum
m. pectoralis profundus
a.v. thoracica interna sinistra

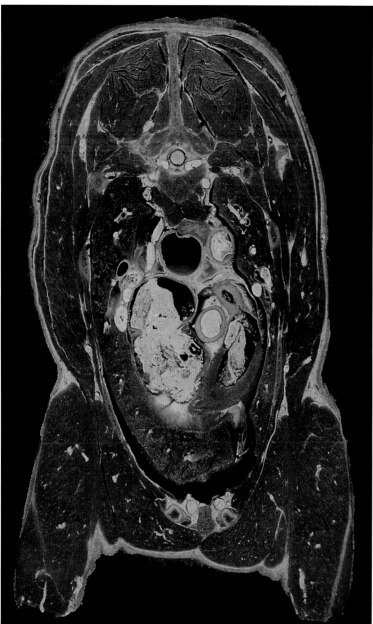

Fig. 5.82 Transverse section (4) through thoracic vertebra 6 and the base of the heart: cranial view. The right atrium and auricle are opened, as is the conus arteriosus of the right ventricle and the beginning of the pulmonary trunk leading from it. Within the lungs numerous vessels are cut through representing the larger ramifications of the pulmonary vessels – blue latex fills branches of the pulmonary artery, pink fills those of the pulmonary veins, contrary to the colors used in the illustrations for arteries (red) and veins (blue).

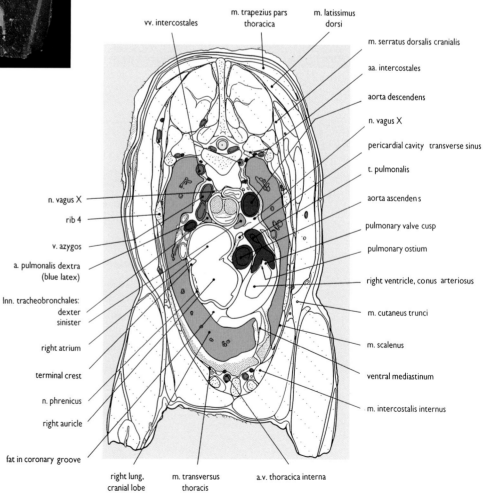

vv. intercostales

m. trapezius pars thoracica

m. latissimus dorsi

m. serratus dorsalis cranialis

aa. intercostales

aorta descendens

n. vagus X

pericardial cavity transverse sinus

t. pulmonalis

aorta ascenden s

pulmonary valve cusp

pulmonary ostium

right ventricle, conus arteriosus

m. cutaneus trunci

m. scalenus

ventral mediastinum

m. intercostalis internus

n. vagus X

rib 4

v. azygos

a. pulmonalis dextra (blue latex)

lnn. tracheobronchales: dexter sinister

right atrium

terminal crest

n. phrenicus

right auricle

fat in coronary groove

right lung, cranial lobe

m. transversus thoracis

a.v. thoracica interna

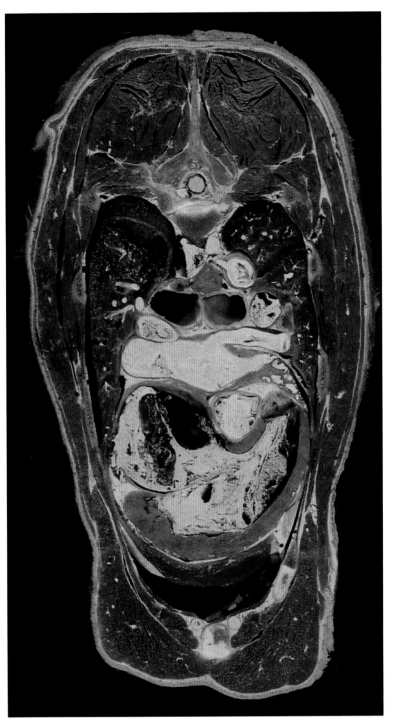

Fig. 5.83 Transverse section (5) through thoracic vertebra 7 and the tracheal bifurcation: cranial view. The bulb of the aorta at the base of the ascending component is flanked by the right atrium and the conus arteriosus of the right ventricle. Note the right atrioventricular ostium and valve leading into the right ventricle in the centre of the sectioned heart, and the base of the pulmonary trunk with a single remaining cusp of the pulmonary valve leading off from the right ventricle on the left side of the heart. This section passes through the root of the lung on either side.

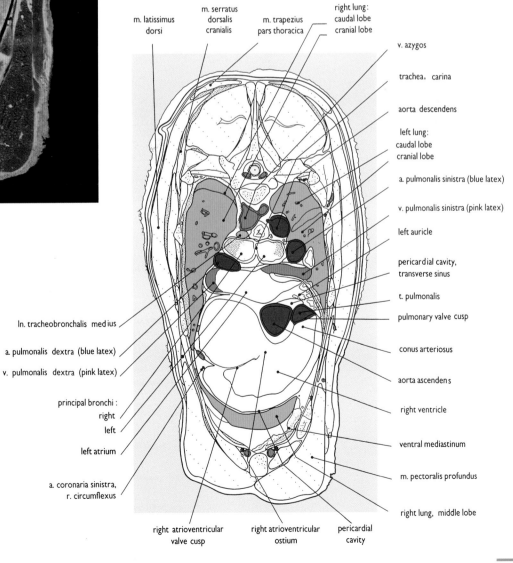

m. latissimus dorsi

m. serratus dorsalis cranialis

m. trapezius pars thoracica

right lung: caudal lobe cranial lobe

v. azygos

trachea, carina

aorta descendens

left lung: caudal lobe cranial lobe

a. pulmonalis sinistra (blue latex)

v. pulmonalis sinistra (pink latex)

left auricle

pericardial cavity, transverse sinus

t. pulmonalis

pulmonary valve cusp

conus arteriosus

aorta ascendens

right ventricle

ventral mediastinum

m. pectoralis profundus

right lung, middle lobe

ln. tracheobronchalis medius

a. pulmonalis dextra (blue latex)

v. pulmonalis dextra (pink latex)

principal bronchi: right left

left atrium

a. coronaria sinistra, r. circumflexus

right atrioventricular valve cusp

right atrioventricular ostium

pericardial cavity

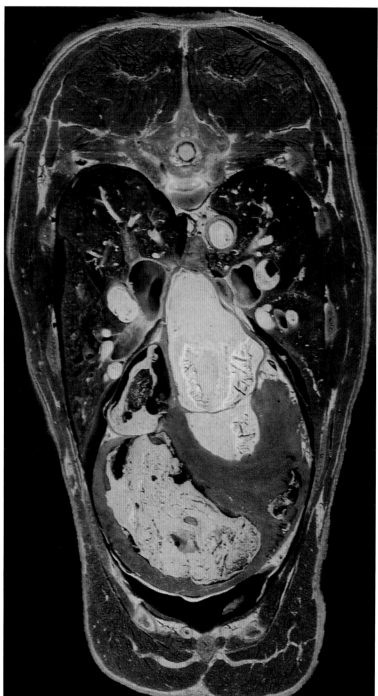

Fig. 5.84 Transverse section (6) through thoracic vertebra 8 and the left atrium: cranial view. This section passes through the heart at the entry of the caudal vena cava into the right atrium. The left atrium, filled with pink latex, occupies the mid-dorsal region of the heart, flanked on either side by the diverging principal bronchi, as well as the middle tracheobronchial lymph node on its left. Left and right ventricles are cut through and the left atrioventricular valve appears in the centre of the section. The pericardial cavity almost completely encircles the heart.

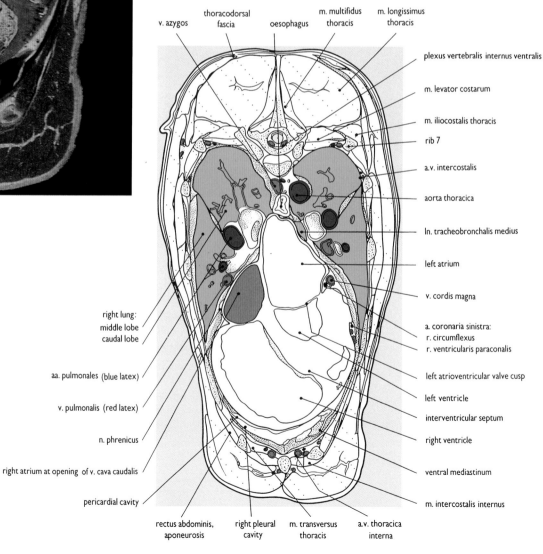

v. azygos

thoracodorsal fascia

oesophagus

m. multifidus thoracis

m. longissimus thoracis

plexus vertebralis internus ventralis

m. levator costarum

m. iliocostalis thoracis

rib 7

a.v. intercostalis

aorta thoracica

ln. tracheobronchalis medius

left atrium

v. cordis magna

a. coronaria sinistra:
r. circumflexus
r. ventricularis paraconalis

left atrioventricular valve cusp

left ventricle

interventricular septum

right ventricle

ventral mediastinum

m. intercostalis internus

right lung:
middle lobe
caudal lobe

aa. pulmonales (blue latex)

v. pulmonalis (red latex)

n. phrenicus

right atrium at opening of v. cava caudalis

pericardial cavity

rectus abdominis, aponeurosis

right pleural cavity

m. transversus thoracis

a.v. thoracica interna

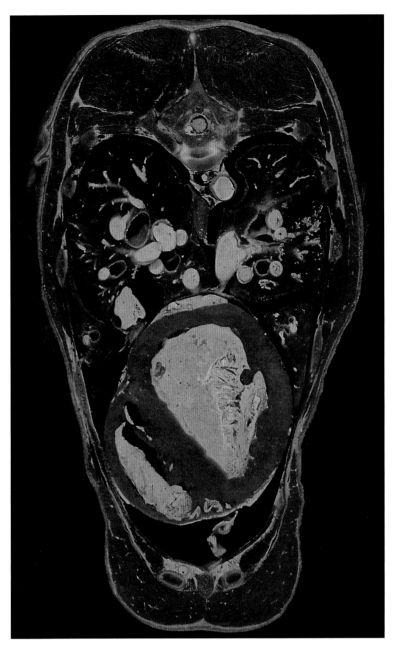

Fig. 5.85 Transverse section (7) through thoracic vertebra 9, the accessory lobe of the right lung and the caudal vena cava: cranial view. The accessory lobe of the right lung is bordered by the attenuated dorsal part of the caudal mediastinum and by the caudal vena cava supported in its own pleural fold (plica). Pulmonary ligaments from both caudal lobes are visible – in the vicinity of the azygos vein on the right and ventral to the esophagus on the left.

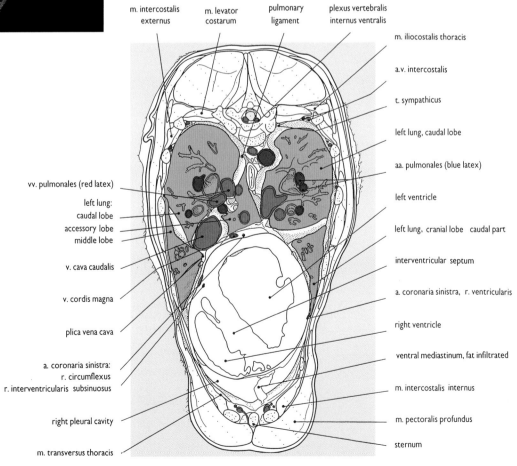

m. intercostalis externus

m. levator costarum

pulmonary ligament

plexus vertebralis internus ventralis

m. iliocostalis thoracis

a.v. intercostalis

t. sympathicus

left lung, caudal lobe

aa. pulmonales (blue latex)

left ventricle

left lung, cranial lobe caudal part

interventricular septum

a. coronaria sinistra, r. ventricularis

right ventricle

ventral mediastinum, fat infiltrated

m. intercostalis internus

m. pectoralis profundus

sternum

vv. pulmonales (red latex)

left lung:
caudal lobe
accessory lobe
middle lobe

v. cava caudalis

v. cordis magna

plica vena cava

a. coronaria sinistra:
r. circumflexus
r. interventricularis subsinuosus

right pleural cavity

m. transversus thoracis

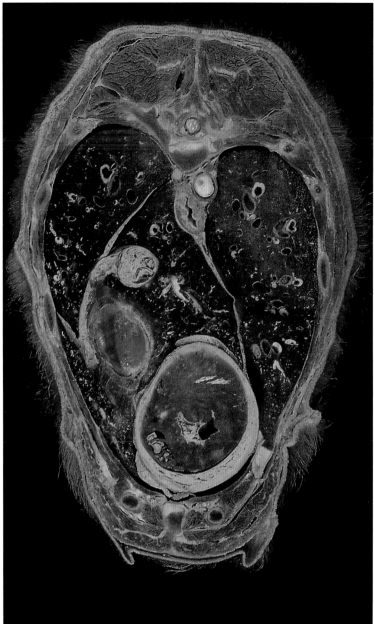

Fig. 5.86 Transverse section (8) through thoracic vertebra 9, the accessory lobe of the right lung, the caudal vena cava and the diaphragm: cranial view. The diaphragm just appears in this section. Its cranial-most extent has been 'shaved off' during sectioning where it appeared lateral to the accessory lobe of the lung. The small portion of the diaphragm removed was replaced in position. The caudal vena cava is sectioned immediately dorsal to this area of the diaphragm indenting the accessory lobe of the right lung. Its supporting plica of pleura from the mediastinum reflects onto the surface of the diaphragm and is visible on the muscular periphery, extending ventrally to the pericardium. The mediastinum is very thin ventral to the esophagus.

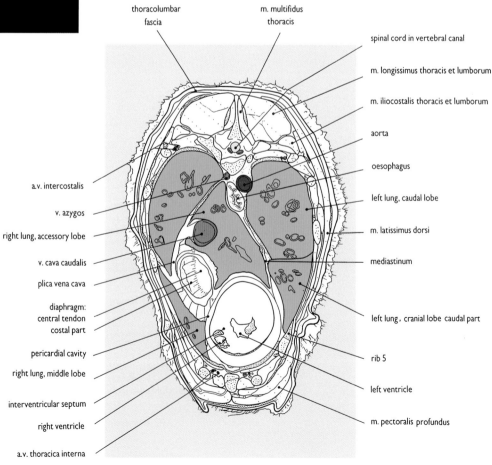

thoracolumbar fascia

m. multifidus thoracis

spinal cord in vertebral canal

m. longissimus thoracis et lumborum

m. iliocostalis thoracis et lumborum

aorta

oesophagus

left lung, caudal lobe

m. latissimus dorsi

mediastinum

left lung, cranial lobe caudal part

rib 5

left ventricle

m. pectoralis profundus

a.v. intercostalis

v. azygos

right lung, accessory lobe

v. cava caudalis

plica vena cava

diaphragm: central tendon costal part

pericardial cavity

right lung, middle lobe

interventricular septum

right ventricle

a.v. thoracica interna

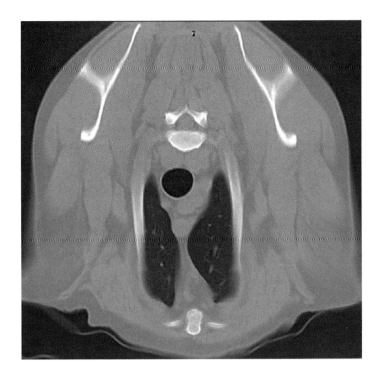

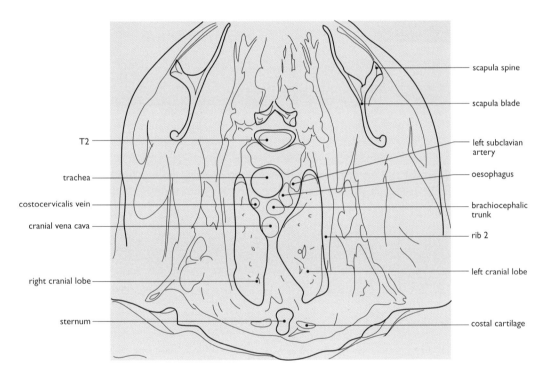

scapula spine

scapula blade

T2

left subclavian
artery

trachea

oesophagus

costocervicalis vein

brachiocephalic
trunk

cranial vena cava

rib 2

right cranial lobe

left cranial lobe

sternum

costal cartilage

Fig. 5.87 Computed tomography image of the thorax: transverse plane, at the level of the 2nd intercostal space.

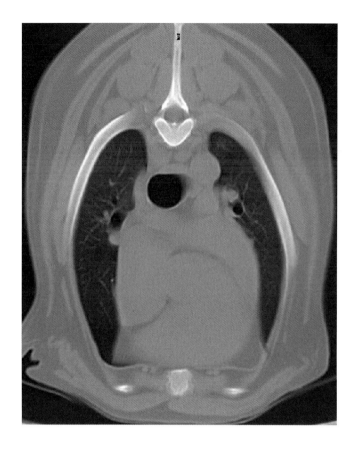

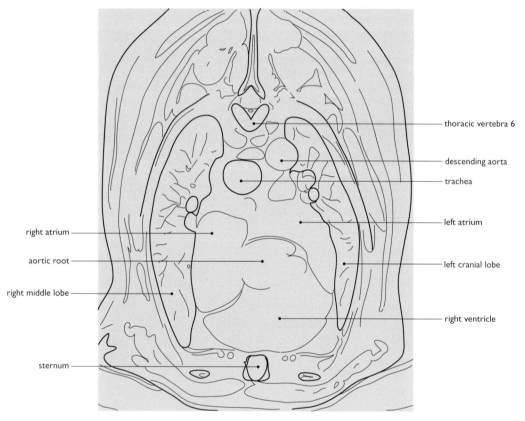

thoracic vertebra 6

descending aorta

trachea

left atrium

right atrium

aortic root

left cranial lobe

right middle lobe

right ventricle

sternum

Fig. 5.88 Computed tomography image of the thorax: transverse plane, at the level of the heart base.

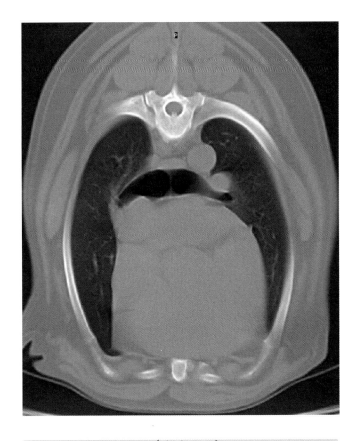

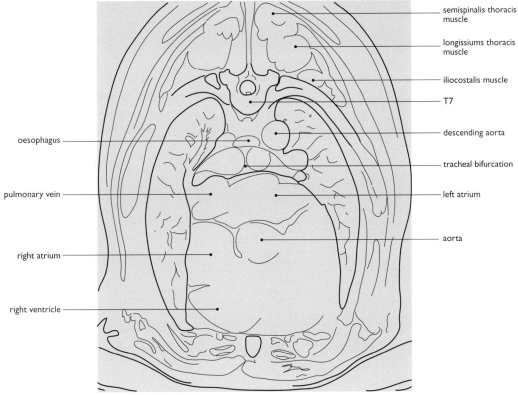

semispinalis thoracis muscle

longissiums thoracis muscle

iliocostalis muscle

T7

descending aorta

tracheal bifurcation

left atrium

aorta

oesophagus

pulmonary vein

right atrium

right ventricle

Fig. 5.89 Computed tomography image of the thorax: transverse plane, at the level of the tracheal bifurcation.

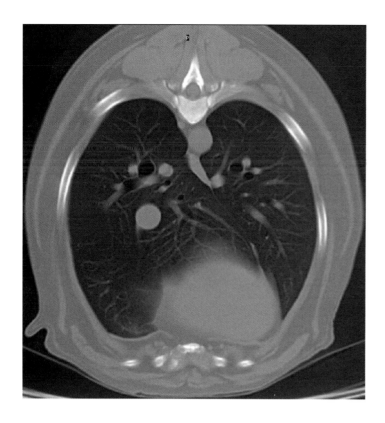

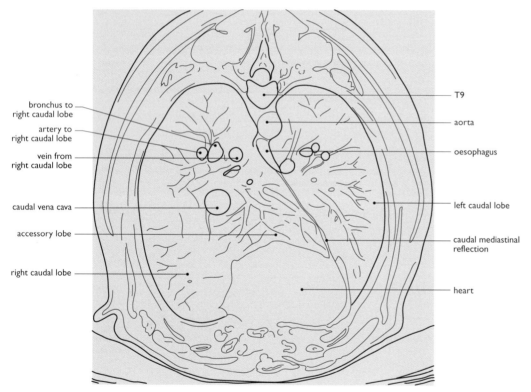

bronchus to
right caudal lobe

artery to
right caudal lobe

vein from
right caudal lobe

caudal vena cava

accessory lobe

right caudal lobe

T9

aorta

oesophagus

left caudal lobe

caudal mediastinal
reflection

heart

Fig. 5.90 Computed tomography image of the thorax: transverse plane, at the level of the caudal mediastinal reflection.

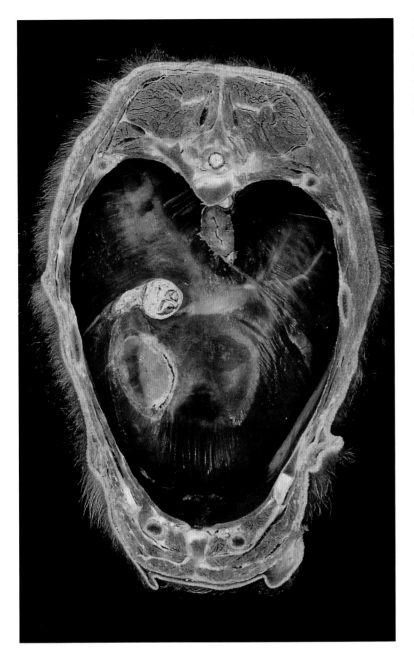

Fig. 5.91 Diaphragm: cranial view. The lobes of the lung, the heart and the remains of the pericardium have been removed. The cranial surface of the diaphragm is now exposed and shows the shape and extent of the central tendon, the position of the mediastinum and plica vena cava, and the relative positions of the diaphragmatic openings. Lumbar crura surround the aorta and esophagus although the two hiatuses so formed are more clearly shown in caudal view (see Chapter 6).

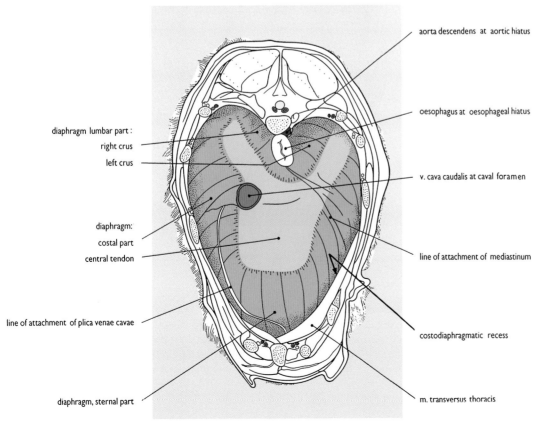

aorta descendens at aortic hiatus

oesophagus at oesophageal hiatus

v. cava caudalis at caval foramen

line of attachment of mediastinum

costodiaphragmatic recess

m. transversus thoracis

diaphragm lumbar part :
right crus
left crus

diaphragm:
costal part
central tendon

line of attachment of plica venae cavae

diaphragm, sternal part

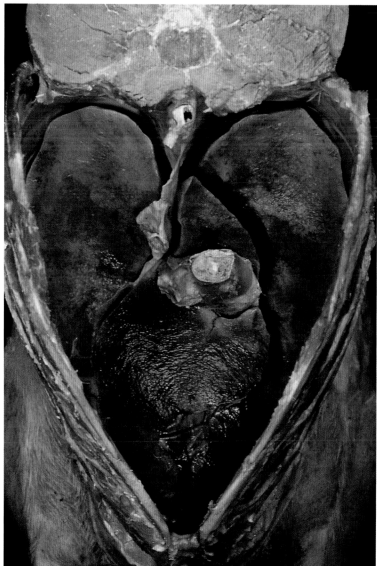

Fig. 5.92 Lungs *in situ* after removal of the diaphragm: caudal view. The diaphragmatic surfaces of the caudal lobes of both lungs, and the accessory and middle lobes of the right lung, are exposed following diaphragmatic removal.

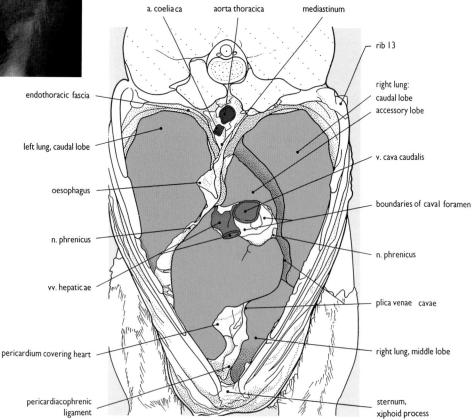

a. coeliaca

aorta thoracica

mediastinum

rib 13

endothoracic fascia

right lung:
caudal lobe
accessory lobe

left lung, caudal lobe

v. cava caudalis

oesophagus

boundaries of caval foramen

n. phrenicus

n. phrenicus

vv. hepaticae

plica venae cavae

pericardium covering heart

right lung, middle lobe

pericardiacophrenic
ligament

sternum,
xiphoid process

6. THE ABDOMEN

The symmetry, size and shape of the abdomen varies considerably from breed to breed. In the bitch, the mammary glands are an important pre- and post-natal feature and in the pregnant bitch the topography may be altered and caesarean section required. This is carried out as for any abdominal laparotomy described below.

The abdomen has basically three regions; cranial abdominal, middle and caudal abdominal, with hyposplanchnic and xiphoid regions. The region is limited by the diaphragm, iliocostal line and pelvic brim. It contains a wide range of organ systems with plenty of opportunity for these to go wrong and require surgery. Many of these surgical interventions are carried out through a midline laparotomy anywhere along a line from the xiphisternum to the umbilicus, although most extend much further caudally than the umbilicus even in males where the penis deflected and the incision continued. This is along the *linea alba* (white line) and the incision here once through the skin can be accomplished with minimum bleeding, as this is the junction of the aponeuroses of the ventral abdominal musculature. The tissue or organ that requires surgery can then be brought to the exterior without damage to other structures and allows them to be kept moist. This site also produces a strong tissue for suturing.

An exploratory laparotomy is carried out to see what is going on and to possibly make a definitive diagnosis, otherwise this site may be used for: ovarohysterectomy (spaying) of the bitch, and for pyometra (uterus fills with a pus-like material), often in nulliparous, aged, and usually post-season bitches. This requires complete surgical removal. Likewise, ovarian cysts and tumours are similarly removed. The same site can also give good access for removal of intestinal neoplasia; enterotomies for foreign body removal such as bones, fish hooks or bouncing rubber balls; enterectomy for intussusception (bowel telescopes into bowel) with subsequent end-to-end anastomoses of the bowel after removal of necrotic portions. Gastric dilation and torsion can be approached through the same site. Here needle decompression to release gas is necessary and a stomach tube tightly in place will remove gas and fluid, and then the re-positioned stomach can be held in place by stitches. This midline ventral laparotomy can also be used for partial gastrectomy for tumours and for operations on the pylorus – particularly pyloric stenosis. Torsion of the spleen may be relieved and splenic tumours can also be removed via a midline ventral incision and good exposure of the kidneys is also achievable. The ventral midline approach also gives good exposure to repair rupture of the diaphragm. The midline laparotomy is used in some circumstances to inject into the intestinal veins for the purpose of portography so that the circulation through the liver can be visualized.

Portosystemic shunts are a not uncommon condition in the dog and require diagnosis by catheterization of the celiac or cranial mesenteric artery via the mesenteric vessels. Surgical correction of the shunt is the only specific treatment. Structures in the upper abdomen (kidneys, thoracolumbar vertebrae) can also be reached by flank laparotomy. This involves cutting the abdominal musculature along the direction of their fibers and therefore there is considerably more potential hemorrhage because the incisions run three ways in the muscle layers (exterior abdominal oblique, interior abdominal oblique and transverse). The exposure is not as good as in a straight midline incision. The other problem is that the ventral branches of the spinal nerves innervating the ventral abdomen, mammary and inguinal region run over the transverse muscles and they should be avoided.

Nowadays, many surgeons use the laparoscopic techniques to routinely spay bitches. Some people, particularly in former times, have always recommended 'spaying' bitches from the right flank as the left ovarian ligament is longer than the right and therefore the left ovary is more easily exteriorized for ligation across the abdomen. Lateral thoracolumbar fenestration for disc problems over the large iliocostal muscle is also a possibility. I have left the discussion of the urogenital system to a discussion of the pelvis, but the mammary glands are an important abdominal feature. They are a frequent site of both benign and malignant tumours requiring surgical incision of single glands or sometimes both complete lines of glands. Each has a good segmental blood supply which requires careful ligation. It is important to note the lymphatic drainage when tumours may be seeded or infection spread as the cranial glands drain to the axillary (possible palpable) and sternal lymph nodes (inside thorax) – caudal abdominal glands drain to both the cranial glands and caudal to the inguinal glands and the inguinal mammary glands to the inguinal (mammary) lymph nodes, which again may be palpable.

Laparoscopy using a fibroscope to investigate the abdominal contents can also be used through the ventral midline incision. Abdominocentesis, which is the withdrawal of fluid from the peritoneal cavity, can be performed at a site 1 to 2 cm caudal to the umbilicus. In younger animals, it may be necessary to repair a hernia at the umbilicus, and in these cases the falciform fat or even small intestine may fill the cavity of the umbilicus, possibly leading later to strangulated hernia.

Other abdominal diagnostic techniques include liver biopsy. This used to be done from the left side of the abdomen to avoid damage to the right-sided gall bladder, large vessels and bile ducts at the hilus of the liver, i.e. dog is in right lateral recumbency after fasting, as it is not easy with a full stomach. To take just liver cells, it is possible to carry out a fine-needle biopsy in the 10th intercostal space on the right hand side, at the level of the costochondral junction. Nowadays, many surgeons tend to do this using ultrasound or laparoscope.

The last area that may require surgery is the inguinal region, with incisions over the inguinal canal to repair either an inguinal hernia or to search for a retained testicle somewhere between the internal inguinal ring and the caudal pole of the kidney from where in embryological terms the testicle originates before its traverse to the scrotum.

The vaginal process of the peritoneum in males exits from the inguinal region through the deep and superficial inguinal rings; 80% of female dogs also have a peritoneal vaginal process. The round ligament of the uterus passes through the inguinal canal and is contained within the vaginal process, and the canal itself is filled with connective tissue.

In 'open' castration of the dog, the parietal layer of the vaginal tunic is incised and thus the potential space of the peritoneal cavity is invaded.

Surgery of the bladder for removal of bladder stones or debris is also carried out through a caudal midline intervention with the incision avoiding the dorsal bladder surface where the ureters enter the bladder. Removal of kidney or ureteric stones may also be required.

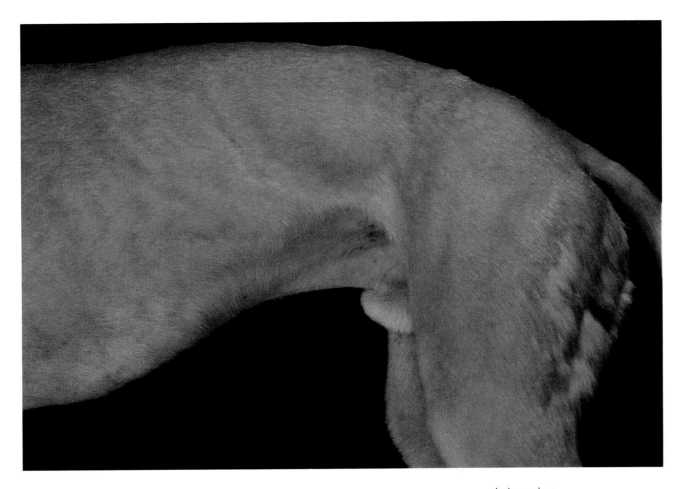

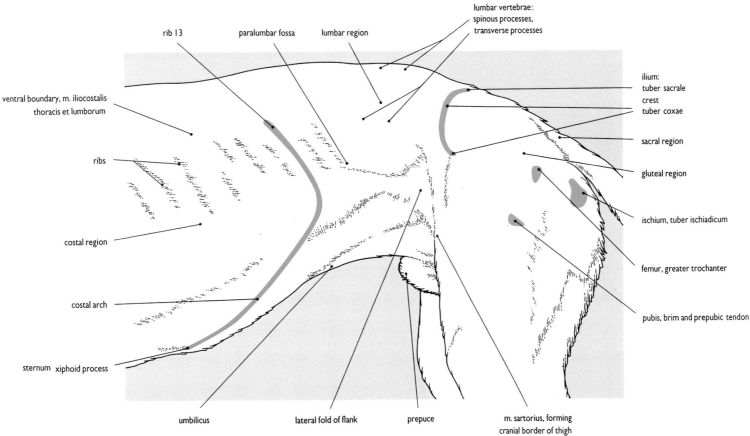

lumbar vertebrae:
spinous processes,
transverse processes

rib 13   paralumbar fossa   lumbar region

ilium:
tuber sacrale
crest
tuber coxae

ventral boundary, m. iliocostalis
thoracis et lumborum

sacral region

gluteal region

ribs

costal region

ischium, tuber ischiadicum

femur, greater trochanter

costal arch

pubis, brim and prepubic tendon

sternum xiphoid process

umbilicus   lateral fold of flank   prepuce   m. sartorius, forming
cranial border of thigh

Fig. 6.1 Surface features of the abdomen and hip: left lateral view. The bony 'landmarks' that are palpable around the borders of the abdomen are shown in this figure. In a normal standing position the femur and its covering thigh muscles obscure the rear end of the abdomen. The caudal border of the abdomen is marked by the tuber coxae dorsolaterally and the pubis ventrally. The inguinal ligament, marking the caudal border of the muscular abdominal wall, is palpable between these two points in the fold of the groin (see also Fig. 6.67 of the abdomen in ventral view).

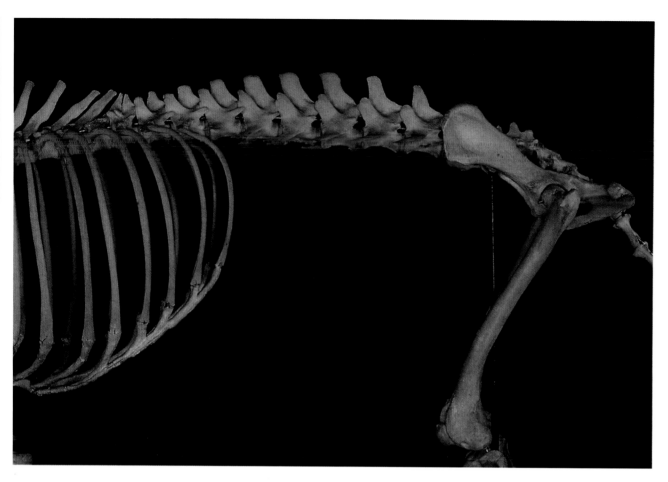

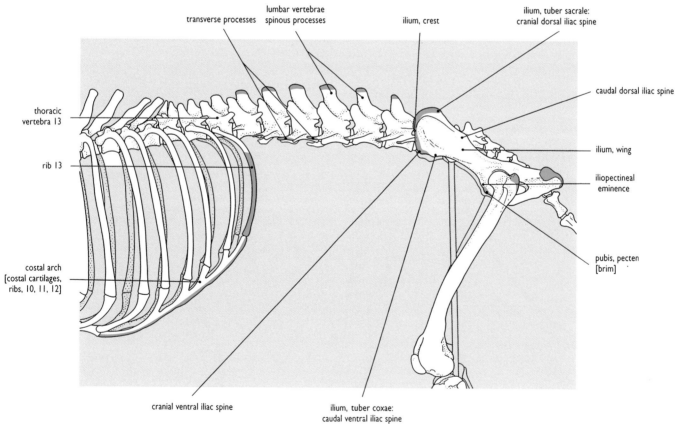

lumbar vertebrae
spinous processes

transverse processes

ilium, crest

ilium, tuber sacrale:
cranial dorsal iliac spine

caudal dorsal iliac spine

thoracic
vertebra 13

ilium, wing

rib 13

iliopectineal
eminence

costal arch
[costal cartilages,
ribs, 10, 11, 12]

pubis, pecten
[brim]

cranial ventral iliac spine

ilium, tuber coxae:
caudal ventral iliac spine

Fig. 6.2 Skeleton related to the abdomen: left lateral view. The palpable bony features shown bordering the abdomen in the surface view on Fig. 6.1 are colored green for reference. It should be noted that caudal to the large thoracic outlet (bounded by the xiphoid cartilage of the sternum, the costal arches and floating ribs) the abdominal wall is entirely muscular. The considerably restricted pelvic inlet, bounded by the sacrum above and pelvic bones bilaterally, marks the caudal boundary of the abdomen.

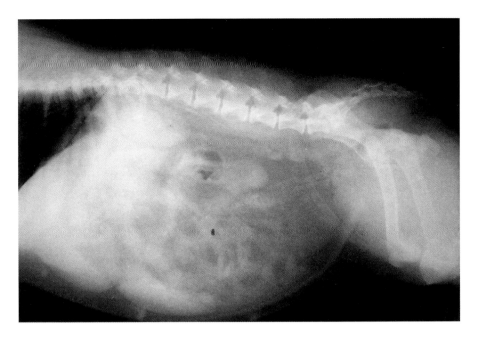

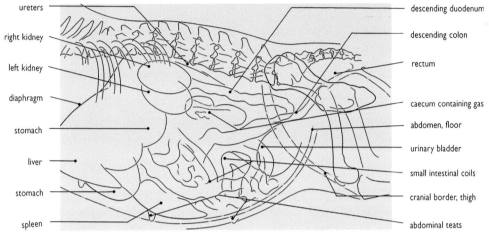

ureters — — descending duodenum

right kidney — — descending colon

left kidney — — rectum

diaphragm — — caecum containing gas

stomach — — abdomen, floor

liver — — urinary bladder

stomach — — small intestinal coils

spleen — — cranial border, thigh

— abdominal teats

Fig. 6.3 Radiograph of the abdomen: left lateral view. The normal features of the abdomen and its contents are shown in this picture. The position and appearance of the viscera do vary considerably with the amount of fat present. The animal used for this radiograph was actually obese, the contrast made possible by its fat clarifying soft tissue to some extent.

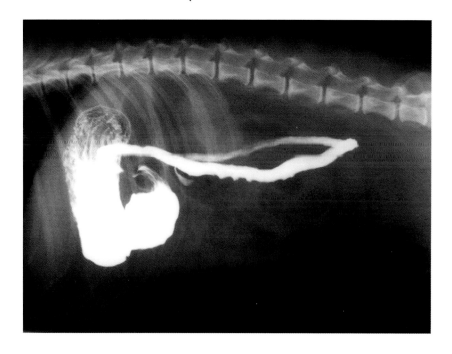

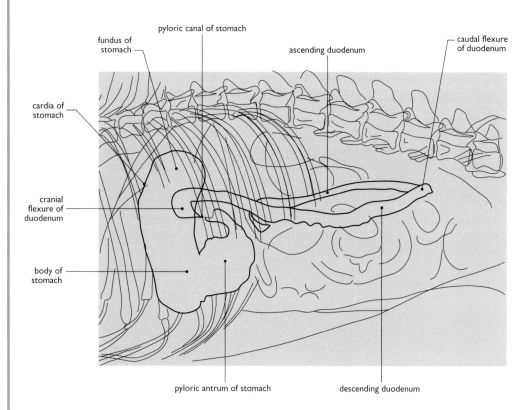

fundus of
stomach

pyloric canal of stomach

ascending duodenum

caudal flexure
of duodenum

cardia of
stomach

cranial
flexure of
duodenum

body of
stomach

pyloric antrum of stomach

descending duodenum

Fig. 6.4 Radiograph of the abdomen: lateral view, 20 minutes after oral administration of barium. Barium can be seen highlighting the stomach and duodenum. Rugal folds are visible in the gastric fundus. Irregularities on the ventral aspect of the descending duodenum represent regions of mucosal thinning over submucosal lymphoid accumulations.

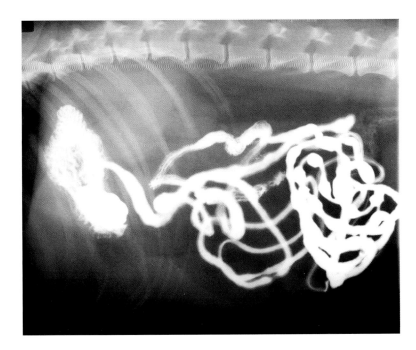

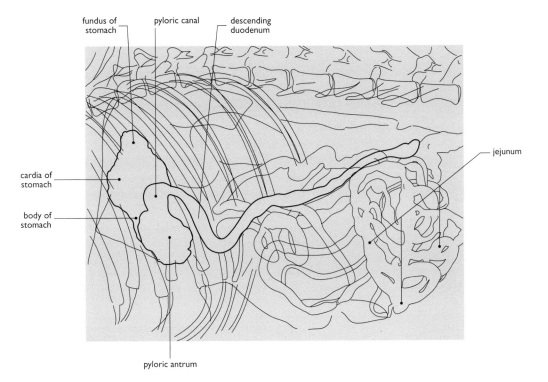

fundus of stomach
pyloric canal
descending duodenum
jejunum
cardia of stomach
body of stomach
pyloric antrum

Fig. 6.5 Radiograph of the abdomen: lateral view, 45 minutes after oral administration of barium. Barium can be seen highlighting the stomach and small intestine. The small intestines occupy the centre of the abdomen.

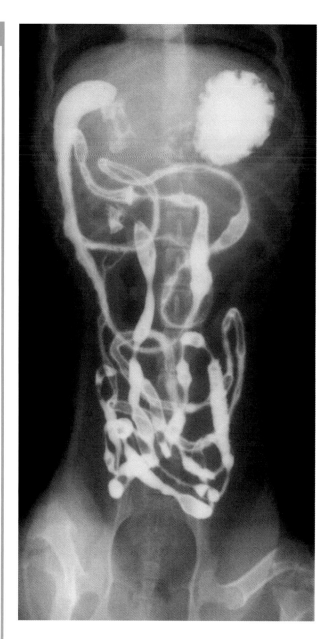

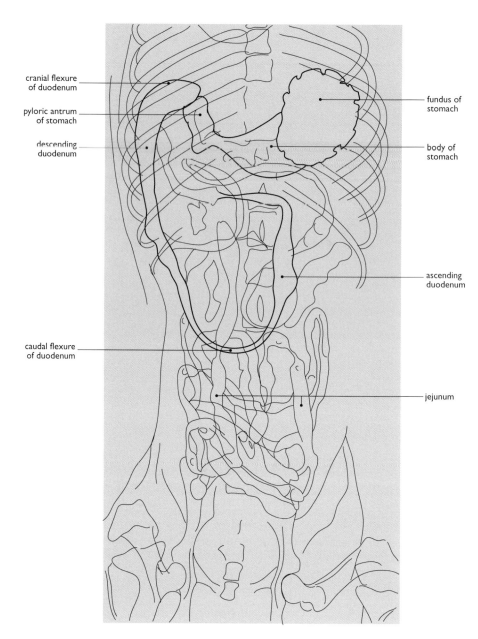

cranial flexure
of duodenum

pyloric antrum
of stomach

descending
duodenum

caudal flexure
of duodenum

fundus of
stomach

body of
stomach

ascending
duodenum

jejunum

Fig. 6.6 Radiograph of the abdomen: ventrodorsal view, 45 minutes after oral administration of barium. Barium can be seen highlighting the stomach and small intestine. The small intestines occupy the centre of the abdomen.

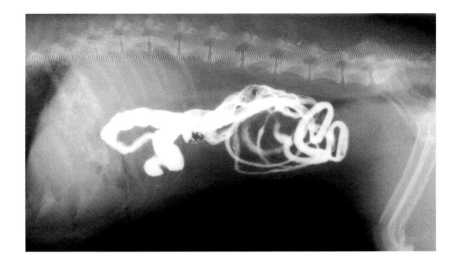

Fig. 6.7 Radiograph of the abdomen: lateral view, 4 hours after oral administration of barium. The barium can be seen highlighting parts of the jejunum and ileum, the caecum and the colon.

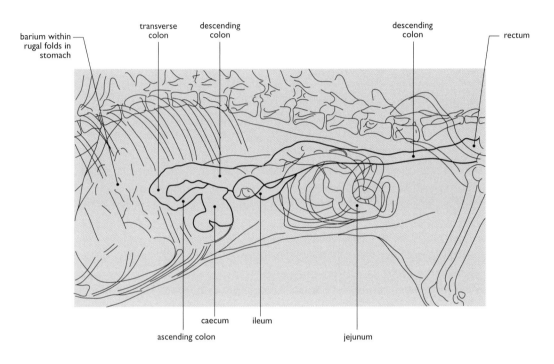

barium within rugal folds in stomach

transverse colon

descending colon

descending colon

rectum

caecum

ileum

ascending colon

jejunum

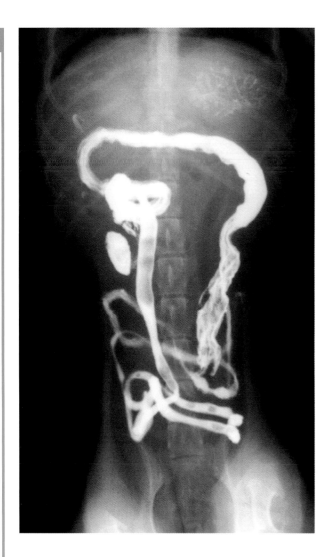
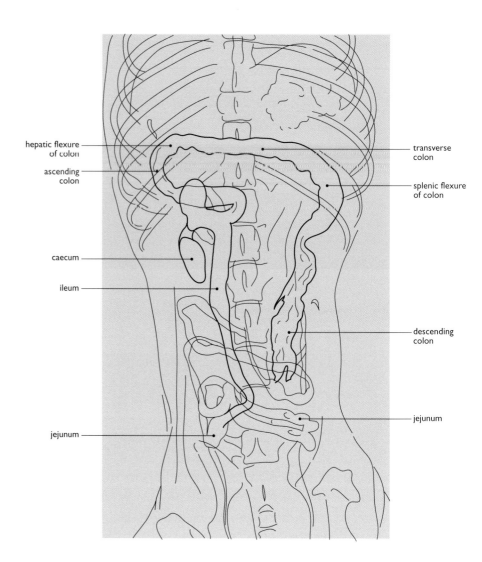

Fig. 6.8 Radiograph of the abdomen: ventrodorsal view, 4 hours after oral administration of barium. The barium can be seen highlighting parts of the jejunum and ileum, the caecum and the colon.

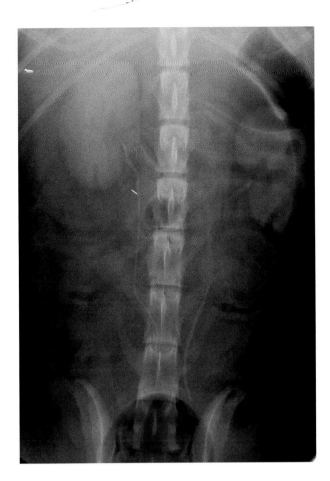
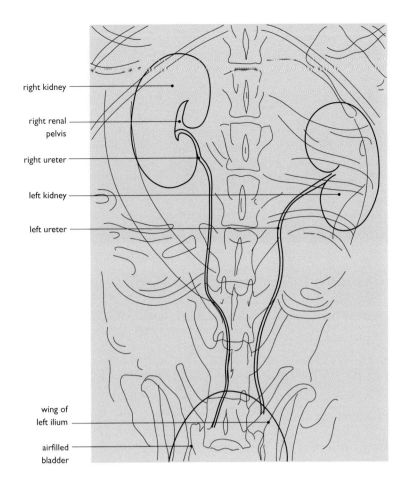

right kidney

right renal pelvis

right ureter

left kidney

left ureter

wing of left ilium

airfilled bladder

Fig. 6.9 Radiograph of the abdomen: ventrodorsal view, 5 minutes after intravenous injection of water-soluble iodine-containing contrast medium. The contrast medium can be seen highlighting the kidney parenchyma, the renal pelves and parts of the ureters. Ureters are rarely highlighted by continuous contrast columns in the normal dog due to their peristaltic movements. The bladder has been filled with air as part of the contrast study to enable greater visualization of the ureters.

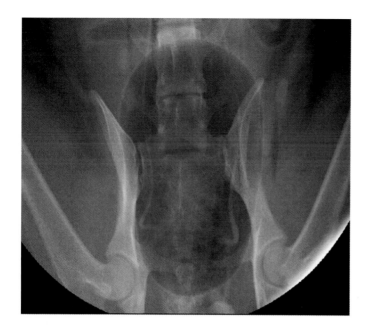

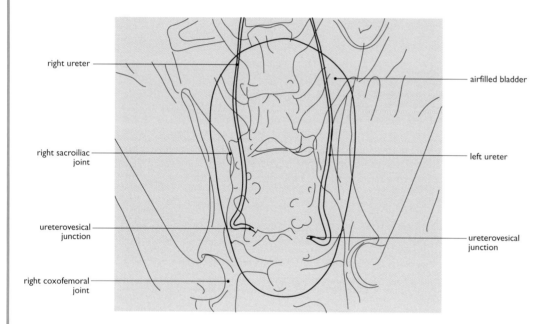

Fig. 6.10 Radiograph of the abdomen: ventrodorsal view, 15 minutes after intravenous injection of water-soluble iodine-containing contrast medium. The bladder has been filled with air to highlight the ureterovesical junctions.

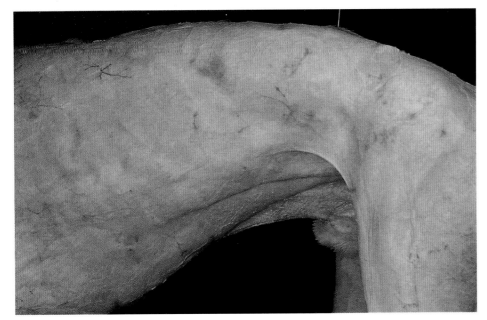

Fig. 6.11 Superficial fascia of the abdomen and hip: left lateral view. The skin has been removed displaying the superficial fascia, a thick subcutaneous covering of loose connective tissue rich in elastic fibers and usually containing variable quantities of fat. The cutaneous muscle of the trunk, located in the superficial fascia, extends cranioventrally and converges into the axilla. It is absent from the skin over the rump and thigh.

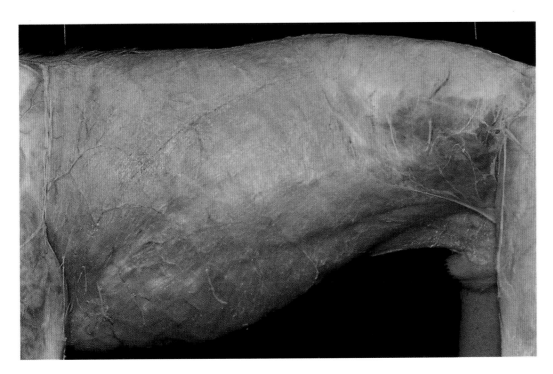

Fig. 6.12 Cutaneous muscle of the trunk and cutaneous nerves of the abdomen and cranial thigh: left lateral view. Limited cleaning of the superficial fascia has exposed the cutaneous muscle of the trunk. It has been cut into and partially removed from the caudodorsal abdomen and loin, a procedure which has exposed two lateral series of cutaneous nerves with accompanying cutaneous vessels.

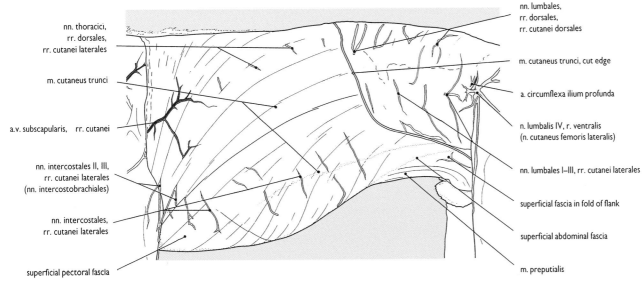

nn. thoracici,
rr. dorsales,
rr. cutanei laterales

m. cutaneus trunci

a.v. subscapularis,   rr. cutanei

nn. intercostales II, III,
rr. cutanei laterales
(nn. intercostobrachiales)

nn. intercostales,
rr. cutanei laterales

superficial pectoral fascia

nn. lumbales,
rr. dorsales,
rr. cutanei dorsales

m. cutaneus trunci, cut edge

a. circumflexa ilium profunda

n. lumbalis IV, r. ventralis
(n. cutaneus femoris lateralis)

nn. lumbales I–III, rr. cutanei laterales

superficial fascia in fold of flank

superficial abdominal fascia

m. preputialis

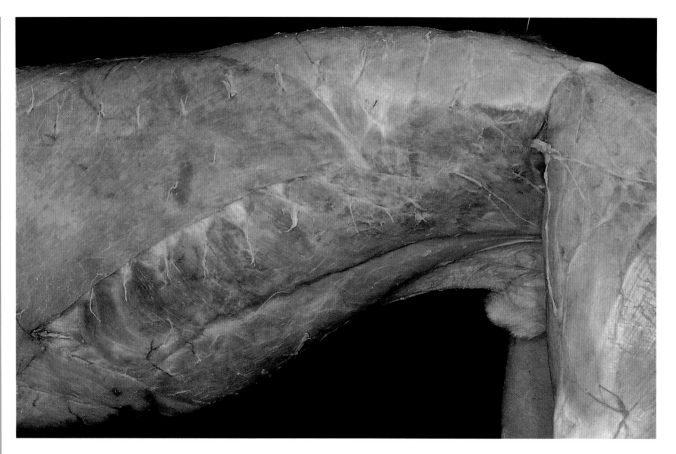

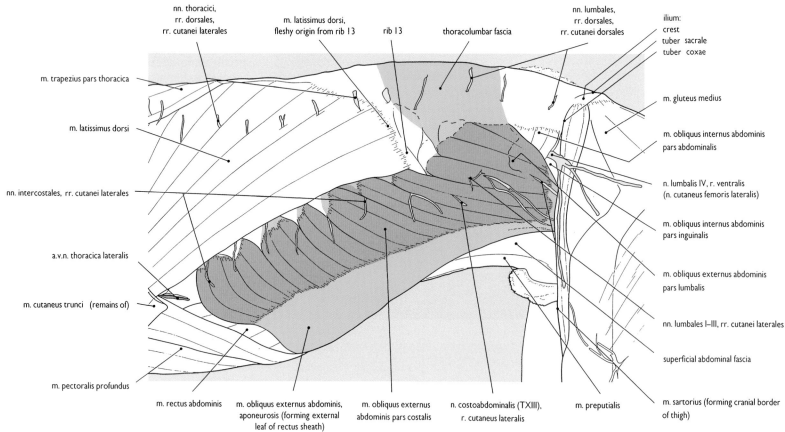

nn. thoracici,
rr. dorsales,
rr. cutanei laterales

m. latissimus dorsi,
fleshy origin from rib 13

rib 13

thoracolumbar fascia

nn. lumbales,
rr. dorsales,
rr. cutanei dorsales

ilium:
crest
tuber sacrale
tuber coxae

m. trapezius pars thoracica

m. gluteus medius

m. latissimus dorsi

m. obliquus internus abdominis
pars abdominalis

nn. intercostales, rr. cutanei laterales

n. lumbalis IV, r. ventralis
(n. cutaneus femoris lateralis)

m. obliquus internus abdominis
pars inguinalis

a.v.n. thoracica lateralis

m. obliquus externus abdominis
pars lumbalis

m. cutaneus trunci (remains of)

nn. lumbales I–III, rr. cutanei laterales

superficial abdominal fascia

m. pectoralis profundus

m. sartorius (forming cranial border
of thigh)

m. rectus abdominis

m. obliquus externus abdominis,
aponeurosis (forming external
leaf of rectus sheath)

m. obliquus externus
abdominis pars costalis

n. costoabdominalis (TXIII),
r. cutaneus lateralis

m. preputialis

Fig. 6.13 Superficial structures of the abdomen – cutaneous nerves: left lateral view. The remaining superficial fascia has been cleaned from the trunk along with most of the cutaneous muscle. On the underside of the abdominal wall the glans of the penis and its enclosing prepuce are suspended by a fold of skin. This fold has been removed from the left side exposing the preputial muscle radiating caudally into the prepuce, and the preputial components of the external pudendal vessels extending cranially from the inguinal region (see also Figs 6.14, 6.46 and 6.101).

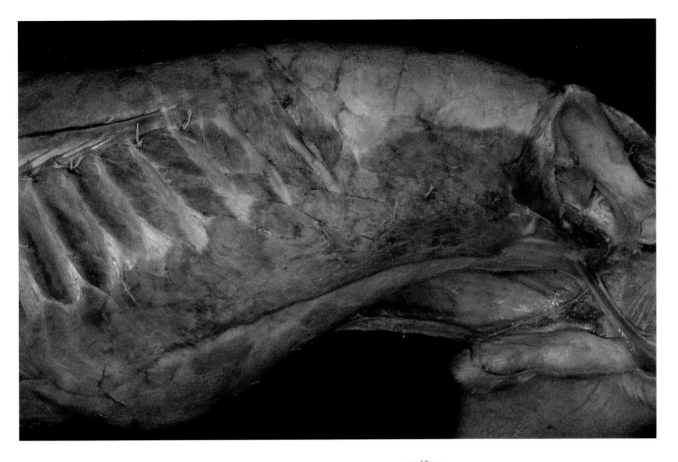

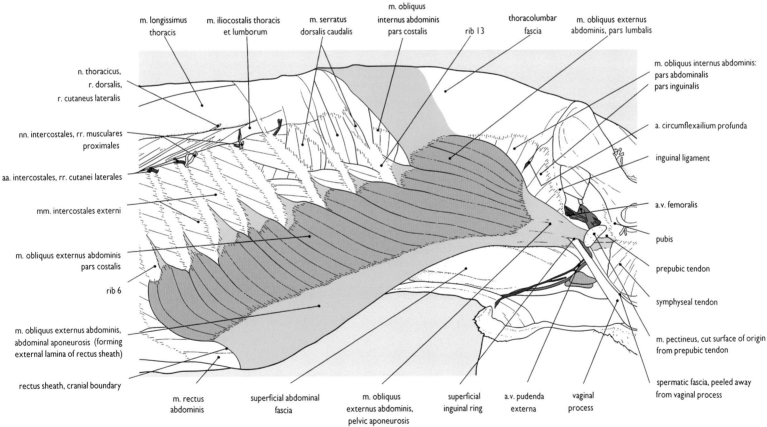

m. longissimus
thoracis

m. iliocostalis thoracis
et lumborum

m. serratus
dorsalis caudalis

m. obliquus
internus abdominis
pars costalis

rib 13

thoracolumbar
fascia

m. obliquus externus
abdominis, pars lumbalis

n. thoracicus,
r. dorsalis,
r. cutaneus lateralis

m. obliquus internus abdominis:
pars abdominalis
pars inguinalis

nn. intercostales, rr. musculares
proximales

a. circumflexailium profunda

inguinal ligament

aa. intercostales, rr. cutanei laterales

a.v. femoralis

mm. intercostales externi

pubis

m. obliquus externus abdominis
pars costalis

prepubic tendon

rib 6

symphyseal tendon

m. obliquus externus abdominis,
abdominal aponeurosis (forming
external lamina of rectus sheath)

m. pectineus, cut surface of origin
from prepubic tendon

rectus sheath, cranial boundary

spermatic fascia, peeled away
from vaginal process

m. rectus
abdominis

superficial abdominal
fascia

m. obliquus
externus abdominis,
pelvic aponeurosis

superficial
inguinal ring

a.v. pudenda
externa

vaginal
process

Fig. 6.14 Abdominal wall (1). External abdominal oblique muscle after removal of the hindlimb: left lateral view. Removal of the left hindlimb exposes the overall extent of the muscular abdominal wall. The latissimus dorsi and pectoral muscles have also been removed from the thorax which exposes the origin of the external oblique muscle. The caudal limit of the muscular abdominal wall, the inguinal ligament, is visible on the surface of the iliopsoas muscle. Ventrally the aponeurosis of the external oblique forms a major component of the external layer of the rectus sheath (see also Figs 6.69–6.71).

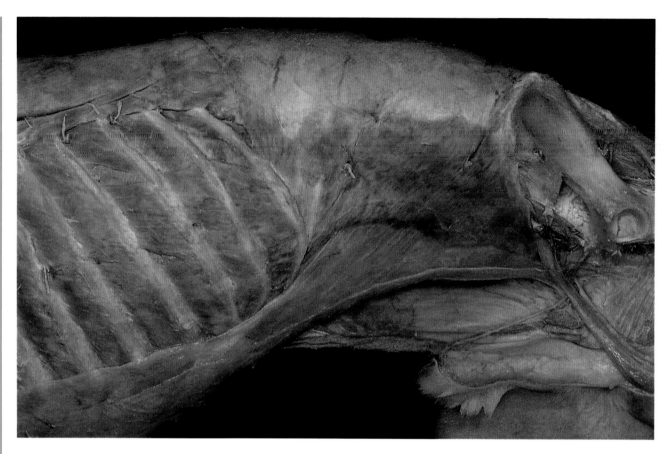

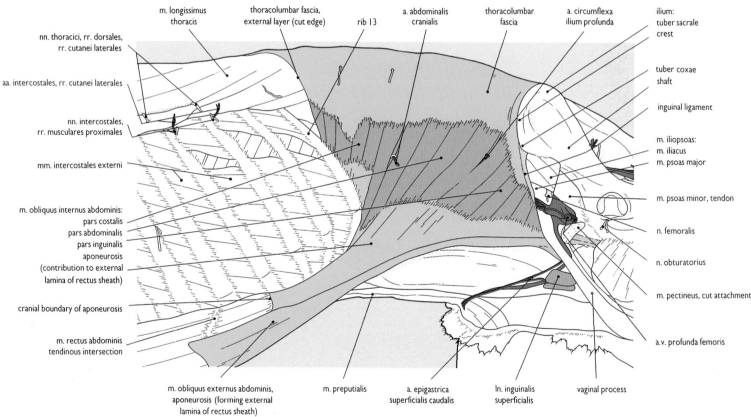

m. longissimus thoracis

thoracolumbar fascia, external layer (cut edge)

rib 13

a. abdominalis cranialis

thoracolumbar fascia

a. circumflexa ilium profunda

ilium: tuber sacrale crest

nn. thoracici, rr. dorsales, rr. cutanei laterales

aa. intercostales, rr. cutanei laterales

nn. intercostales, rr. musculares proximales

mm. intercostales externi

m. obliquus internus abdominis:
pars costalis
pars abdominalis
pars inguinalis
aponeurosis
(contribution to external lamina of rectus sheath)

cranial boundary of aponeurosis

m. rectus abdominis tendinous intersection

tuber coxae shaft

inguinal ligament

m. iliopsoas:
m. iliacus
m. psoas major

m. psoas minor, tendon

n. femoralis

n. obturatorius

m. pectineus, cut attachment

a.v. profunda femoris

m. obliquus externus abdominis, aponeurosis (forming external lamina of rectus sheath)

m. preputialis

a. epigastrica superficialis caudalis

ln. inguinalis superficialis

vaginal process

Fig. 6.15 Abdominal wall (2). Internal abdominal oblique muscle: left lateral view. The external oblique has been removed except where it forms part of the external layer of the rectus sheath. Here it is inseparable from the underlying aponeurosis of the internal oblique (see also Figs 6.69–6.71). The pelvic tendon of the external oblique has also been removed, in consequence the inguinal canal is completely opened on its cranial and lateral aspects. Cranially the contribution of the aponeurosis of the internal oblique to both deep and superficial layers of the rectus sheath is exposed. This relationship is shown to advantage in the next few figures and in Figs 5.16–5.19.

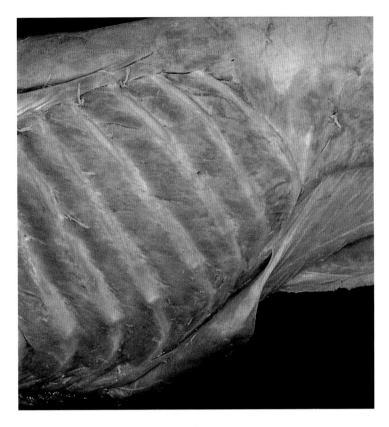

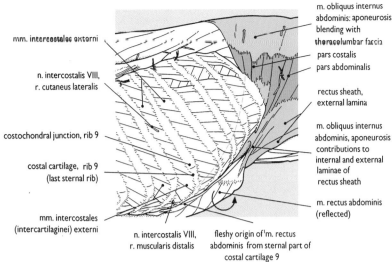

mm. intercostales externi

n. intercostalis VIII,
r. cutaneus lateralis

costochondral junction, rib 9

costal cartilage, rib 9
(last sternal rib)

mm. intercostales
(intercartilaginei) externi

n. intercostalis VIII,
r. muscularis distalis

m. obliquus internus
abdominis: aponeurosis
blending with
thoracolumbar fascia
pars costalis
pars abdominalis

rectus sheath,
external lamina

m. obliquus internus
abdominis, aponeurosis
contributions to
internal and external
laminae of
rectus sheath

m. rectus abdominis
(reflected)

fleshy origin of m. rectus
abdominis from sternal part of
costal cartilage 9

Fig. 6.16 Abdominal wall (3). Internal abdominal oblique muscle and rectus sheath: left lateral view (1). Reflection of the cranial part of the rectus abdominis muscle from the thorax exposes the costal cartilages and the fleshy origin of the rectus from costal cartilage 9. The position internally of the costodiaphragmatic line of pleural reflection (broken line) demonstrates the caudal-most extent of the thoracic cavity and therefore penetration caudal to this line will enter the abdomen.

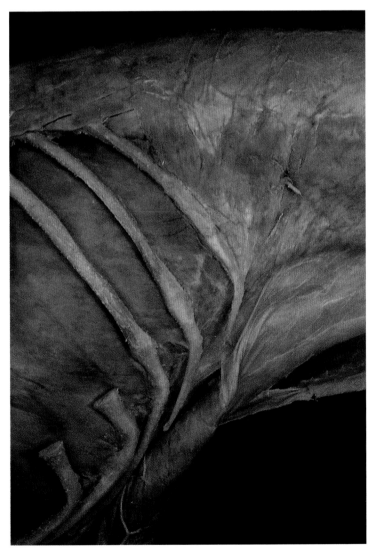

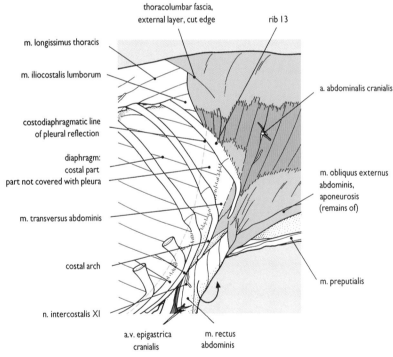

thoracolumbar fascia,
external layer, cut edge   rib 13

m. longissimus thoracis

m. iliocostalis lumborum

a. abdominalis cranialis

costodiaphragmatic line
of pleural reflection

diaphragm:
costal part
part not covered with pleura

m. obliquus externus
abdominis,
aponeurosis
(remains of)

m. transversus abdominis

costal arch

m. preputialis

n. intercostalis XI

a.v. epigastrica
cranialis

m. rectus
abdominis

Fig. 6.17 Abdominal wall (4). Internal abdominal oblique muscle and rectus sheath: left lateral view (2). Further reflection of the rectus muscle has been accomplished after severance of its fleshy attachment to costal cartilage 9. The costal arch is now displayed and the intercostal/interchondral spaces are completely cleared of intercostal musculature. Caudal to the costodiaphragmatic line of pleural reflection (broken line), diaphragmatic muscle is attached to the internal surfaces of costal cartilages except that of rib 13 whose costal cartilage remains free.

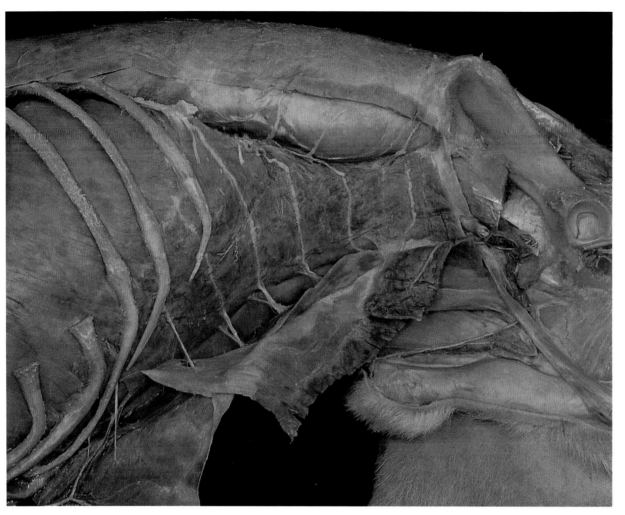

Fig. 6.18 Abdominal wall (5). Transverse abdominal muscle and nerves of the abdominal wall: left lateral view. The internal oblique muscle has been cut through longitudinally close to its origin from the thoracolumbar fascia, and from its association with the inguinal ligament. The muscle is reflected ventrally and is left hanging down from the ventrolateral aspect of the abdomen. The rectus abdominis has also been reflected away from the transverse abdominal aponeurosis stretching the nerves which enter it dorsally. In the upper part of the abdominal wall, caudal to rib 13, a rudimentary rib 14 is visible. This extra rib is only cartilaginous and has fascial connective tissue attachments to both internal oblique and transverse muscles.

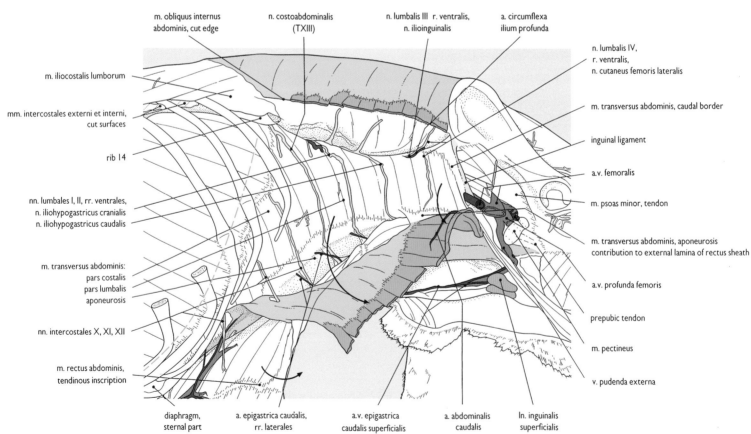

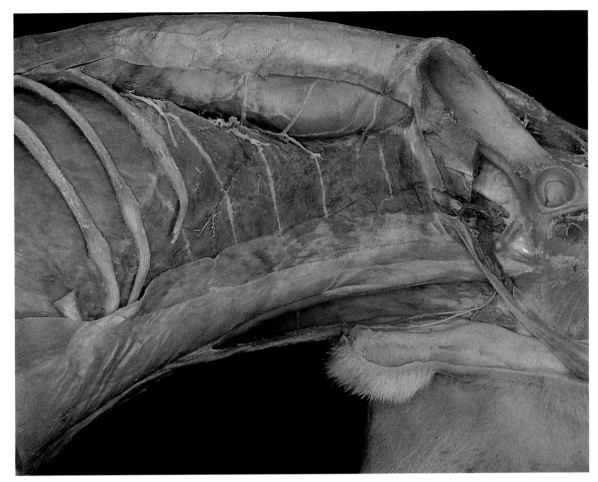

Fig. 6.19 Abdominal wall (6). Rectus abdominis muscle and rectus sheath external layer: left lateral view. The internal oblique muscle has been almost completely removed. Only the ventral part of its aponeurosis remains on the surface of the rectus abdominis muscle where it forms the external layer of the rectus sheath together with the aponeurosis of the external oblique. The two are inseparably fused down to the linea alba in the midventral line. The rudimentary rib 14 has been removed and the series of nerves entering the upper part of the abdominal wall are displayed on the surface of the transverse muscle (see also Fig. 6.72).

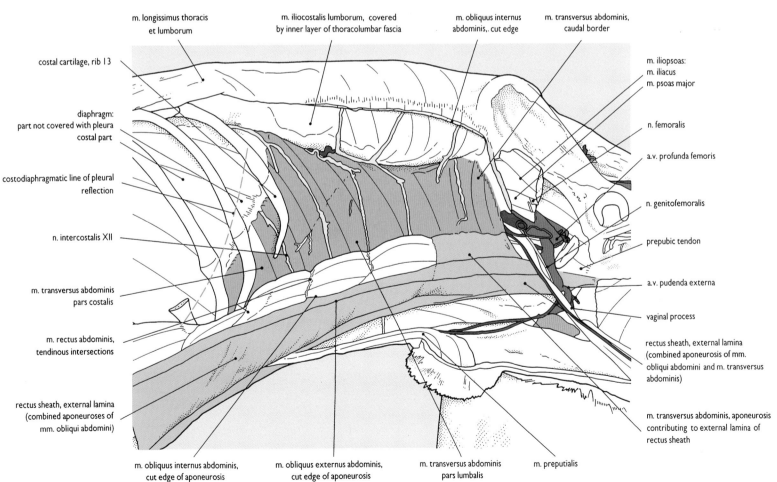

m. longissimus thoracis et lumborum

m. iliocostalis lumborum, covered by inner layer of thoracolumbar fascia

m. obliquus internus abdominis,. cut edge

m. transversus abdominis, caudal border

costal cartilage, rib 13

diaphragm: part not covered with pleura costal part

costodiaphragmatic line of pleural reflection

n. intercostalis XII

m. transversus abdominis pars costalis

m. rectus abdominis, tendinous intersections

rectus sheath, external lamina (combined aponeuroses of mm. obliqui abdomini)

m. iliopsoas: m. iliacus m. psoas major

n. femoralis

a.v. profunda femoris

n. genitofemoralis

prepubic tendon

a.v. pudenda externa

vaginal process

rectus sheath, external lamina (combined aponeurosis of mm. obliqui abdomini and m. transversus abdominis)

m. transversus abdominis, aponeurosis contributing to external lamina of rectus sheath

m. obliquus internus abdominis, cut edge of aponeurosis

m. obliquus externus abdominis, cut edge of aponeurosis

m. transversus abdominis pars lumbalis

m. preputialis

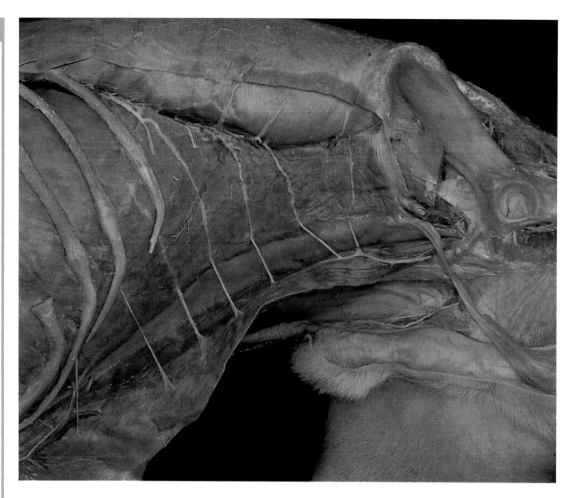

Fig. 6.20 Abdominal wall (7). Rectus abdominis muscle and rectus sheath internal layer: left lateral view. Severing of the caudal part of the transverse abdominal aponeurosis where it contributed to the external layer of the rectus sheath has allowed the rectus abdominis muscle to be reflected ventrally away from the underlying transverse muscle and aponeurosis. The dorsal surface of the rectus is exposed with the terminations of abdominal wall nerves entering it in series. The internal layer of the rectus sheath is represented here by the aponeurosis of the transverse muscle, except caudal to the caudal iliohypogastric nerve branch where it consists solely of transverse fascia (see also Figs 6.72 and 6.101).

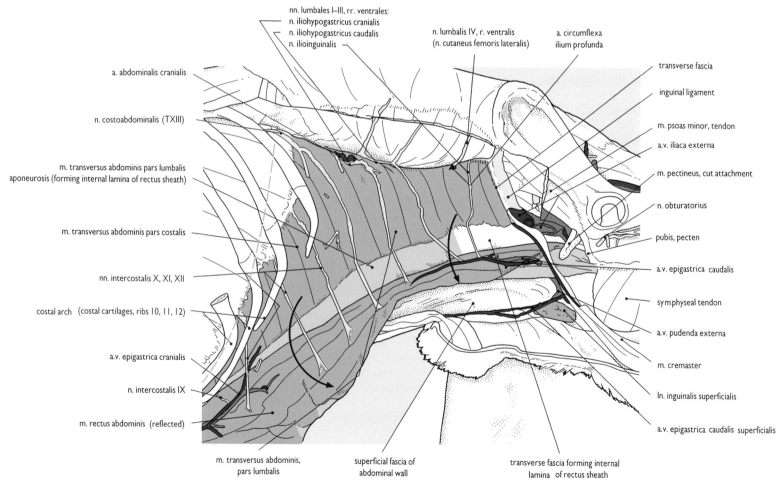

nn. lumbales I–III, rr. ventrales:
n. iliohypogastricus cranialis
n. iliohypogastricus caudalis
n. ilioinguinalis

n. lumbalis IV, r. ventralis
(n. cutaneus femoris lateralis)

a. circumflexa ilium profunda

a. abdominalis cranialis

transverse fascia

inguinal ligament

n. costoabdominalis (TXIII)

m. psoas minor, tendon

a.v. iliaca externa

m. transversus abdominis pars lumbalis aponeurosis (forming internal lamina of rectus sheath)

m. pectineus, cut attachment

m. transversus abdominis pars costalis

n. obturatorius

pubis, pecten

nn. intercostalis X, XI, XII

a.v. epigastrica caudalis

costal arch (costal cartilages, ribs 10, 11, 12)

symphyseal tendon

a.v. epigastrica cranialis

a.v. pudenda externa

m. cremaster

n. intercostalis IX

ln. inguinalis superficialis

m. rectus abdominis (reflected)

a.v. epigastrica caudalis superficialis

m. transversus abdominis, pars lumbalis

superficial fascia of abdominal wall

transverse fascia forming internal lamina of rectus sheath

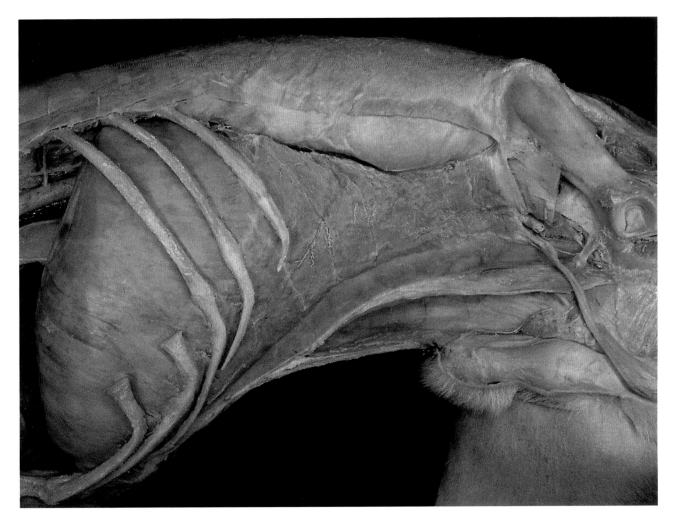

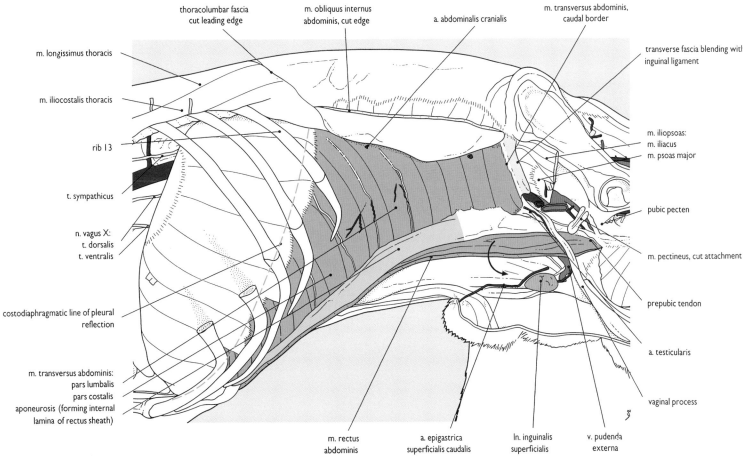

thoracolumbar fascia
cut leading edge

m. obliquus internus
abdominis, cut edge

a. abdominalis cranialis

m. transversus abdominis,
caudal border

m. longissimus thoracis

transverse fascia blending with
inguinal ligament

m. iliocostalis thoracis

m. iliopsoas:
m. iliacus
m. psoas major

rib 13

t. sympathicus

pubic pecten

n. vagus X:
t. dorsalis
t. ventralis

m. pectineus, cut attachment

prepubic tendon

costodiaphragmatic line of pleural
reflection

a. testicularis

m. transversus abdominis:
pars lumbalis
pars costalis
aponeurosis (forming internal
lamina of rectus sheath)

vaginal process

m. rectus
abdominis

a. epigastrica
superficialis caudalis

ln. inguinalis
superficialis

v. pudenda
externa

Fig. 6.21 Abdominal wall (8). Transverse abdominal muscle and diaphragm: left lateral view. The transverse abdominal muscle is exposed in its entirety after removal of the rectus abdominis muscle and the nerves of the abdominal wall. The costal part is seen arising from the internal face of the costal arch interdigitating with fibers of the diaphragm immediately caudal to the costodiaphragmatic line of pleural reflection. The lumbar part emerges from beneath the iliocostalis lumborum. The extensive aponeurosis ventrally provides the internal lamina of the rectus sheath and extends down to the linea alba (see also Figs 6.70, 6.72). The caudal border of the transverse muscle does not extend to the caudal end of the abdominal wall.

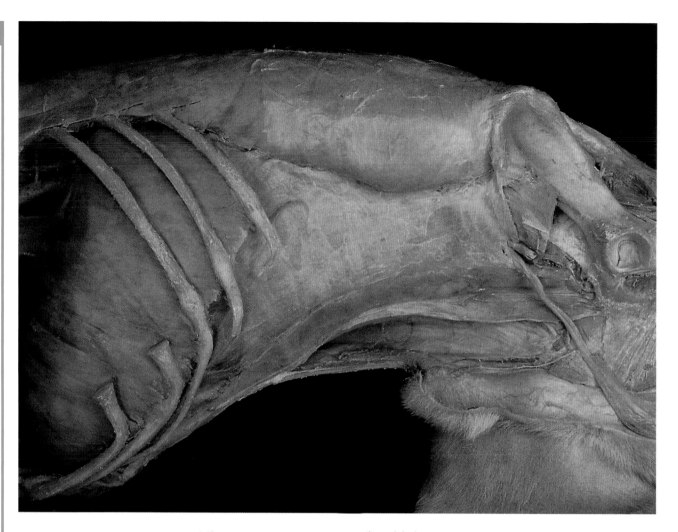

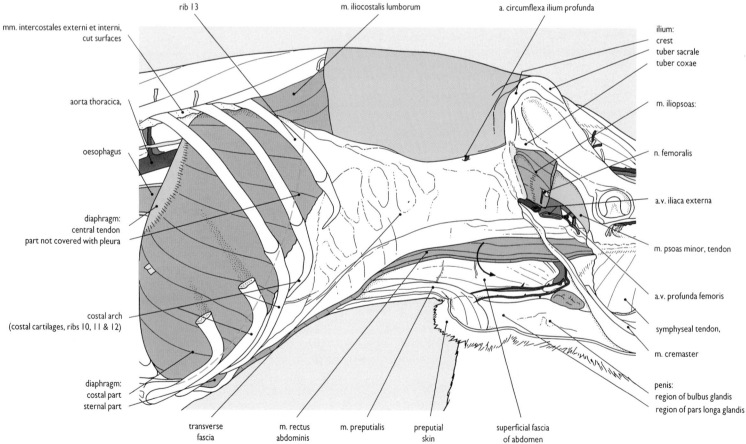

mm. intercostales externi et interni, cut surfaces

rib 13

m. iliocostalis lumborum

a. circumflexa ilium profunda

aorta thoracica,

oesophagus

diaphragm:
central tendon
part not covered with pleura

costal arch
(costal cartilages, ribs 10, 11 & 12)

diaphragm:
costal part
sternal part

transverse
fascia

m. rectus
abdominis

m. preputialis

preputial
skin

superficial fascia
of abdomen

ilium:
crest
tuber sacrale
tuber coxae

m. iliopsoas:

n. femoralis

a.v. iliaca externa

m. psoas minor, tendon

a.v. profunda femoris

symphyseal tendon,

m. cremaster

penis:
region of bulbus glandis
region of pars longa glandis

Fig. 6.22 Abdominal wall (9). Transverse fascia: left lateral view. The transverse abdominal muscle has been carefully removed and the transverse fascia lining the internal face of the abdominal wall is exposed. This clear layer supports the parietal peritoneum internally and blends with the iliac fascia on the iliopsoas muscle and with the pelvic fascia at the pelvic inlet ventrally. Cranially the transverse fascia is continued onto the rear surface of the diaphragm medial to the costal arch.

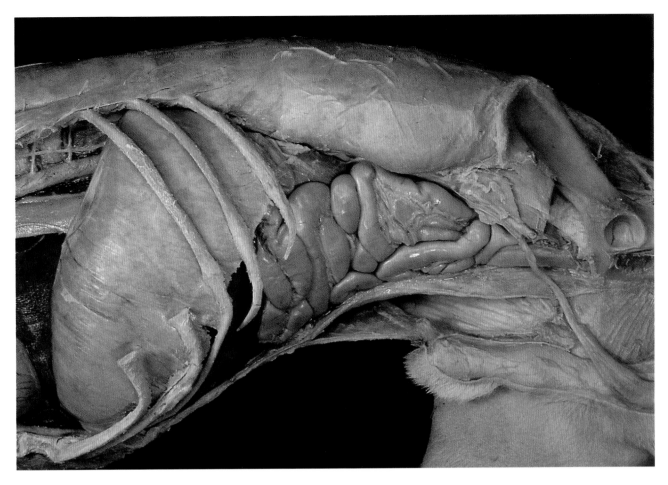

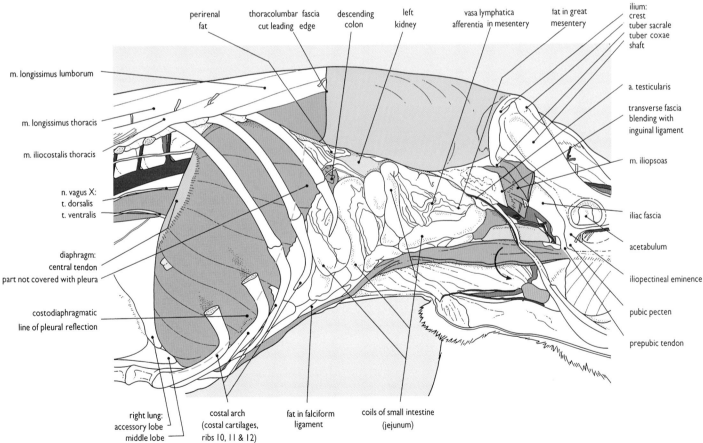

perirenal fat	thoracolumbar fascia cut leading edge	descending colon	left kidney	vasa lymphatica afferentia in mesentery	fat in great mesentery

ilium:
crest
tuber sacrale
tuber coxae
shaft

m. longissimus lumborum

m. longissimus thoracis

m. iliocostalis thoracis

a. testicularis

transverse fascia blending with inguinal ligament

m. iliopsoas

n. vagus X:
t. dorsalis
t. ventralis

iliac fascia

diaphragm:
central tendon
part not covered with pleura

acetabulum

iliopectineal eminence

costodiaphragmatic
line of pleural reflection

pubic pecten

prepubic tendon

right lung:
accessory lobe
middle lobe

costal arch
(costal cartilages,
ribs 10, 11 & 12)

fat in falciform
ligament

coils of small intestine
(jejunum)

Fig. 6.23 Abdominal viscera in situ (1). After removal of the abdominal wall: left lateral view. Removal of the transverse fascia and the closely applied parietal peritoneum opens the peritoneal cavity and exposes jejunal coils. Several areas where fat is deposited beneath the peritoneum are apparent; viz. great mesentery associated with the jejunal coils, around the kidney (perirenal fat), and in the falciform ligament ventrally (see also Figs 6.74 and 6.75 for fat deposits in the abdomen). Also visible in the great mesentery are clearly defined opaque strips which represent afferent lymphatic channels. Compare this view with equivalent views from the right (Fig. 6.47) and ventrally (Fig. 6.73).

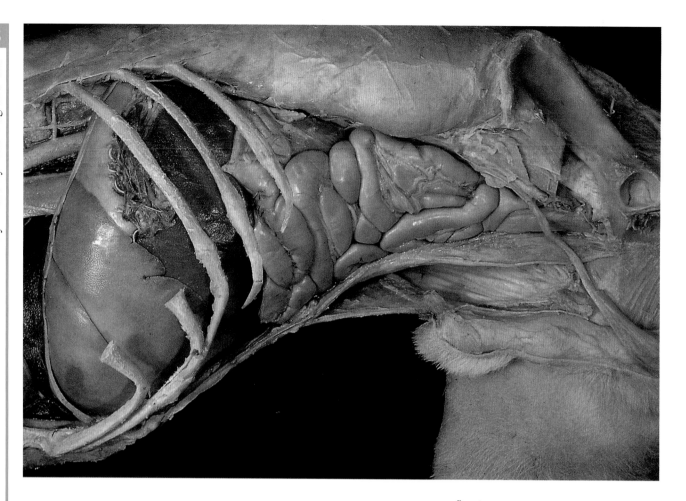

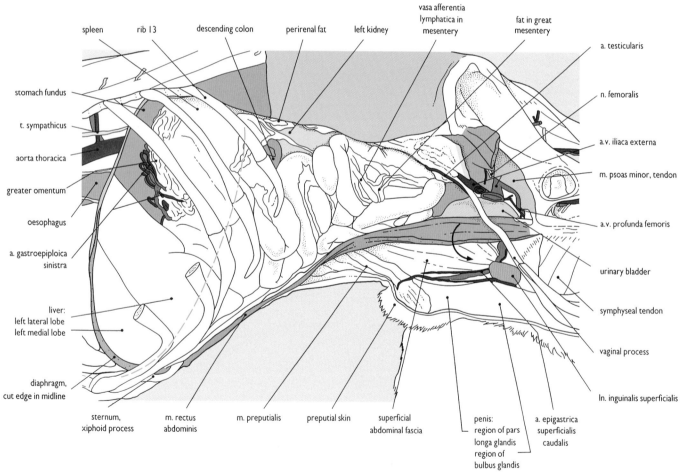

spleen   rib 13   descending colon   perirenal fat   left kidney   vasa afferentia lymphatica in mesentery   fat in great mesentery

stomach fundus

t. sympathicus

aorta thoracica

greater omentum

oesophagus

a. gastroepiploica sinistra

liver:
left lateral lobe
left medial lobe

diaphragm,
cut edge in midline

a. testicularis

n. femoralis

a.v. iliaca externa

m. psoas minor, tendon

a.v. profunda femoris

urinary bladder

symphyseal tendon

vaginal process

ln. inguinalis superficialis

sternum,
xiphoid process   m. rectus abdominis   m. preputialis   preputial skin   superficial abdominal fascia   penis:
region of pars longa glandis
region of bulbus glandis   a. epigastrica superficialis caudalis

Fig. 6.24 Abdominal viscera in situ (2). After removal of the abdominal wall and diaphragm: left lateral view. The left half of the diaphragm has been removed, the cut edge of the diaphragmatic cupola in the midline now indicates the most cranial extent of the abdominal cavity. The costal arch is left in place and the position of the costodiaphragmatic line of pleural reflection is still indicated by the broken line in advance of it. Compare this view with equivalent views from the right side (Fig. 6.48) and ventrally (Fig. 6.76).

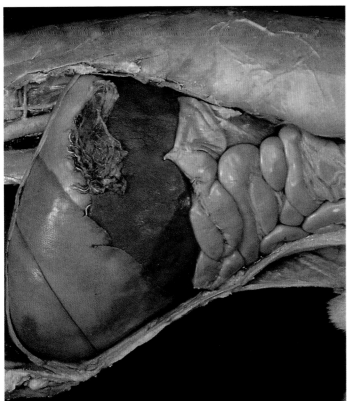

Fig. 6.25 Viscera of the cranial abdomen *in situ* after removal of the abdominal wall, ribs and diaphragm: left lateral view. At the cranial end of the abdomen the remaining ribs and costal arch have been removed. The spleen is abnormally enlarged following barbiturate narcosis, and extends right down to the belly floor in the xiphoid region (see also Figs 6.77, 6.78 in ventral view, Figs 6.88–6.90 in caudal view, and Figs 6.96, 6.97 in section).

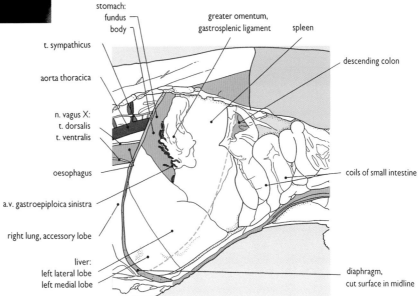

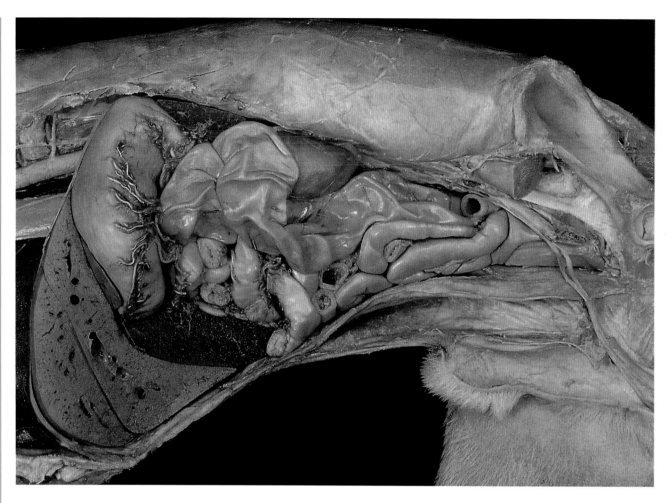

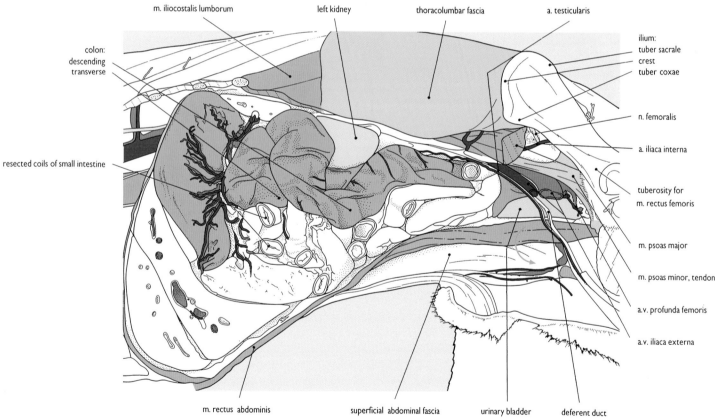

m. iliocostalis lumborum   left kidney   thoracolumbar fascia   a. testicularis

colon:
descending
transverse

ilium:
tuber sacrale
crest
tuber coxae

n. femoralis

a. iliaca interna

resected coils of small intestine

tuberosity for
m. rectus femoris

m. psoas major

m. psoas minor, tendon

a.v. profunda femoris

a.v. iliaca externa

m. rectus abdominis   superficial abdominal fascia   urinary bladder   deferent duct

Fig. 6.26 Descending colon: left lateral view (1). The transverse and much of the descending part of the colon have been exposed following removal of the deep layer of the greater omentum and a number of jejunal coils. The colon in this specimen is somewhat enlarged and appears sacculated. For a more 'normal' appearance see Fig. 6.61 from a right medial view and Figs 6.80 and 6.82 from a ventral view. Dorsal to the colon the left kidney is exposed further by removal of perirenal fat. In the caudal abdomen the iliacus component of the iliopsoas muscle has been removed, and the psoas major has been additionally trimmed as far cranially as the tuber coxae.

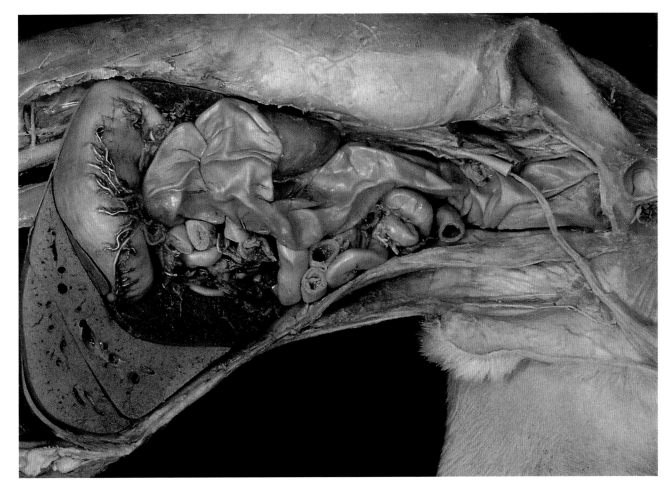

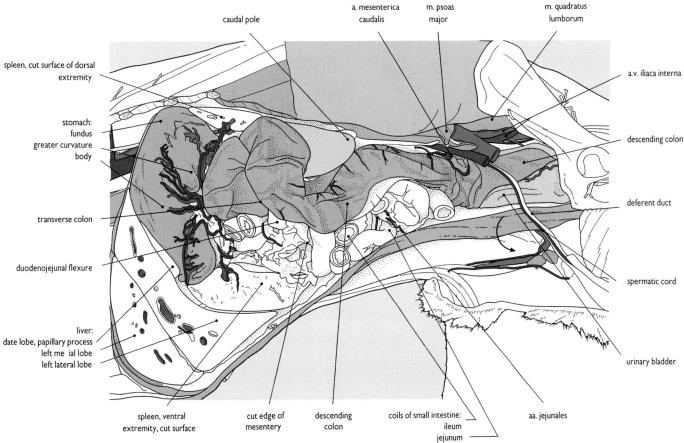

caudal pole

a. mesenterica caudalis

m. psoas major

m. quadratus lumborum

spleen, cut surface of dorsal extremity

a.v. iliaca interna

stomach: fundus greater curvature body

descending colon

transverse colon

deferent duct

duodenojejunal flexure

spermatic cord

liver: date lobe, papillary process left me ial lobe left lateral lobe

urinary bladder

spleen, ventral extremity, cut surface

cut edge of mesentery

descending colon

coils of small intestine: ileum jejunum

aa. jejunales

Fig. 6.27 Descending colon: left lateral view (2). More jejunal coils have been removed from the ventral abdomen and the cut ends are clearly displayed. The jejunum has actually been severed close to its commencement at the duodenojejunal flexure which is visible immediately ventral to the initial part of the descending colon. Caudally, removal of more of the psoas major and the flattened tendon of the psoas minor muscle has exposed the most caudal extent of the descending colon as it enters the pelvis. Removal of the iliopsoas muscle has also exposed both internal and external iliac vessels, a medial iliac lymph node and the quadratus lumborum muscle.

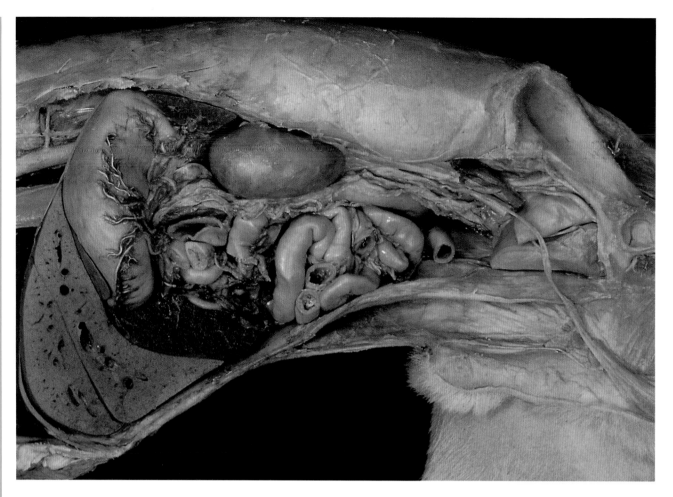

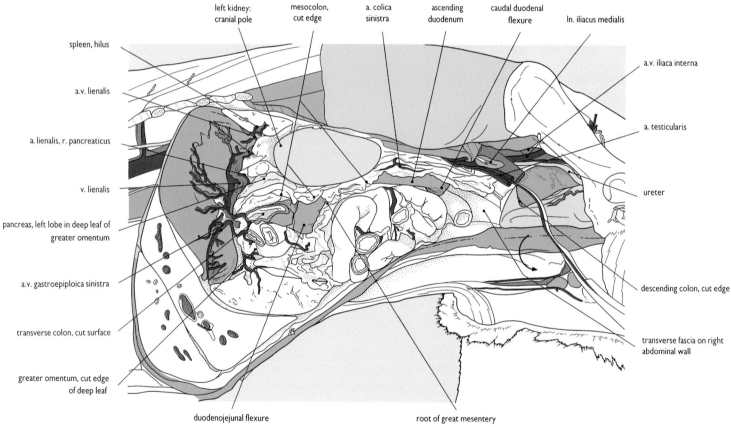

spleen, hilus

a.v. lienalis

a. lienalis, r. pancreaticus

v. lienalis

pancreas, left lobe in deep leaf of
greater omentum

a.v. gastroepiploica sinistra

transverse colon, cut surface

greater omentum, cut edge
of deep leaf

left kidney:
cranial pole

mesocolon,
cut edge

a. colica
sinistra

ascending
duodenum

caudal duodenal
flexure

ln. iliacus medialis

a.v. iliaca interna

a. testicularis

ureter

descending colon, cut edge

transverse fascia on right
abdominal wall

duodenojejunal flexure

root of great mesentery

Fig. 6.28 Left kidney and mesocolon: left lateral view. The descending colon has been removed except for its terminal part dorsal to the bladder. Cranially, the cut surface of the transverse colon is clearly observed immediately cranial to the duodenojejunal flexure (its position is shown to advantage in section in Fig. 6.97). Extending caudally from the transverse colon, below the kidney, the fat infiltrated mesocolon and its cut edge are visible. Medial to the duodenojejunal flexure and caudal to the transverse colon the mesenteric root is just exposed. The relationship of structures to the root is shown to advantage in ventral view (Figs 6.80, 6.81) and in section (Figs 6.98, 6.99).

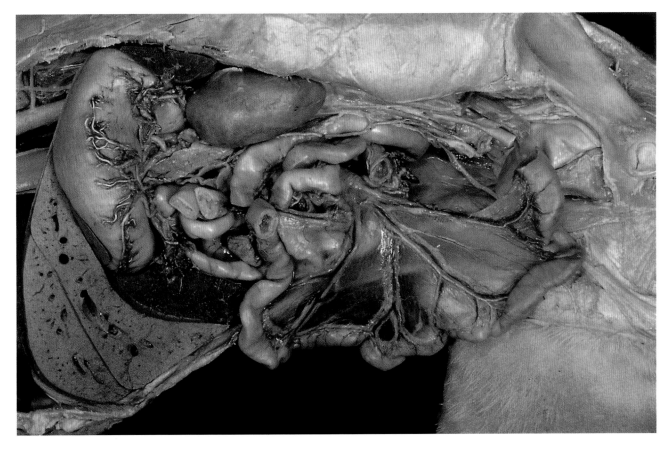

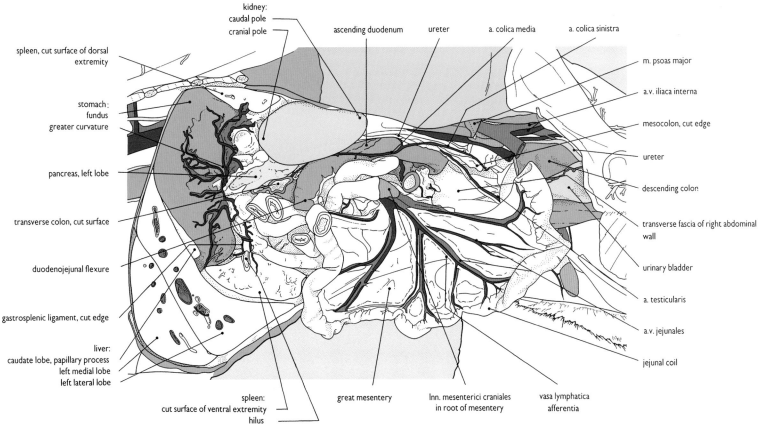

spleen, cut surface of dorsal extremity

stomach:
fundus
greater curvature

pancreas, left lobe

transverse colon, cut surface

duodenojejunal flexure

gastrosplenic ligament, cut edge

liver:
caudate lobe, papillary process
left medial lobe
left lateral lobe

kidney:
caudal pole
cranial pole

ascending duodenum

ureter

a. colica media

a. colica sinistra

m. psoas major

a.v. iliaca interna

mesocolon, cut edge

ureter

descending colon

transverse fascia of right abdominal wall

urinary bladder

a. testicularis

a.v. jejunales

jejunal coil

spleen:
cut surface of ventral extremity
hilus

great mesentery

lnn. mesenterici craniales
in root of mesentery

vasa lymphatica
afferentia

Fig. 6.29 Vessels and lymphatics of the great mesentery: left lateral view. The mesocolon has been removed from below the left kidney to expose the ascending duodenum from caudal duodenal to duodenojejunal flexure. Some of the remaining jejunal coils have been pulled out of the abdominal cavity in order to spread out and display a large fan of the great mesentery. Jejunal arteries and veins are paralleled by opaque stripes representing afferent lymphatic channels. All vessels converge on the mesenteric root, evident as a prominent 'knot' of tissue thickened up considerably by a number of cranial mesenteric lymph nodes.

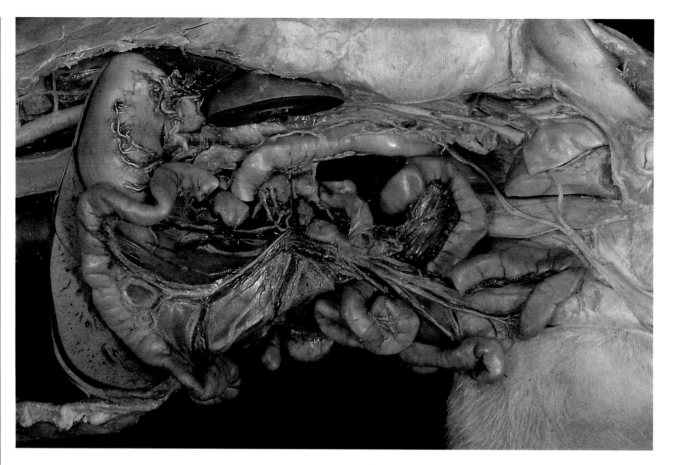

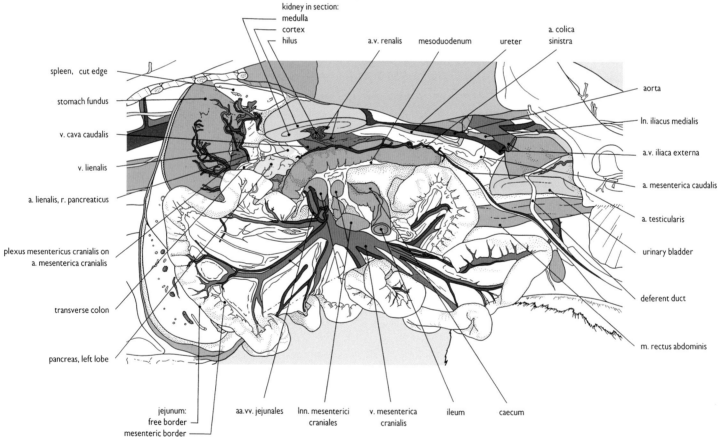

kidney in section:
medulla
cortex
hilus

a.v. renalis   mesoduodenum   ureter

a. colica
sinistra

spleen, cut edge

stomach fundus

v. cava caudalis

v. lienalis

a. lienalis, r. pancreaticus

plexus mesentericus cranialis on
a. mesenterica cranialis

transverse colon

pancreas, left lobe

aorta

ln. iliacus medialis

a.v. iliaca externa

a. mesenterica caudalis

a. testicularis

urinary bladder

deferent duct

m. rectus abdominis

jejunum:
free border
mesenteric border

aa.vv. jejunales   lnn. mesenterici
cranialis

v. mesenterica
cranialis

ileum   caecum

Fig. 6.30 Mesenteric lymph nodes and the root of the mesentery: left lateral view (1). Considerably more of the remaining jejunal coils are spread out ventrally. This has pulled the caecum and ileum ventrally to some extent; they 'return' to a more normal position in Fig. 6.34 *et seq*. Horizontal sectioning of the kidney has exposed the renal artery and vein and the ureter, all entering the hilus. Considerable amounts of fat and peritoneal tissue have been removed from the mesenteric root exposing the cranial mesenteric lymph nodes. The relationship of the gut tube to mesenteric root is shown in Figs 6.80 and 6.81 from a ventral view, and Figs 6.97–6.99 in section.

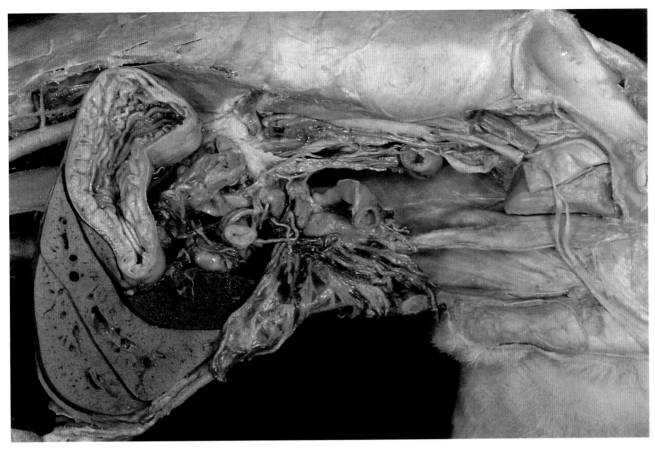

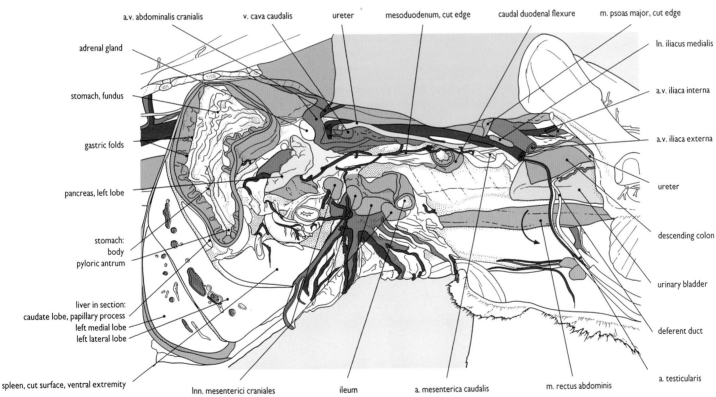

a.v. abdominalis cranialis · v. cava caudalis · ureter · mesoduodenum, cut edge · caudal duodenal flexure · m. psoas major, cut edge

adrenal gland

stomach, fundus

gastric folds

pancreas, left lobe

stomach:
body
pyloric antrum

liver in section:
caudate lobe, papillary process
left medial lobe
left lateral lobe

spleen, cut surface, ventral extremity

ln. iliacus medialis

a.v. iliaca interna

a.v. iliaca externa

ureter

descending colon

urinary bladder

deferent duct

a. testicularis

lnn. mesenterici craniales · ileum · a. mesenterica caudalis · m. rectus abdominis

Fig. 6.31 Mesenteric lymph nodes and the root of the mesentery: left lateral view (2). The ascending duodenum has been removed, exposing the root of the great mesentery and the left pancreatic lobe. The stomach has been sectioned vertically so that the fundus and body have been opened as far as the pyloric antrum. In the abdominal roof the remnants of the left kidney and spleen have been removed. Kidney removal involved severing renal vessels and ureter; the cut ends are visible. Ventrally most of the remaining jejunal coils have been taken out leaving only a coil or two cranial to the mesenteric root, and a mass of mesenteric tissue 'hanging' ventrally out of the abdomen.

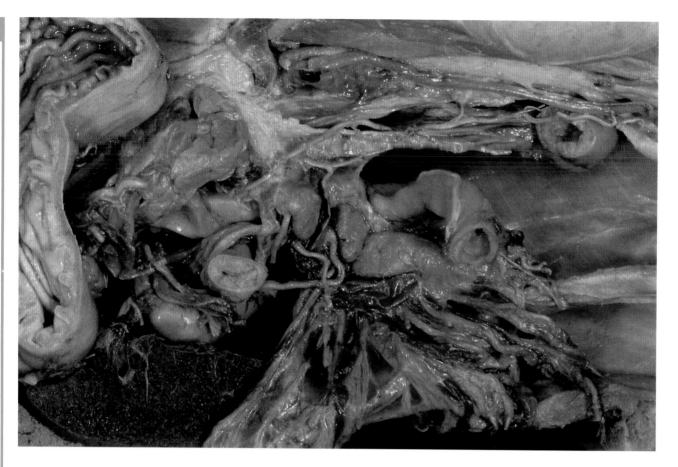

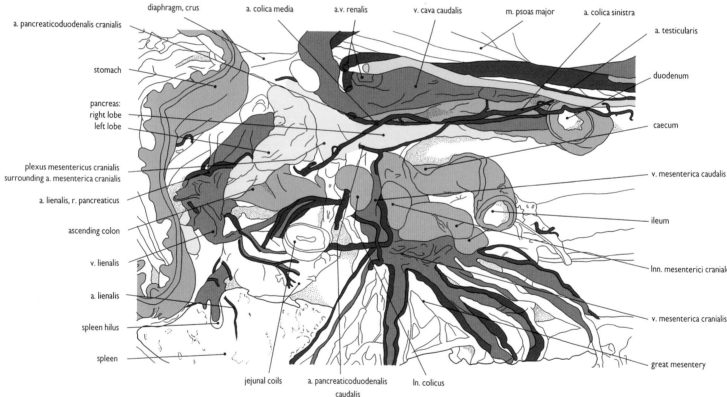

a. pancreaticoduodenalis cranialis

diaphragm, crus

a. colica media

a.v. renalis

v. cava caudalis

m. psoas major

a. colica sinistra

a. testicularis

stomach

duodenum

pancreas:
right lobe
left lobe

caecum

plexus mesentericus cranialis
surrounding a. mesenterica cranialis

v. mesenterica caudalis

a. lienalis, r. pancreaticus

ileum

ascending colon

v. lienalis

lnn. mesenterici craniales

a. lienalis

v. mesenterica cranialis

spleen hilus

spleen

great mesentery

jejunal coils

a. pancreaticoduodenalis
caudalis

ln. colicus

Fig. 6.32 Mesenteric lymph nodes and the root of the mesentery: left lateral view (3). This figure is an enlargement of part of the dissection shown in Fig. 6.31. The cranial mesenteric artery is still obscured by its surrounding plexus of autonomic nerves. Cranial to the root the pancreas lies dorsal to the remnant of the colon; caudal to it and looking through onto the right side of the abdomen the right pancreatic lobe and descending duodenum lie dorsal to the caecum and terminal end of the ileum (see also Figs 6.80, 6.81). Dorsal to the lymph nodes the middle colic artery has been left in position following earlier removal of the descending colon and its supporting mesocolon (see Figs 6.28, 6.29).

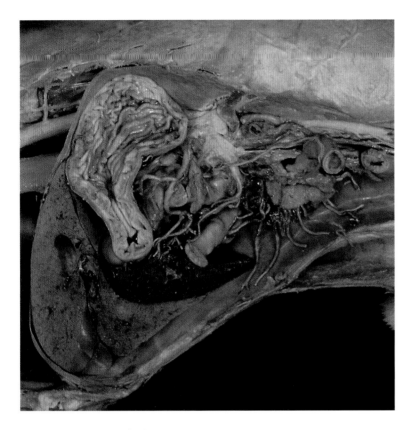

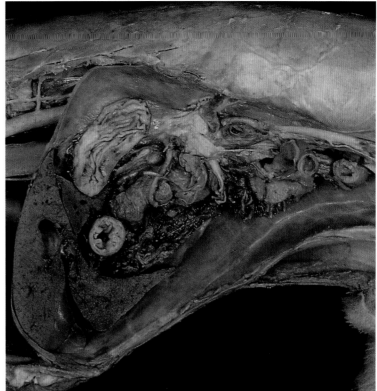

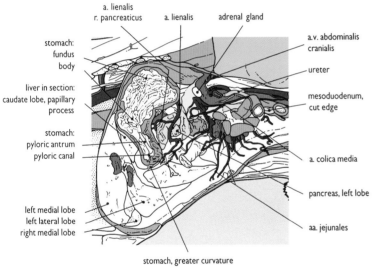

a. lienalis
r. pancreaticus · a. lienalis · adrenal gland

stomach:
fundus
body

liver in section:
caudate lobe, papillary
process

stomach:
pyloric antrum
pyloric canal

left medial lobe
left lateral lobe
right medial lobe

a.v. abdominalis
cranialis

ureter

mesoduodenum,
cut edge

a. colica media

pancreas, left lobe

aa. jejunales

stomach, greater curvature

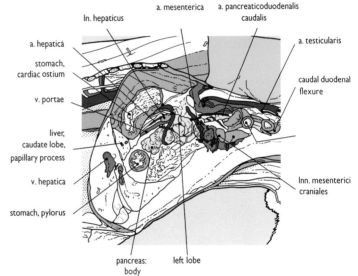

a. mesenterica · a. pancreaticoduodenalis
caudalis

ln. hepaticus

a. hepatica

stomach,
cardiac ostium

v. portae

liver,
caudate lobe,
papillary process

v. hepatica

stomach, pylorus

a. testicularis

caudal duodenal
flexure

lnn. mesenterici
craniales

pancreas:
body

left lobe

Fig. 6.33 Cranial mesenteric artery and coeliacomesenteric plexus: left lateral view (1). Continued clearing of tissues from the mesenteric root, particularly cranial to it, has involved removing part of the left pancreatic lobe. The pylorus has been opened up to show the pyloric canal while further sectioning of the liver has exposed the right medial lobe. After removal of much of the remaining fan of mesentery and the mesenteric lymph nodes, the caecum and terminal end of the ileum have been replaced in a more 'normal' position closer to the abdominal roof.

Fig. 6.34 Cranial mesenteric artery and coeliacomesenteric plexus: left lateral view (2). Considerably more of the fundus has been removed and practically all of the body, so that the cardia is separated from the pylorus. A remnant of the papillary process of the liver is located between the two in what was the lesser curvature. More pancreatic tissue has been removed from caudal to the stomach and the remnant of the ventral extremity of the spleen has been removed, along with the gastrosplenic ligament.

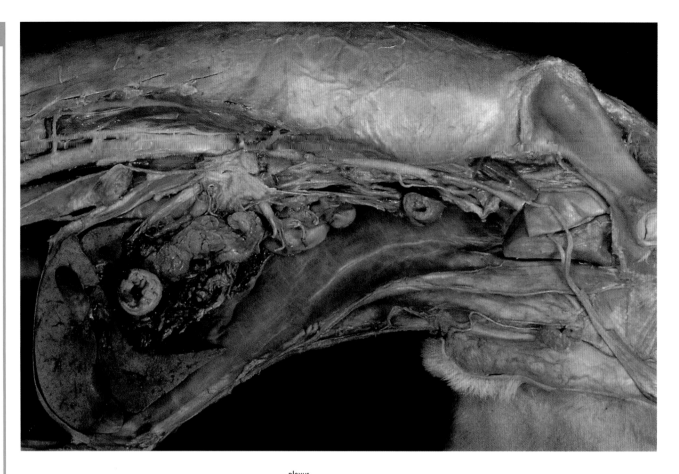

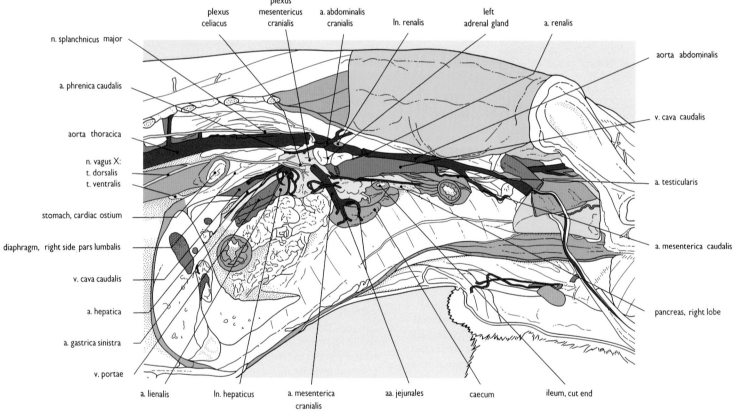

plexus
celiacus

plexus
mesentericus
cranialis

a. abdominalis
cranialis

ln. renalis

left
adrenal gland

a. renalis

n. splanchnicus major

aorta abdominalis

a. phrenica caudalis

v. cava caudalis

aorta thoracica

n. vagus X:
t. dorsalis
t. ventralis

a. testicularis

stomach, cardiac ostium

diaphragm, right side pars lumbalis

a. mesenterica caudalis

v. cava caudalis

a. hepatica

pancreas, right lobe

a. gastrica sinistra

v. portae

a. lienalis

ln. hepaticus

a. mesenterica
cranialis

aa. jejunales

caecum

ileum, cut end

Fig. 6.35 Autonomic nervous supply to the abdominal viscera: left lateral view (1). The fundus and body of the stomach have been removed, leaving only the cardia and pylorus and severing the left gastric artery. The costal and lumbar parts of the diaphragm have been removed, the left lumbar crus having been cut through dorsal to the adrenal gland and cranial to the cranial abdominal artery. Both esophageal and aortic hiatuses have consequently been destroyed (see also Figs 6.63, 6.64, 6.86, 6.87 and 6.91). The cranial abdominal vein has been removed and the caudal phrenic artery is visible passing cranially from the phrenicoabdominal artery dorsal to the adrenal gland (see also Fig. 6.87).

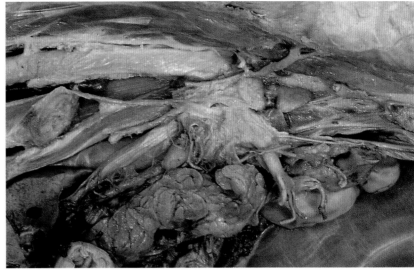

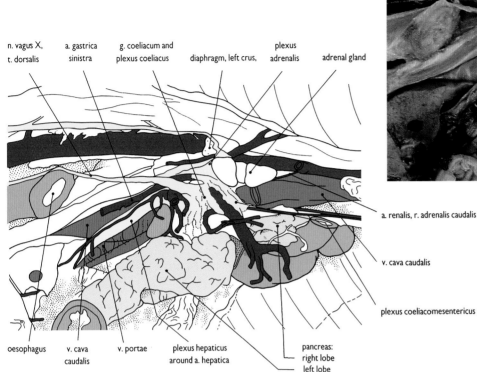

n. vagus X,   a. gastrica   g. coeliacum and   plexus
t. dorsalis   sinistra   plexus coeliacus   diaphragm, left crus,   adrenalis   adrenal gland

a. renalis, r. adrenalis caudalis

v. cava caudalis

plexus coeliacomesentericus

oesophagus   v. cava   v. portae   plexus hepaticus   pancreas:
            caudalis   around a. hepatica   right lobe
                                                     left lobe

Fig. 6.36 Autonomic nervous supply to the abdominal viscera: left lateral view (2). This figure is an enlarged view of part of the dissection shown in Fig. 6.35. The splenic and left gastric branches of the coeliac artery are cut short following spleen and stomach removal; an hepatic plexus of autonomic nerves surrounds the hepatic branch.

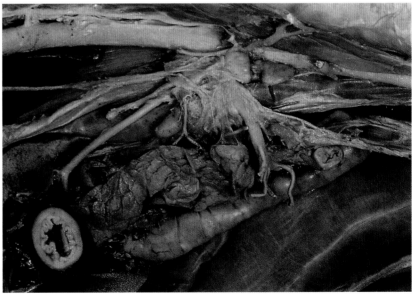

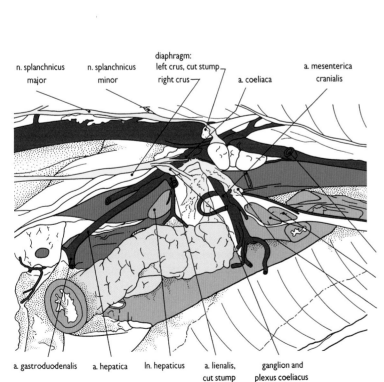

n. splanchnicus   n. splanchnicus   diaphragm: a. mesenterica
major   minor   left crus, cut stump   cranialis
                              right crus   a. coeliaca

a. renalis

lnn. mesenterici craniales

plexus mesentericus cranialis

a. gastroduodenalis   a. hepatica   ln. hepaticus   a. lienalis,   ganglion and
                                              cut stump   plexus coeliacus

Fig. 6.37 Coeliac and cranial mesenteric arteries: left lateral view. Cleaning of mesenteric tissue and fascia round the coeliacomesenteric plexus has removed much of the meshwork of autonomic fibers, exposing both coeliac and cranial mesenteric arteries. The splanchnic nerves together arch lateroventrally around the cut stump of the left diaphragmatic crus and disappear beneath the adrenal gland en route for the coeliacomesenteric plexus. Compare this figure with Fig. 6.62 from the right side.

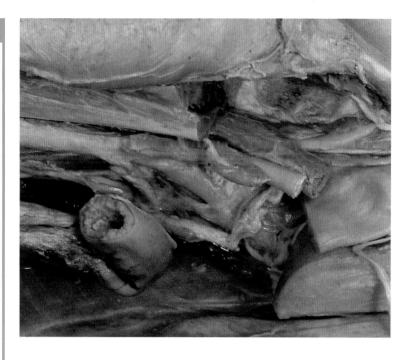

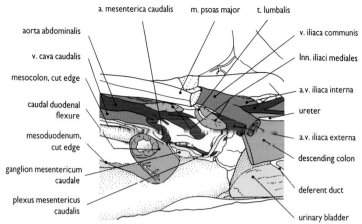

Fig. 6.38 Caudal mesenteric artery: left lateral view. This is an enlarged view of the caudal end of the abdomen after removal of more of the iliopsoas muscle. The diameter of the caudal mesenteric artery in its somewhat tortuous course is increased by a surrounding caudal mesenteric plexus in which a caudal mesenteric ganglion is clearly apparent.

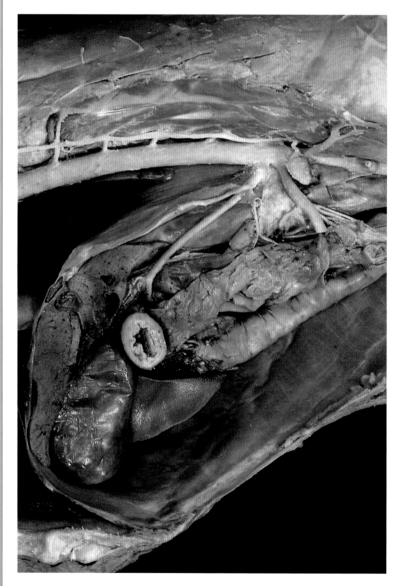

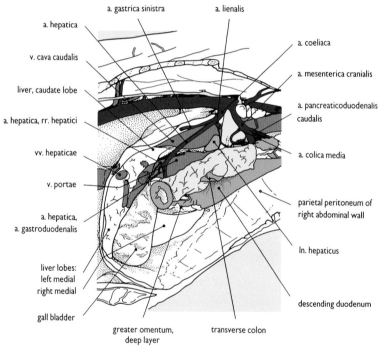

Fig. 6.39 Hepatic artery, hepatic portal vein and gall bladder: left lateral view. Additional cleaning of tissue has exposed the coeliac artery at its origin from the aorta, and its three branches are clearly demonstrated. The esophagus and cardia of the stomach have been removed and more diaphragmatic and liver tissue has been cut away. Within sectioned liver tissue close to the diaphragm and its caval foramen, large hepatic veins are apparent. Compare this figure with Fig. 6.63 from the right side.

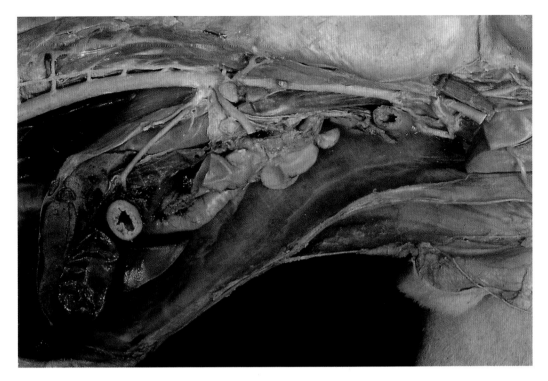

Fig. 6.40 Ileum, caecum and ascending colon: medial view of the right side. The left lobe of the pancreas has been removed to expose in medial view structures lying on the right side of the abdomen. Immediately to the right of the cranial mesenteric artery, the ascending colon, caecum and terminal end of the ileum are exposed along with several colic lymph nodes. Further over on the right side the right pancreatic lobe is visible with the descending duodenum (see also Figs 6.80, 6.81 from a ventral view, and Fig. 6.98 in section). Compare this figure with Fig. 6.55 from the right lateral aspect.

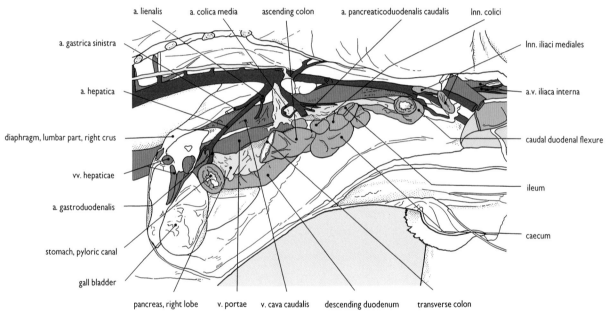

a. lienalis — a. colica media — ascending colon — a. pancreaticoduodenalis caudalis — lnn. colici

a. gastrica sinistra

a. hepatica

diaphragm, lumbar part, right crus

vv. hepaticae

a. gastroduodenalis

stomach, pyloric canal

gall bladder

pancreas, right lobe — v. portae — v. cava caudalis — descending duodenum — transverse colon

lnn. iliaci mediales

a.v. iliaca interna

caudal duodenal flexure

ileum

caecum

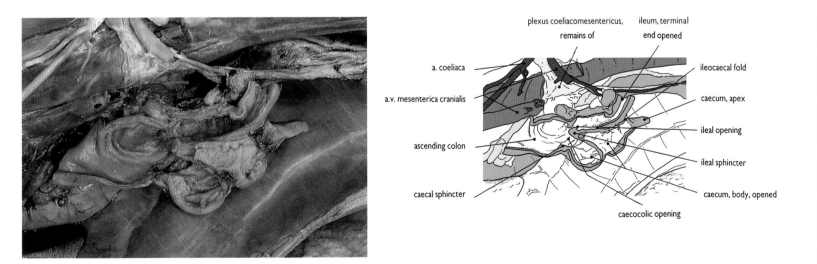

plexus coeliacomesentericus, remains of — ileum, terminal end opened

a. coeliaca

a.v. mesenterica cranialis

ascending colon

caecal sphincter

ileocaecal fold

caecum, apex

ileal opening

ileal sphincter

caecum, body, opened

caecocolic opening

Fig. 6.41 Caecum opened to display caeccocolic and ileocolic openings: medial view of the right side. The ends of the colon and ileum have been opened and the ileocolic opening is displayed in the centre of the figure. The body of the caecum has also been opened and the caeccocolic opening lies directly ventral to the ileocolic. Compare this figure with Figs 6.56 and 6.57 of the caecum opened from the right lateral aspect.

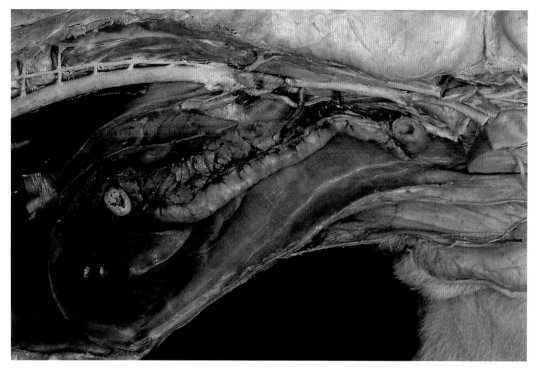

Fig. 6.42 Descending duodenum, right lobe of the pancreas and the right kidney: medial view. The remains of the colon, caecum and ileum and their associated lymph nodes have been removed; the coeliac and cranial mesenteric arteries have been cut back to the aorta, and much of the hepatic portal vein is removed. Compare this figure with Fig. 6.51 from the right lateral aspect. Practically all of the caudal vena cava has been removed, except close to the caval foramen where some of the right wall of the vena cava remains and the entry of a hepatic vein from the right lobe of the liver is apparent.

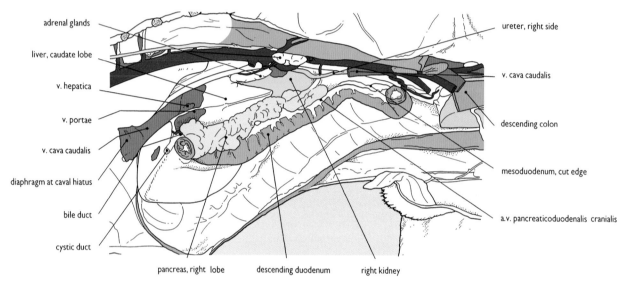

adrenal glands

liver, caudate lobe

v. hepatica

v. portae

v. cava caudalis

diaphragm at caval hiatus

bile duct

cystic duct

ureter, right side

v. cava caudalis

descending colon

mesoduodenum, cut edge

a.v. pancreaticoduodenalis cranialis

pancreas, right lobe   descending duodenum   right kidney

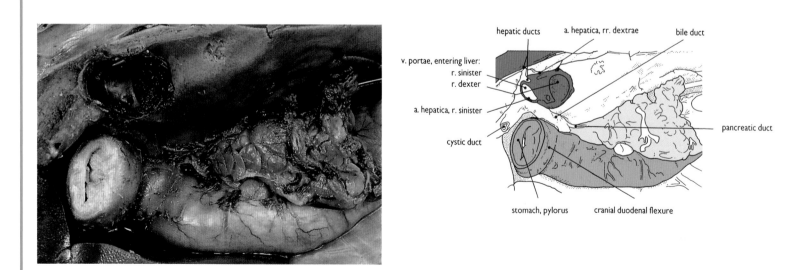

hepatic ducts   a. hepatica, rr. dextrae   bile duct

v. portae, entering liver:
r. sinister
r. dexter

a. hepatica, r. sinister

cystic duct

pancreatic duct

stomach, pylorus   cranial duodenal flexure

Fig. 6.43 Bile duct and porta of the liver: medial view. This is an enlarged view of the bile duct and porta of the liver. The cystic and hepatic ducts are also exposed and a pancreatic duct joins the bile duct. The two main branches of the portal vein are shown entering the liver and three branches of the proper hepatic arteries are also visible in section at the periphery of the porta (see also Fig. 6.95 in section).

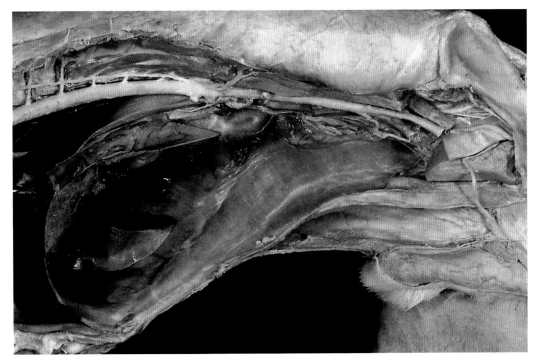

Fig. 6.44 Right kidney and caudate lobe of the liver: medial view. Removal of the descending duodenum and right pancreatic lobe exposes the right kidney and the caudate lobe of the liver which caps its cranial pole. Compare this figure with Fig. 6.50 from the right lateral aspect (see also Figs 6.84, 6.88 and 6.97). Diaphragmatic musculature is covered by internal abdominal fascia supporting the glistening peritoneum which is continued back on the inside of the abdominal wall.

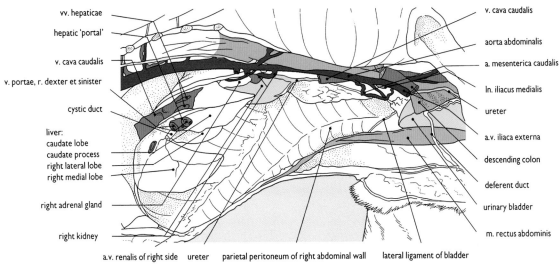

vv. hepaticae
hepatic 'portal'
v. cava caudalis
v. portae, r. dexter et sinister
cystic duct
liver:
caudate lobe
caudate process
right lateral lobe
right medial lobe
right adrenal gland
right kidney

a.v. renalis of right side   ureter   parietal peritoneum of right abdominal wall

v. cava caudalis
aorta abdominalis
a. mesenterica caudalis
ln. iliacus medialis
ureter
a.v. iliaca externa
descending colon
deferent duct
urinary bladder
m. rectus abdominis

lateral ligament of bladder

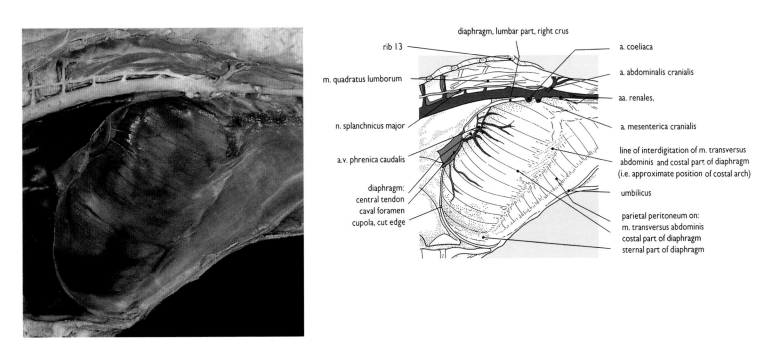

rib 13
m. quadratus lumborum
n. splanchnicus major
a.v. phrenica caudalis
diaphragm:
central tendon
caval foramen
cupola, cut edge

diaphragm, lumbar part, right crus

a. coeliaca
a. abdominalis cranialis
aa. renales,
a. mesenterica cranialis
line of interdigitation of m. transversus abdominis and costal part of diaphragm (i.e. approximate position of costal arch)
umbilicus
parietal peritoneum on:
m. transversus abdominis
costal part of diaphragm
sternal part of diaphragm

Fig. 6.45 Abdominal wall and diaphragm of the right side: medial view. After removal of the cranial abdominal viscera the parietal peritoneum is exposed lining the abdomen. The 'line' at which the costal and sternal parts of the diaphragmatic musculature interdigitate with transverse abdominal muscle is clearly visible through it and will mark the approximate position of the costal arch (see also Figs 6.21, 6.22 from lateral view).

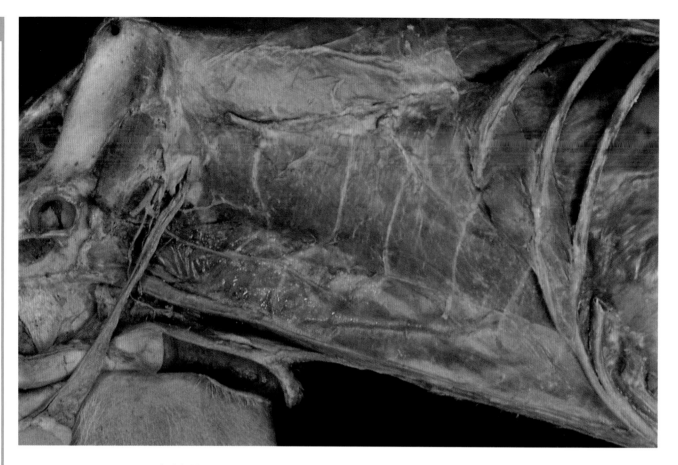

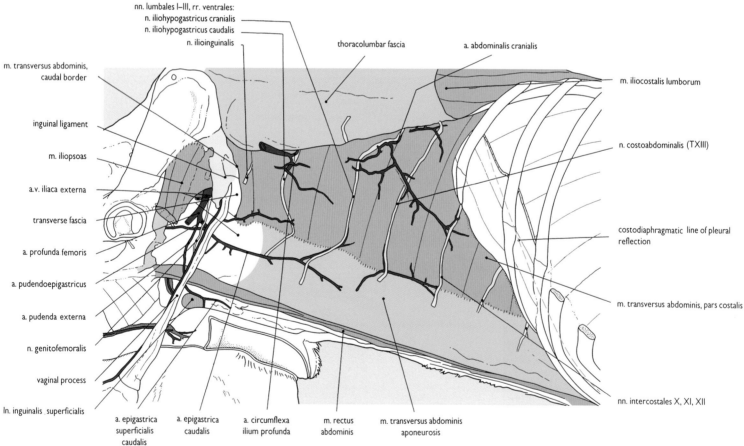

nn. lumbales I–III, rr. ventrales:
n. iliohypogastricus cranialis
n. iliohypogastricus caudalis
n. ilioinguinalis

thoracolumbar fascia

a. abdominalis cranialis

m. transversus abdominis, caudal border

inguinal ligament

m. iliopsoas

a.v. iliaca externa

transverse fascia

a. profunda femoris

a. pudendoepigastricus

a. pudenda externa

n. genitofemoralis

vaginal process

ln. inguinalis superficialis

a. epigastrica superficialis caudalis

a. epigastrica caudalis

a. circumflexa ilium profunda

m. rectus abdominis

m. transversus abdominis aponeurosis

m. iliocostalis lumborum

n. costoabdominalis (TXIII)

costodiaphragmatic line of pleural reflection

m. transversus abdominis, pars costalis

nn. intercostales X, XI, XII

Fig. 6.46 Transverse abdominal muscle, nerves and arteries of the abdominal wall: right lateral view. This view of the right abdominal wall is comparable in most respects with that of the left side already shown in Fig. 6.20. The right hindlimb has been removed in much the same manner as the left and the oblique muscles and rectus abdominis have been removed to expose the transverse abdominal muscle with the nerves to the wall displayed on its surface. As distinct from Fig. 6.21 this specimen does show clearly the pudendoepigastric trunk giving rise to the caudal epigastric and external pudendal arteries.

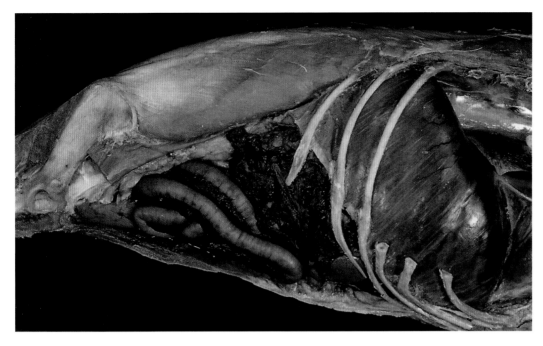

Fig. 6.47 Abdominal viscera in situ after removal of the abdominal wall: right lateral view (1). The abdominal contents have been displayed after removal of the abdominal wall, and this view should be compared with Fig. 6.23 of the left side. On this right side more of the greater omentum (colored black) is visible than on the left, extending caudally between the abdominal wall and intestines. In many instances it would completely cover the intestines back to the urinary bladder (see also ventral view; Fig. 6.73).

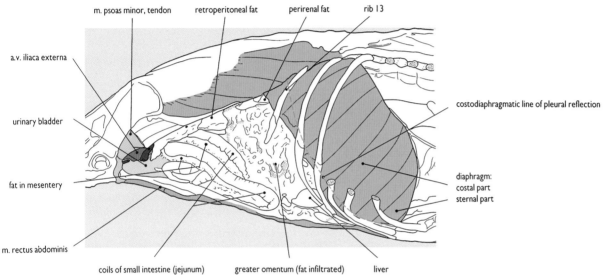

m. psoas minor, tendon   retroperitoneal fat   perirenal fat   rib 13

a.v. iliaca externa

urinary bladder

costodiaphragmatic line of pleural reflection

fat in mesentery

diaphragm:
costal part
sternal part

m. rectus abdominis

coils of small intestine (jejunum)   greater omentum (fat infiltrated)   liver

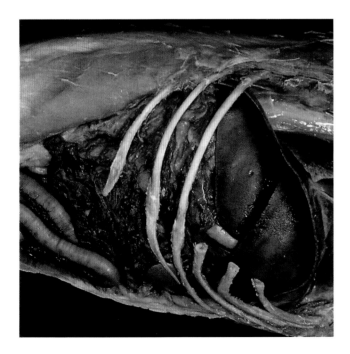

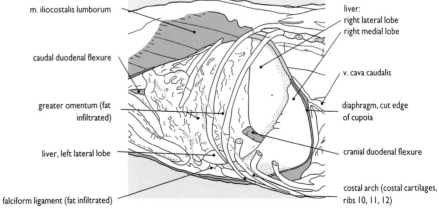

m. iliocostalis lumborum

liver:
right lateral lobe
right medial lobe

caudal duodenal flexure

v. cava caudalis

greater omentum (fat infiltrated)

diaphragm, cut edge of cupoia

liver, left lateral lobe

cranial duodenal flexure

falciform ligament (fat infiltrated)

costal arch (costal cartilages, ribs 10, 11, 12)

Fig. 6.48 Viscera of the cranial abdomen after removal of the diaphragm: right lateral view. The right half of the diaphragm has been removed whilst leaving the caudal three ribs and the costal arch intact. The line of diaphragmatic attachment to the ribs is indicated by the broken line.

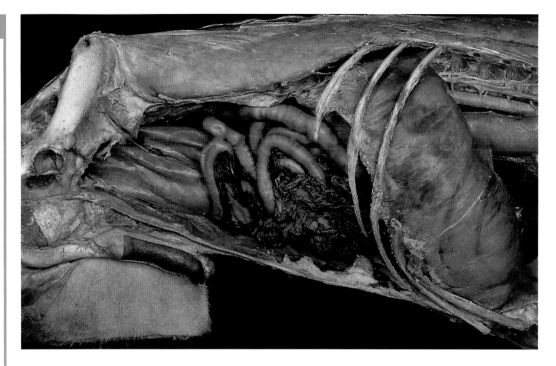

Fig. 6.49 Abdominal viscera in situ after removal of the abdominal wall: right lateral view (2). This additional specimen has been included specifically to indicate how extensive the urinary bladder may be. Compare this with Fig. 6.47 which has a relatively small bladder. In this specimen practically the entire caudal one-third of the abdominal cavity is occupied by the distended bladder

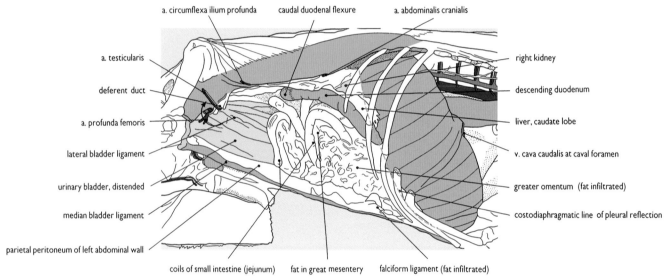

a. circumflexa ilium profunda
caudal duodenal flexure
a. abdominalis cranialis

a. testicularis

deferent duct

a. profunda femoris

lateral bladder ligament

urinary bladder, distended

median bladder ligament

parietal peritoneum of left abdominal wall

right kidney

descending duodenum

liver, caudate lobe

v. cava caudalis at caval foramen

greater omentum (fat infiltrated)

costodiaphragmatic line of pleural reflection

coils of small intestine (jejunum)
fat in great mesentery
falciform ligament (fat infiltrated)

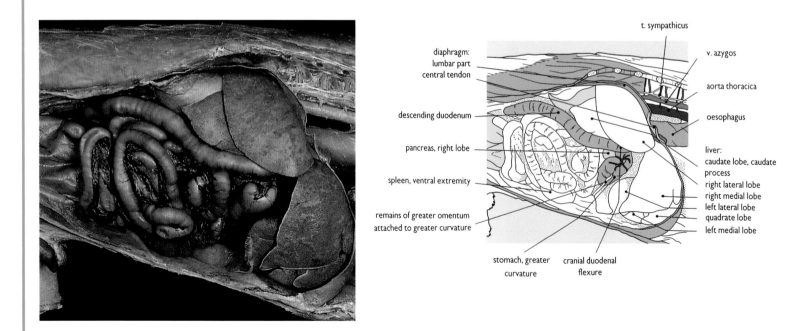

diaphragm:
lumbar part
central tendon

descending duodenum

pancreas, right lobe

spleen, ventral extremity

remains of greater omentum
attached to greater curvature

t. sympathicus

v. azygos

aorta thoracica

oesophagus

liver:
caudate lobe, caudate
process
right lateral lobe
right medial lobe
left lateral lobe
quadrate lobe
left medial lobe

stomach, greater
curvature
cranial duodenal
flexure

Fig. 6.50 Viscera of the cranial abdomen after removal of the diaphragm and ribs: right lateral view. The right half of the diaphragm, caudal ribs and costal arch have been removed and the greater omentum has been cut away.

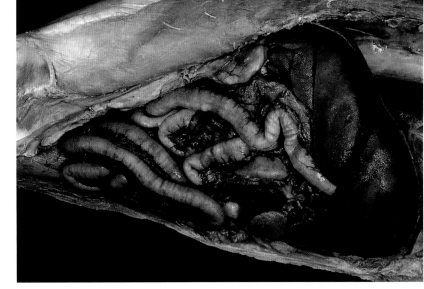

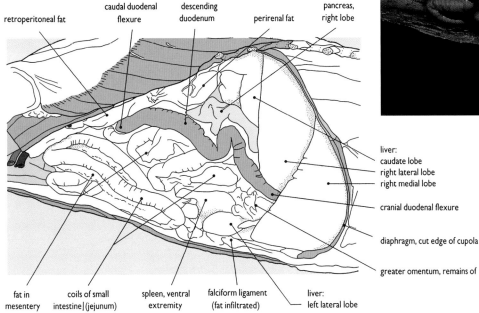

retroperitoneal fat

caudal duodenal flexure

descending duodenum

perirenal fat

pancreas, right lobe

liver:
caudate lobe
right lateral lobe
right medial lobe

cranial duodenal flexure

diaphragm, cut edge of cupola

greater omentum, remains of

fat in mesentery

coils of small intestine|(jejunum)

spleen, ventral extremity

falciform ligament (fat infiltrated)

liver:
left lateral lobe

Fig. 6.51 Abdominal viscera after removal of the greater omentum: right lateral view. The greater omentum has been removed and a view of the abdomen is obtained much like Fig. 6.50 of a different specimen. Additional deposits of fat are visible in the great mesentery and as a continuous strand in a retroperitoneal position in the abdominal roof.

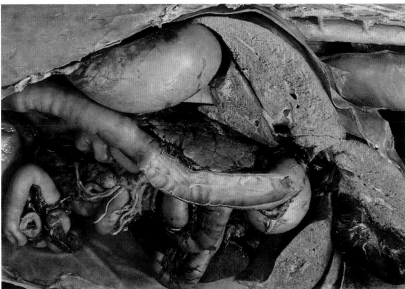

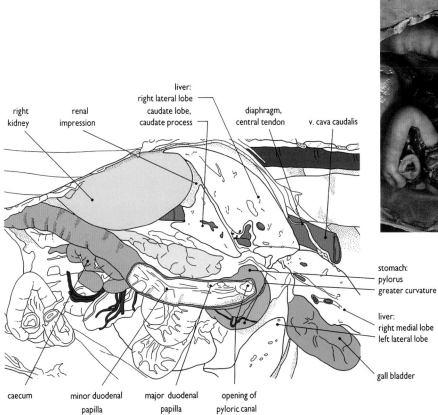

right kidney

renal impression

liver:
right lateral lobe
caudate lobe, caudate process

diaphragm, central tendon

v. cava caudalis

stomach:
pylorus
greater curvature

liver:
right medial lobe
left lateral lobe

gall bladder

caecum

minor duodenal papilla

major duodenal papilla

opening of pyloric canal

Fig. 6.52 Bile duct and duodenal papillae of the descending duodenum: right lateral view. The liver has been resected to expose the initial part of the descending duodenum. A section of the right lateral wall of the duodenum is removed and its internal mucosal lining has been scraped clean. The opening of the pyloric canal is visible and both major and minor duodenal papillae are exposed. Removal of the right lateral and parts of the right medial lobes of the liver has exposed the gall bladder and its cystic duct.

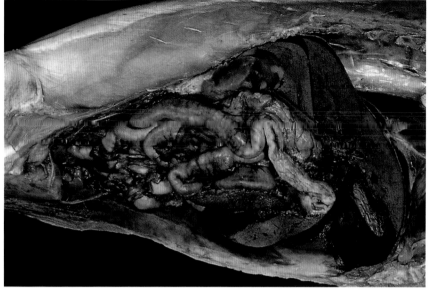

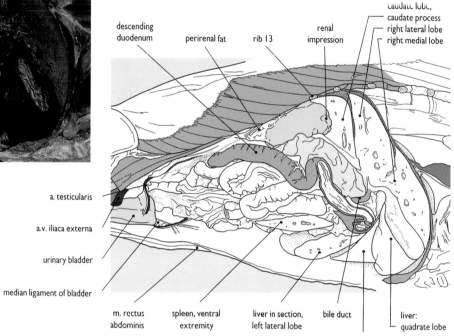

Fig. 6.53 Descending duodenum, right lobe of the pancreas and right kidney: right lateral view. Removal of much of the right lateral and medial lobes of the liver has exposed the gall bladder, cystic duct and bile duct. Sectioning of the caudate process of the caudate lobe of the liver has exposed the cranial pole of the right kidney located in the renal fossa (see also Figs 6.88, 6.96).

descending duodenum · perirenal fat · rib 13 · renal impression · caudate lobe, caudate process · right lateral lobe · right medial lobe

a. testicularis

a.v. iliaca externa

urinary bladder

median ligament of bladder

m. rectus abdominis · spleen, ventral extremity · liver in section, left lateral lobe · bile duct · liver: quadrate lobe

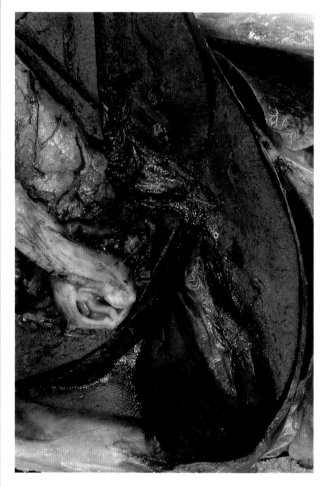

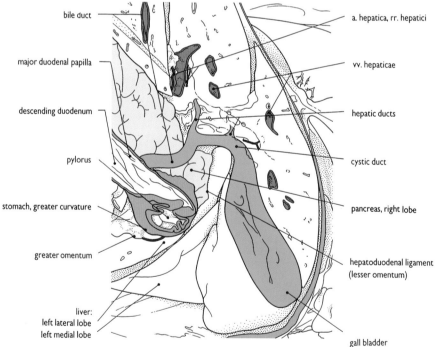

bile duct · a. hepatica, rr. hepatici

major duodenal papilla · vv. hepaticae

descending duodenum · hepatic ducts

pylorus · cystic duct

stomach, greater curvature · pancreas, right lobe

greater omentum · hepatoduodenal ligament (lesser omentum)

liver: left lateral lobe left medial lobe · gall bladder

Fig. 6.54 Gall bladder, cystic, hepatic and bile ducts: right lateral view. This is an enlarged view of part of the dissection shown in Fig. 6.53 and shows a similar dissection to that shown in Fig. 6.52. In the sectioned surfaces of the liver large hepatic veins are visible, and two proper hepatic artery radicles are evident in the right lateral lobe dorsally.

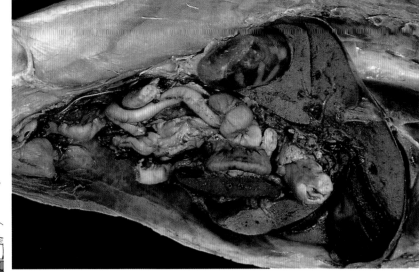

descending colon | mesocolon | caudal duodenal flexure | ileum | caecum | right kidney | mesoduodenum, cut edge

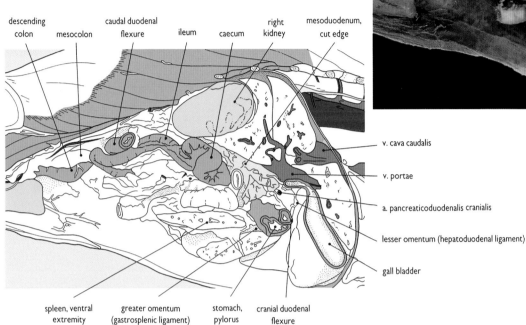

v. cava caudalis

v. portae

a. pancreaticoduodenalis cranialis

lesser omentum (hepatoduodenal ligament)

gall bladder

spleen, ventral extremity | greater omentum (gastrosplenic ligament) | stomach, pylorus | cranial duodenal flexure

Fig. 6.55 Ileum, caecum and ascending colon: right lateral view. The descending duodenum and right pancreatic lobe have been removed, exposing the caecum and the ileum extending caudally from it ventral to the cut edge of the mesoduodenum. More caudally a number of jejunal coils have been removed and the descending colon and mesocolon are exposed craniodorsal to the bladder. The spleen has also been cut through at its ventral extremity and the gastrosplenic ligament is visible.

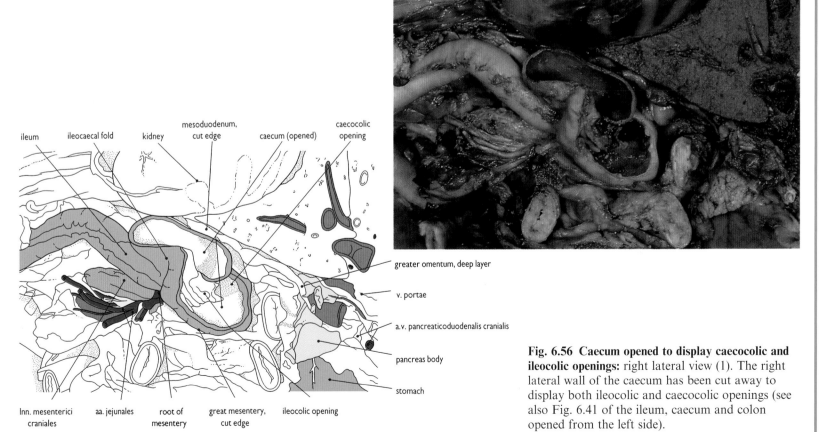

ileum | ileocaecal fold | kidney | mesoduodenum, cut edge | caecum (opened) | caecocolic opening

greater omentum, deep layer

v. portae

a.v. pancreaticoduodenalis cranialis

pancreas body

stomach

lnn. mesenterici craniales | aa. jejunales | root of mesentery | great mesentery, cut edge | ileocolic opening

Fig. 6.56 Caecum opened to display caecocolic and ileocolic openings: right lateral view (1). The right lateral wall of the caecum has been cut away to display both ileocolic and caecocolic openings (see also Fig. 6.41 of the ileum, caecum and colon opened from the left side).

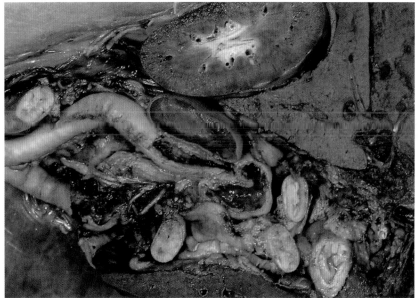

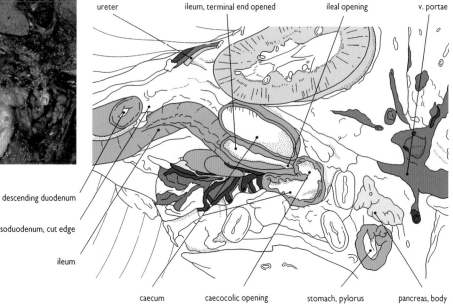

Fig. 6.57 Caecum opened to display caecocolic and ileocolic openings: right lateral view (2). More of the wall of the caecum has been removed so that the terminal end of the ileum is exposed and opened to show the ileocolic opening to greater advantage.

ureter

ileum, terminal end opened

ileal opening

v. portae

descending duodenum

mesoduodenum, cut edge

ileum

caecum

caecocolic opening

stomach, pylorus

pancreas, body

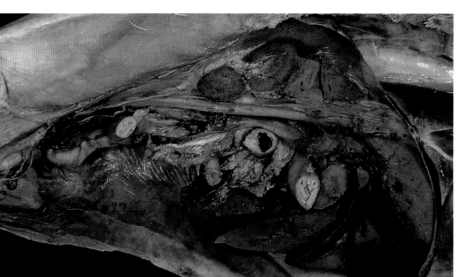

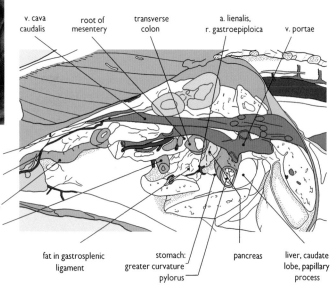

Fig. 6.58 Caudal vena cava and hepatic portal vein: right lateral view. The remaining jejunal coils and the ileum and the caecum which lay to the right of the mesenteric root have been removed. Removal of considerably more liver tissue exposes the caudal vena cava right to the diaphragm. The pylorus has been cut through and the cranial duodenal flexure removed along with the lesser omentum, exposing the papillary process of the caudate lobe of the liver in the lesser curvature (see also liver in caudal view, Fig. 6.92, and in section in Fig. 6.95).

v. cava caudalis

root of mesentery

transverse colon

a. lienalis, r. gastroepiploica

v. portae

ureter

a. testicularis

descending colon

duodenojejunal flexure

fat in gastrosplenic ligament

stomach: greater curvature

pylorus

pancreas

liver, caudate lobe, papillary process

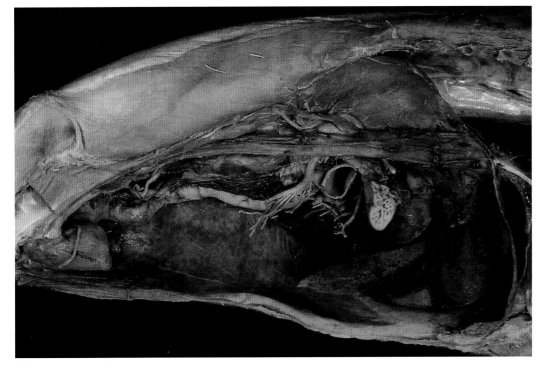

Fig. 6.59 Caudal vena cava, cranial and caudal mesenteric arteries and descending colon: right lateral view. The ascending duodenum has been removed and the descending colon and mesocolon are exposed on the left side. Removal of mesenteric tissues and lymph nodes from the mesenteric root has exposed the cranial mesenteric artery caudal to the transverse colon. The hepatic portal vein has been removed and liver tissue has been cut away from above the caudal vena cava. Additional trimming of the spleen has revealed the branches of the splenic artery: some enter the hilus at the dorsal extremity of the spleen; a larger single branch immediately caudal to the stomach travels to the hilus at the ventral extremity. Removal of the remains of the right kidney and ureter have revealed the adrenal gland and cranial abdominal vessels but also some autonomic splanchnic nerves passing over the lumbocostal arch.

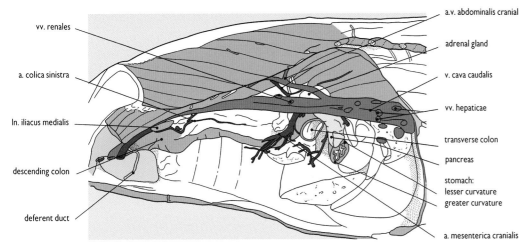

- vv. renales
- a. colica sinistra
- ln. iliacus medialis
- descending colon
- deferent duct

- a.v. abdominalis cranial
- adrenal gland
- v. cava caudalis
- vv. hepaticae
- transverse colon
- pancreas
- stomach:
  lesser curvature
  greater curvature
- a. mesenterica cranialis

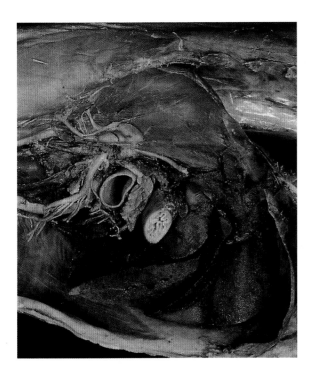

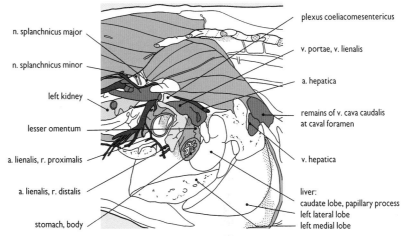

- n. splanchnicus major
- n. splanchnicus minor
- left kidney
- lesser omentum
- a. lienalis, r. proximalis
- a. lienalis, r. distalis
- stomach, body

- plexus coeliacomesentericus
- v. portae, v. lienalis
- a. hepatica
- remains of v. cava caudalis at caval foramen
- v. hepatica
- liver:
  caudate lobe, papillary process
  left lateral lobe
  left medial lobe

Fig. 6.60 Splanchnic nerves and adrenal gland of the right side: right lateral view. Removal of the caudal vena cava and the cranial abdominal vein has revealed little more of the cranial mesenteric artery since the large left renal vein remains in position. The hepatic artery has been exposed more fully and the remains of the caudal vena cava mark the position of the caval foramen in the diaphragm.

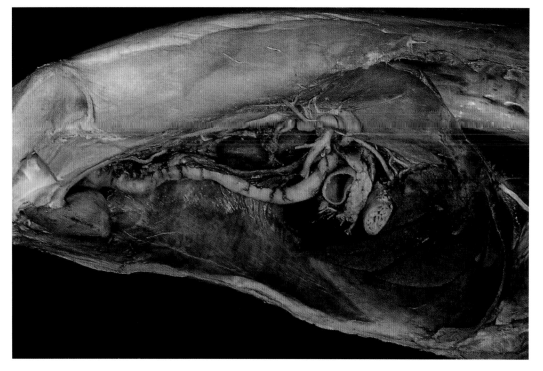

Fig. 6.61 Adrenal glands, left kidney and descending colon: medial view. Removal of the left renal vein and cleaning of perirenal fat has exposed the left kidney and adrenal gland. Trimming of the cranial mesenteric artery has exposed the entire length of the descending colon which in this specimen does not have the abnormally sacculated appearance seen in the colon of the specimen viewed from the left side (see also Figs 6.26, 6.27 from the left lateral aspect). Removal of more of the portal vein and additional cleaning of the lesser omentum from around the papillary process of the liver and the lesser curvature of the stomach reveals the left gastric artery.

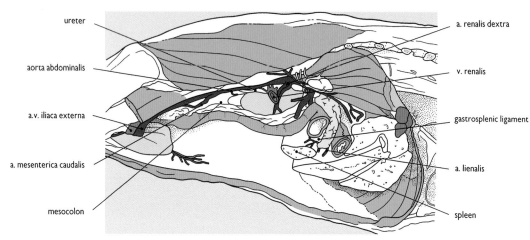

ureter

aorta abdominalis

a.v. iliaca externa

a. mesenterica caudalis

mesocolon

a. renalis dextra

v. renalis

gastrosplenic ligament

a. lienalis

spleen

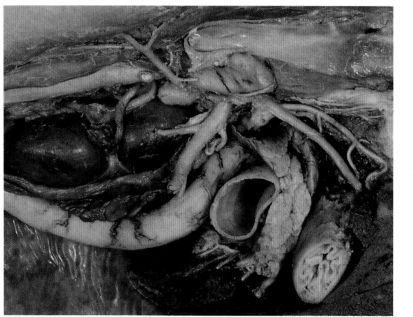

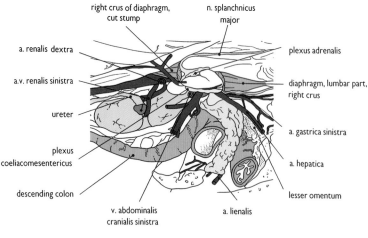

right crus of diaphragm, cut stump

n. splanchnicus major

a. renalis dextra

a.v. renalis sinistra

ureter

plexus coeliacomesentericus

descending colon

v. abdominalis cranialis sinistra

a. lienalis

plexus adrenalis

diaphragm, lumbar part, right crus

a. gastrica sinistra

a. hepatica

lesser omentum

Fig. 6.62 Splanchnic nerves and aortic branches in the cranial abdomen: right lateral view. The costal part of the diaphragm, and consequently the lumbocostal arch, has been removed and a section of the right diaphragmatic crus has been taken out from beneath the adrenal gland. The cut stumps remain in position cranial and caudal to the adrenal gland, and the connection of the splanchnic nerves with an adrenal plexus is displayed above the gland.

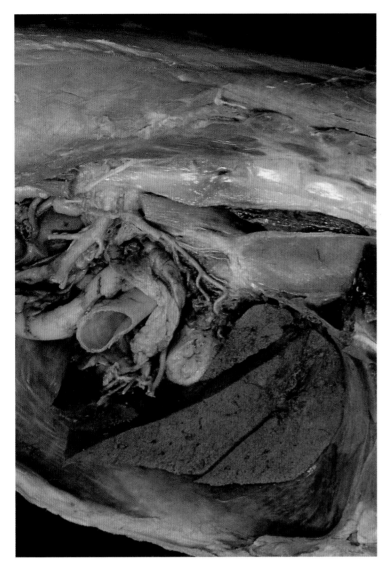

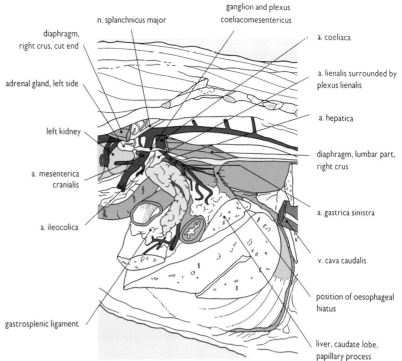

ganglion and plexus
coeliacomestericus

n. splanchnicus major

diaphragm,
right crus, cut end

a. coeliaca

a. lienalis surrounded by
plexus lienalis

adrenal gland, left side

a. hepatica

left kidney

diaphragm, lumbar part,
right crus

a. mesenterica
cranialis

a. gastrica sinistra

a. ileocolica

v. cava caudalis

position of oesophageal
hiatus

gastrosplenic ligament

liver, caudate lobe,
papillary process

Fig. 6.63 Coeliacomesenteric plexus and branching of the cranial mesenteric and coeliac arteries: right lateral view. The right adrenal gland and cranial abdominal artery have been removed and the splanchnic nerves have been pulled ventrally somewhat. The autonomic arterial plexuses have been cleaned although the splenic autonomic plexus is still apparent, making this vessel appear considerably larger than the others. More of the right lumbar part of the diaphragm has been removed to open the esophageal hiatus, and most of the lesser omentum has been cleared from the lesser stomach curvature.

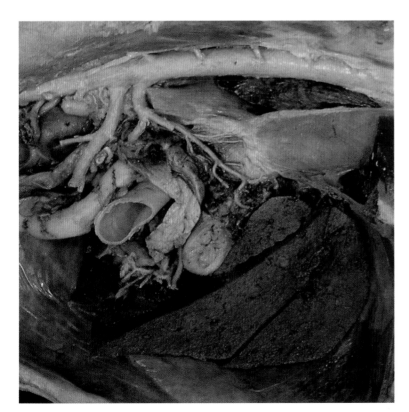

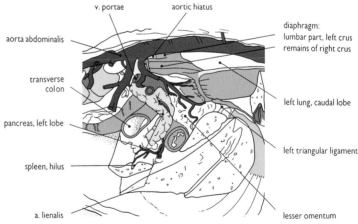

v. portae

aortic hiatus

aorta abdominalis

diaphragm:
lumbar part, left crus
remains of right crus

transverse
colon

left lung, caudal lobe

pancreas, left lobe

left triangular ligament

spleen, hilus

a. lienalis

lesser omentum

Fig. 6.64 Left lobe of the pancreas and transverse colon: medial view. The remaining caudal part of the right diaphragmatic crus has been removed, as have the splanchnic nerves and autonomic nerve plexuses from around the roots of the cranial mesenteric and coeliac arteries. Cleaning of fat, fascia and pleura from around the descending aorta has exposed its full extent and the position of the aortic hiatus is especially well displayed in advance of the coeliac artery (see also Figs 6.86, 6.96, 6.97).

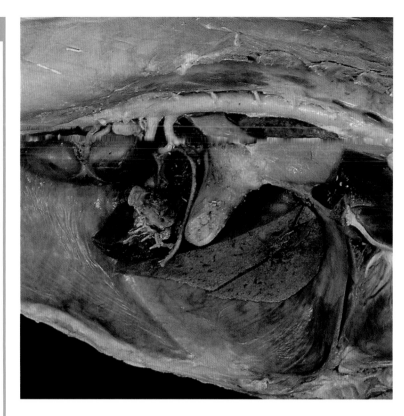

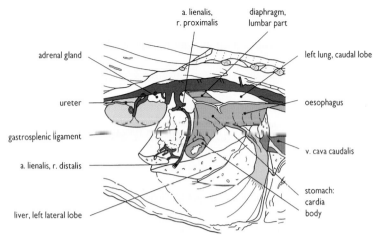

a. lienalis, r. proximalis

diaphragm, lumbar part

adrenal gland

left lung, caudal lobe

ureter

oesophagus

gastrosplenic ligament

a. lienalis, r. distalis

v. cava caudalis

liver, left lateral lobe

stomach: cardia body

Fig. 6.65 Esophagus, cardia and dorsal extremity of the spleen: medial view of left side. The remnants of the right half of the diaphragm have been removed and the coeliac and cranial mesenteric arteries have both been cut back to stumps from the aorta. The lesser omentum and papillary process of the caudate lobe of the liver are completely removed, exposing the cardia and remains of the body of the stomach. Removal of the diaphragmatic crus of the left side has destroyed the esophageal hiatus of the diaphragm and the esophagus is exposed entering the abdomen. More caudally the remains of the colon have been removed and the left kidney is completely exposed.

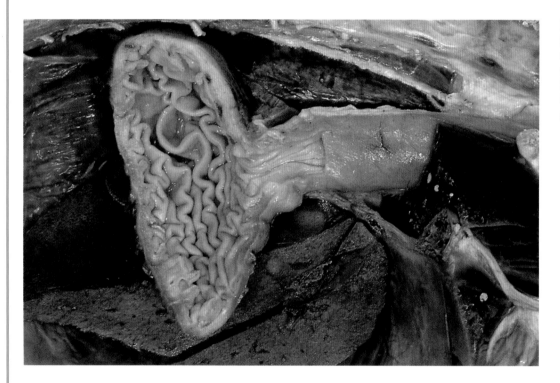

Fig. 6.66 Interior of the esophagus, cardia and fundus of the stomach: medial view. Practically all of the viscera have been removed from the cranial end of the abdomen except for the fundus of the stomach and the cardia. The interior of the fundus exhibits numerous gastric folds.

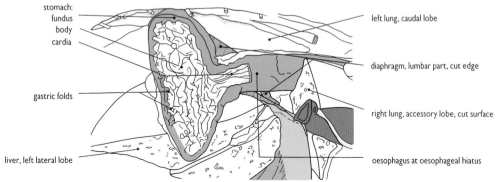

stomach:
fundus
body
cardia

left lung, caudal lobe

diaphragm, lumbar part, cut edge

gastric folds

right lung, accessory lobe, cut surface

liver, left lateral lobe

oesophagus at oesophageal hiatus

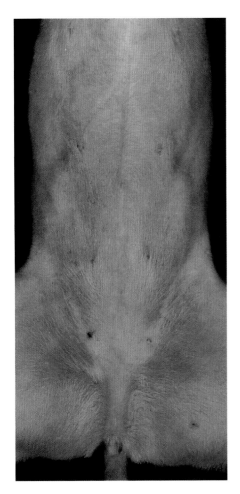

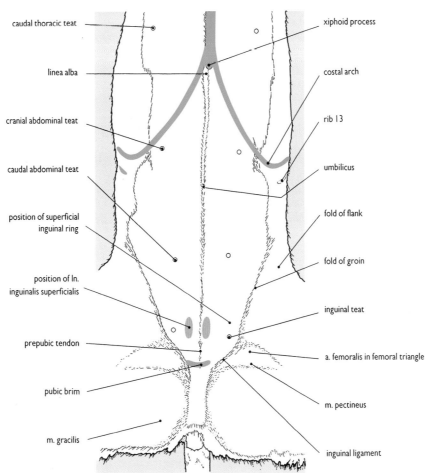

caudal thoracic teat

linea alba

cranial abdominal teat

caudal abdominal teat

position of superficial inguinal ring

position of ln. inguinalis superficialis

prepubic tendon

pubic brim

m. gracilis

xiphoid process

costal arch

rib 13

umbilicus

fold of flank

fold of groin

inguinal teat

a. femoralis in femoral triangle

m. pectineus

inguinal ligament

Fig. 6.67 Surface features of the abdomen and inner thigh of the bitch: ventral view. The bony 'landmarks' that are palpable at the cranial and caudal limits of the abdomen are shown in this figure. In addition a number of 'soft' structures are clearly palpable in the inguinal region and femoral triangle, and the femoral artery may be used to take a pulse.

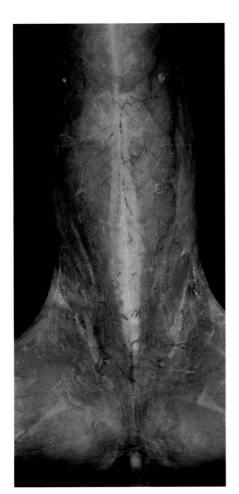

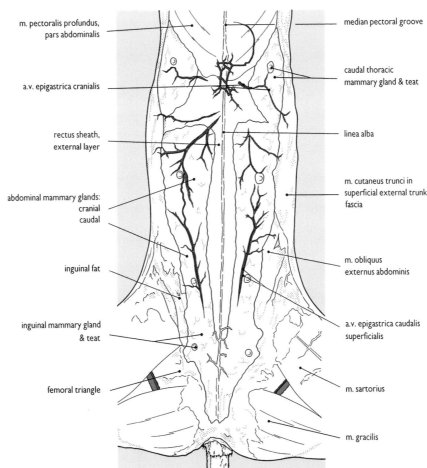

m. pectoralis profundus, pars abdominalis

a.v. epigastrica cranialis

rectus sheath, external layer

abdominal mammary glands: cranial caudal

inguinal fat

inguinal mammary gland & teat

femoral triangle

median pectoral groove

caudal thoracic mammary gland & teat

linea alba

m. cutaneus trunci in superficial external trunk fascia

m. obliquus externus abdominis

a.v. epigastrica caudalis superficialis

m. sartorius

m. gracilis

Fig. 6.68 Superficial fascia of the abdomen and mammary glands of the bitch: ventral view. Removal of the skin has displayed the superficial fascia containing, in this bitch, well developed mammary glands covering much of the ventral surface of the abdominal wall.

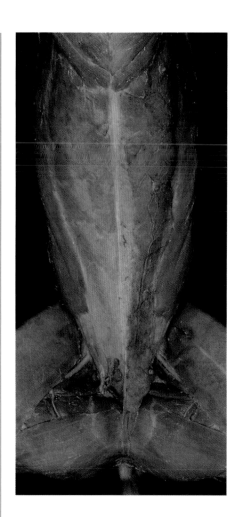

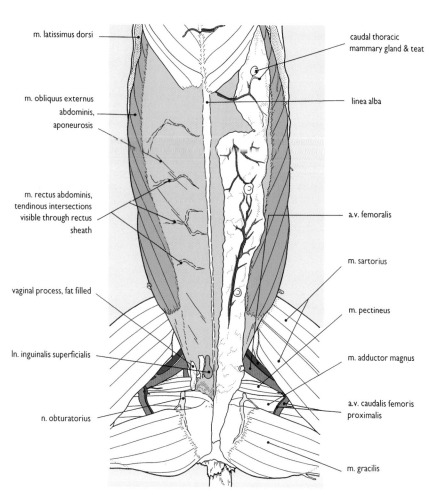

m. latissimus dorsi

m. obliquus externus abdominis, aponeurosis

m. rectus abdominis, tendinous intersections visible through rectus sheath

vaginal process, fat filled

ln. inguinalis superficialis

n. obturatorius

caudal thoracic mammary gland & teat

linea alba

a.v. femoralis

m. sartorius

m. pectineus

m. adductor magnus

a.v. caudalis femoris proximalis

m. gracilis

Fig. 6.69 Abdominal wall of the bitch (1). External abdominal oblique muscle: ventral view. The superficial fascia and cutaneous muscle have been removed from both sides and the mammary glands from the right. Fat and fascia in the groin and femoral triangle have also been cleaned away.

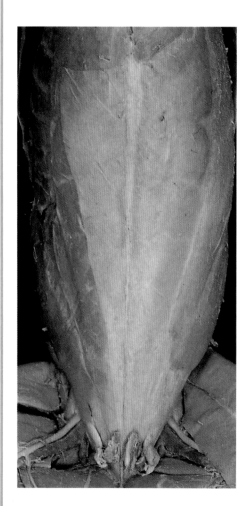

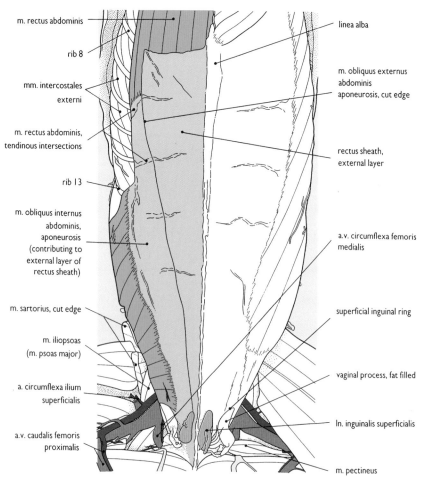

m. rectus abdominis

rib 8

mm. intercostales externi

m. rectus abdominis, tendinous intersections

rib 13

m. obliquus internus abdominis, aponeurosis (contributing to external layer of rectus sheath)

m. sartorius, cut edge

m. iliopsoas (m. psoas major)

a. circumflexa ilium superficialis

a.v. caudalis femoris proximalis

linea alba

m. obliquus externus abdominis aponeurosis, cut edge

rectus sheath, external layer

a.v. circumflexa femoris medialis

superficial inguinal ring

vaginal process, fat filled

ln. inguinalis superficialis

m. pectineus

Fig. 6.70 Abdominal wall of the bitch (2). Internal abdominal oblique muscle and rectus sheath: ventral view. The entire abdominal wall has been cleaned of fascia, cutaneous muscle and mammary tissue. On the right side the external oblique has been removed except for the most ventral part of its aponeurosis of attachment to the linea alba (see also Fig. 6.15). Removal of the external oblique aponeurosis has removed much of the ventral and lateral wall of the inguinal canal so that the fat-filled vaginal process appears more prominent caudal to the rear border of the internal oblique muscle.

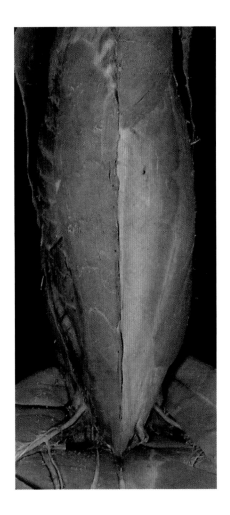

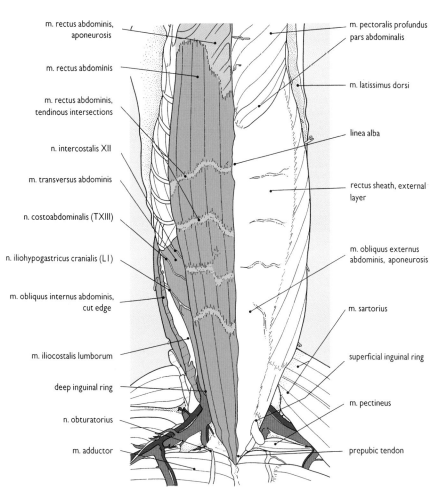

m. rectus abdominis, aponeurosis

m. rectus abdominis

m. rectus abdominis, tendinous intersections

n. intercostalis XII

m. transversus abdominis

n. costoabdominalis (TXIII)

n. iliohypogastricus cranialis (LI)

m. obliquus internus abdominis, cut edge

m. iliocostalis lumborum

deep inguinal ring

n. obturatorius

m. adductor

m. pectoralis profundus pars abdominalis

m. latissimus dorsi

linea alba

rectus sheath, external layer

m. obliquus externus abdominis, aponeurosis

m. sartorius

superficial inguinal ring

m. pectineus

prepubic tendon

Fig. 6.71 Abdominal wall of the bitch (3). Rectus abdominis and transverse abdominal muscles: ventral view. The internal oblique muscle has been removed from the right side along with the external layer of the rectus sheath. Although the vaginal process has been removed, the caudal boundary of the transverse muscle forms the cranial limit of the inguinal canal marking the approximate position of the deep inguinal ring. For a consideration of inguinal canal structure see Chapter 8.

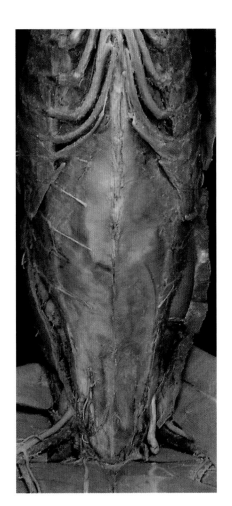

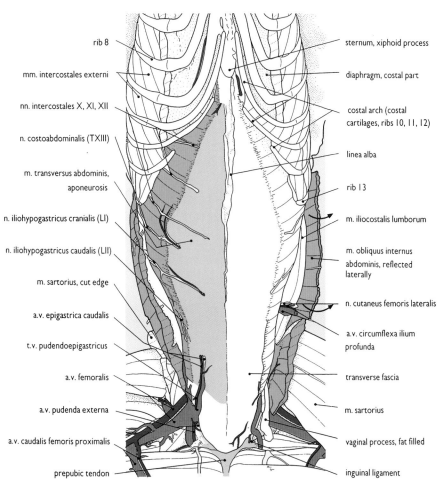

rib 8

mm. intercostales externi

nn. intercostales X, XI, XII

n. costoabdominalis (TXIII)

m. transversus abdominis, aponeurosis

n. iliohypogastricus cranialis (LI)

n. iliohypogastricus caudalis (LII)

m. sartorius, cut edge

a.v. epigastrica caudalis

t.v. pudendoepigastricus

a.v. femoralis

a.v. pudenda externa

a.v. caudalis femoris proximalis

prepubic tendon

sternum, xiphoid process

diaphragm, costal part

costal arch (costal cartilages, ribs 10, 11, 12)

linea alba

rib 13

m. iliocostalis lumborum

m. obliquus internus abdominis, reflected laterally

n. cutaneus femoris lateralis

a.v. circumflexa ilium profunda

transverse fascia

m. sartorius

vaginal process, fat filled

inguinal ligament

Fig. 6.72 Abdominal wall of the bitch (4). Transverse abdominal muscles and nerves of the abdominal wall: ventral view. Removal of the oblique and rectus muscles from both sides of the abdominal wall has exposed the transverse abdominal muscles and linea alba (see also Fig. 6.21). The deep inguinal ring, vaginal process and inguinal ligament are all more clearly displayed on the left side. However, the pudendoepigastric vessels and their terminal branches are present on the right side following rectus removal (see also Fig. 6.46).

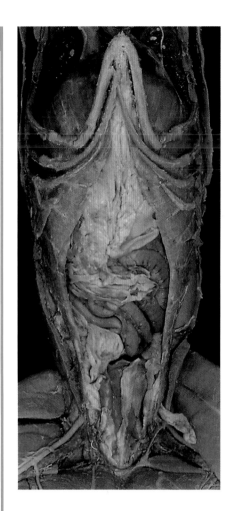
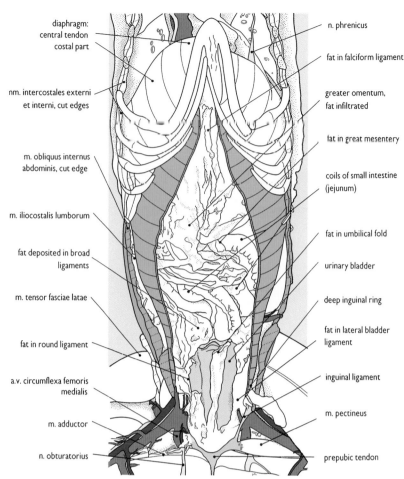

diaphragm:
central tendon
costal part

nm. intercostales externi
et interni, cut edges

m. obliquus internus
abdominis, cut edge

m. iliocostalis lumborum

fat deposited in broad
ligaments

m. tensor fasciae latae

fat in round ligament

a.v. circumflexa femoris
medialis

m. adductor

n. obturatorius

n. phrenicus

fat in falciform ligament

greater omentum,
fat infiltrated

fat in great mesentery

coils of small intestine
(jejunum)

fat in umbilical fold

urinary bladder

deep inguinal ring

fat in lateral bladder
ligament

inguinal ligament

m. pectineus

prepubic tendon

Fig. 6.73 Abdominal viscera of the bitch in situ after removal of the aponeuroses of the transverse abdominal muscles: ventral view. The abdominal cavity has been opened by removing the aponeuroses of both transverse muscles. Large masses of subperitoneal fat are present in the falciform ligament, the umbilical fold and lateral ligaments of the bladder, the greater omentum, the great mesentery, and the broad ligaments (see also Figs 6.23, 6.47).

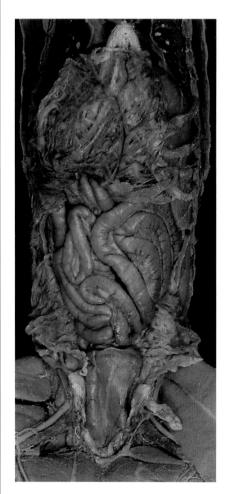
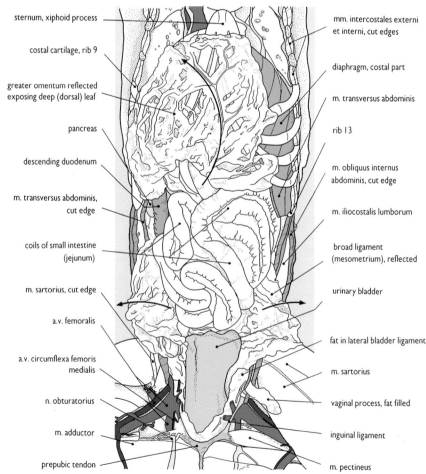

sternum, xiphoid process

costal cartilage, rib 9

greater omentum reflected
exposing deep (dorsal) leaf

pancreas

descending duodenum

m. transversus abdominis,
cut edge

coils of small intestine
(jejunum)

m. sartorius, cut edge

a.v. femoralis

a.v. circumflexa femoris
medialis

n. obturatorius

m. adductor

prepubic tendon

mm. intercostales externi
et interni, cut edges

diaphragm, costal part

m. transversus abdominis

rib 13

m. obliquus internus
abdominis, cut edge

m. iliocostalis lumborum

broad ligament
(mesometrium), reflected

urinary bladder

fat in lateral bladder ligament

m. sartorius

vaginal process, fat filled

inguinal ligament

m. pectineus

Fig. 6.74 Abdominal viscera of the bitch after reflection of the greater omentum and broad ligaments: ventral view. The transverse abdominal muscles have been removed, the greater omentum has been reflected cranially as far as the present dissection allows, the broad ligaments have been reflected laterally, and the umbilical fold has been removed from the bladder.

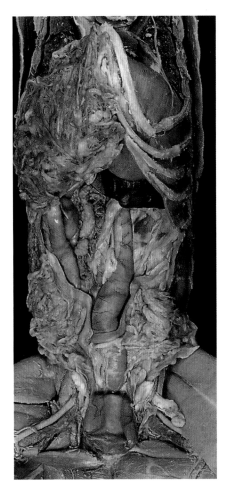

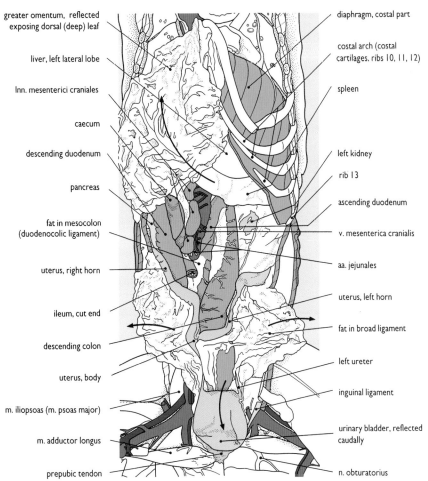

greater omentum, reflected exposing dorsal (deep) leaf

liver, left lateral lobe

lnn. mesenterici craniales

caecum

descending duodenum

pancreas

fat in mesocolon (duodenocolic ligament)

uterus, right horn

ileum, cut end

descending colon

uterus, body

m. iliopsoas (m. psoas major)

m. adductor longus

prepubic tendon

diaphragm, costal part

costal arch (costal cartilages, ribs 10, 11, 12)

spleen

left kidney

rib 13

ascending duodenum

v. mesenterica cranialis

aa. jejunales

uterus, left horn

fat in broad ligament

left ureter

inguinal ligament

urinary bladder, reflected caudally

n. obturatorius

Fig. 6.75 Abdominal viscera of the bitch after removal of the jejunum and reflection of the bladder: ventral view. The jejunum and the fat-laden great mesentery have been removed en masse by severing: the ileum close to the ileocolic junction; the jejunum close to the duodenojejunal flexure; and the great mesentery close to its root. Some of the fat in the mesenteric root was cleared and the bladder was reflected caudally.

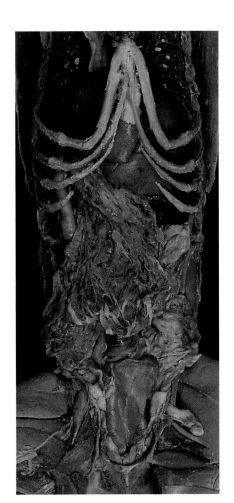

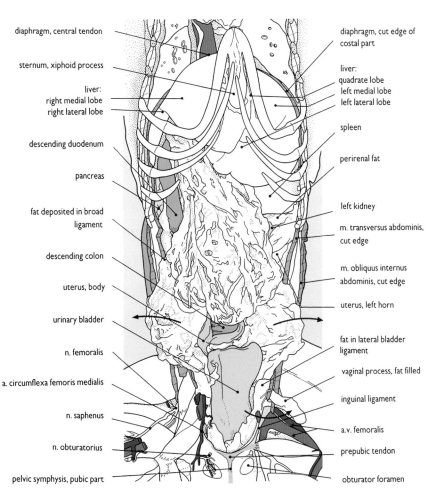

diaphragm, central tendon

sternum, xiphoid process

liver:
right medial lobe
right lateral lobe

descending duodenum

pancreas

fat deposited in broad ligament

descending colon

uterus, body

urinary bladder

n. femoralis

a. circumflexa femoris medialis

n. saphenus

n. obturatorius

pelvic symphysis, pubic part

diaphragm, cut edge of costal part

liver:
quadrate lobe
left medial lobe
left lateral lobe

spleen

perirenal fat

left kidney

m. transversus abdominis, cut edge

m. obliquus internus abdominis, cut edge

uterus, left horn

fat in lateral bladder ligament

vaginal process, fat filled

inguinal ligament

a.v. femoralis

prepubic tendon

obturator foramen

Fig. 6.76 Liver, spleen and greater omentum of the bitch after removal of the diaphragm: ventral view. The ventral part of the diaphragm has been removed by cutting horizontally through central tendon and muscular periphery, exposing the diaphragmatic surface of the liver with the costal arches and caudal ribs still in position (see also Figs 6.24, 6.48). The liver extends into the xiphoid region between the left and right costal arches (see also Fig. 6.67).

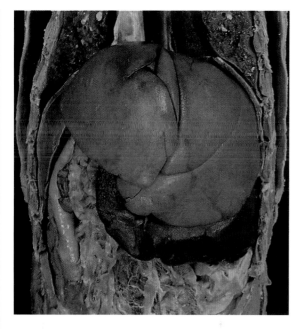

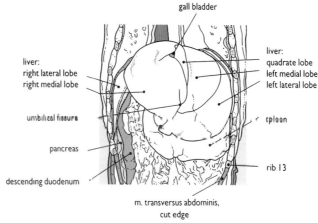

Fig. 6.77 **Liver, spleen and greater omentum after removal of the ribs and costal arch:** ventral view. Removal of the remaining ribs and costal arch exposes the diaphragmatic surface of the liver and the spleen. The spleen is enlarged and its ventral extremity extends considerably beyond the midventral line onto the right side of the abdomen (see also Figs 6.25, 6.89, 6.90, 6.96, 6.97).

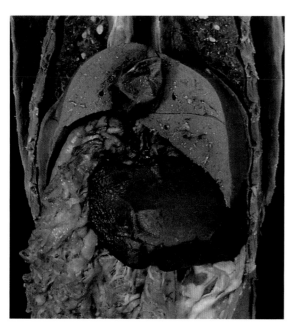

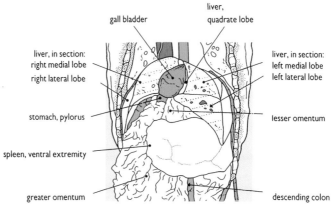

Fig. 6.78 **Gall bladder after horizontal sectioning of the liver:** ventral view. Sectioning and removal of liver tissue has exposed the gall bladder in its fossa between right medial and quadrate lobes of the liver.

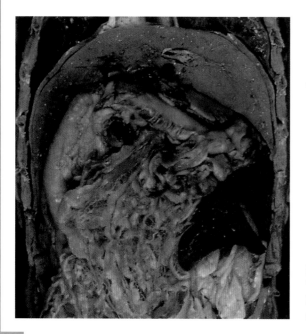

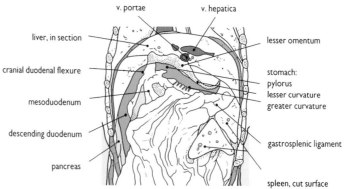

Fig. 6.79 **Stomach and greater omentum after resection of the liver and spleen:** ventral view. The caudal ribs, costal arch, liver and spleen have been cut down to the same horizontal level as the previously cut diaphragm. The curvature of the spleen, and its greatly increased size consequent upon barbiturate anesthesia, means that it has in fact been sectioned twice.

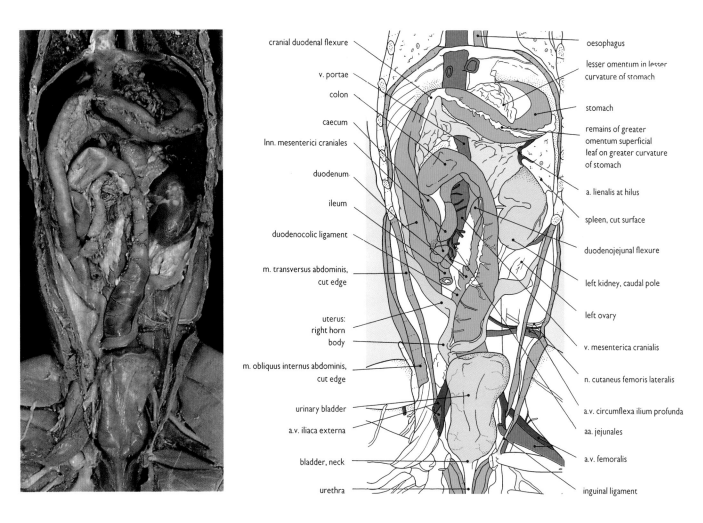

cranial duodenal flexure

v. portae

colon

caecum

lnn. mesenterici craniales

duodenum

ileum

duodenocolic ligament

m. transversus abdominis, cut edge

uterus:
right horn
body

m. obliquus internus abdominis, cut edge

urinary bladder

a.v. iliaca externa

bladder, neck

urethra

oesophagus

lesser omentum in lesser curvature of stomach

stomach

remains of greater omentum superficial leaf on greater curvature of stomach

a. lienalis at hilus

spleen, cut surface

duodenojejunal flexure

left kidney, caudal pole

left ovary

v. mesenterica cranialis

n. cutaneus femoris lateralis

a.v. circumflexa ilium profunda

aa. jejunales

a.v. femoralis

inguinal ligament

Fig. 6.80 Duodenum, caecum, colon and mesenteric lymph nodes of the bitch: ventral view. Removal of much of the liver exposes the stomach and the lesser omentum gathered up in the lesser curvature. The greater omentum has been cut from its attachment to the greater curvature of the stomach and cut at its attachment to the left lobe and body of the pancreas (see also Fig. 6.89).

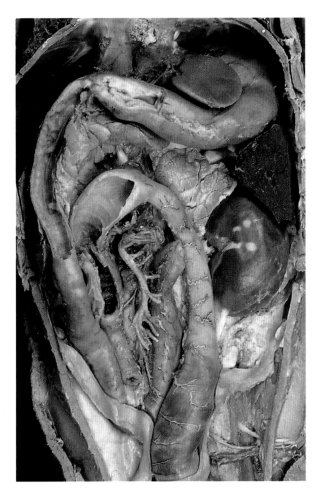

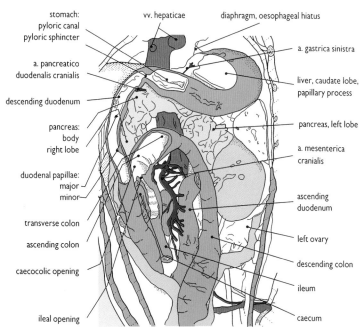

stomach:
pyloric canal
pyloric sphincter

a. pancreatico duodenalis cranialis

descending duodenum

pancreas:
body
right lobe

duodenal papillae:
major
minor

transverse colon

ascending colon

caecocolic opening

ileal opening

vv. hepaticae

diaphragm, oesophageal hiatus

a. gastrica sinistra

liver, caudate lobe, papillary process

pancreas, left lobe

a. mesenterica cranialis

ascending duodenum

left ovary

descending colon

ileum

caecum

Fig. 6.81 Duodenum, pancreas, caecum and colon of the bitch: ventral view. Opening the pylorus of the stomach and the commencement of the descending duodenum displays the pyloric canal and sphincter and the duodenal papillae (see also Figs 6.52, 6.54). Opening of the terminal end of the ileum and ascending colon has exposed the ileocolic opening; the caecocolic opening is also visible, although much of the caecum is hidden dorsal to the descending colon (see also Figs 6.41, 6.56, 6.57).

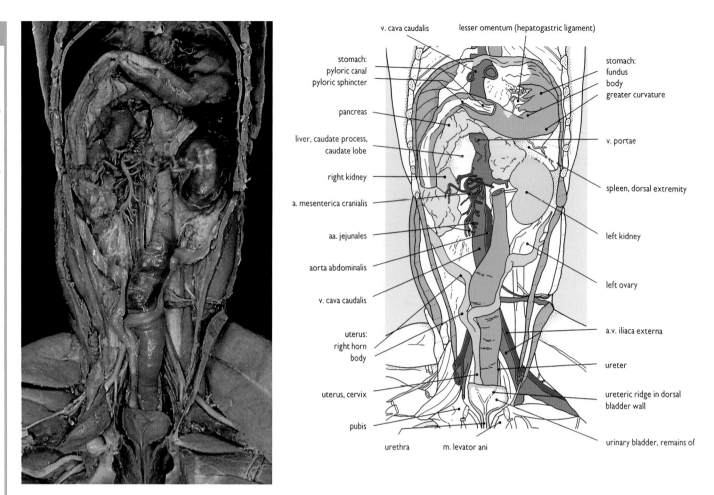

stomach:
pyloric canal
pyloric sphincter

pancreas

liver, caudate process,
caudate lobe

right kidney

a. mesenterica cranialis

aa. jejunales

aorta abdominalis

v. cava caudalis

uterus:
right horn
body

uterus, cervix

pubis

urethra   m. levator ani

v. cava caudalis   lesser omentum (hepatogastric ligament)

stomach:
fundus
body
greater curvature

v. portae

spleen, dorsal extremity

left kidney

left ovary

a.v. iliaca externa

ureter

ureteric ridge in dorsal
bladder wall

urinary bladder, remains of

Fig. 6.82 Descending colon and uterus of the bitch: ventral view. Removal of the caecum and much of the duodenum and colon exposes the pancreas, whilst removal of the mesenteric lymph nodes has exposed the cranial mesenteric artery. The bladder is opened and trimmed in size and fat has been cleaned from the abdominal roof to expose the uterine horns and body. The urethra is visible following removal of the pubic bones.

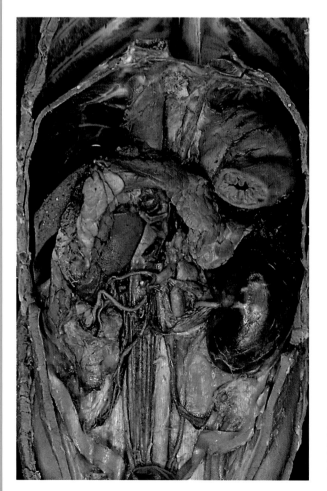

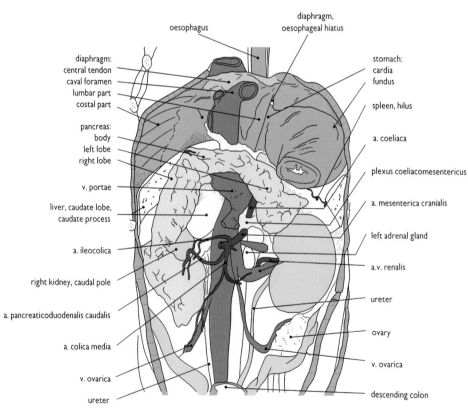

oesophagus

diaphragm,
oesophageal hiatus

diaphragm:
central tendon
caval foramen
lumbar part
costal part

pancreas:
body
left lobe
right lobe

v. portae

liver, caudate lobe,
caudate process

a. ileocolica

right kidney, caudal pole

a. pancreaticoduodenalis caudalis

a. colica media

v. ovarica

ureter

stomach:
cardia
fundus

spleen, hilus

a. coeliaca

plexus coeliacomesentericus

a. mesenterica cranialis

left adrenal gland

a.v. renalis

ureter

ovary

v. ovarica

descending colon

Fig. 6.83 Pancreas of the bitch: ventral view. Removal of the descending colon, the remaining part of the duodenum, the pylorus of the stomach and some of its body has exposed the entire pancreas (see also Figs 6.88, 6.89). Also exposed more clearly are the hepatic portal vein and the cranial mesenteric artery with a caudal pancreaticoduodenal branch.

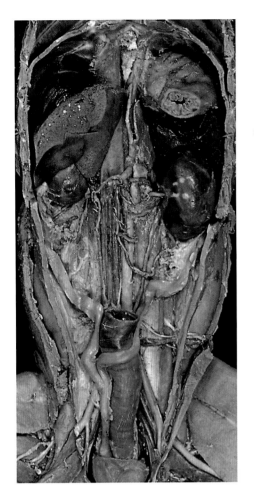

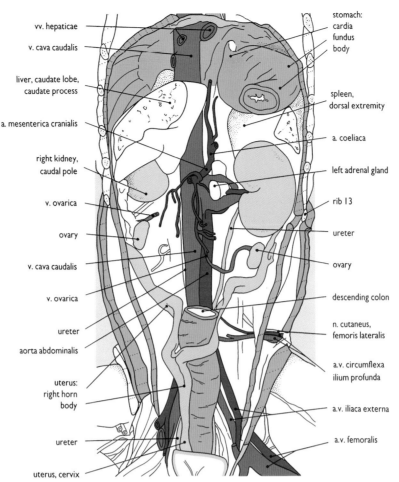

vv. hepaticae
v. cava caudalis
liver, caudate lobe, caudate process
a. mesenterica cranialis
right kidney, caudal pole
v. ovarica
ovary
v. cava caudalis
v. ovarica
ureter
aorta abdominalis
uterus: right horn body
ureter
uterus, cervix

stomach: cardia fundus body
spleen, dorsal extremity
a. coeliaca
left adrenal gland
rib 13
ureter
ovary
descending colon
n. cutaneus, femoris lateralis
a.v. circumflexa ilium profunda
a.v. iliaca externa
a.v. femoralis

Fig. 6.84 Uterus of the bitch: ventral view. The pancreas and hepatic portal vein have been removed and some attempt has been made to clear the extensive amounts of retroperitoneal fat located in the abdominal roof. However, extensive fat deposits in and around the ovarian bursa and ovary have obscured detail. The uterine horns and body are shown and a slight swelling close to the cut edge of the bladder denotes the position of the cervix.

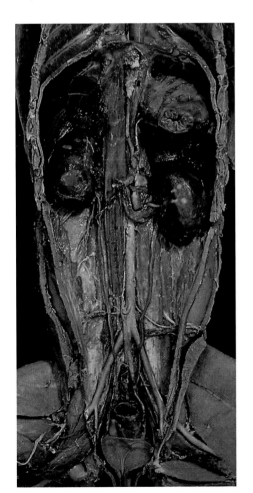

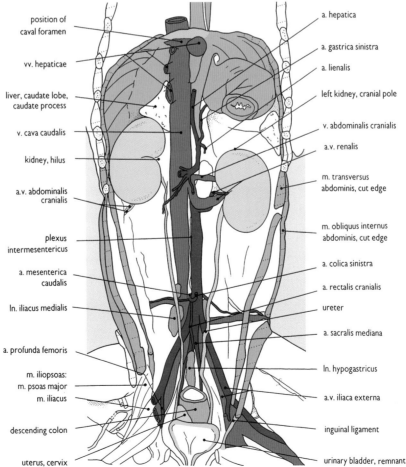

position of caval foramen
vv. hepaticae
liver, caudate lobe, caudate process
v. cava caudalis
kidney, hilus
a.v. abdominalis cranialis
plexus intermesentericus
a. mesenterica caudalis
ln. iliacus medialis
a. profunda femoris
m. iliopsoas: m. psoas major m. iliacus
descending colon
uterus, cervix

a. hepatica
a. gastrica sinistra
a. lienalis
left kidney, cranial pole
v. abdominalis cranialis
a.v. renalis
m. transversus abdominis, cut edge
m. obliquus internus abdominis, cut edge
a. colica sinistra
a. rectalis cranialis
ureter
a. sacralis mediana
ln. hypogastricus
a.v. iliaca externa
inguinal ligament
urinary bladder, remnant

Fig. 6.85 Kidneys, ureters and blood vessels in the abdominal roof of the bitch: ventral view. Removal of practically all of the caudate lobe of the liver has exposed the right kidney and the full extent of the caudal vena cava. Removal of most of the descending colon, the ovaries and the uterus has exposed the ureters, the abdominal aorta and the external iliac vessels in the roof.

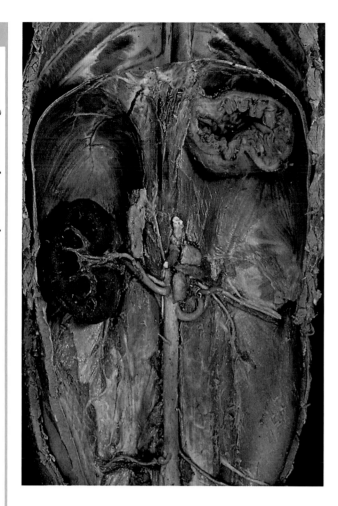

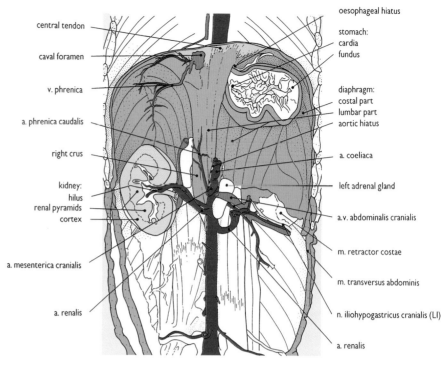

central tendon

caval foramen

v. phrenica

a. phrenica caudalis

right crus

kidney:
hilus
renal pyramids
cortex

a. mesenterica cranialis

a. renalis

oesophageal hiatus

stomach:
cardia
fundus

diaphragm:
costal part
lumbar part
aortic hiatus

a. coeliaca

left adrenal gland

a.v. abdominalis cranialis

m. retractor costae

m. transversus abdominis

n. iliohypogastricus cranialis (LI)

a. renalis

Fig. 6.86 Adrenal glands and diaphragmatic crura of the bitch: ventral view. The caudal vena cava has been removed and the coeliac and cranial mesenteric arteries have been trimmed to stumps. The left kidney has been removed while the right has been sectioned horizontally. Most of the remains of the stomach have also been removed, only leaving part of the fundus and the cardia.

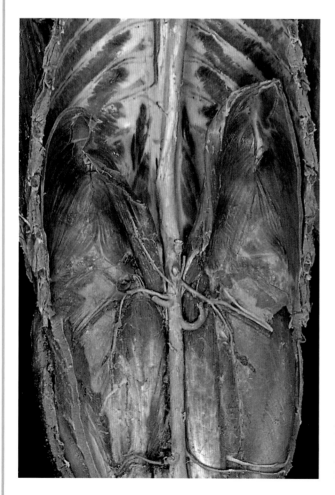

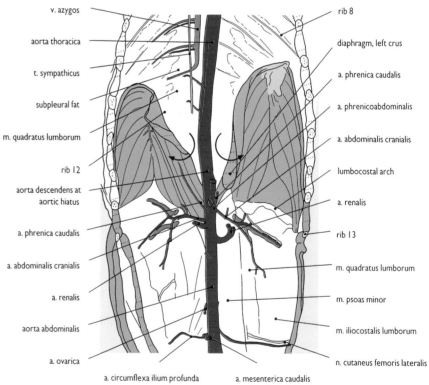

v. azygos

aorta thoracica

t. sympathicus

subpleural fat

m. quadratus lumborum

rib 12

aorta descendens at
aortic hiatus

a. phrenica caudalis

a. abdominalis cranialis

a. renalis

aorta abdominalis

a. ovarica

a. circumflexa ilium profunda

rib 8

diaphragm, left crus

a. phrenica caudalis

a. phrenicoabdominalis

a. abdominalis cranialis

lumbocostal arch

a. renalis

rib 13

m. quadratus lumborum

m. psoas minor

m. iliocostalis lumborum

n. cutaneus femoris lateralis

a. mesenterica caudalis

Fig. 6.87 Descending aorta and diaphragmatic crura of the bitch: ventral view. The remains of the right kidney, both adrenal glands and the stomach and esophagus have all been removed. The diaphragm is cut through, allowing the lumbar parts to be reflected laterally opening the aortic hiatus.

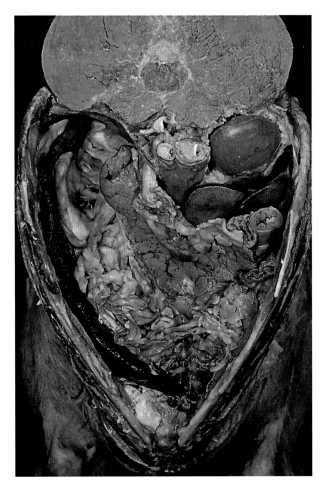

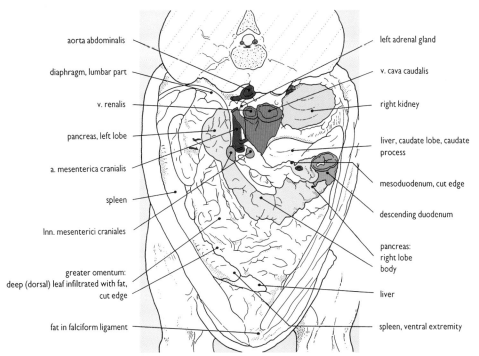

aorta abdominalis
diaphragm, lumbar part
v. renalis
pancreas, left lobe
a. mesenterica cranialis
spleen
lnn. mesenterici craniales
greater omentum:
deep (dorsal) leaf infiltrated with fat,
cut edge
fat in falciform ligament

left adrenal gland
v. cava caudalis
right kidney
liver, caudate lobe, caudate process
mesoduodenum, cut edge
descending duodenum
pancreas: right lobe body
liver
spleen, ventral extremity

Fig. 6.88 Viscera of the cranial abdomen (1). After sectioning of the body and removal of the intestines: caudal view. The body shown in this picture was sectioned transversely through lumbar vertebra 2. The intestines were removed after cutting through the descending duodenum and mesoduodenum, consequently part of the right lobe of the pancreas was also removed. Other structures which have been cut through and are visible include the aorta, caudal vena cava, hepatic portal vein, cranial mesenteric artery and the greater omentum.

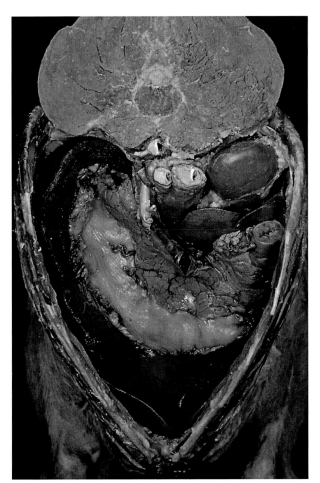

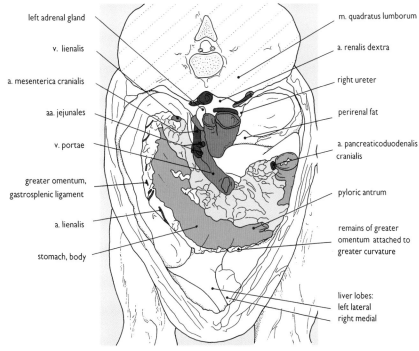

left adrenal gland
v. lienalis
a. mesenterica cranialis
aa. jejunales
v. portae
greater omentum, gastrosplenic ligament
a. lienalis
stomach, body

m. quadratus lumborum
a. renalis dextra
right ureter
perirenal fat
a. pancreaticoduodenalis cranialis
pyloric antrum
remains of greater omentum attached to greater curvature
liver lobes: left lateral right medial

Fig. 6.89 Viscera of the cranial abdomen (2). Pancreas, stomach and spleen: caudal view. Superficial and deep layers of the greater omentum have been removed and tissue has been cleared from around the cranial mesenteric artery and hepatic portal vein. The spleen is confined to the left side of the body and is of more 'normal' size when compared with other dissections (see also Figs 6.25, 6.77, 6.96, 6.97).

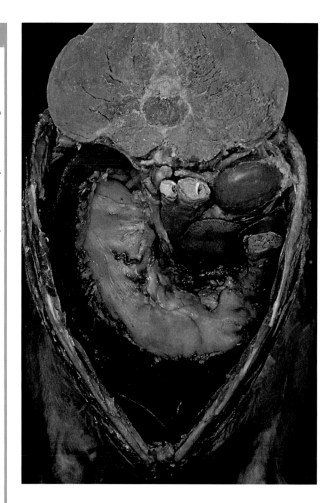

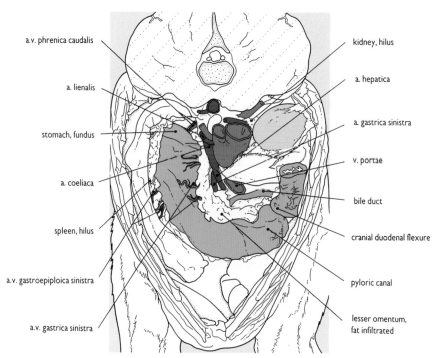

a.v. phrenica caudalis

a. lienalis

stomach, fundus

a. coeliaca

spleen, hilus

a.v. gastroepiploica sinistra

a.v. gastrica sinistra

kidney, hilus

a. hepatica

a. gastrica sinistra

v. portae

bile duct

cranial duodenal flexure

pyloric canal

lesser omentum,
fat infiltrated

Fig. 6.90 Viscera of the cranial abdomen (3). Stomach, spleen and right kidney: caudal view. The pancreas has been removed exposing the visceral surface of the stomach from fundus on the left to cranial duodenal flexure on the right. Stomach position and relationships are also demonstrated ventrally in Figs 6.79–6.82 and in section, Figs 6.94, 6.95.

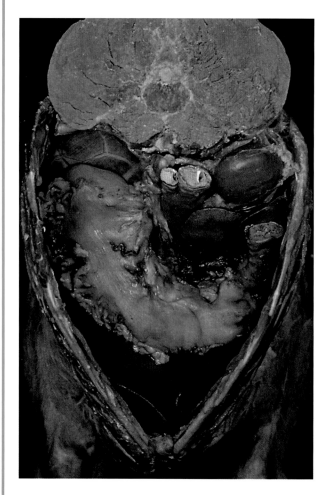

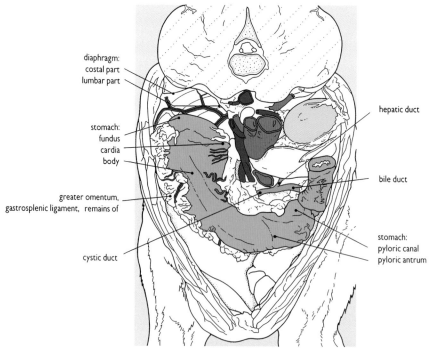

diaphragm:
costal part
lumbar part

stomach:
fundus
cardia
body

greater omentum,
gastrosplenic ligament, remains of

cystic duct

hepatic duct

bile duct

stomach:
pyloric canal
pyloric antrum

Fig. 6.91 Viscera of the cranial abdomen (4). Stomach and liver: caudal view. Removal of the spleen, combined with limited clearing of the lesser omentum, has exposed the entire stomach *in situ* against the visceral surface of the liver. A remnant of the gastrosplenic ligament is still attached to the greater curvature on the fundus and body; the cardia is exposed to the left of the coeliac artery.

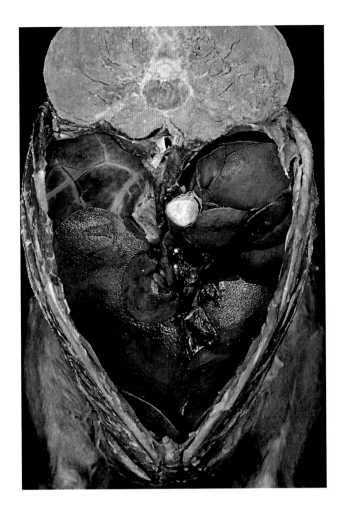

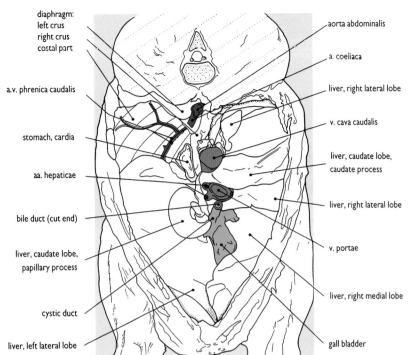

diaphragm:
left crus
right crus
costal part

aorta abdominalis

a. coeliaca

a.v. phrenica caudalis

liver, right lateral lobe

v. cava caudalis

stomach, cardia

liver, caudate lobe,
caudate process

aa. hepaticae

liver, right lateral lobe

bile duct (cut end)

v. portae

liver, caudate lobe,
papillary process

liver, right medial lobe

cystic duct

liver, left lateral lobe

gall bladder

Fig. 6.92 Liver and diaphragm: caudal view. The stomach has been removed after cutting through at the cardia and the remains of the lesser omentum have been cleared from the porta of the liver. The right kidney has been removed from its fossa in the caudate lobe of the liver. Trimming of the caudal vena cava has removed the renal veins and cutting back the coeliac artery has also removed its branches. The bile duct has been severed close to the porta.

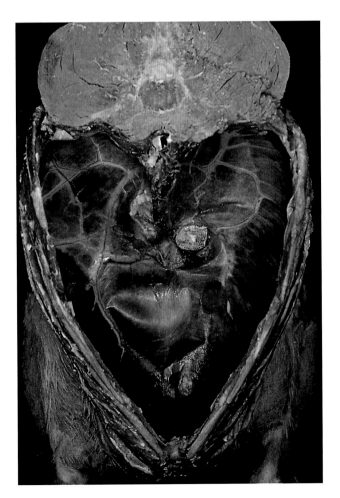

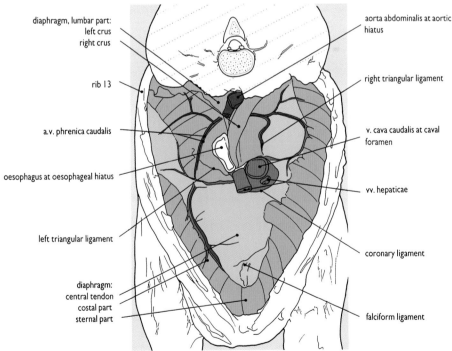

diaphragm, lumbar part:
left crus
right crus

aorta abdominalis at aortic
hiatus

rib 13

right triangular ligament

a.v. phrenica caudalis

v. cava caudalis at caval
foramen

oesophagus at oesophageal hiatus

vv. hepaticae

left triangular ligament

coronary ligament

diaphragm:
central tendon
costal part
sternal part

falciform ligament

Fig. 6.93 Diaphragm: caudal view. Removal of the liver and additional trimming of both caudal vena cava and cardia of the stomach has exposed the caudal face of the diaphragm (see also Fig. 5.91 for a cranial view). The caval foramen in the central tendon is surrounded by the remains of the coronary ligament and triangular ligaments are evident on the central tendon on both sides.

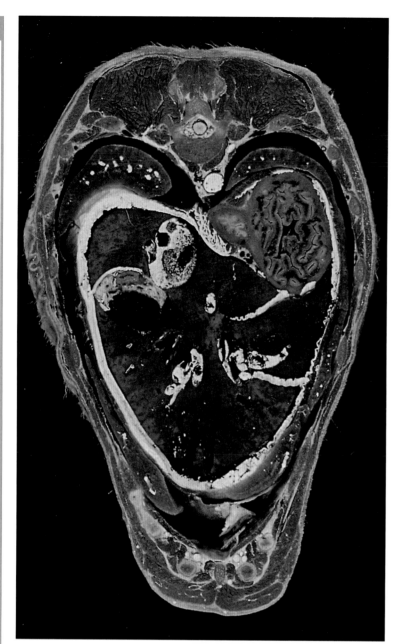

Fig. 6.94 Transverse section (1). Through the liver and diaphragm at the esophageal hiatus: cranial view. This and the following seven sections through the abdomen were made at approximately the levels shown in the accompanying sketch and are all viewed from the cranial aspect. They continue the sequence of transverse sections through the thorax (Chapter 5) and are continued by the sections through the pelvis (Chapter 7). In this first section the esophageal hiatus of the diaphragm is apparent with diaphragmatic crura flanking the cardia of the stomach. The fundus of the stomach bulges out onto the left side (see also Figs 6.81, 6.91). The cranial-most part of the liver is cut through as it lies against the visceral surface of the diaphragm and at this level the liver is incompletely subdivided into lobes.

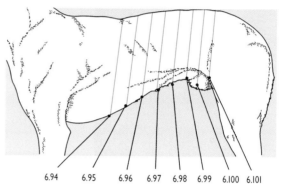

6.94   6.95   6.96   6.97   6.98   6.99   6.100   6.101

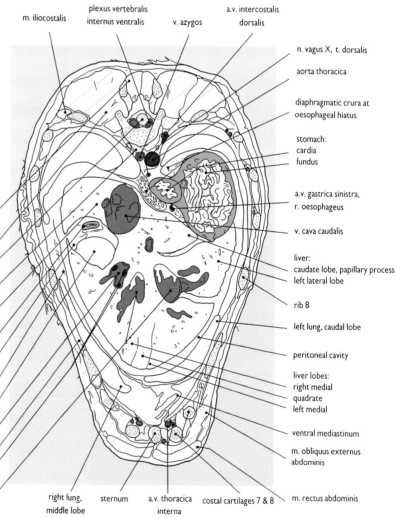

m. iliocostalis

plexus vertebralis
internus ventralis

v. azygos

a.v. intercostalis
dorsalis

n. vagus X, t. dorsalis

aorta thoracica

diaphragmatic crura at
oesophageal hiatus

stomach:
cardia
fundus

a.v. gastrica sinistra,
r. oesophageus

v. cava caudalis

liver:
caudate lobe, papillary process
left lateral lobe

rib 8

left lung, caudal lobe

peritoneal cavity

liver lobes:
right medial
quadrate
left medial

ventral mediastinum

m. obliquus externus
abdominis

m. rectus abdominis

m. multifidus

m. longissimus

spinal cord in spinal canal

m. quadratus lumborum

liver, right lateral lobe

cranial duodenal flexure

greater omentum

diaphragm, costal part

spleen

v. portae

costodiaphragmatic recess

aa. hepaticae

vv. hepaticae

right lung,
middle lobe

sternum

a.v. thoracica
interna

costal cartilages 7 & 8

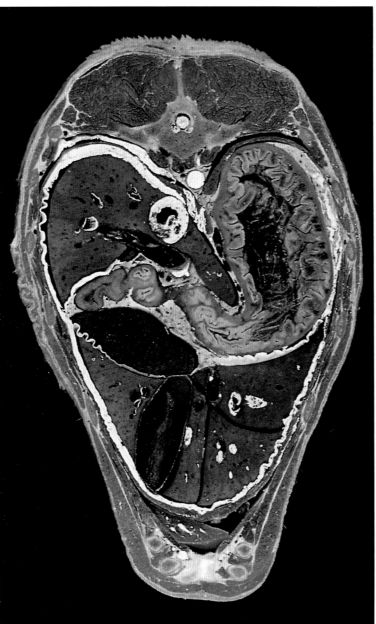

Fig. 6.95 Transverse section (2). Through the liver, gall bladder, stomach and cranial duodenal flexure: cranial view. This section passes through the stomach and liver. It demonstrates the almost transverse orientation of the long axis of the stomach with fundus on the left side and pylorus on the right (see also Figs 6.80, 6.91). The liver lobes are clearly separated from each other and the large gall bladder is sectioned. A section through the ventral extremity of the spleen also lies on the right side, an abnormal relationship occasioned by splenic swelling consequent upon barbiturate anesthesia (see also Figs 6.25, 6.51, 6.77, 6.96). The costal parts of the diaphragm are sectioned and the costodiaphragmatic recesses of the pleural cavities are opened. Some lung tissue (right lung, caudal lobe) is still present ventrally and the ventral mediastinum remains intact.

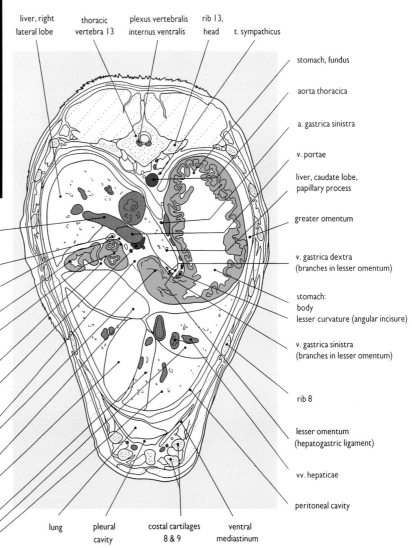

liver, right lateral lobe

thoracic vertebra 13

plexus vertebralis internus ventralis

rib 13, head

t. sympathicus

stomach, fundus

aorta thoracica

a. gastrica sinistra

v. portae

liver, caudate lobe, papillary process

greater omentum

v. portae, r. dexter

bile duct

lesser omentum (hepatoduodenal ligament)

descending duodenum

cranial duodenal flexure

greater omentum

a. hepatica, rr. hepatici

stomach: pyloric canal pyloric antrum

spleen

gall bladder

liver lobes: quadrate left lateral left medial

lung

pleural cavity

costal cartilages 8 & 9

ventral mediastinum

v. gastrica dextra (branches in lesser omentum)

stomach: body lesser curvature (angular incisure)

v. gastrica sinistra (branches in lesser omentum)

rib 8

lesser omentum (hepatogastric ligament)

vv. hepaticae

peritoneal cavity

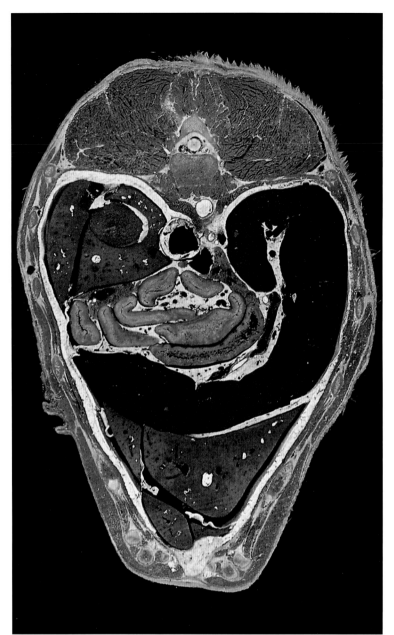

Fig. 6.96 Transverse section (3). Through the spleen, right kidney and aortic hiatus of the diaphragm: cranial view. The enormously enlarged spleen occupies considerably more of this section than would be the case normally. It is usually confined to the left side of the body, only its ventral extremity lying against the body wall close to the midventral line (see also Fig. 6.90). Ventral to the jejunum, separating its coils from the spleen, is the greater omentum. Left and right lobes of the pancreas have been cut through and the descending duodenum occupies its characteristic position against the right flank. Diaphragmatic crura are sectioned where they flank the descending aorta at the approximate position of the aortic hiatus.

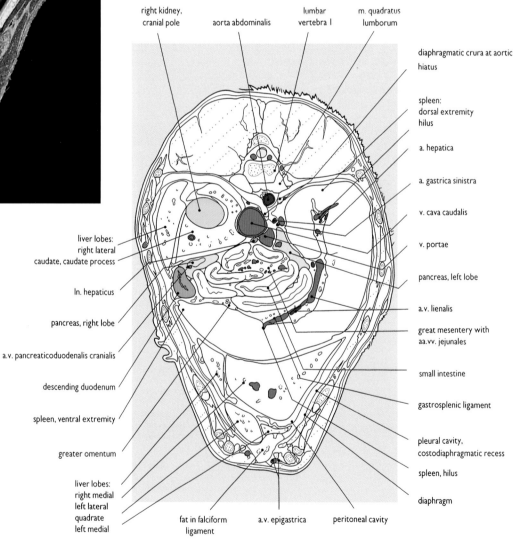

right kidney, cranial pole

aorta abdominalis

lumbar vertebra I

m. quadratus lumborum

diaphragmatic crura at aortic hiatus

spleen: dorsal extremity hilus

a. hepatica

a. gastrica sinistra

v. cava caudalis

v. portae

pancreas, left lobe

a.v. lienalis

great mesentery with aa.vv. jejunales

small intestine

gastrosplenic ligament

pleural cavity, costodiaphragmatic recess

spleen, hilus

diaphragm

liver lobes: right lateral caudate, caudate process

ln. hepaticus

pancreas, right lobe

a.v. pancreaticoduodenalis cranialis

descending duodenum

spleen, ventral extremity

greater omentum

liver lobes: right medial left lateral quadrate left medial

fat in falciform ligament

a.v. epigastrica

peritoneal cavity

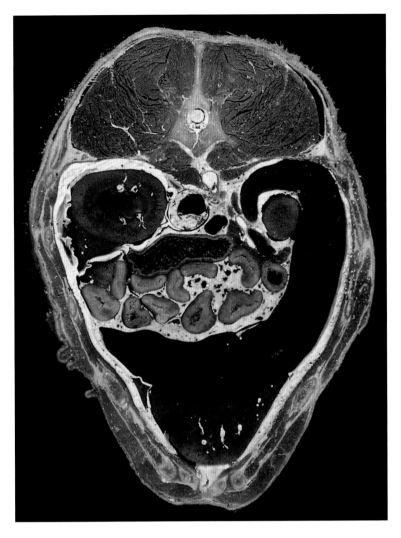

Fig. 6.97 Transverse section (4). Through the spleen, kidneys and the transverse colon: cranial view. This section still includes the greatly enlarged spleen and some remnants of the liver. Medial to the dorsal extremity of the spleen the coeliac artery is visible, as are the ganglia of the coeliacomesenteric plexus (see also Figs 6.36, 6.62). Ventral to the caudal vena cava and hepatic portal vein, the transverse colon is sectioned as it passes from right to left, 'hooking' around the cranial aspect of the mesenteric root (see also Figs 6.59, 6.81). The great mesentery supporting jejunal coils is infiltrated with fat and contains numerous jejunal vessels. The greater omentum lies ventral to the jejunum and its separation into deep and superficial laminae is apparent, the omental bursa is therefore visible.

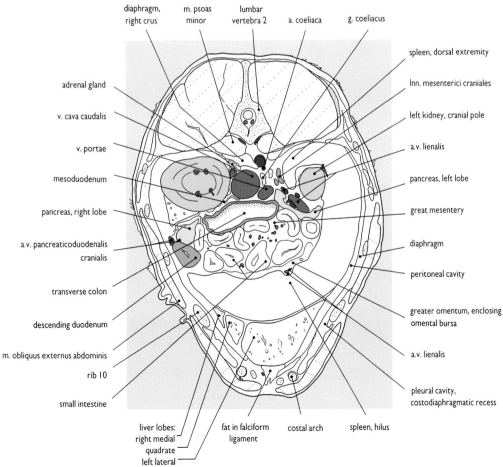

diaphragm, right crus

m. psoas minor

lumbar vertebra 2

a. coeliaca

g. coeliacus

adrenal gland

v. cava caudalis

v. portae

mesoduodenum

pancreas, right lobe

a.v. pancreaticoduodenalis cranialis

transverse colon

descending duodenum

m. obliquus externus abdominis

rib 10

small intestine

spleen, dorsal extremity

lnn. mesenterici craniales

left kidney, cranial pole

a.v. lienalis

pancreas, left lobe

great mesentery

diaphragm

peritoneal cavity

greater omentum, enclosing omental bursa

a.v. lienalis

pleural cavity, costodiaphragmatic recess

liver lobes:
right medial
quadrate
left lateral

fat in falciform ligament

costal arch

spleen, hilus

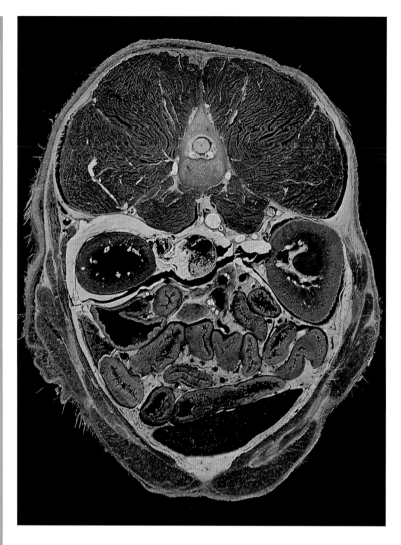

Fig. 6.98 Transverse section (5). Through the caecum and root of the great mesentery: cranial view. This section actually passes through the cranial part of the mesenteric root and cuts through mesenteric lymph nodes and the cranial mesenteric artery and vein. To the right of the root lie the ileum, caecum and ascending colon and against the right flank the descending duodenum and right lobe of the pancreas. To the left of the root lie the ascending duodenum and descending colon (see also Figs 6.80, 6.81). Apparent in this section, as it is in all the abdominal and pelvic slices, is the blue latex which has burst through one of the veins in the abdominal roof during injection and has infiltrated the peritoneal cavity quite extensively. In the sections so far (Figs 6.94–6.97) it will have been of some assistance in outlining and therefore identifying abdominal viscera. However, in this and the more caudal sections through abdomen and pelvis, the quantities of blue latex building up, especially in the abdominal roof, have become sufficient to distort relationships to some extent, and to make venous identification obscure.

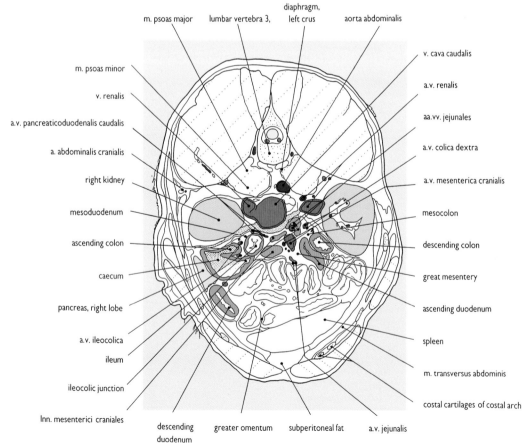

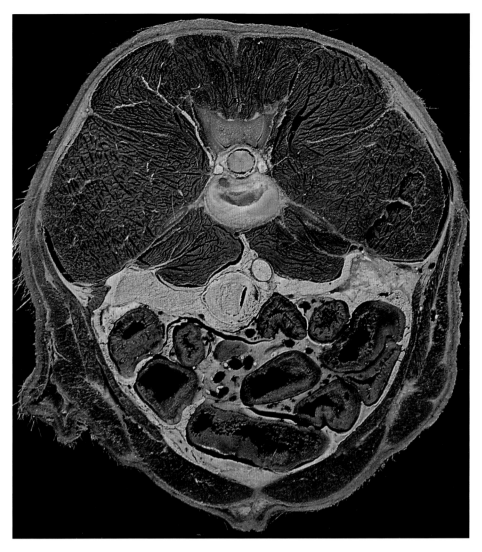

Fig. 6.99 Transverse section (6). Through the duodenal loop, jejunum, ileum and descending colon at lumbar vertebra 4: cranial view. This section passes just caudal to the mesenteric root. Consequently the ascending duodenum lies close to the midline on the left side and the ileum on the right. Further laterally the descending colon lies on the left and the descending duodenum on the right (see also Figs 6.80, 6.81 in ventral view). The section has passed through the intervertebral disc between lumbar vertebrae 3 and 4 (see also Chapter 9). Sublumbar musculature (quadratus and psoas muscles) has reached considerable proportions at this level and the abdominal aorta and caudal vena cava are sunk to some extent in the groove between muscle blocks of left and right sides. Unfortunately the excess blue latex has altered this relationship to some extent.

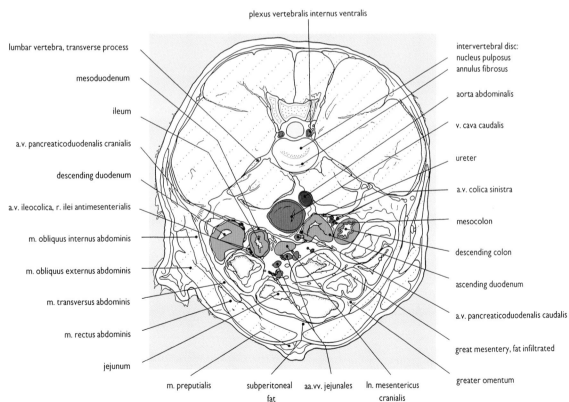

plexus vertebralis internus ventralis

lumbar vertebra, transverse process

mesoduodenum

ileum

a.v. pancreaticoduodenalis cranialis

descending duodenum

a.v. ileocolica, r. ilei antimesenterialis

m. obliquus internus abdominis

m. obliquus externus abdominis

m. transversus abdominis

m. rectus abdominis

jejunum

intervertebral disc:
nucleus pulposus
annulus fibrosus

aorta abdominalis

v. cava caudalis

ureter

a.v. colica sinistra

mesocolon

descending colon

ascending duodenum

a.v. pancreaticoduodenalis caudalis

great mesentery, fat infiltrated

greater omentum

m. preputialis   subperitoneal   aa.vv. jejunales   ln. mesentericus
                          fat   cranialis

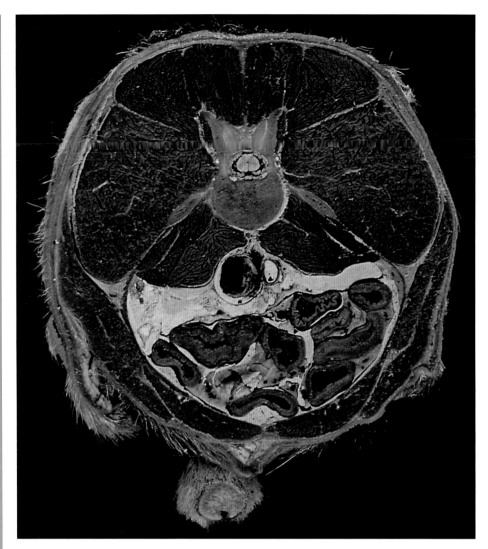

Fig. 6.100 Transverse section (7). Through the caudal duodenal flexure and descending colon at lumbar vertebra 5: cranial view. This section passes through the caudal duodenal flexure at the caudal end of the duodenal loop. Testicular blood vessels and a ureter are exposed on both sides in the abdominal root. However, the mass of blue latex has infiltrated the peritoneal cavity and has forced these structures away from their contact in life with the sublumbar muscles. The abdominal aorta and caudal vena cava are 'isolated' within this latex mass but clearly lie within the groove between sublumbar muscle blocks. Unfortunately traces of the cisterna chyli could not be positively identified in the abdominal roof of this or any of the preceding sections through the abdomen.

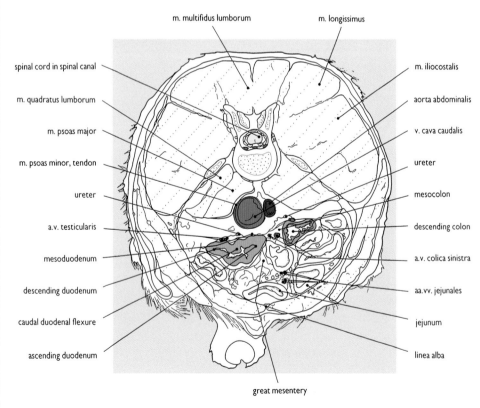

m. multifidus lumborum

m. longissimus

spinal cord in spinal canal

m. iliocostalis

m. quadratus lumborum

aorta abdominalis

m. psoas major

v. cava caudalis

m. psoas minor, tendon

ureter

ureter

mesocolon

a.v. testicularis

descending colon

mesoduodenum

a.v. colica sinistra

descending duodenum

aa.vv. jejunales

caudal duodenal flexure

jejunum

ascending duodenum

linea alba

great mesentery

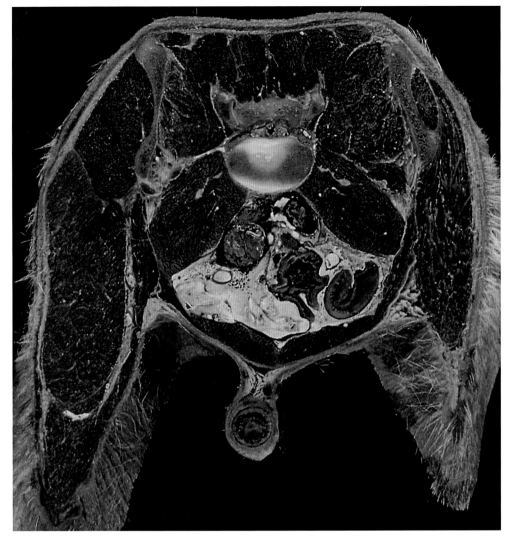

Fig. 6.101 Transverse section (8). Through lumbar vertebra 7, the iliac wings and the external iliac arteries: cranial view. This section passes through the caudal end of the abdomen. The descending colon is cut through although somewhat distorted by the mass of blue latex occupying the right side of the abdominal cavity. On the left a last remaining coil of jejunum remains in place. In the roof both internal and external iliac vessels are displayed with a single hypogastric lymph node dorsal to the descending colon. Both ureters are visible although the left is considerably displaced by the leaked latex. In the belly wall the rectus abdominis muscles are particularly prominent with caudal epigastric vessels on their internal surfaces (see also Figs 6.20, 6.46). Superficial epigastric vessels are visible in the superficial abdominal fascia dorsal to the penis. The section through the penis passes through the more cranial part of the penile body and displays the pars longa glandis surrounding an os penis. The sectioned prepuce surrounds a preputial cavity.

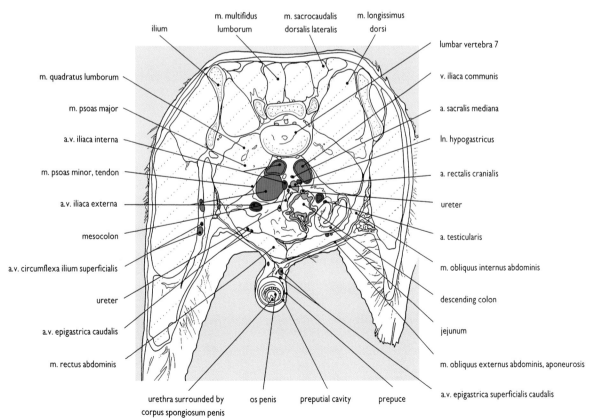

ilium — m. multifidus lumborum — m. sacrocaudalis dorsalis lateralis — m. longissimus dorsi

lumbar vertebra 7

m. quadratus lumborum

v. iliaca communis

m. psoas major

a. sacralis mediana

a.v. iliaca interna

ln. hypogastricus

m. psoas minor, tendon

a. rectalis cranialis

a.v. iliaca externa

ureter

mesocolon

a. testicularis

a.v. circumflexa ilium superficialis

m. obliquus internus abdominis

ureter

descending colon

a.v. epigastrica caudalis

jejunum

m. rectus abdominis

m. obliquus externus abdominis, aponeurosis

a.v. epigastrica superficialis caudalis

urethra surrounded by corpus spongiosum penis — os penis — preputial cavity — prepuce

7. THE HINDLIMB

The hindlimb has gluteal, perineal, thigh, knee or stifle, crural, tarsal, metatarsal and phalangeal regions. Bony prominences are readily identifiable: these include the cranial dorsal iliac spine, the greater trochanter and the ischiatic tuberosity. An assessment of the relative positions of left and right hindlimbs allows assessment of fractures of the ossa coxae or hip dislocation. The once thought hereditary condition of hip dysplasia is now thought to be multifactorial in origin, resulting in an overall incongruity of the hip joint rather than just the lack of a proper acetabulum. The degree of abnormality can be assessed by placing the animal in dorsal recumbency and then abducting stifles to see how far they approach the horizontal i.e. the amount of congruency in the hip joint. The Ortalani sign is also used and in this the animal is laid on its side, the stifle abducted and proximal pressure is applied to the hip – the hip can be felt to click as it pops back into the acetabulum.

Where there is complete instability of the joint, several repair techniques are available. These include total hip replacement, triple pelvic osteotomy, Steinman pins and femoral head and neck excision arthroplasty. This technique is used for repairing long-standing or recurrent dislocations of the hip joint. Incisions are made over the greater trochanter and continue distally over the femur to the mid-shaft region.

The first stage in helping hip dysplasia used to be pectineal myotomy, when a piece of pectineus muscle was removed from each side thereby reducing the adductor forces on the legs. This is rarely used nowadays. In a dorsal surgical approach to the hip joint, it is necessary to section the tendons of insertion of the gluteal muscles taking care not to damage the sciatic nerve (which lies alongside the sacrotuberous ligament). In essence, there is a curved incision over the gluteal muscles just cranial to the greater trochanter with dissection between the middle gluteal and the tensor fasciae latae to create a triangle to work in. Nowadays, many dogs are treated medically using NSAIDs, correct nutrition (particularly in large, young dogs), weight control, glucosamine chondroitin and appropriate exercise.

Major trauma can occur to the stifle (knee) joint in that the joint is very easily damaged when dogs turn with one hind leg on the ground and all the weight (i.e. torque) on this leg. This may result in damage to menisci, but it is usually the medial meniscus (classic bucket handle type of tear) in the joint or particularly the collateral ligaments or cranial cruciate ligaments that are damaged. The cranial cruciate in the femoropatellar joint is the most likely casualty. It is the result of too much movement in the fibia in relation to the stabilized femur.

One can grasp the femur and the tibia and if there is too much forward movement it indicates rupture of the cranial cruciate ligament. Too much caudal movement indicates that it is the caudal cruciate ligament. Caudal cruciate problems are rarely recognized. The main tests to assess the joint stability are direct cranial drawer and tibial compression. The cranial cruciate ligament is repaired by many different methods but the most likely one is the use of extra-capsule sutures.

Surgical repair of fractures of femur is by incising along the fusion of the fasciae latae and caudal edge of biceps femoris muscles. A combination of pins, coerciage wires, external fixators and particularly bone plates may be used. Pins are inserted normograde through the trochanteric fossa or retrograde. There are a number of different methods depending on the nature of the fracture.

Patella luxation may occur in small breeds and in these it is usually lateral, whereas the medial luxation may occur in larger breeds but less commonly. In these cases repair is by deepening the trochlear groove and moving the tibial tuberosity and then tightening the lateral patellar ligaments. This technique of tibial crest transplantation is used for medial luxation of the patella but there are many other techniques. including groove deepening or tightening of the joint. There are many anatomical causes of this condition including varus deformity, bowing of the distal femur, medial condyle hypoplasia and shallow trochlear sulcus.

The tibial crest has its own centre of ossification separated from the body of the tibia by a growth plate and it can be pulled off by the straight patellar ligament. If this is so, it may require screwing back into place. The calcaneal tuberosity also has its own centre of ossification with a separate epiphyseal line and can then be pulled off, as the common calcaneal tendon inserts here.

The lymph nodes associated with the hindlimb are not normally palpable. Rostral to the hindlimb, the subiliac (prefemoral) drains the lateral region of the hip and thigh. The popliteal, situated between the heads of the gastrocnemius, is more important in draining the lower limb. Infection or neoplasia will make both lymph nodes more easily palpable.

The lateral saphenous vein can be used for blood sample collection if necessary. The pulse can be taken from the femoral artery in the femoral triangle which comprises the femoral artery and vein and saphenous nerve.

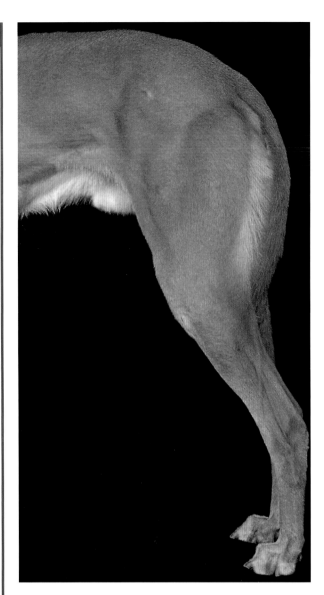

Fig. 7.1 Surface features of the hindlimb: left lateral view. The palpable bony prominences of the hindlimb are shown in this picture. In addition the position of a number of muscles that are readily palpable and/or whose outlines are clearly visible are shown. Although nonpalpable from the surface, the position of the hip joint is indicated by the greater trochanter of the femur which lies lateral to it. In the lower part of the leg the common calcaneal tendon is a well-defined cord terminating on the calcaneal tuberosity ('point of the hock'). Its three components – gastrocnemius tendon, superficial digital flexor tendon, and accessory tendon from the hamstring muscles – might be distinguishable if the paw is raised, removing tension from the tendon. Fig. 7.1A shows the main topographical regions of the hindlimb based on internal osteological components: the subsidiary topographical regions are related to the underlying joints between segments.

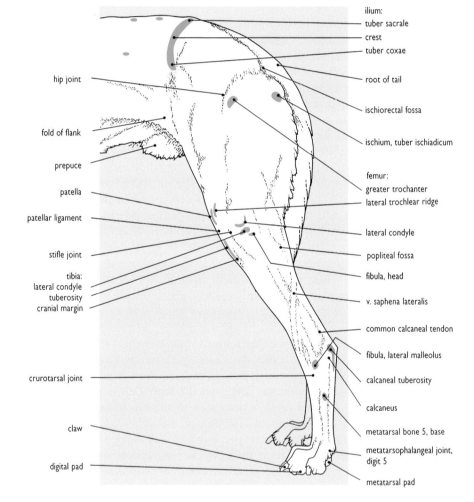

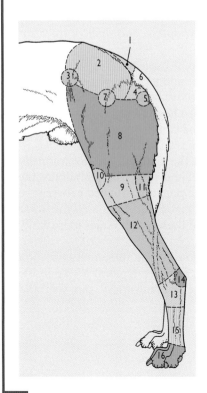

Fig. 7.1A Topographical regions of the hindlimb: left lateral view. **1–6** Pelvic Regions. **1** Sacral Region. **2** Gluteal Region. **3** Coxal Tuber Region. **4** Ischiorectal Fossa. **5** Ischiadic Tuber Region. **6** Caudal Region. **7** Hip Joint Region. **8** Femoral Region. **9** Genual (Stifle Joint) Region. **10** Patellar Region. **11** Popliteal Region. **12** Crural Region. **13** Tarsal Region. **14** Calcaneal Region. **15** Metatarsal Region. **16** Phalangeal (Digital) Region.

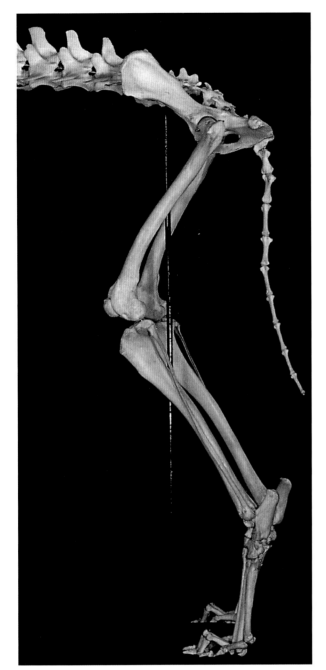

Fig. 7.2 Skeleton of the hindlimb: left lateral view. The palpable bony features shown in the surface view in Fig. 7.1 are colored in the drawing. The adjacent bones of the vertebral column are included in the picture to show the topographical relationships between the two in the normal standing posture. Unlike the forelimb there is a firm bony union between hindlimb and trunk – left and right pelvic bones are joined in a pelvic girdle which is united with the vertebral column through strong sacroiliac joints situated caudomedial to the sacral tuberosities. Each pelvic bone has four developmental components fusing at an early age (2–3 months). The three obvious components (ilium, ischium and pubis) each have palpable features shown here. The fourth component (acetabular bone) is small and located within the acetabular fossa of the hip joint.

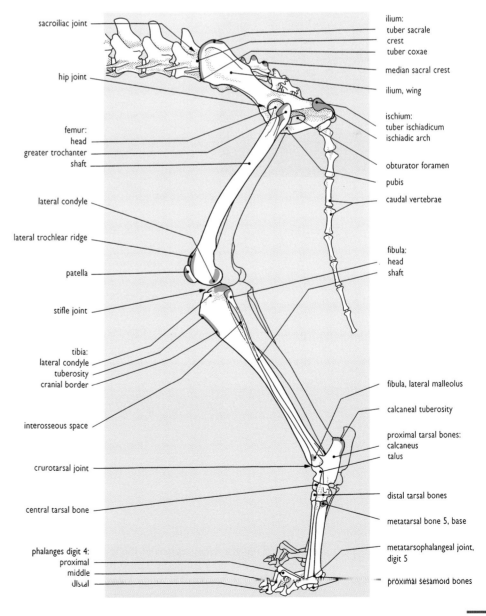

sacroiliac joint

hip joint

femur:
head
greater trochanter
shaft

lateral condyle

lateral trochlear ridge

patella

stifle joint

tibia:
lateral condyle
tuberosity
cranial border

interosseous space

crurotarsal joint

central tarsal bone

phalanges digit 4:
proximal
middle
distal

ilium:
tuber sacrale
crest
tuber coxae

median sacral crest

ilium, wing

ischium:
tuber ischiadicum
ischiadic arch

obturator foramen

pubis

caudal vertebrae

fibula:
head
shaft

fibula, lateral malleolus

calcaneal tuberosity

proximal tarsal bones:
calcaneus
talus

distal tarsal bones

metatarsal bone 5, base

metatarsophalangeal joint,
digit 5

proximal sesamoid bones

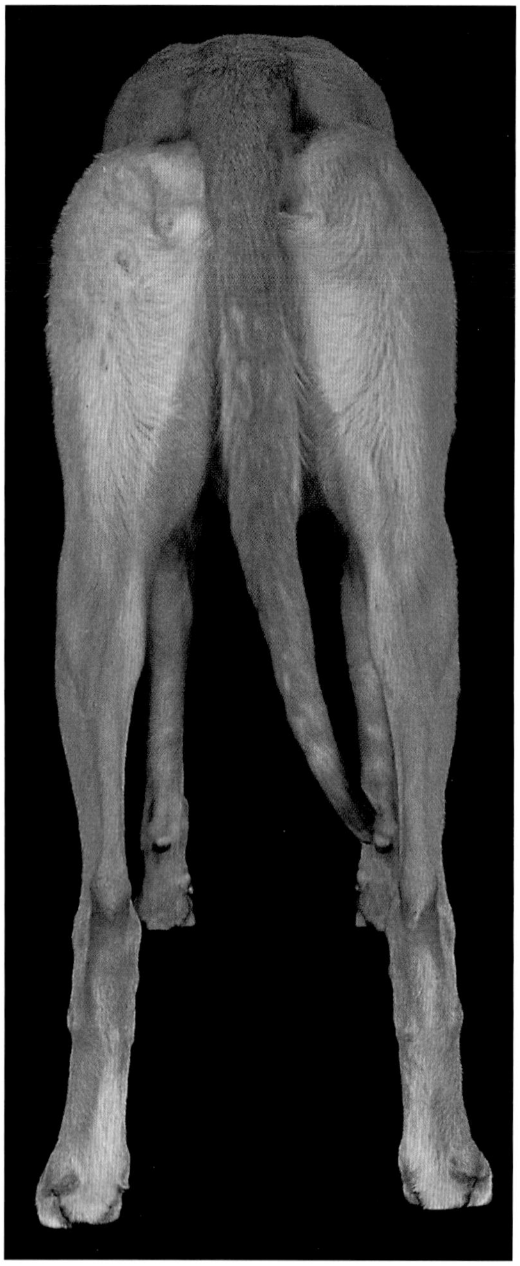

Fig. 7.3 Surface features of the hindlimb: caudal view. The major palpable bony features and topographical regions already noticed in the lateral view of the limb are shown again as reference points and are indicated in the drawing. One or two additional bony prominences palpable on the medial aspect of the limb are also shown. The ischiorectal fossa is a clearly visible and palpable depression lateral to the root of the tail. Lying alongside the anal canal it is normally padded out with fat and would not be quite as readily apparent as it is in the greyhound. A second clearly visible and palpable depression, the popliteal fossa, is caudal to the stifle joint between the diverging lower ends of the hamstring muscles. The large popliteal lymph node can be felt within the fossa. Fig. 7.3A shows the main topographical regions of the hindlimb.

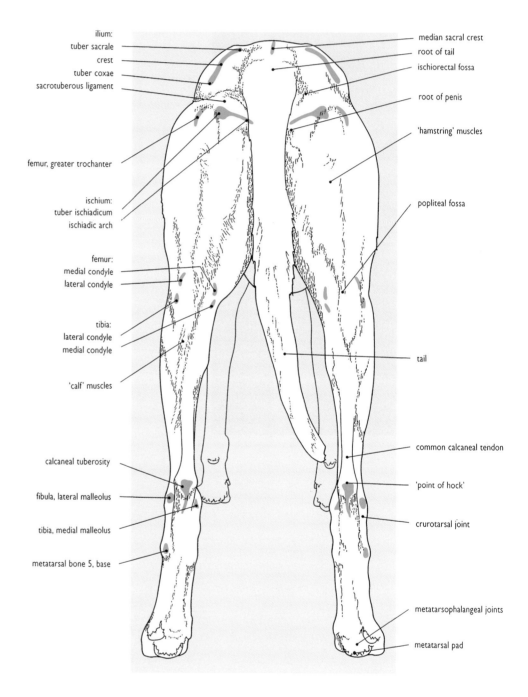

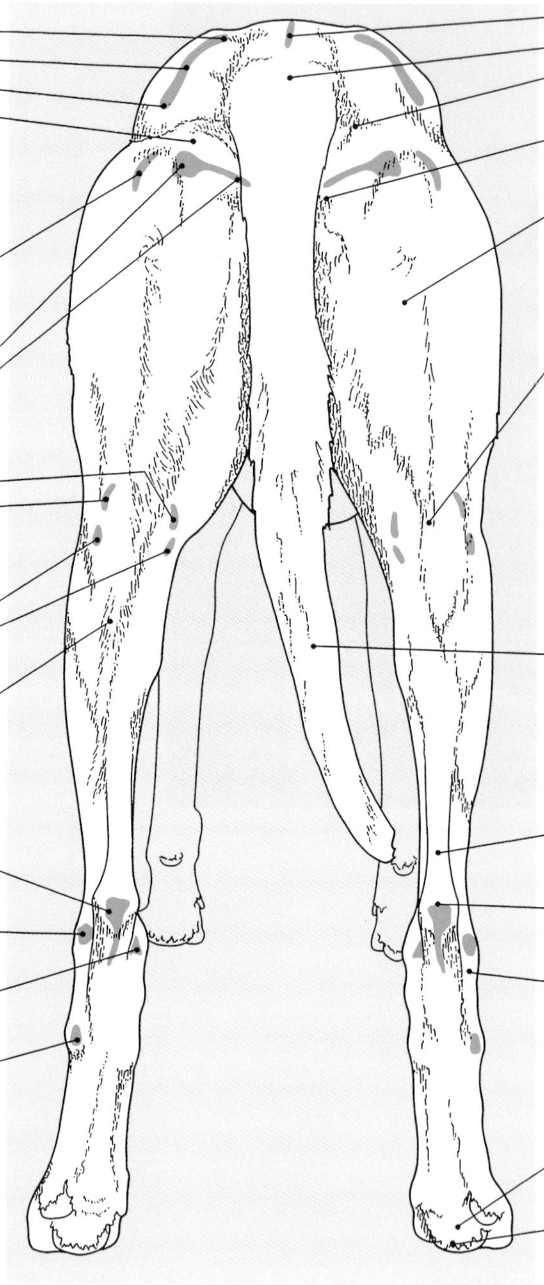
ilium:
tuber sacrale
crest
tuber coxae
sacrotuberous ligament
femur, greater trochanter
ischium:
tuber ischiadicum
ischiadic arch
femur:
medial condyle
lateral condyle
tibia:
lateral condyle
medial condyle
'calf' muscles
calcaneal tuberosity
fibula, lateral malleolus
tibia, medial malleolus
metatarsal bone 5, base
median sacral crest
root of tail
ischiorectal fossa
root of penis
'hamstring' muscles
popliteal fossa
tail
common calcaneal tendon
'point of hock'
crurotarsal joint
metatarsophalangeal joints
metatarsal pad

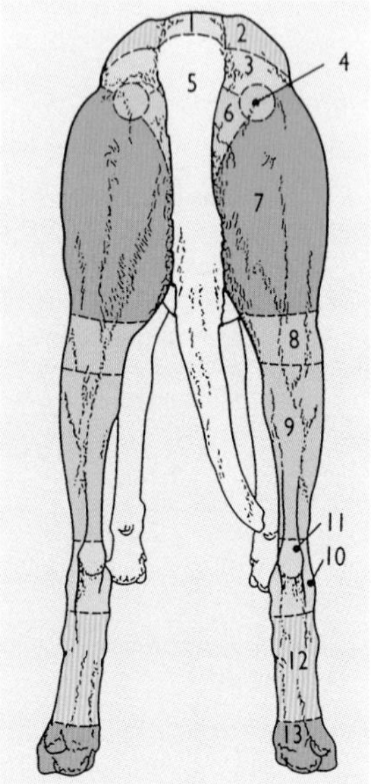
2
3
4
5
6
7
8
9
11
10
12
13

Fig. 7.3A Topographical regions of the hindlimb: caudal view. **1–6** Pelvic Regions. **1** Sacral Region. **2** Gluteal Region. **3** Ischiorectal Fossa. **4** Ischiadic Tuber Region. **5** Caudal Region. **6** Perineal Region. **7** Femoral Region. **8** Popliteal Region. **9** Crural Region. **10** Tarsal Region. **11** Calcaneal Region. **12** Metatarsal Region. **13** Phalangeal (Digital) Region.

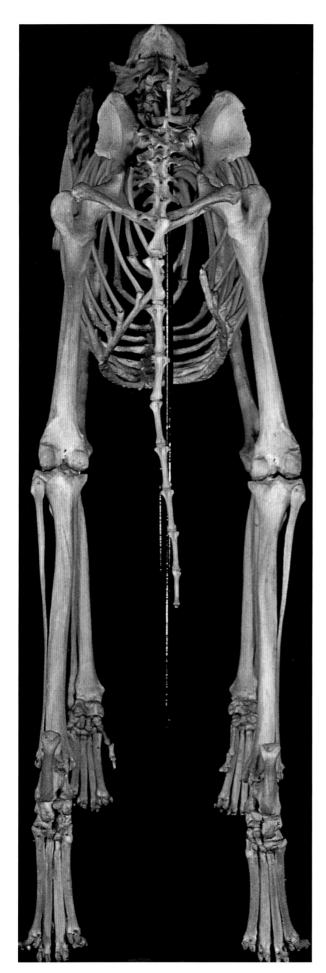

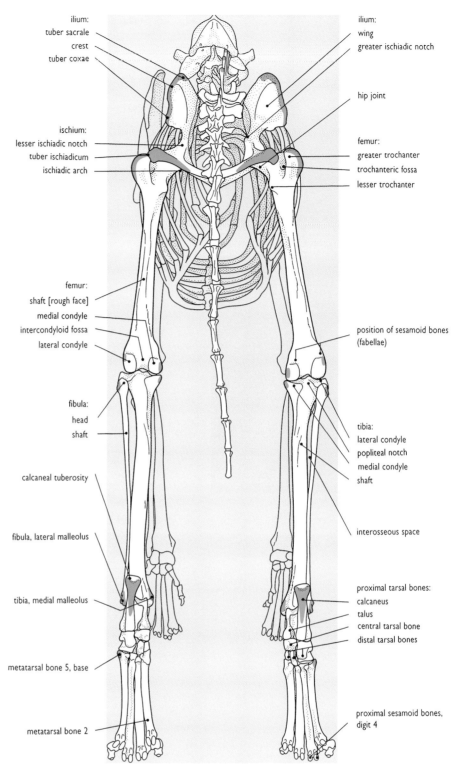

ilium:
tuber sacrale
crest
tuber coxae

ilium:
wing
greater ischiadic notch

hip joint

ischium:
lesser ischiadic notch
tuber ischiadicum
ischiadic arch

femur:
greater trochanter
trochanteric fossa
lesser trochanter

femur:
shaft [rough face]
medial condyle
intercondyloid fossa
lateral condyle

position of sesamoid bones
(fabellae)

fibula:
head
shaft

tibia:
lateral condyle
popliteal notch
medial condyle
shaft

calcaneal tuberosity

interosseous space

fibula, lateral malleolus

tibia, medial malleolus

proximal tarsal bones:
calcaneus
talus
central tarsal bone
distal tarsal bones

metatarsal bone 5, base

metatarsal bone 2

proximal sesamoid bones,
digit 4

Fig. 7.4 Skeleton of the hindlimb: caudal view. The palpable bony features shown on the surface view are colored in the drawing. In this skeletal preparation the fabellae – sesamoid bones located in the gastrocnemius muscle tendons caudal to the stifle joints – have been lost. The position they would have occupied is shown by smooth articular facets on the caudodorsal aspect of the prominent femoral condyles, and they are clearly displayed radiographically in Fig. 7.10. In the crural region the tibia and much reduced fibula lie side by side, an arrangement in marked contrast to the forearm where radius and ulna, equally well developed, cross over one another. The limited degree of mobility that this forearm orientation imparts to the forepaw is completely lacking in the hindpaw.

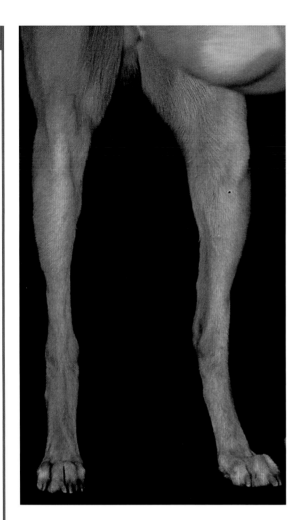

Fig. 7.5 Surface features of the hindlimb: cranial view. The major palpable bony features already noticed in lateral and caudal views are shown again as reference points and are indicated in the drawing. In addition, much of the medial surface of the tibia is subcutaneous from medial tibial condyle at its proximal end down to medial malleolus at its distal end. The position of the crurotarsal joint is identifiable since the ridges and grooves of the trochlea of the talus are palpable alongside the tarsal flexor and digital extensor tendons. Slightly farther distally pulsation within the dorsal pedal artery may be felt at the base of the metatarsal region towards the medial side. Fig. 7.5A shows the main topographical regions of the hindlimb.

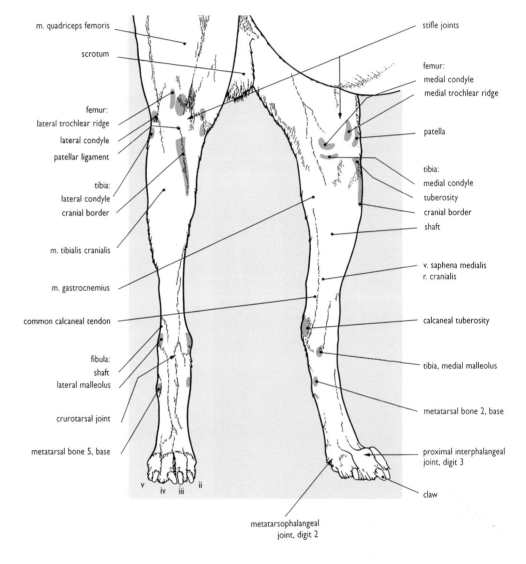

m. quadriceps femoris

scrotum

femur:
lateral trochlear ridge
lateral condyle
patellar ligament

tibia:
lateral condyle
cranial border

m. tibialis cranialis

m. gastrocnemius

common calcaneal tendon

fibula:
shaft
lateral malleolus

crurotarsal joint

metatarsal bone 5, base

metatarsophalangeal
joint, digit 2

stifle joints

femur:
medial condyle
medial trochlear ridge

patella

tibia:
medial condyle
tuberosity
cranial border
shaft

v. saphena medialis
r. cranialis

calcaneal tuberosity

tibia, medial malleolus

metatarsal bone 2, base

proximal interphalangeal
joint, digit 3

claw

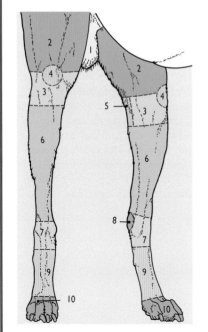

Fig. 7.5A Topographical regions of the hindlimb: cranial view. **1** Perineal (Scrotal) Region. **2** Femoral Region. **3** Genual (Stifle Joint) Region. **4** Patellar Region. **5** Popliteal Region. **6** Crural Region. **7** Tarsal Region. **8** Calcaneal Region. **9** Metatarsal Region. **10** Phalangeal (Digital) Region.

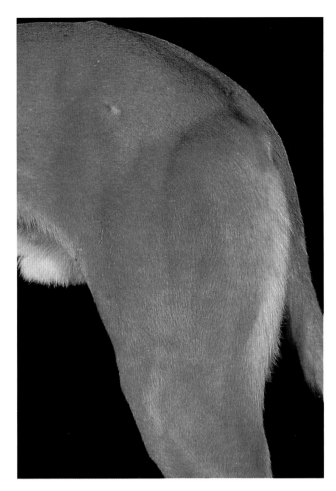

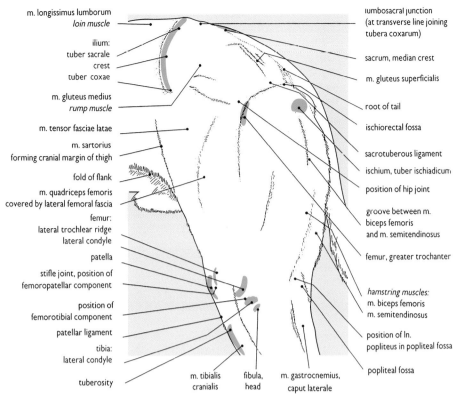

m. longissimus lumborum
loin muscle

ilium:
tuber sacrale
crest
tuber coxae

m. gluteus medius
rump muscle

m. tensor fasciae latae

m. sartorius
forming cranial margin of thigh

fold of flank

m. quadriceps femoris
covered by lateral femoral fascia

femur:
lateral trochlear ridge
lateral condyle

patella

stifle joint, position of
femoropatellar component

position of
femorotibial component

patellar ligament

tibia:
lateral condyle

tuberosity

m. tibialis
cranialis

fibula,
head

m. gastrocnemius,
caput laterale

lumbosacral junction
(at transverse line joining
tubera coxarum)

sacrum, median crest

m. gluteus superficialis

root of tail

ischiorectal fossa

sacrotuberous ligament

ischium, tuber ischiadicum

position of hip joint

groove between m.
biceps femoris
and m. semitendinosus

femur, greater trochanter

hamstring muscles:
m. biceps femoris
m. semitendinosus

position of ln.
popliteus in popliteal fossa

popliteal fossa

Fig. 7.6 Surface features of pelvic and femoral regions: left lateral view. Palpable and visible features are indicated.

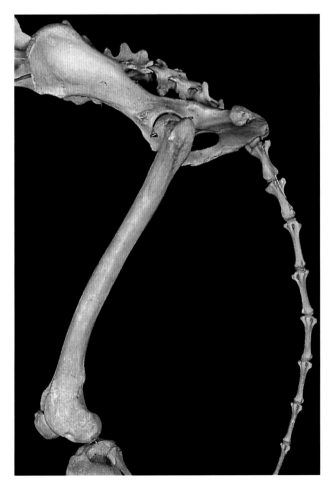

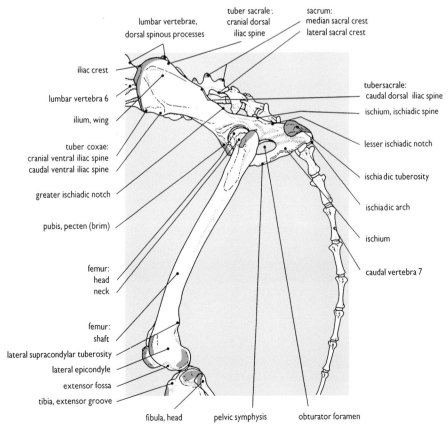

lumbar vertebrae,
dorsal spinous processes

tuber sacrale:
cranial dorsal
iliac spine

sacrum:
median sacral crest
lateral sacral crest

iliac crest

lumbar vertebra 6

ilium, wing

tuber coxae:
cranial ventral iliac spine
caudal ventral iliac spine

greater ischiadic notch

pubis, pecten (brim)

femur:
head
neck

femur:
shaft

lateral supracondylar tuberosity

lateral epicondyle

extensor fossa

tibia, extensor groove

tubersacrale:
caudal dorsal iliac spine

ischium, ischiadic spine

lesser ischiadic notch

ischiadic tuberosity

ischiadic arch

ischium

caudal vertebra 7

fibula, head

pelvic symphysis

obturator foramen

Fig. 7.7 Skeleton of pelvic and femoral regions. left lateral view. The features colored green correspond to the palpable bony features shown in Fig. 7.6.

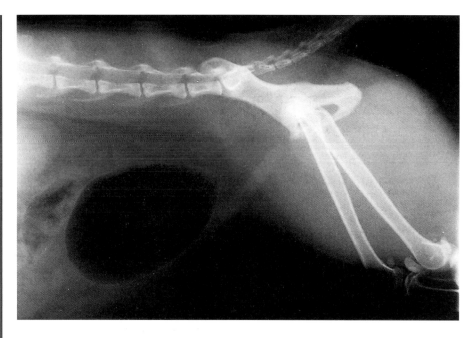

Fig. 7.8 Radiograph of the pelvis and hip joint: left lateral view. The hip joint and pelvis in lateral view is potentially of less anatomical value than the ventrodorsal view (fig. 7.9) since the femoral heads and hip joints are superimposed. However, such a view as this with the hindlimbs pulled caudally demonstrates the considerable overall mobility available to the hindlimbs. This is the sum total of movements at the caudal lumbar, lumbosacral and sacroiliac joints as well as the hip joints themselves.

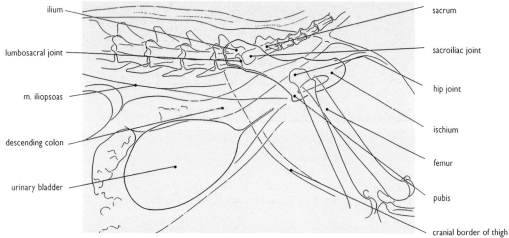

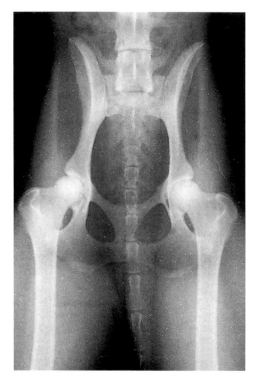

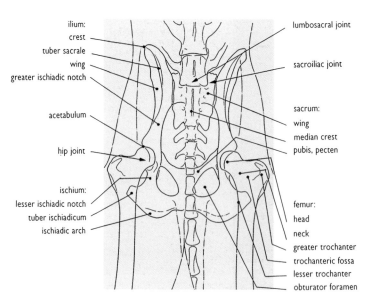

Fig. 7.9 Radiograph of the pelvis and hip joints: ventrodorsal view. The hip joint has a more fully enclosed femoral head in an extensive acetabular fossa than is seen in the shoulder joint. The acetabulum is deepened further by a fibrocartilaginous rim (radiolucent and so not apparent). Hip movement is potentially considerable; here both hindlegs have been pulled caudally, placing the hip joints in extreme extension. This radiographic position is often used to assess the hip joints for dysplasia.

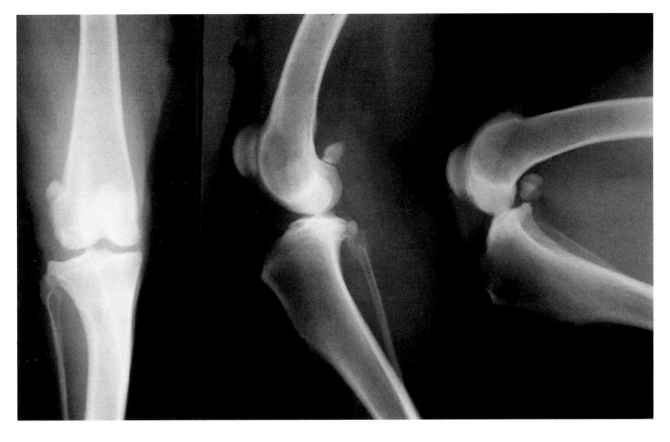

(a)   (b)   (c)

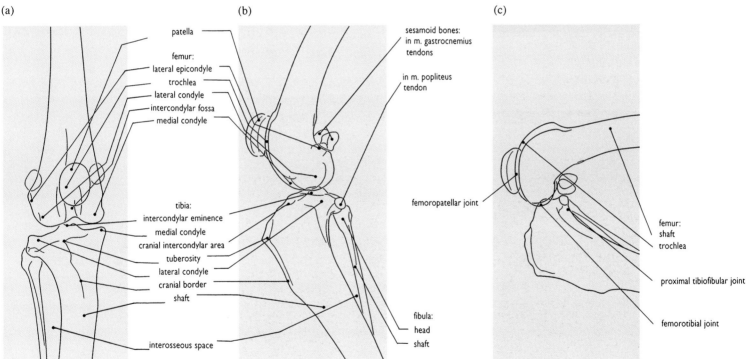

Fig. 7.10 Radiographs of the stifle joint: craniocaudal and lateral views. The major osteological features of the stifle joint are shown in these three radiographs. In the craniocaudal view (a) the composite nature of the joint is clearly shown. In the lateral view the stifle joint is extended (b) and in the normal standing position highlighting the restricted area of contact between femoral and tibial condyles. The marked incongruity of joint surfaces is rendered more congruent by the paired meniscal cartilages which are radiolucent. The patellar tendon although palpable as a firm almost bone-like surface feature, is not radio-opaque, just like the parapatellar fibrocartilages engaging on the lips of the femoral trochlea. The paired fabellae (absent from the skeletal pictures) are visible at the rear of the joint, as is the small sesamoid bone in the popliteal muscle tendon. Stifle joint flexion (c) and extension is regulated by a pair of cruciate ligaments lying in the centre of the joint between the condyles. Like the meniscal cartilages they are radiolucent and hence invisible.

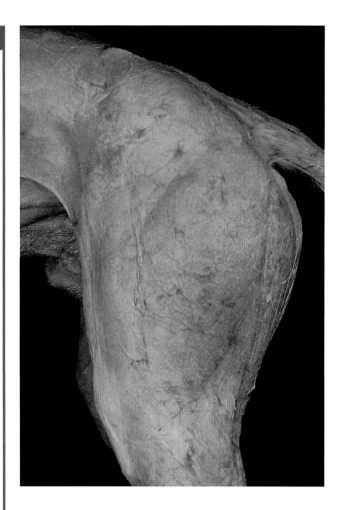

Fig. 7.11 Superficial fascia of rump and thigh: left lateral view. Only the skin has been removed. The superficial gluteal fascia and the superficial lateral fascia of the thigh are continuous with the superficial fascia of the trunk and with the superficial coccygeal fascia over the tail. The superficial and deep fascia are united over the biceps femoris muscle. The deep gluteal fascia is thick and firmly covers the middle gluteal muscle. The gluteal fascia continues as the strong lateral femoral fascia, or fascia lata, over the lateral thigh. The aponeurosis of the tensor fasciae latae creates a two-leaved fascia lata for some distance. The fascia lata is continuous with the medial femoral fascia. The deep femoral fascia is attached to the lateral and medial lips of the femur as well as to the patella and to the condyles of the femur. Fat is contained within the ischiorectal fossa.

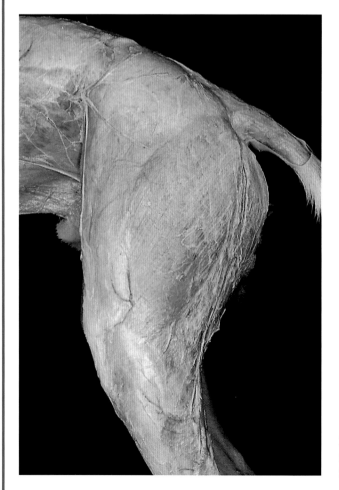

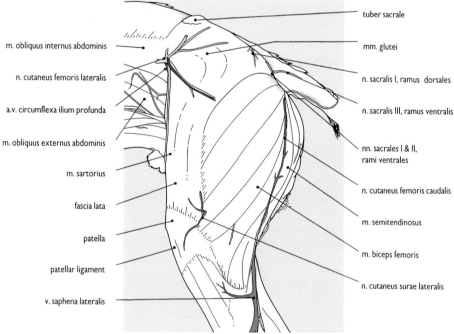

m. obliquus internus abdominis

n. cutaneus femoris lateralis

a.v. circumflexa ilium profunda

m. obliquus externus abdominis

m. sartorius

fascia lata

patella

patellar ligament

v. saphena lateralis

tuber sacrale

mm. glutei

n. sacralis I, ramus dorsales

n. sacralis III, ramus ventralis

nn. sacrales I & II, rami ventrales

n. cutaneus femoris caudalis

m. semitendinosus

m. biceps femoris

n. cutaneus surae lateralis

Fig. 7.12 Superficial structures of rump and thigh: left lateral view. Some clearing of superficial fascia has exposed superficial nerves and blood vessels. All of the deep fascia is intact.

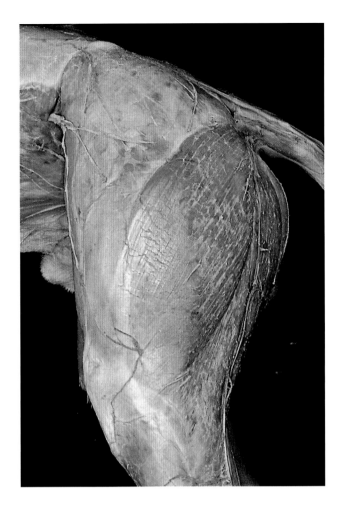

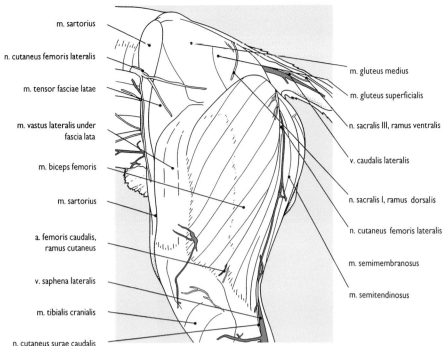

m. sartorius
n. cutaneus femoris lateralis
m. tensor fasciae latae
m. vastus lateralis under fascia lata
m. biceps femoris
m. sartorius
a. femoris caudalis, ramus cutaneus
v. saphena lateralis
m. tibialis cranialis
n. cutaneus surae caudalis

m. gluteus medius
m. gluteus superficialis
n. sacralis III, ramus ventralis
v. caudalis lateralis
n. sacralis I, ramus dorsalis
n. cutaneus femoris lateralis
m. semimembranosus
m. semitendinosus

Fig. 7.13 Superficial muscles and deep fascia of rump and thigh: left lateral view. All of the superficial fascia and associated fat has been removed.

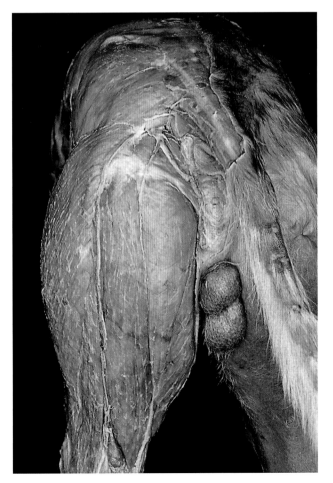

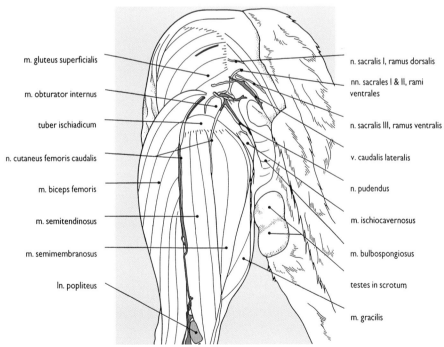

m. gluteus superficialis
m. obturator internus
tuber ischiadicum
n. cutaneus femoris caudalis
m. biceps femoris
m. semitendinosus
m. semimembranosus
ln. popliteus

n. sacralis I, ramus dorsalis
nn. sacrales I & II, rami ventrales
n. sacralis III, ramus ventralis
v. caudalis lateralis
n. pudendus
m. ischiocavernosus
m. bulbospongiosus
testes in scrotum
m. gracilis

Fig. 7.14 Superficial muscles of left rump and thigh: caudal view. Fat has been removed from the ischiorectal fossa to expose many small nerves and blood vessels. The superficial position of the popliteal lymph node may also be seen.

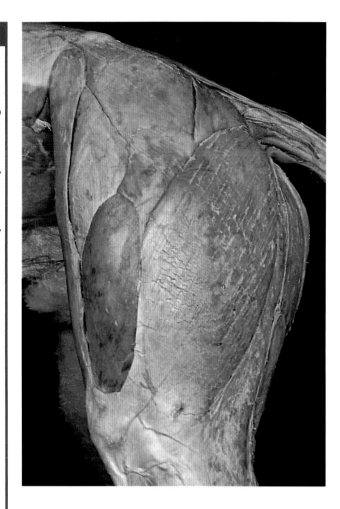

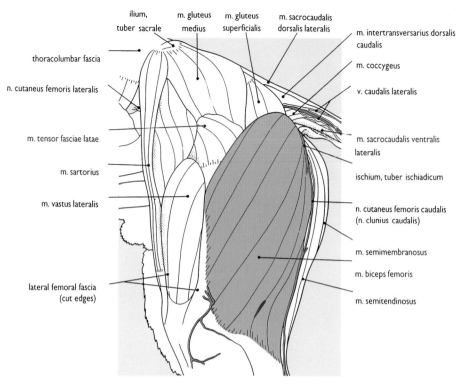

ilium, tuber sacrale
m. gluteus medius
m. gluteus superficialis
m. sacrocaudalis dorsalis lateralis
m. intertransversarius dorsalis caudalis

thoracolumbar fascia

n. cutaneus femoris lateralis

m. coccygeus

v. caudalis lateralis

m. tensor fasciae latae

m. sartorius

m. sacrocaudalis ventralis lateralis

ischium, tuber ischiadicum

m. vastus lateralis

n. cutaneus femoris caudalis (n. clunius caudalis)

m. semimembranosus

m. biceps femoris

lateral femoral fascia (cut edges)

m. semitendinosus

Fig. 7.15 Rump and thigh after removal of gluteal fascia and the exposed lateral femoral fascia: left lateral view. Superficial nerves and blood vessels have also been removed.

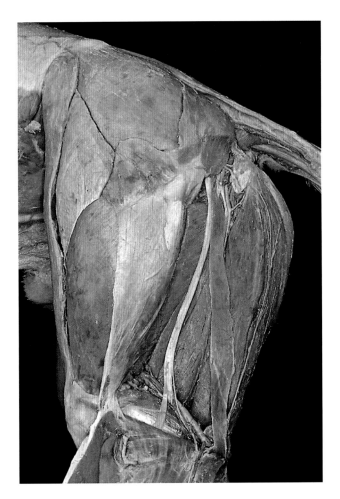

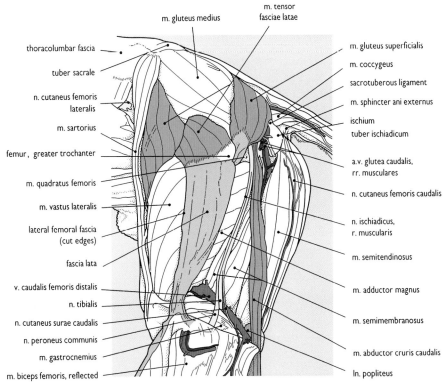

m. gluteus medius
m. tensor fasciae latae

thoracolumbar fascia
tuber sacrale
n. cutaneus femoris lateralis
m. sartorius
femur, greater trochanter
m. quadratus femoris
m. vastus lateralis
lateral femoral fascia (cut edges)
fascia lata
v. caudalis femoris distalis
n. tibialis
n. cutaneus surae caudalis
n. peroneus communis
m. gastrocnemius
m. biceps femoris, reflected

m. gluteus superficialis
m. coccygeus
sacrotuberous ligament
m. sphincter ani externus
ischium tuber ischiadicum
a.v. glutea caudalis, rr. musculares
n. cutaneus femoris caudalis
n. ischiadicus, r. muscularis
m. semitendinosus
m. adductor magnus
m. semimembranosus
m. abductor cruris caudalis
ln. popliteus

Fig. 7.16 Rump and thigh after reflection of biceps femoris muscle: left lateral view. Biceps femoris muscle has been reflected distally leaving the caudal crural abductor muscle in position. The large sciatic nerve is now exposed.

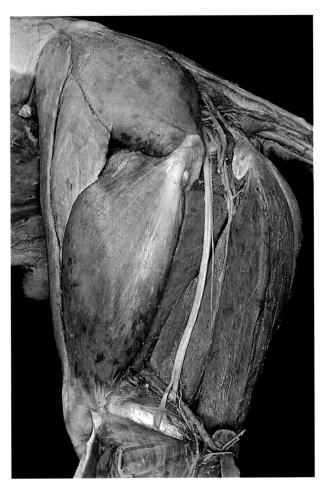

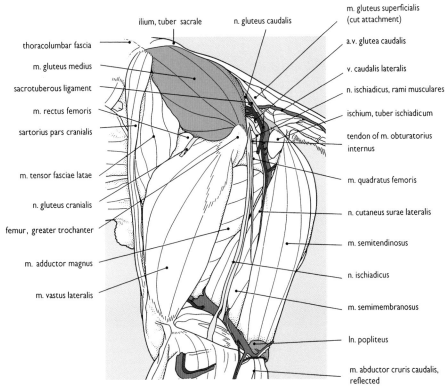

ilium, tuber sacrale
n. gluteus caudalis

thoracolumbar fascia
m. gluteus medius
sacrotuberous ligament
m. rectus femoris
sartorius pars cranialis
m. tensor fasciae latae
n. gluteus cranialis
femur, greater trochanter
m. adductor magnus
m. vastus lateralis

m. gluteus superficialis (cut attachment)
a.v. glutea caudalis
v. caudalis lateralis
n. ischiadicus, rami musculares
ischium, tuber ischiadicum
tendon of m. obturatorius internus
m. quadratus femoris
n. cutaneus surae lateralis
m. semitendinosus
n. ischiadicus
m. semimembranosus
ln. popliteus
m. abductor cruris caudalis, reflected

Fig. 7.17 Rump and thigh after removal of the superficial gluteal muscle and the remaining fascia lata: left lateral view. The caudal crural abductor muscle has also been reflected distally. The sacrotuberous ligament can now be seen.

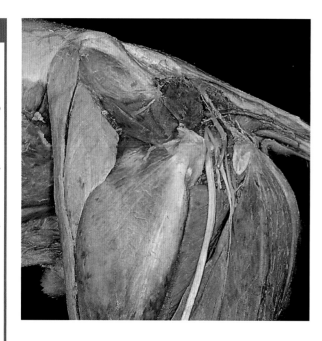

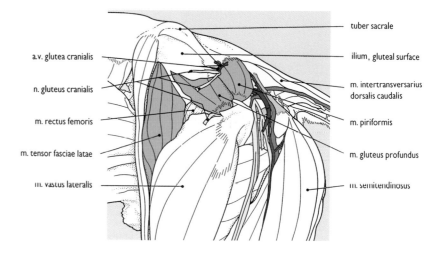

a.v. glutea cranialis

n. gluteus cranialis

m. rectus femoris

m. tensor fasciae latae

m. vastus lateralis

tuber sacrale

ilium, gluteal surface

m. intertransversarius dorsalis caudalis

m. piriformis

m. gluteus profundus

m. semitendinosus

Fig. 7.18 Rump and proximal thigh after removal of the middle gluteal muscle: left lateral view. The deep gluteal muscle is now exposed.

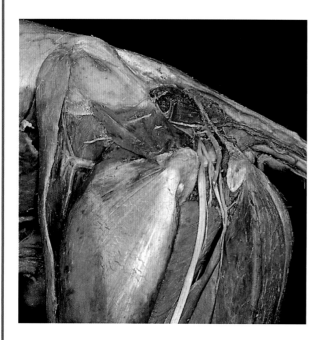

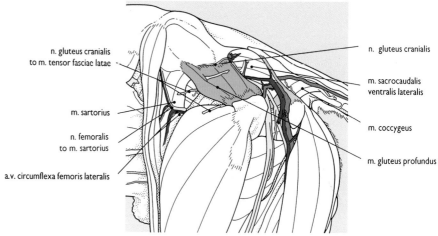

n. gluteus cranialis
to m. tensor fasciae latae

m. sartorius

n. femoralis
to m. sartorius

a.v. circumflexa femoris lateralis

n. gluteus cranialis

m. sacrocaudalis ventralis lateralis

m. coccygeus

m. gluteus profundus

Fig. 7.19 Rump and proximal thigh after removal of the tensor fasciae latae and piriformis muscles: left lateral view.

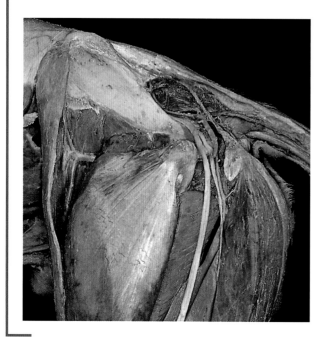

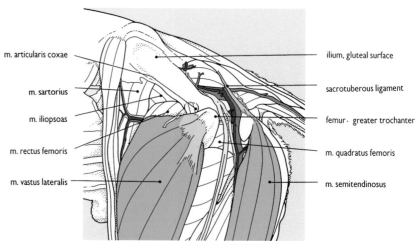

m. articularis coxae

m. sartorius

m. iliopsoas

m. rectus femoris

m. vastus lateralis

ilium, gluteal surface

sacrotuberous ligament

femur, greater trochanter

m. quadratus femoris

m. semitendinosus

Fig. 7.20 Rump and proximal thigh after removal of the deep gluteal muscle: left lateral view.

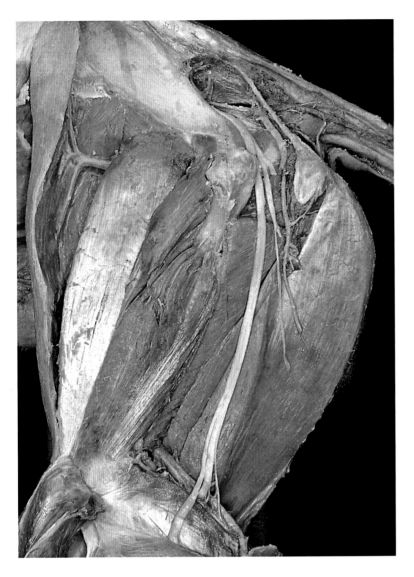

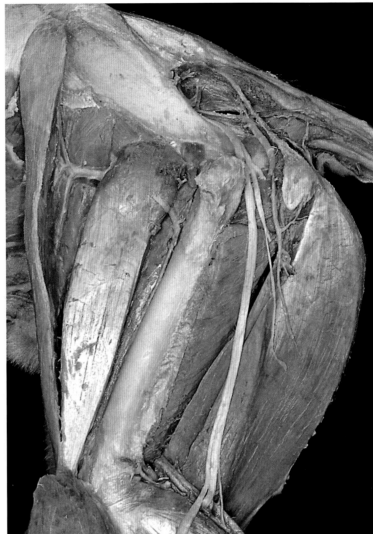

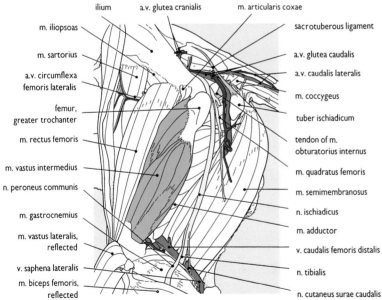

ilium   a.v. glutea cranialis   m. articularis coxae

m. iliopsoas

m. sartorius

a.v. circumflexa
femoris lateralis

femur,
greater trochanter

m. rectus femoris

m. vastus intermedius

n. peroneus communis

m. gastrocnemius

m. vastus lateralis,
reflected

v. saphena lateralis

m. biceps femoris,
reflected

sacrotuberous ligament

a.v. glutea caudalis

a.v. caudalis lateralis

m. coccygeus

tuber ischiadicum

tendon of m.
obturatorius internus

m. quadratus femoris

m. semimembranosus

n. ischiadicus

m. adductor

v. caudalis femoris distalis

n. tibialis

n. cutaneus surae caudalis

Fig. 7.21 Rump and thigh after reflection of the lateral vastus and semitendinosus muscles: left lateral view.

m. sartorius

a.v. circumflexa
femoris lateralis

n. femoralis

a. circumflexa
femoris lateralis
ramus descendens

m. rectus femoris

m. vastus medialis

m. articularis genu

m. articularis coxae

hip joint capsule

femur, greater
trochanter

n. ischiadicus

femur, shaft

m. semimembranosus

femur, lateral
epicondyle

m. vastus intermedius,
reflected

Fig. 7.22 Rump and thigh after reflection of the intermediate vastus muscle: left lateral view. Muscles have been reflected distally.

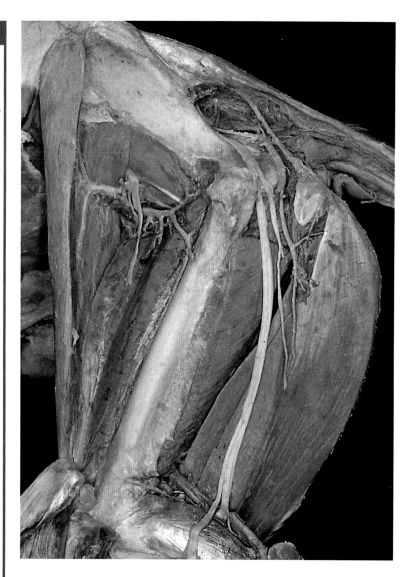

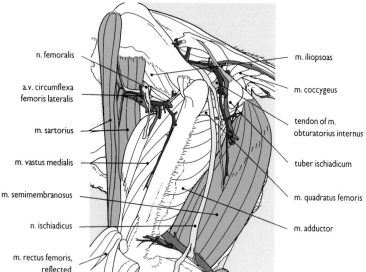

n. femoralis

a.v. circumflexa
femoris lateralis

m. sartorius

m. vastus medialis

m. semimembranosus

n. ischiadicus

m. rectus femoris,
reflected

m. iliopsoas

m. coccygeus

tendon of m.
obturatorius internus

tuber ischiadicum

m. quadratus femoris

m. adductor

Fig. 7.23 Rump and thigh after reflection of the rectus femoris muscle:
left lateral view.

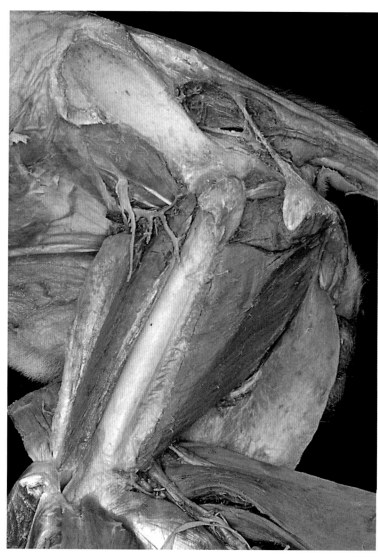

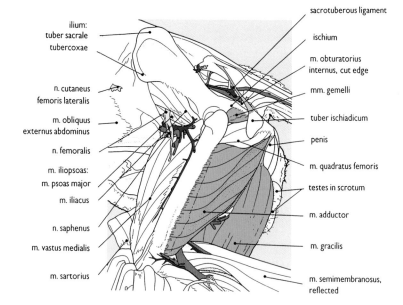

sacrotuberous ligament

ilium:
tuber sacrale
tubercoxae

ischium

m. obturatorius
internus, cut edge

n. cutaneus
femoris lateralis

mm. gemelli

m. obliquus
externus abdominus

tuber ischiadicum

n. femoralis

penis

m. iliopsoas:
m. psoas major

m. quadratus femoris

m. iliacus

testes in scrotum

n. saphenus

m. adductor

m. vastus medialis

m. gracilis

m. sartorius

m. semimembranosus,
reflected

**Fig. 7.24 Rump and thigh after reflection of the sartorius and
semimembranosus muscles:** left lateral view. The sciatic nerve and part of
the internal obturator muscle have been removed to expose the dorsal
border of the ischium and the gemelli muscles. The large adductor
muscle can also be seen as well as the gracilis, which is the most medial
muscle of the thigh in that region.

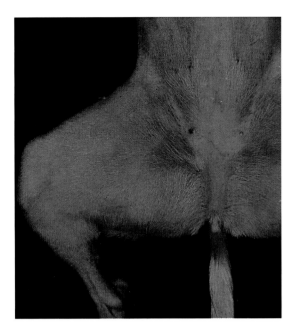

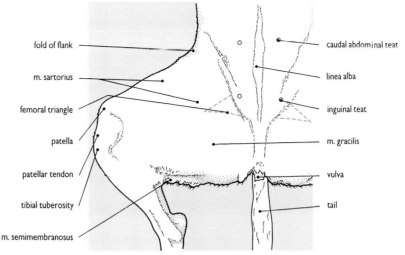

fold of flank
m. sartorius
femoral triangle
patella
patellar tendon
tibial tuberosity
m. semimembranosus

caudal abdominal teat
linea alba
inguinal teat
m. gracilis
vulva
tail

Fig. 7.25 Surface features of the right thigh: medial view. Palpable and visible features are indicated. It should be noted that Figs 7.25–7.34, showing the medial view of the thigh, were produced whilst the dog was fixed on its back with the thighs fully abducted and the stifles flexed.

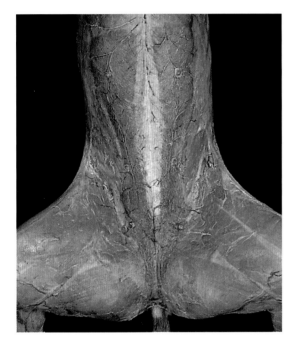

Fig. 7.26 Superficial fascia of the right thigh: medial view. The superficial fascia contains many small blood vessels and nerves including the medial saphenous vein and its accompanying artery and nerve. The deep medial femoral fascia joins with the lateral femoral fascia to form a cylinder arrangement around the thigh.

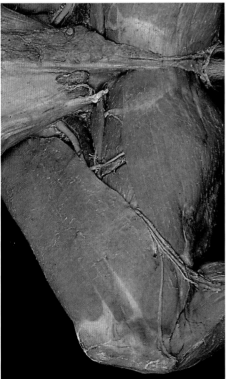

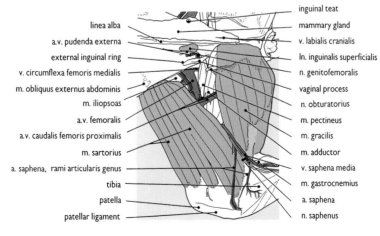

linea alba
a.v. pudenda externa
external inguinal ring
v. circumflexa femoris medialis
m. obliquus externus abdominis
m. iliopsoas
a.v. femoralis
a.v. caudalis femoris proximalis
m. sartorius
a. saphena, rami articularis genus
tibia
patella
patellar ligament

inguinal teat
mammary gland
v. labialis cranialis
ln. inguinalis superficialis
n. genitofemoralis
vaginal process
n. obturatorius
m. pectineus
m. gracilis
m. adductor
v. saphena media
m. gastrocnemius
a. saphena
n. saphenus

Fig. 7.27 Superficial muscles of the right thigh: medial view. All superficial and deep fascia has been removed, as has fat from the femoral triangle. The mammary gland on the right side has also been removed. The boundaries of the femoral triangle can now be clearly seen. It should be noted that the sartorius muscle is usually better delineated into a cranial and caudal part than in this specimen.

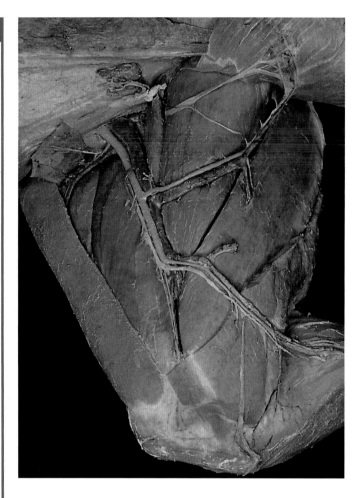

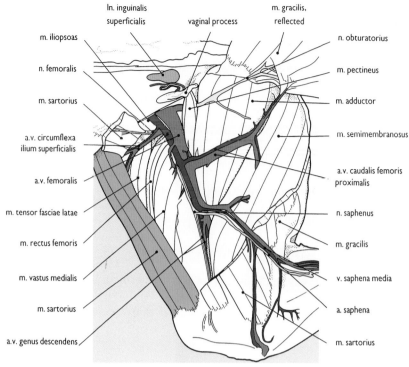

ln. inguinalis superficialis

vaginal process

m. gracilis, reflected

m. iliopsoas

n. obturatorius

n. femoralis

m. pectineus

m. sartorius

m. adductor

a.v. circumflexa ilium superficialis

m. semimembranosus

a.v. femoralis

a.v. caudalis femoris proximalis

m. tensor fasciae latae

m. rectus femoris

n. saphenus

m. vastus medialis

m. gracilis

m. sartorius

v. saphena media

a.v. genus descendens

a. saphena

m. sartorius

Fig. 7.28 Right thigh after part removal of caudal sartorius muscle and reflection of gracilis muscle: medial view. Deeper medial thigh muscles are now exposed.

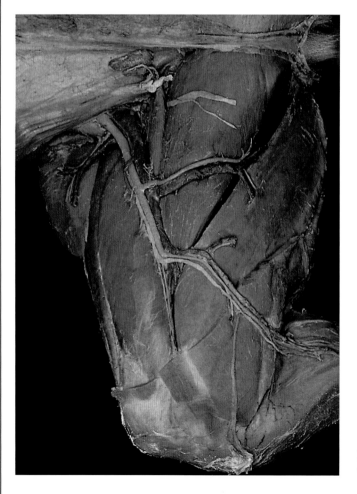

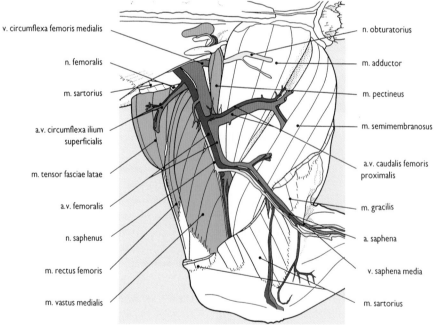

v. circumflexa femoris medialis

n. obturatorius

n. femoralis

m. adductor

m. sartorius

m. pectineus

a.v. circumflexa ilium superficialis

m. semimembranosus

m. tensor fasciae latae

a.v. caudalis femoris proximalis

a.v. femoralis

m. gracilis

n. saphenus

a. saphena

m. rectus femoris

v. saphena media

m. vastus medialis

m. sartorius

Fig. 7.29 Right thigh after removal of cranial sartorius muscle: medial view. The tensor fasciae latae and parts of the quadriceps muscle are now exposed.

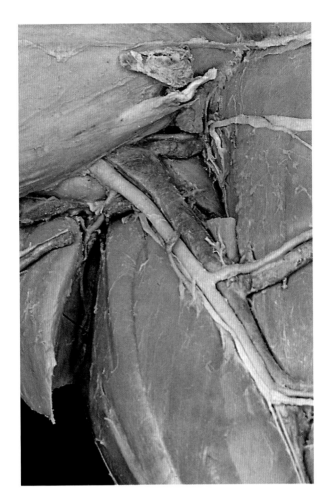

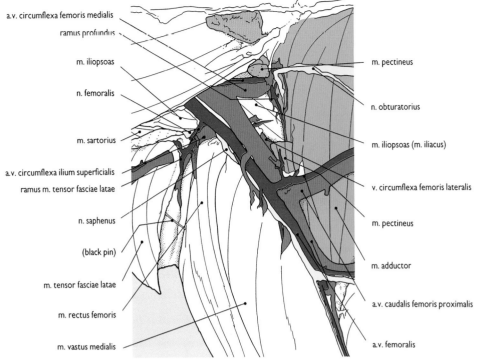

a.v. circumflexa femoris medialis
ramus profundus
m. iliopsoas
n. femoralis
m. sartorius
a.v. circumflexa ilium superficialis
ramus m. tensor fasciae latae
n. saphenus
(black pin)
m. tensor fasciae latae
m. rectus femoris
m. vastus medialis

m. pectineus
n. obturatorius
m. iliopsoas (m. iliacus)
v. circumflexa femoris lateralis
m. pectineus
m. adductor
a.v. caudalis femoris proximalis
a.v. femoralis

Fig. 7.30 Right thigh after removal of the pectineus muscle: medial view. More of the medial circumflex femoral vessels can now be seen.

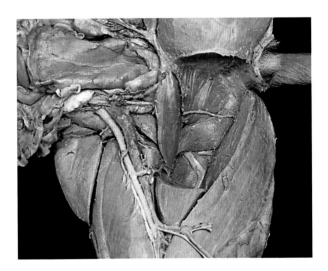

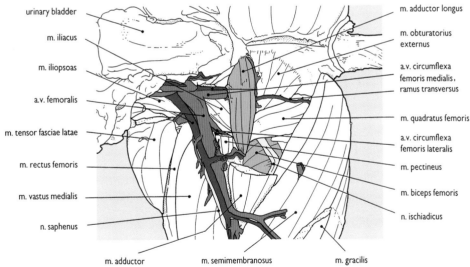

urinary bladder
m. iliacus
m. iliopsoas
a.v. femoralis
m. tensor fasciae latae
m. rectus femoris
m. vastus medialis
n. saphenus

m. adductor longus
m. obturatorius externus
a.v. circumflexa femoris medialis, ramus transversus
m. quadratus femoris
a.v. circumflexa femoris lateralis
m. pectineus
m. biceps femoris
n. ischiadicus

m. adductor   m. semimembranosus   m. gracilis

Fig. 7.31 Right thigh after removal of the adductor magnus muscle: medial view. The abdominal wall has also been removed. The adductor longus muscle has been left in position. Note the location of the sciatic nerve medial to the biceps femoris muscle.

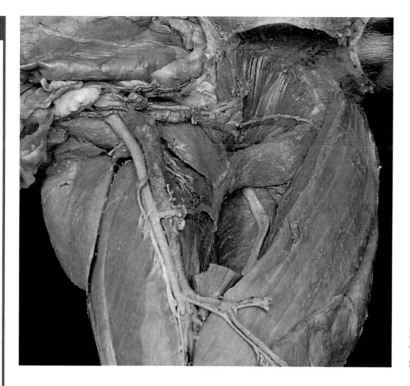

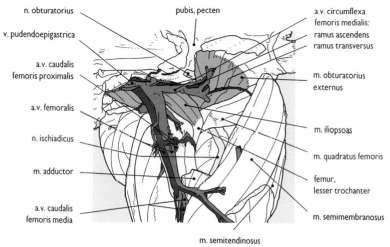

n. obturatorius

v. pudendoepigastrica

a.v. caudalis
femoris proximalis

a.v. femoralis

n. ischiadicus

m. adductor

a.v. caudalis
femoris media

pubis, pecten

a.v. circumflexa
femoris medialis:
ramus ascendens
ramus transversus

m. obturatorius
externus

m. iliopsoas

m. quadratus femoris

femur,
lesser trochanter

m. semimembranosus

m. semitendinosus

Fig. 7.32 Right thigh after removal of the adductor longus muscle: medial view. The insertion of the iliopsoas on the lesser trochanter of the femur is now exposed.

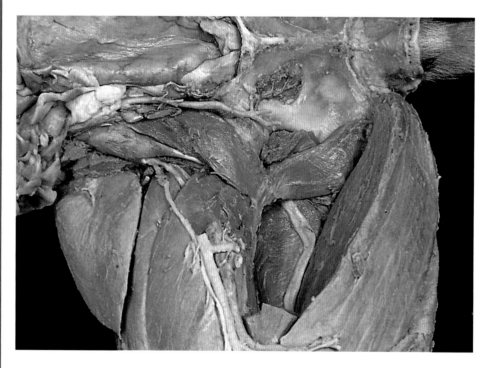

Fig. 7.33 Right thigh after removal of the external obturator muscle: medial view. The femoral artery and vein and the medial circumflex femoral vein have also been removed. The internal obturator muscle which originates on the floor of the pelvis can be seen through the obturator foramen.

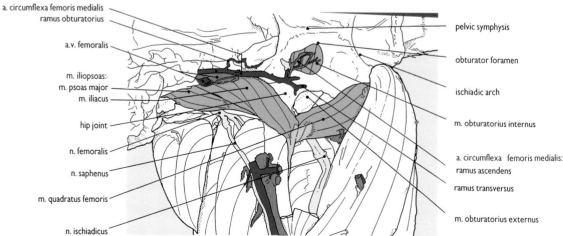

a. circumflexa femoris medialis
ramus obturatorius

a.v. femoralis

m. iliopsoas:
m. psoas major
m. iliacus

hip joint

n. femoralis

n. saphenus

m. quadratus femoris

n. ischiadicus

pelvic symphysis

obturator foramen

ischiadic arch

m. obturatorius internus

a. circumflexa femoris medialis:
ramus ascendens

ramus transversus

m. obturatorius externus

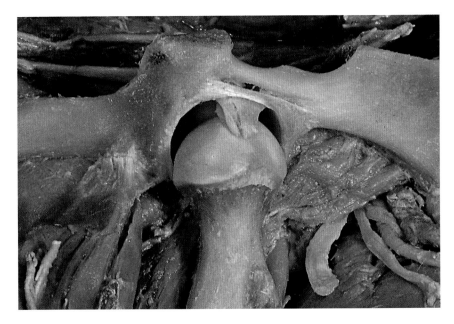

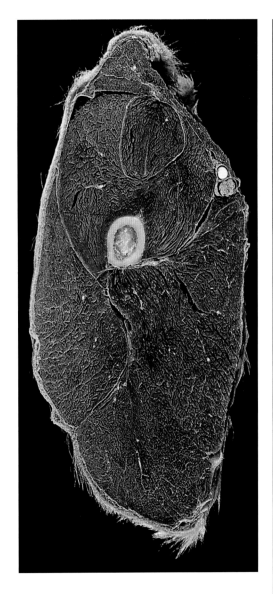

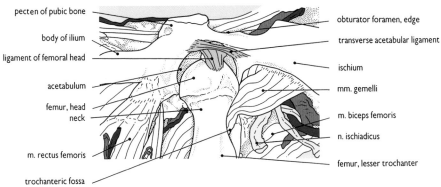

pecten of pubic bone

body of ilium

ligament of femoral head

acetabulum

femur, head
neck

m. rectus femoris

trochanteric fossa

obturator foramen, edge

transverse acetabular ligament

ischium

mm. gemelli

m. biceps femoris

n. ischiadicus

femur, lesser trochanter

Fig. 7.34 Right hip joint: Ventral view. The iliopsoas and quadratus femoris muscles have been removed. The hip joint capsule has also been removed and the head of the femur has been slightly pulled out from the acetabulum to expose the ligament of the femoral head.

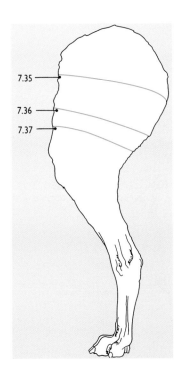

7.35

7.36

7.37

Figs. 7.35–7.37 Transverse sections through left thigh at levels indicated in the accompanying drawing: view of proximal surfaces of sections. Notice the deeper position of the femoral artery and vein as the stifle is approached.

cranial
medial

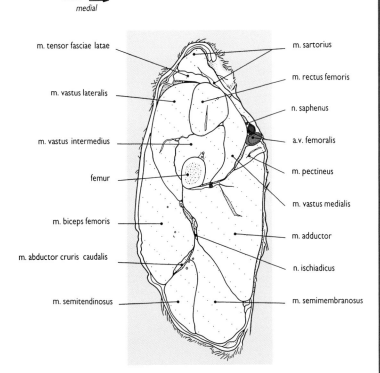

m. tensor fasciae latae

m. vastus lateralis

m. vastus intermedius

femur

m. biceps femoris

m. abductor cruris caudalis

m. semitendinosus

m. sartorius

m. rectus femoris

n. saphenus

a.v. femoralis

m. pectineus

m. vastus medialis

m. adductor

n. ischiadicus

m. semimembranosus

Fig. 7.35

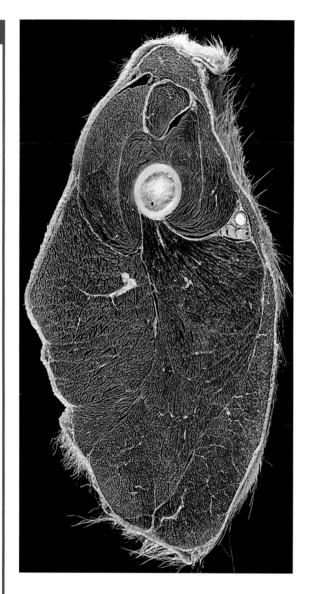

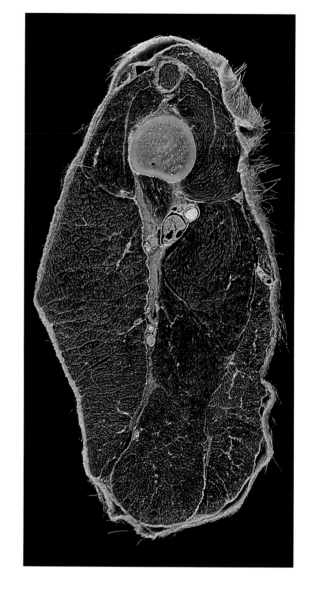

cranial
medial

cranial
medial

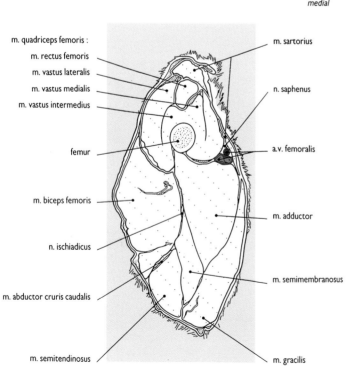

m. quadriceps femoris :
m. rectus femoris
m. vastus lateralis
m. vastus medialis
m. vastus intermedius

femur

m. biceps femoris

n. ischiadicus

m. abductor cruris caudalis

m. semitendinosus

m. sartorius

n. saphenus

a.v. femoralis

m. adductor

m. semimembranosus

m. gracilis

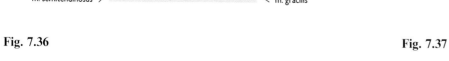

Fig. 7.36

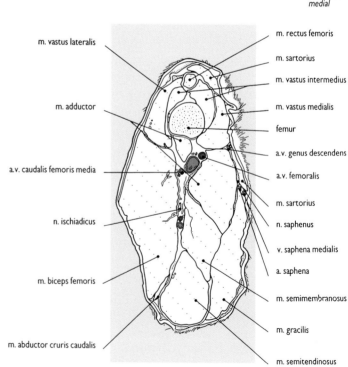

m. vastus lateralis

m. adductor

a.v. caudalis femoris media

n. ischiadicus

m. biceps femoris

m. abductor cruris caudalis

m. rectus femoris

m. sartorius

m. vastus intermedius

m. vastus medialis

femur

a.v. genus descendens

a.v. femoralis

m. sartorius

n. saphenus

v. saphena medialis

a. saphena

m. semimembranosus

m. gracilis

m. semitendinosus

Fig. 7.37

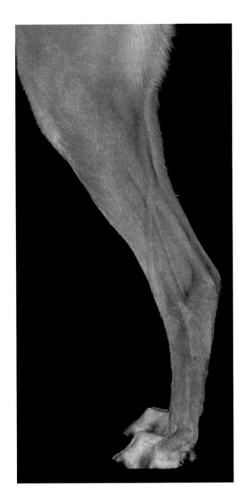

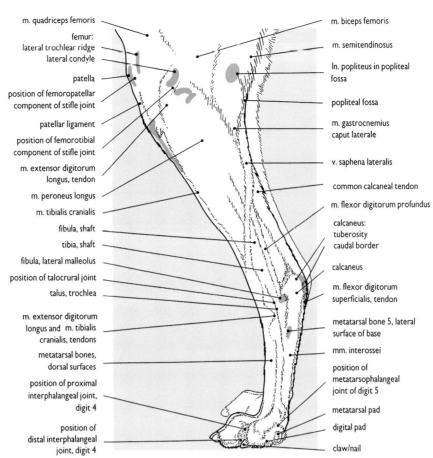

m. quadriceps femoris

femur:
lateral trochlear ridge
lateral condyle

patella

position of femoropatellar
component of stifle joint

patellar ligament

position of femorotibial
component of stifle joint

m. extensor digitorum
longus, tendon

m. peroneus longus

m. tibialis cranialis

fibula, shaft

tibia, shaft

fibula, lateral malleolus

position of talocrural joint

talus, trochlea

m. extensor digitorum
longus and m. tibialis
cranialis, tendons

metatarsal bones,
dorsal surfaces

position of proximal
interphalangeal joint,
digit 4

position of
distal interphalangeal
joint, digit 4

m. biceps femoris

m. semitendinosus

ln. popliteus in popliteal
fossa

popliteal fossa

m. gastrocnemius
caput laterale

v. saphena lateralis

common calcaneal tendon

m. flexor digitorum profundus

calcaneus:
tuberosity
caudal border

calcaneus

m. flexor digitorum
superficialis, tendon

metatarsal bone 5, lateral
surface of base

mm. interossei

position of
metatarsophalangeal
joint of digit 5

metatarsal pad

digital pad

claw/nail

Fig. 7.38 Surface features of crus and pes: left lateral view. Palpable and visible features are indicated.

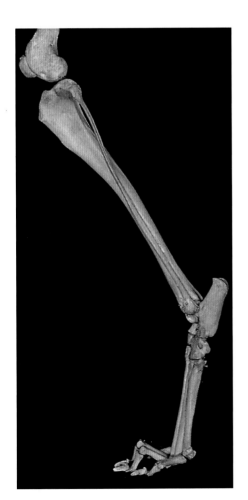

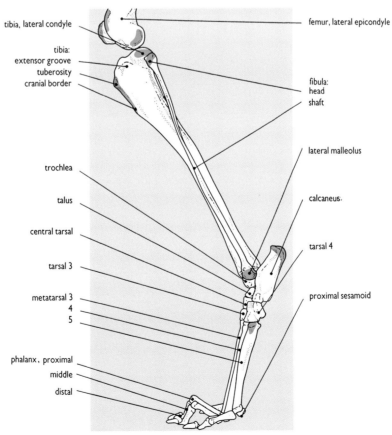

tibia, lateral condyle

tibia:
extensor groove
tuberosity
cranial border

trochlea

talus

central tarsal

tarsal 3

metatarsal 3
4
5

phalanx, proximal
middle
distal

femur, lateral epicondyle

fibula:
head
shaft

lateral malleolus

calcaneus

tarsal 4

proximal sesamoid

Fig. 7.39 Skeleton of crus and pes: left lateral view. The features colored green correspond to the palpable bony features shown in Fig. 7.38.

Veterinary Anatomy: The Dog and Cat

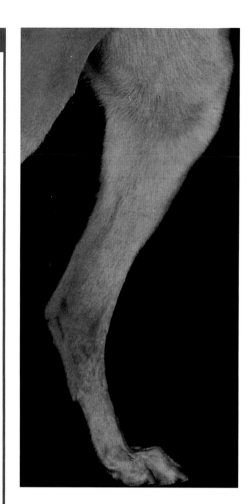

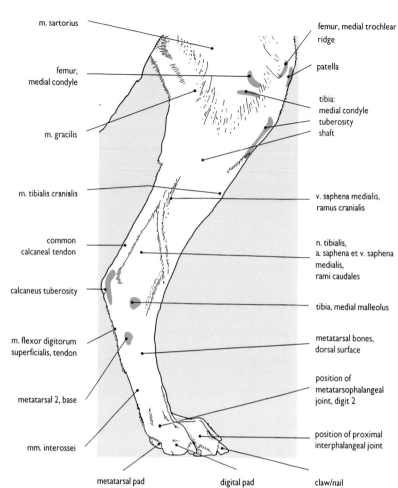

m. sartorius

femur, medial condyle

m. gracilis

m. tibialis cranialis

common calcaneal tendon

calcaneus tuberosity

m. flexor digitorum superficialis, tendon

metatarsal 2, base

mm. interossei

metatarsal pad

digital pad

femur, medial trochlear ridge

patella

tibia:
medial condyle
tuberosity
shaft

v. saphena medialis, ramus cranialis

n. tibialis,
a. saphena et v. saphena medialis,
rami caudales

tibia, medial malleolus

metatarsal bones, dorsal surface

position of metatarsophalangeal joint, digit 2

position of proximal interphalangeal joint

claw/nail

Fig. 7.40 Surface features of crus and pes: left medial view. Palpable and visible features are indicated.

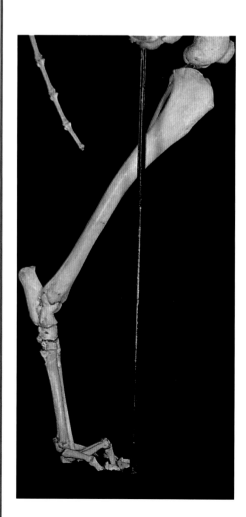

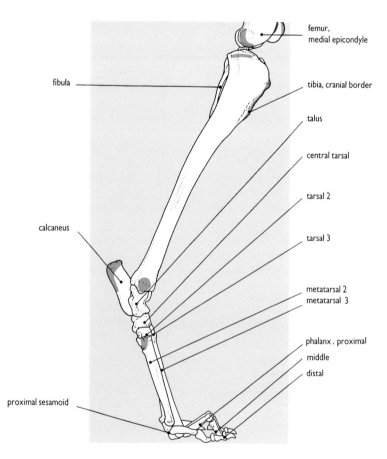

fibula

calcaneus

proximal sesamoid

femur, medial epicondyle

tibia, cranial border

talus

central tarsal

tarsal 2

tarsal 3

metatarsal 2
metatarsal 3

phalanx. proximal
middle
distal

Fig. 7.41 Skeleton of crus and pes: left medial view. The features colored green correspond to the palpable bony features shown in Fig. 7.40.

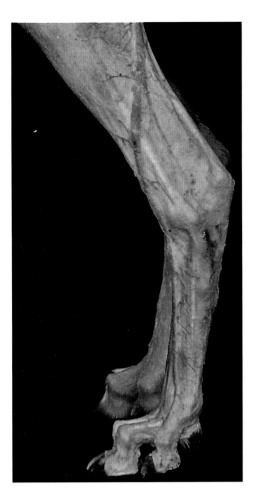

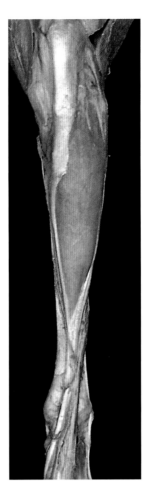

Fig. 7.42 Superficial fascia of crus, tarsus and pes: left lateral view. The superficial fascia envelopes the crus, tarsus and pes, and contains many blood vessels and nerves including the saphenous vessels. The deep fascia of the stifle joint is associated closely with the patellar ligament and is continuous with the femoral fascia proximally and with the crural fascia distally. The crural fascia is two-leaved with the deeper leaf covering muscles and bones and partly providing insertion for the biceps femoris muscle. Towards the foot, the deep fascia is intimately associated with the calcaneal tuber and other bones, tendons and ligaments.

Fig. 7.43 Left leg: cranial view. Only the fascia has been removed.

m. biceps femoris

patella

m. sartorius

patellar ligament

m. tibialis cranialis

v. saphena medialis, ramus cranialis

v. saphena lateralis, ramus cranialis

n. peroneus superficialis

v. tarsea medialis

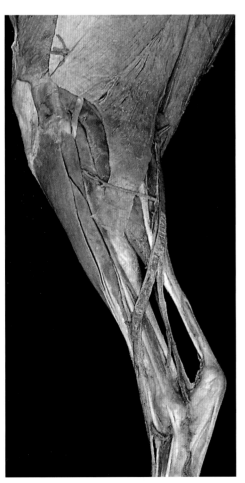

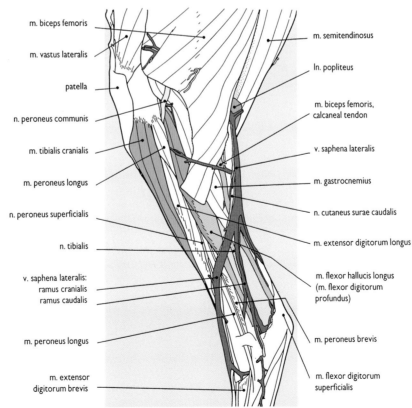

m. biceps femoris

m. vastus lateralis

patella

n. peroneus communis

m. tibialis cranialis

m. peroneus longus

n. peroneus superficialis

n. tibialis

v. saphena lateralis:
ramus cranialis
ramus caudalis

m. peroneus longus

m. extensor
digitorum brevis

m. semitendinosus

ln. popliteus

m. biceps femoris,
calcaneal tendon

v. saphena lateralis

m. gastrocnemius

n. cutaneus surae caudalis

m. extensor digitorum longus

m. flexor hallucis longus
(m. flexor digitorum
profundus)

m. peroneus brevis

m. flexor digitorum
superficialis

Fig. 7.44 Left leg: left lateral view. Only the fascia has been removed.

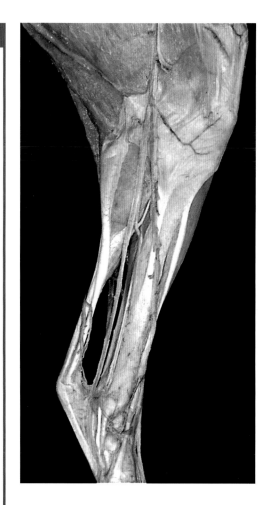

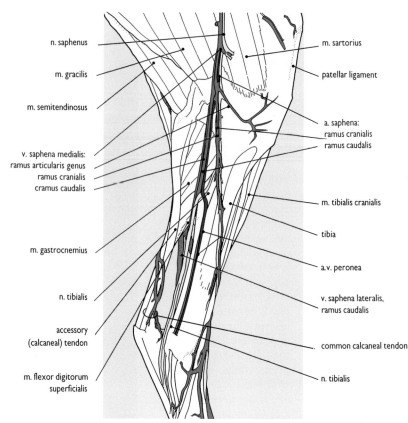

n. saphenus

m. gracilis

m. semitendinosus

v. saphena medialis:
ramus articularis genus
ramus cranialis
cramus caudalis

m. gastrocnemius

n. tibialis

accessory
(calcaneal) tendon

m. flexor digitorum
superficialis

m. sartorius

patellar ligament

a. saphena:
ramus cranialis
ramus caudalis

m. tibialis cranialis

tibia

a.v. peronea

v. saphena lateralis,
ramus caudalis

common calcaneal tendon

n. tibialis

Fig. 7.45 Left leg: medial view. Only the fascia has been removed. The common calcaneal tendon is made up of contributions from the gastrocnemius, superficial digital flexor, biceps femoris, semitendinosus and gracilis muscles.

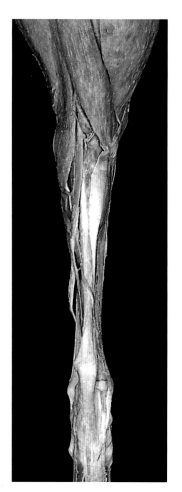

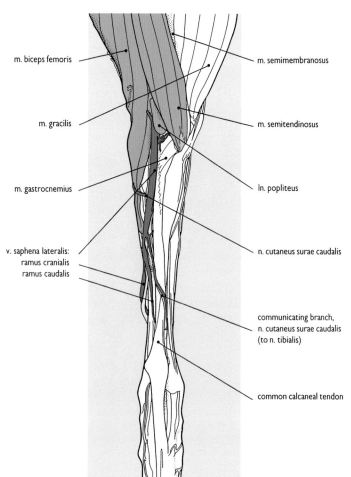

m. biceps femoris

m. gracilis

m. gastrocnemius

v. saphena lateralis:
ramus cranialis
ramus caudalis

m. semimembranosus

m. semitendinosus

ln. popliteus

n. cutaneus surae caudalis

communicating branch,
n. cutaneus surae caudalis
(to n. tibialis)

common calcaneal tendon

Fig. 7.46 Left crus: caudal view. Note the superficial position of the popliteal lymph node in the popliteal fossa between the biceps femoris and semitendinosus muscles.

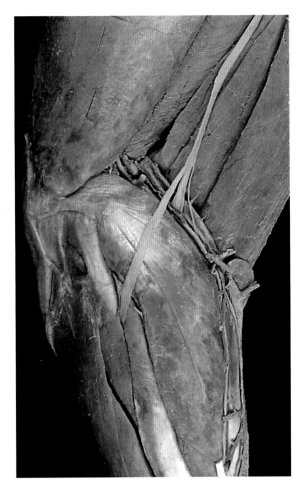

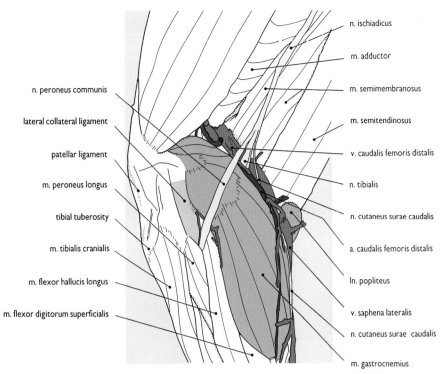

n. ischiadicus

m. adductor

m. semimembranosus

m. semitendinosus

v. caudalis femoris distalis

n. tibialis

n. cutaneus surae caudalis

a. caudalis femoris distalis

ln. popliteus

v. saphena lateralis

n. cutaneus surae caudalis

m. gastrocnemius

n. peroneus communis

lateral collateral ligament

patellar ligament

m. peroneus longus

tibial tuberosity

m. tibialis cranialis

m. flexor hallucis longus

m. flexor digitorum superficialis

Fig. 7.47 Stifle region of left hindlimb: lateral view. The biceps femoris muscle has been removed to expose the proximal part of the gastrocnemius muscle and the bifurcation of the sciatic nerve.

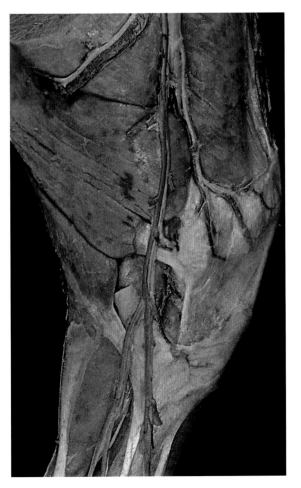

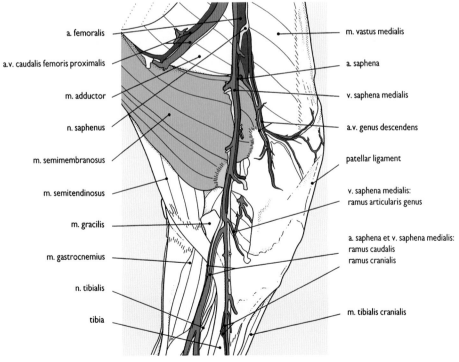

a. femoralis

a.v. caudalis femoris proximalis

m. adductor

n. saphenus

m. semimembranosus

m. semitendinosus

m. gracilis

m. gastrocnemius

n. tibialis

tibia

m. vastus medialis

a. saphena

v. saphena medialis

a.v. genus descendens

patellar ligament

v. saphena medialis:
ramus articularis genus

a. saphena et v. saphena medialis:
ramus caudalis
ramus cranialis

m. tibialis cranialis

Fig. 7.48 Stifle region of left hindlimb: medial view. The gracilis and sartorius muscles have been removed.

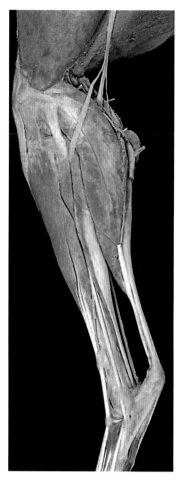

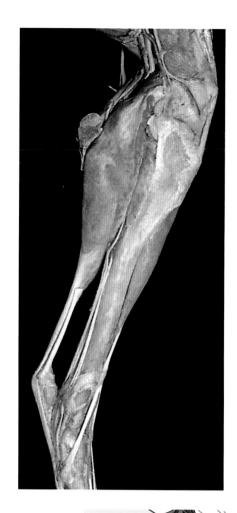

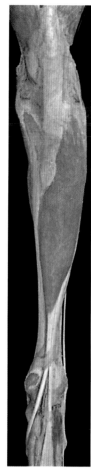

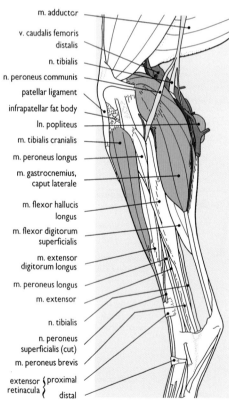

m. adductor

v. caudalis femoris distalis

n. tibialis

n. peroneus communis

patellar ligament

infrapatellar fat body

ln. popliteus

m. tibialis cranialis

m. peroneus longus

m. gastrocnemius, caput laterale

m. flexor hallucis longus

m. flexor digitorum superficialis

m. extensor digitorum longus

m. peroneus longus

m. extensor

n. tibialis

n. peroneus superficialis (cut)

m. peroneus brevis

extensor { proximal
retinacula { distal

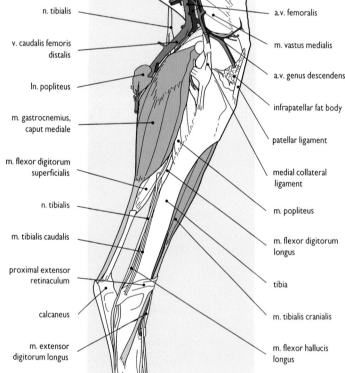

n. tibialis

v. caudalis femoris distalis

ln. popliteus

m. gastrocnemius, caput mediale

m. flexor digitorum superficialis

n. tibialis

m. tibialis caudalis

proximal extensor retinaculum

calcaneus

m. extensor digitorum longus

a.v. femoralis

m. vastus medialis

a.v. genus descendens

infrapatellar fat body

patellar ligament

medial collateral ligament

m. popliteus

m. flexor digitorum longus

tibia

m. tibialis cranialis

m. flexor hallucis longus

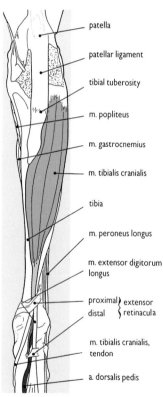

patella

patellar ligament

tibial tuberosity

m. popliteus

m. gastrocnemius

m. tibialis cranialis

tibia

m. peroneus longus

m. extensor digitorum longus

proximal } extensor
distal } retinacula

m. tibialis cranialis, tendon

a. dorsalis pedis

Fig. 7.49 Left crus after removal of the lateral saphenous vein: lateral view. The biceps femoris, semitendinosus and semimembranosus muscles have also been removed.

Fig. 7.50 Left crus after removal of the saphenous artery and nerve and medial saphenous vein: medial view. The gracilis, sartorius, semitendinosus removed and semimembranosus muscles have also been removed.

Fig. 7.51 Left crus after removal of superficial veins and nerves: cranial view.

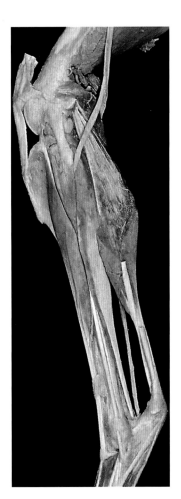

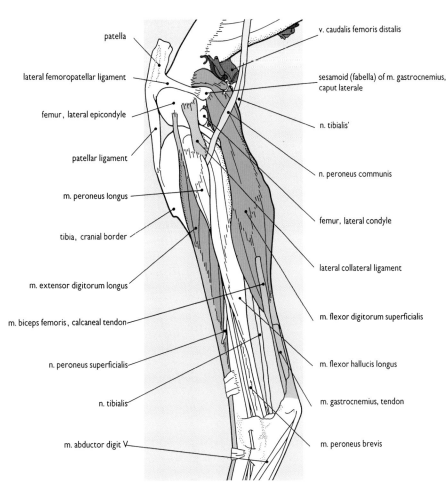

patella

lateral femoropatellar ligament

femur, lateral epicondyle

patellar ligament

m. peroneus longus

tibia, cranial border

m. extensor digitorum longus

m. biceps femoris, calcaneal tendon

n. peroneus superficialis

n. tibialis

m. abductor digit V

v. caudalis femoris distalis

sesamoid (fabella) of m. gastrocnemius, caput laterale

n. tibialis'

n. peroneus communis

femur, lateral condyle

lateral collateral ligament

m. flexor digitorum superficialis

m. flexor hallucis longus

m. gastrocnemius, tendon

m. peroneus brevis

Fig. 7.52 Left crus after removal of the cranial tibial and gastrocnemius muscles: lateral view. The infrapatellar fat body and popliteal lymph node have also been removed. The length of the long digital extensor and the superficial digital flexor muscles are exposed. The next three figures are at the same stage of dissection.

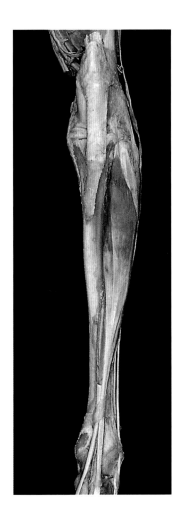

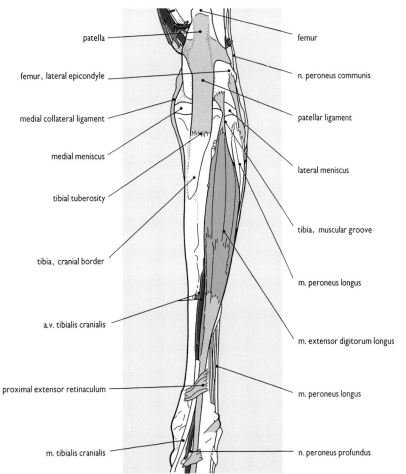

patella

femur, lateral epicondyle

medial collateral ligament

medial meniscus

tibial tuberosity

tibia, cranial border

a.v. tibialis cranialis

proximal extensor retinaculum

m. tibialis cranialis

femur

n. peroneus communis

patellar ligament

lateral meniscus

tibia, muscular groove

m. peroneus longus

m. extensor digitorum longus

m. peroneus longus

n. peroneus profundus

Fig. 7.53 Left crus after removal of the cranial tibial muscle: cranial view.

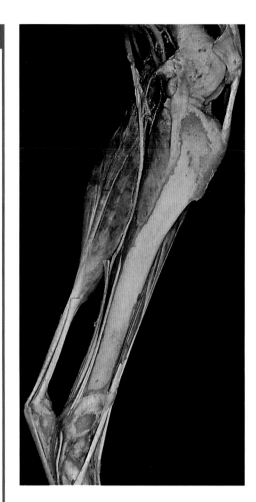

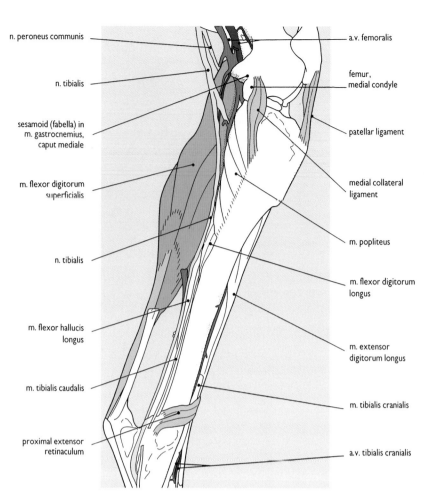

n. peroneus communis

n. tibialis

sesamoid (fabella) in
m. gastrocnemius,
caput mediale

m. flexor digitorum
superficialis

n. tibialis

m. flexor hallucis
longus

m. tibialis caudalis

proximal extensor
retinaculum

a.v. femoralis

femur,
medial condyle

patellar ligament

medial collateral
ligament

m. popliteus

m. flexor digitorum
longus

m. extensor
digitorum longus

m. tibialis cranialis

a.v. tibialis cranialis

**Fig. 7.54 Left crus
after removal of the
cranial tibial and
gastrocnemius
muscle:** medial view.
The course of the
tibial nerve is now
revealed.

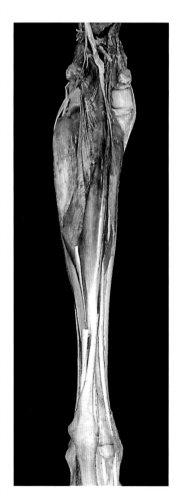

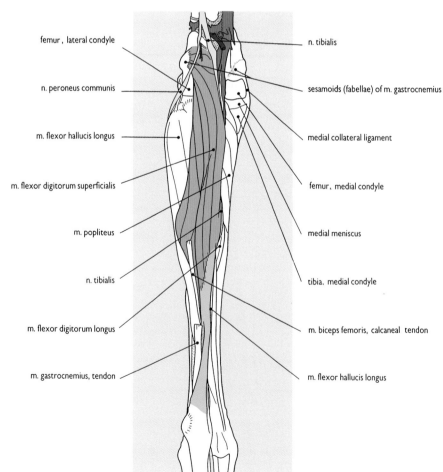

femur , lateral condyle

n. peroneus communis

m. flexor hallucis longus

m. flexor digitorum superficialis

m. popliteus

n. tibialis

m. flexor digitorum longus

m. gastrocnemius, tendon

n. tibialis

sesamoids (fabellae) of m. gastrocnemius

medial collateral ligament

femur, medial condyle

medial meniscus

tibia, medial condyle

m. biceps femoris, calcaneal tendon

m. flexor hallucis longus

**Fig. 7.55 Left crus after
removal of the gastrocnemius
muscle:** caudal view.

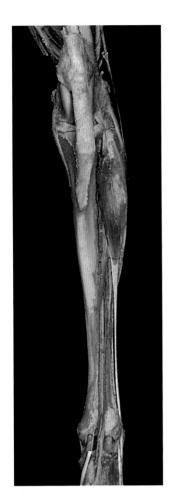
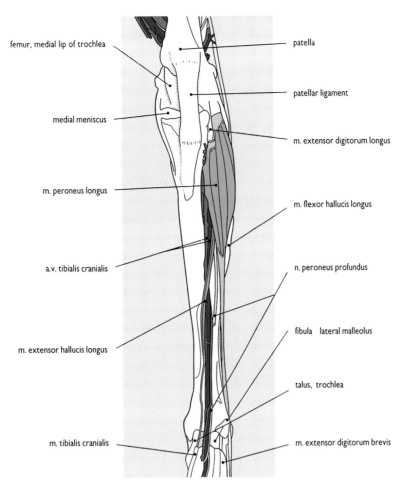

femur, medial lip of trochlea

patella

medial meniscus

patellar ligament

m. extensor digitorum longus

m. peroneus longus

m. flexor hallucis longus

a.v. tibialis cranialis

n. peroneus profundus

fibula   lateral malleolus

m. extensor hallucis longus

talus, trochlea

m. tibialis cranialis

m. extensor digitorum brevis

Fig. 7.56 Left crus after removal of the long digital extensor muscle: cranial view. The cranial tibial vessels and the extensor muscle of the hallux are exposed. This muscle is an extensor of the second digit when the first digit (hallux) is absent.

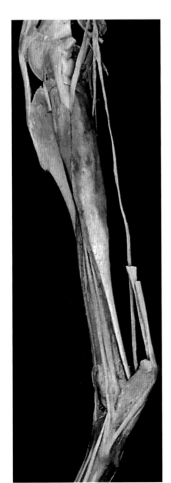
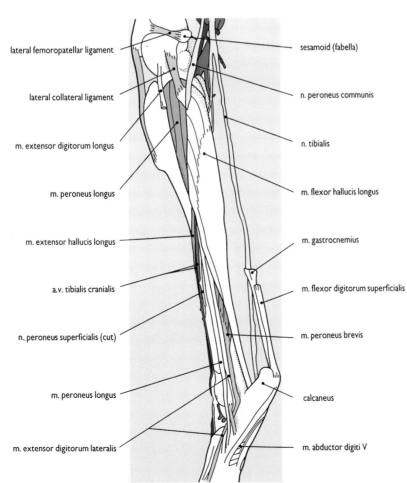

lateral femoropatellar ligament

sesamoid (fabella)

lateral collateral ligament

n. peroneus communis

m. extensor digitorum longus

n. tibialis

m. peroneus longus

m. extensor hallucis longus

m. flexor hallucis longus

m. gastrocnemius

a.v. tibialis cranialis

m. flexor digitorum superficialis

n. peroneus superficialis (cut)

m. peroneus brevis

m. peroneus longus

calcaneus

m. extensor digitorum lateralis

m. abductor digiti V

Fig. 7.57 Left crus after removal of the long digital extensor and superficial digital flexor muscles: lateral view. The next two figures are at the same stage of dissection.

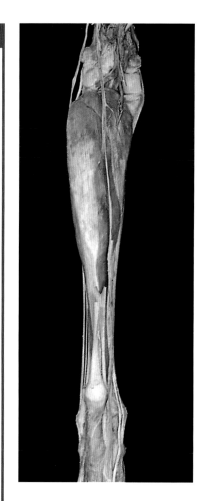

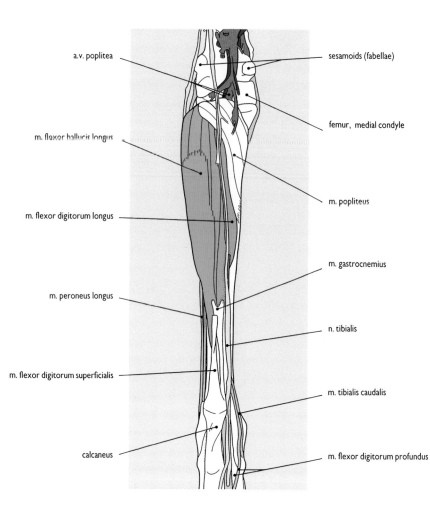

a.v. poplitea

m. flexor hallucis longus

m. flexor digitorum longus

m. peroneus longus

m. flexor digitorum superficialis

calcaneus

sesamoids (fabellae)

femur, medial condyle

m. popliteus

m. gastrocnemius

n. tibialis

m. tibialis caudalis

m. flexor digitorum profundus

Fig. 7.58 Left leg after removal of the superficial digital flexor muscle: caudal view. The long flexor of the hallux and the long digital flexor muscles are the lateral and medial heads, respectively, of the deep digital flexor muscle.

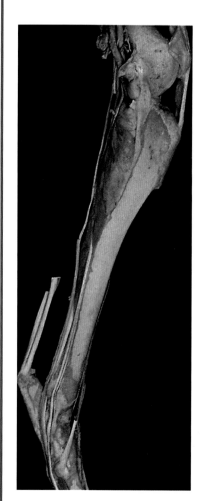

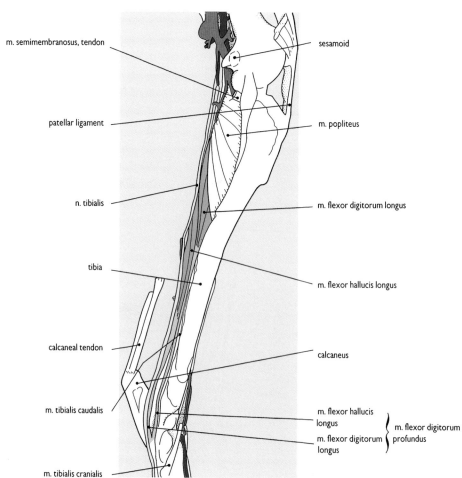

m. semimembranosus, tendon

patellar ligament

n. tibialis

tibia

calcaneal tendon

m. tibialis caudalis

m. tibialis cranialis

sesamoid

m. popliteus

m. flexor digitorum longus

m. flexor hallucis longus

calcaneus

m. flexor hallucis longus

m. flexor digitorum longus

} m. flexor digitorum profundus

Fig. 7.59 Leg after removal of the superficial digital flexor muscle: medial view.

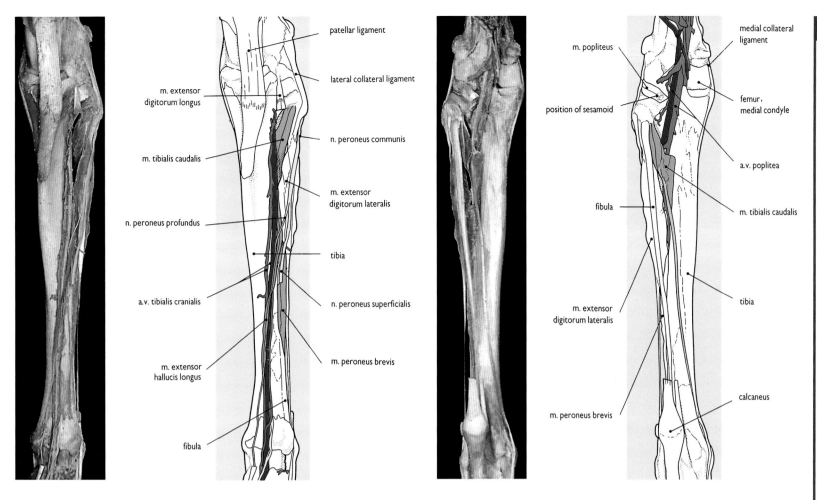

m. extensor
digitorum longus

m. tibialis caudalis

n. peroneus profundus

a.v. tibialis cranialis

m. extensor
hallucis longus

fibula

patellar ligament

lateral collateral ligament

n. peroneus communis

m. extensor
digitorum lateralis

tibia

n. peroneus superficialis

m. peroneus brevis

m. popliteus

position of sesamoid

fibula

m. extensor
digitorum lateralis

m. peroneus brevis

medial collateral
ligament

femur,
medial condyle

a.v. poplitea

m. tibialis caudalis

tibia

calcaneus

Fig. 7.60 Left crus after removal of the long peroneal muscle: cranial view. The cranial tibial vessels can be seen in their cranial position on the tibia having emerged between the tibia and fibula. The cranial tibial artery does not contain red latex in this specimen.

Fig. 7.61 Left crus after removal of the deep digital flexor and popliteal muscles: caudal view. The small caudal tibial muscle is exposed.

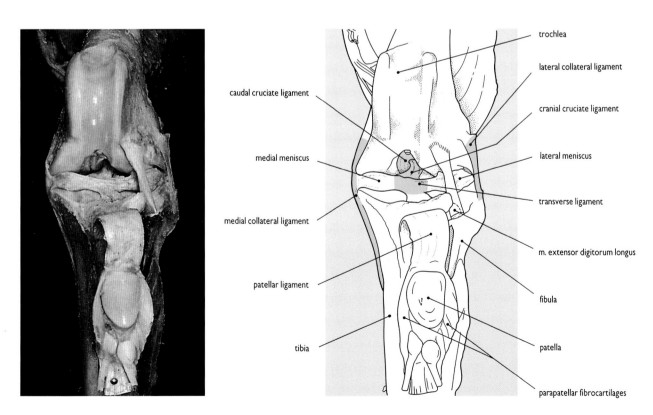

caudal cruciate ligament

medial meniscus

medial collateral ligament

patellar ligament

tibia

trochlea

lateral collateral ligament

cranial cruciate ligament

lateral meniscus

transverse ligament

m. extensor digitorum longus

fibula

patella

parapatellar fibrocartilages

Fig. 7.62 Left stifle joint: cranial view. The patella and its ligament have been reflected distally to expose the cruciate ligaments. The stifle is partly flexed.

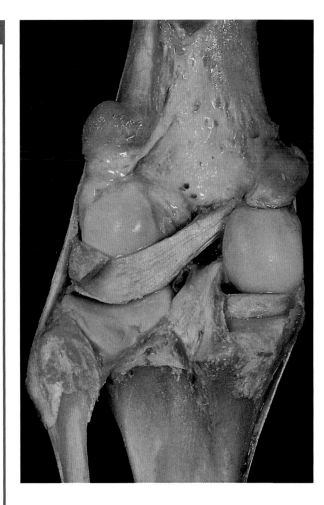

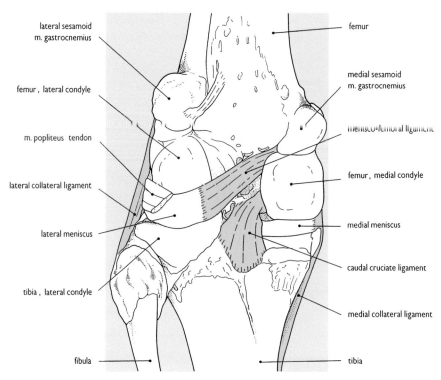

Fig. 7.63 Left stifle joint: caudal view.

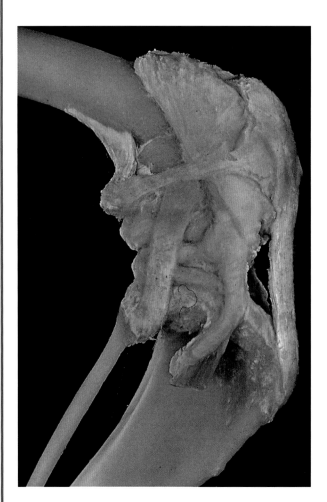

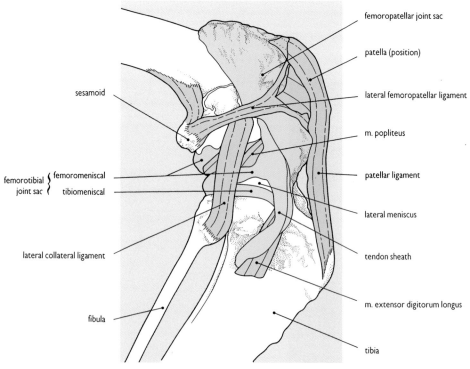

Fig. 7.64 Right stifle joint with joint cavity injected with yellow resin: lateral view. Note the tendon sheath of the long digital extensor tendon and the proximal extent of the femoropatellar joint sac.

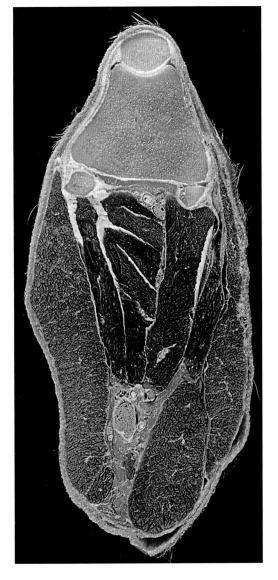

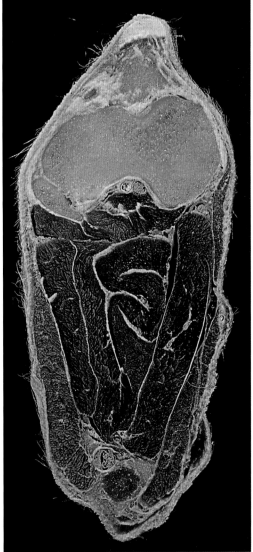

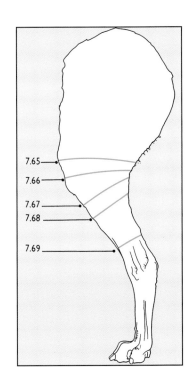

7.65
7.66
7.67
7.68
7.69

Figs. 7.65–7.69 Transverse sections through the left stifle and crural regions at the levels, indicated in the accompanying drawing: view of proximal surfaces of sections.

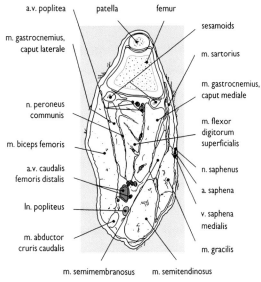

a.v. poplitea — patella — femur — sesamoids — m. sartorius — m. gastrocnemius, caput mediale — m. flexor digitorum superficialis — n. saphenus — a. saphena — v. saphena medialis — m. gracilis — m. semitendinosus — m. semimembranosus — m. abductor cruris caudalis — ln. popliteus — a.v. caudalis femoris distalis — m. biceps femoris — n. peroneus communis — m. gastrocnemius, caput laterale

Fig. 7.65

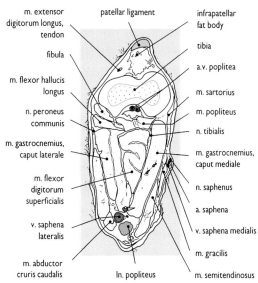

m. extensor digitorum longus, tendon — patellar ligament — infrapatellar fat body — tibia — a.v. poplitea — m. sartorius — m. popliteus — n. tibialis — m. gastrocnemius, caput mediale — n. saphenus — a. saphena — v. saphena medialis — m. gracilis — m. semitendinosus — ln. popliteus — m. abductor cruris caudalis — v. saphena lateralis — m. flexor digitorum superficialis — m. gastrocnemius, caput laterale — n. peroneus communis — m. flexor hallucis longus — fibula

Fig. 7.66

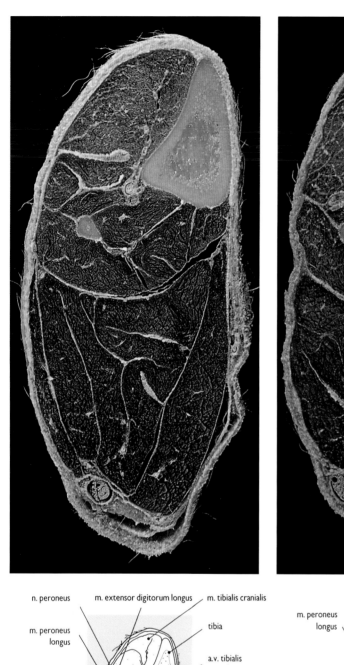
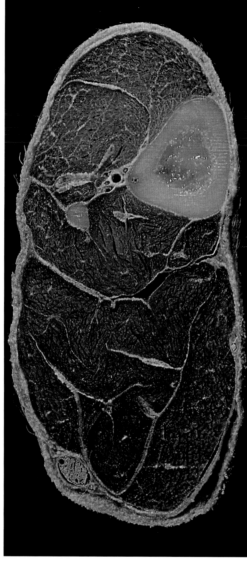
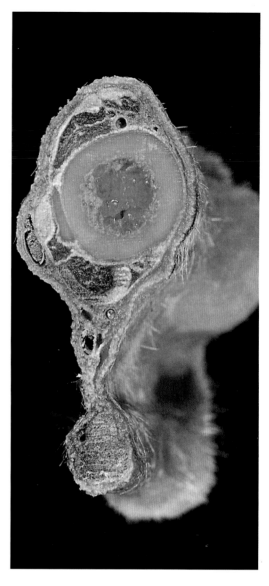

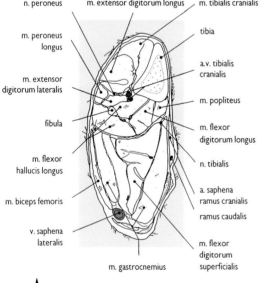

n. peroneus — m. extensor digitorum longus — m. tibialis cranialis

m. peroneus longus

m. extensor digitorum lateralis

fibula

m. flexor hallucis longus

m. biceps femoris

v. saphena lateralis

m. gastrocnemius

tibia

a.v. tibialis cranialis

m. popliteus

m. flexor digitorum longus

n. tibialis

a. saphena ramus cranialis

ramus caudalis

m. flexor digitorum superficialis

cranial
medial

Fig. 7.67

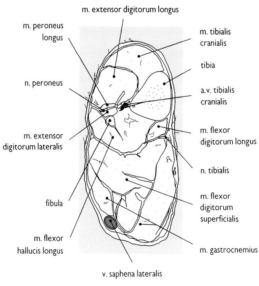

m. extensor digitorum longus

m. peroneus longus

n. peroneus

m. extensor digitorum lateralis

fibula

m. flexor hallucis longus

v. saphena lateralis

m. tibialis cranialis

tibia

a.v. tibialis cranialis

m. flexor digitorum longus

n. tibialis

m. flexor digitorum superficialis

m. gastrocnemius

Fig. 7.68

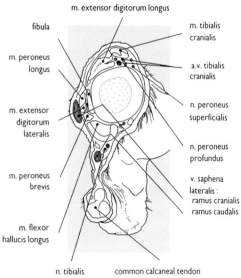

m. extensor digitorum longus

fibula

m. peroneus longus

m. extensor digitorum lateralis

m. peroneus brevis

m. flexor hallucis longus

n. tibialis

common calcaneal tendon

m. tibialis cranialis

a.v. tibialis cranialis

n. peroneus superficialis

n. peroneus profundus

v. saphena lateralis : ramus cranialis ramus caudalis

Fig. 7.69

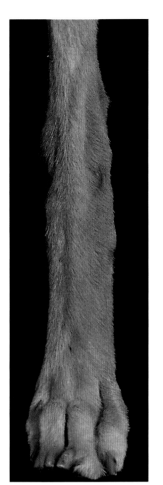

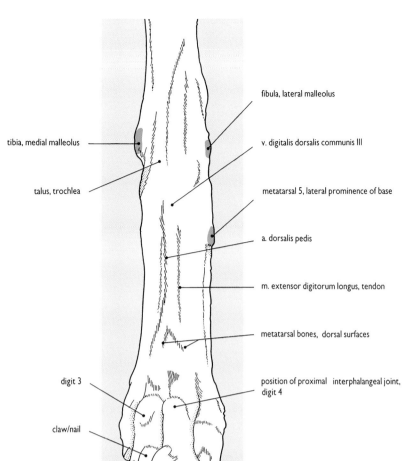

Fig. 7.70 Surface features of left tarsus and pes: dorsal view. Palpable and visible features are indicated.

tibia, medial malleolus

talus, trochlea

digit 3

claw/nail

fibula, lateral malleolus

v. digitalis dorsalis communis III

metatarsal 5, lateral prominence of base

a. dorsalis pedis

m. extensor digitorum longus, tendon

metatarsal bones, dorsal surfaces

position of proximal interphalangeal joint, digit 4

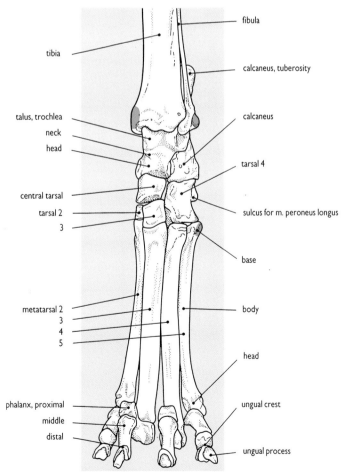

Fig. 7.71 Skeleton of left tarsus and pes: dorsal view. The features colored green correspond to the palpable bony features shown in Fig. 7.70.

tibia

talus, trochlea
neck
head

central tarsal

tarsal 2
3

metatarsal 2
3
4
5

phalanx, proximal
middle
distal

fibula

calcaneus, tuberosity

calcaneus

tarsal 4

sulcus for m. peroneus longus

base

body

head

ungual crest

ungual process

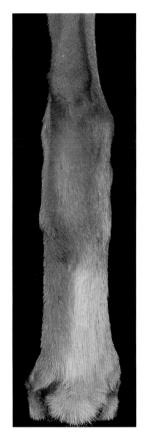

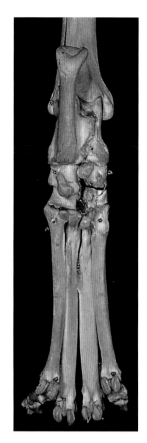

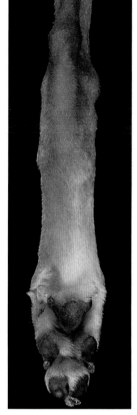

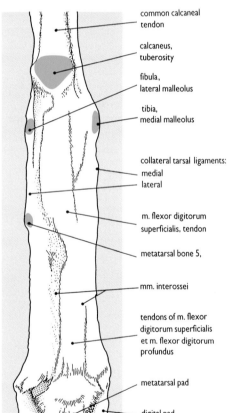

common calcaneal tendon

calcaneus, tuberosity

fibula, lateral malleolus

tibia, medial malleolus

collateral tarsal ligaments:
medial
lateral

m. flexor digitorum superficialis, tendon

metatarsal bone 5,

mm. interossei

tendons of m. flexor digitorum superficialis et m. flexor digitorum profundus

metatarsal pad

digital pad

Fig. 7.72 Surface features of left tarsus and pes: plantar view. Palpable and visible features are indicated.

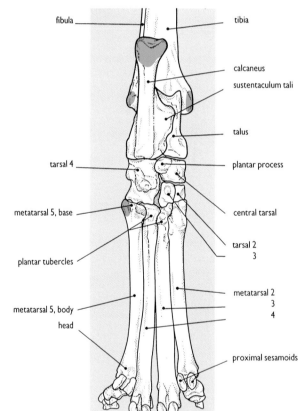

fibula

tibia

calcaneus

sustentaculum tali

talus

plantar process

tarsal 4

central tarsal

metatarsal 5, base

tarsal 2
3

plantar tubercles

metatarsal 2
3
4

metatarsal 5, body

head

proximal sesamoids

Fig. 7.73 Skeleton of left tarsus and pes: plantar view. The features colored green correspond to the palpable bony features shown in Fig. 7.72.

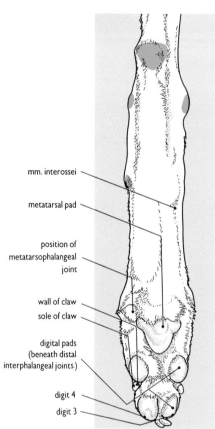

mm. interossei

metatarsal pad

position of metatarsophalangeal joint

wall of claw
sole of claw

digital pads (beneath distal interphalangeal joints)

digit 4
digit 3

Fig. 7.74 Surface features of left tarsus and pes (pes off the ground): plantar view. Palpable and visible features are indicated.

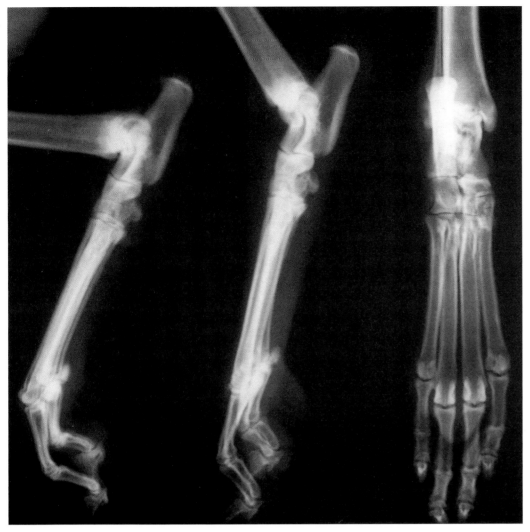

Fig. 7.75 Radiographs of the tarsus and hindpaw: dorsoplantar and lateral views. The major osteological features of the pes are shown in these three radiographs. The detailed osteology of the hindpaw below the tarsus does not differ significantly from the forepaw aside from the normal absence of digit 1 and the longer and somewhat narrower metatarsal region. The dorsoplantar view of the tarsus (c) shows a central tarsal bone without a counterpart in the carpus of the forepaw. The lateral views (a – with tarsal joint flexed; b – with tarsal joint extended) give a clear appreciation of joints between tarsal bones. The major joint and that at which practically all movement occurs is the crurotarsal joint and the prominent rounded trochlear surface is a dominant radiographic feature. The ridges and troughs of the joint conform closely and show why the joint is a strictly confined hinge in its action with little if any lateral or medial movement. Joints more distally in the tarsus exhibit very restricted degrees of movement, especially the tarsometatarsal joints.

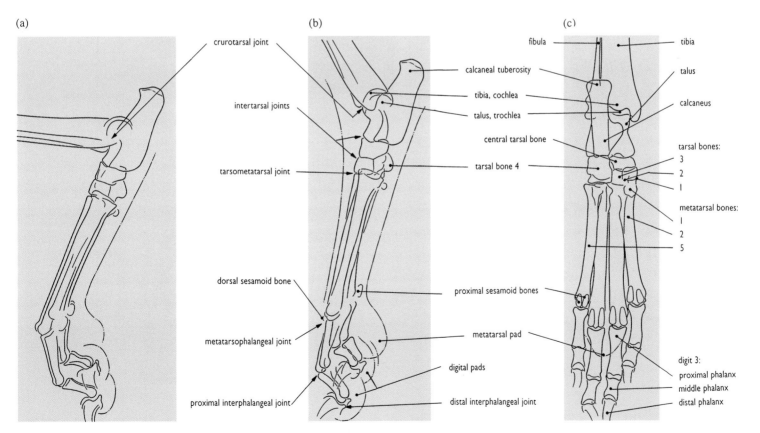

(a)

(b)

(c)

crurotarsal joint

intertarsal joints

tarsometatarsal joint

dorsal sesamoid bone

metatarsophalangeal joint

proximal interphalangeal joint

fibula

calcaneal tuberosity

tibia, cochlea

talus, trochlea

central tarsal bone

tarsal bone 4

proximal sesamoid bones

metatarsal pad

digital pads

distal interphalangeal joint

tibia

talus

calcaneus

tarsal bones:
3
2
1

metatarsal bones:
1
2
5

digit 3:
proximal phalanx
middle phalanx
distal phalanx

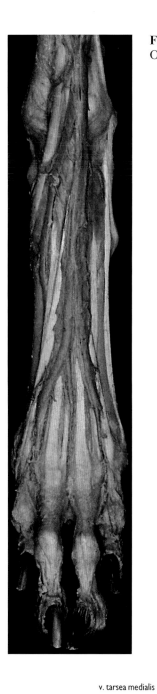

Fig. 7.76 Left tarsus and pes: dorsal view. Only the fascia has been removed.

Fig. 7.77 Left tarsus and pes: plantar view. Only the fascia has been removed. The metatarsal pad has been removed but the digital pads remain in place.

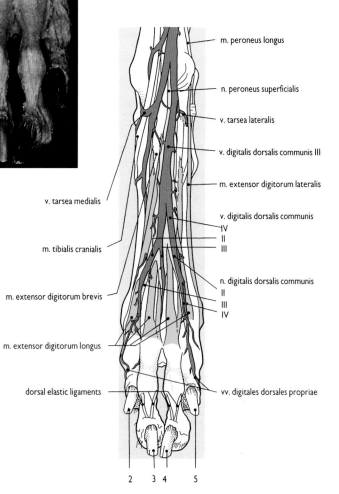

m. peroneus longus

n. peroneus superficialis

v. tarsea lateralis

v. digitalis dorsalis communis III

m. extensor digitorum lateralis

v. tarsea medialis

v. digitalis dorsalis communis
IV
II
III

m. tibialis cranialis

n. digitalis dorsalis communis
II
III
IV

m. extensor digitorum brevis

m. extensor digitorum longus

dorsal elastic ligaments

vv. digitales dorsales propriae

2   3 4   5

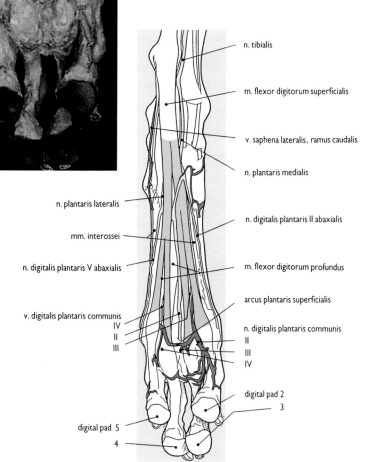

n. tibialis

m. flexor digitorum superficialis

v. saphena lateralis, ramus caudalis

n. plantaris medialis

n. plantaris lateralis

n. digitalis plantaris II abaxialis

mm. interossei

n. digitalis plantaris V abaxialis

m. flexor digitorum profundus

arcus plantaris superficialis

v. digitalis plantaris communis
IV
II
III

n. digitalis plantaris communis
II
III
IV

digital pad 2

3

digital pad 5

4

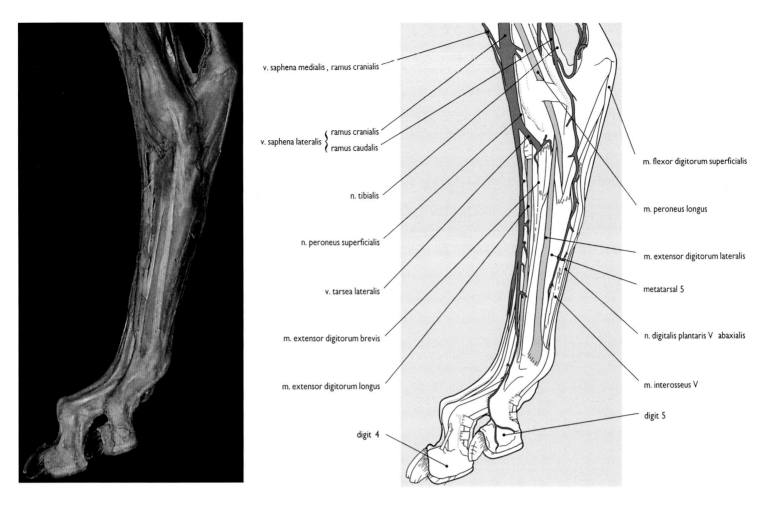

v. saphena medialis , ramus cranialis

v. saphena lateralis { ramus cranialis / ramus caudalis }

n. tibialis

n. peroneus superficialis

v. tarsea lateralis

m. extensor digitorum brevis

m. extensor digitorum longus

digit 4

m. flexor digitorum superficialis

m. peroneus longus

m. extensor digitorum lateralis

metatarsal 5

n. digitalis plantaris V abaxialis

m. interosseus V

digit 5

Fig. 7.78 Left tarsus and pes: lateral view. Only the fascia has been removed.

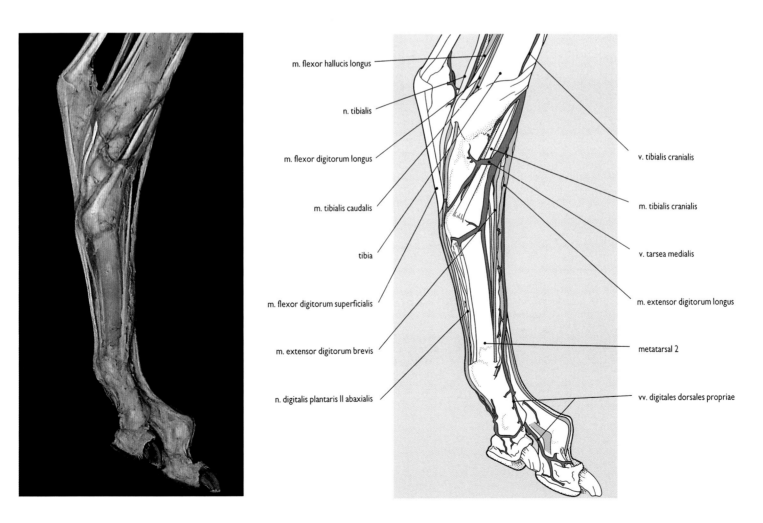

m. flexor hallucis longus

n. tibialis

m. flexor digitorum longus

m. tibialis caudalis

tibia

m. flexor digitorum superficialis

m. extensor digitorum brevis

n. digitalis plantaris II abaxialis

v. tibialis cranialis

m. tibialis cranialis

v. tarsea medialis

m. extensor digitorum longus

metatarsal 2

vv. digitales dorsales propriae

Fig. 7.79 Left tarsus and pes: medial view. Only the fascia has been removed.

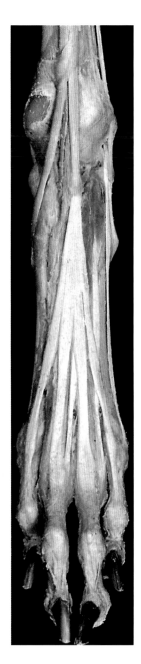

Fig. 7.80 Left tarsus and pes after removal of superficial veins and nerves: dorsal view. The digital divisions of the long digital extensor tendon can now be seen as well as the extensor retinaculum holding the tendon in position.

Fig. 7.81 Left tarsus and pes after removal of superficial veins and nerves: plantar view. The digital divisions of the superficial digital flexor have been exposed. Digital pads have been removed.

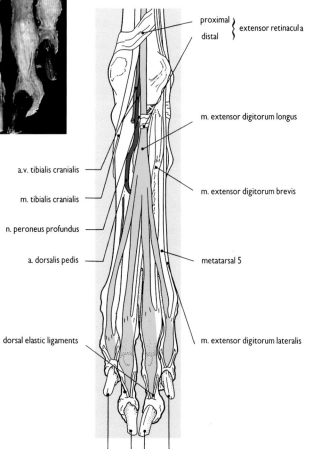

proximal
distal } extensor retinacula

m. extensor digitorum longus

a.v. tibialis cranialis

m. tibialis cranialis

n. peroneus profundus

a. dorsalis pedis

m. extensor digitorum brevis

metatarsal 5

dorsal elastic ligaments

m. extensor digitorum lateralis

2   3 4   5

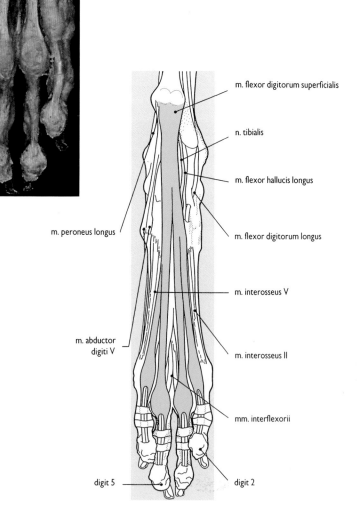

m. flexor digitorum superficialis

n. tibialis

m. flexor hallucis longus

m. peroneus longus

m. flexor digitorum longus

m. interosseus V

m. abductor
digiti V

m. interosseus II

mm. interflexorii

digit 5

digit 2

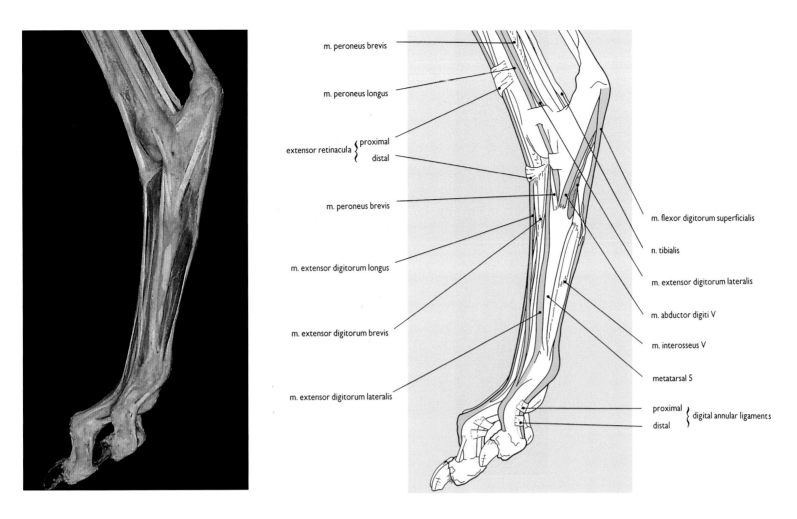

- m. peroneus brevis
- m. peroneus longus
- extensor retinacula { proximal / distal }
- m. peroneus brevis
- m. extensor digitorum longus
- m. extensor digitorum brevis
- m. extensor digitorum lateralis
- m. flexor digitorum superficialis
- n. tibialis
- m. extensor digitorum lateralis
- m. abductor digiti V
- m. interosseus V
- metatarsal 5
- proximal { digital annular ligaments / distal }

Fig. 7.82 Left tarsus and pes after removal of superficial veins and nerves: lateral view. In this specimen some muscle is associated with the normally entirely collagenous abductor of the fifth digit.

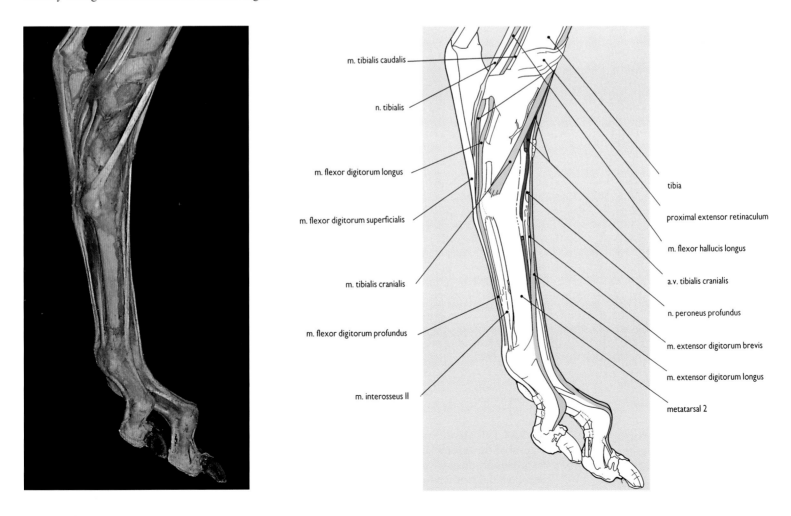

- m. tibialis caudalis
- n. tibialis
- m. flexor digitorum longus
- m. flexor digitorum superficialis
- m. tibialis cranialis
- m. flexor digitorum profundus
- m. interosseus II
- tibia
- proximal extensor retinaculum
- m. flexor hallucis longus
- a.v. tibialis cranialis
- n. peroneus profundus
- m. extensor digitorum brevis
- m. extensor digitorum longus
- metatarsal 2

Fig. 7.83 Left tarsus and pes after removal of superficial veins and nerves: medial view.

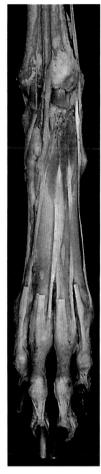
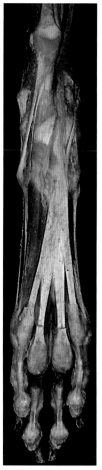
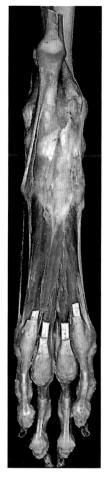

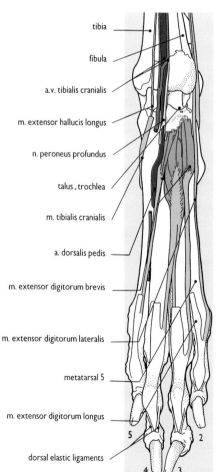

tibia

fibula

a.v. tibialis cranialis

m. extensor hallucis longus

n. peroneus profundus

talus , trochlea

m. tibialis cranialis

a. dorsalis pedis

m. extensor digitorum brevis

m. extensor digitorum lateralis

metatarsal 5

m. extensor digitorum longus

dorsal elastic ligaments

5   2

4   3

Fig. 7.84 Left tarsus and pes after removal of the long digital extensor and cranial tibial muscles: dorsal view. The short digital extensor muscle is exposed. Note also the continuation of the cranial tibial artery into the foot as the dorsal pedal artery.

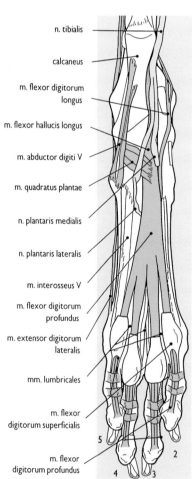

n. tibialis

calcaneus

m. flexor digitorum longus

m. flexor hallucis longus

m. abductor digiti V

m. quadratus plantae

n. plantaris medialis

n. plantaris lateralis

m. interosseus V

m. flexor digitorum profundus

m. extensor digitorum lateralis

mm. lumbricales

m. flexor digitorum superficialis

5   2

4   3

m. flexor digitorum profundus

Fig. 7.85 Left tarsus and pes after removal of the superficial digital flexor muscle: plantar view. The deep digital flexor tendons are exposed. The medial and lateral plantar nerves can be seen as the termination of the tibial nerve.

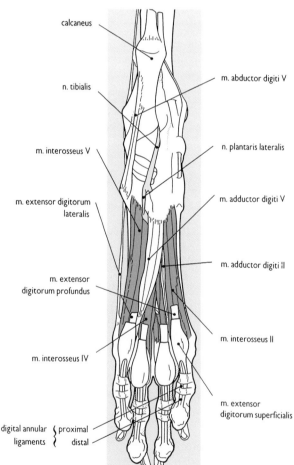

calcaneus

n. tibialis

m. interosseus V

m. extensor digitorum lateralis

m. extensor digitorum profundus

m. interosseus IV

digital annular { proximal
ligaments { distal

m. abductor digiti V

n. plantaris lateralis

m. adductor digiti V

m. adductor digiti II

m. interosseus II

m. extensor digitorum superficialis

Fig. 7.86 Left tarsus and pes after removal of the deep digital flexor muscle: plantar view.

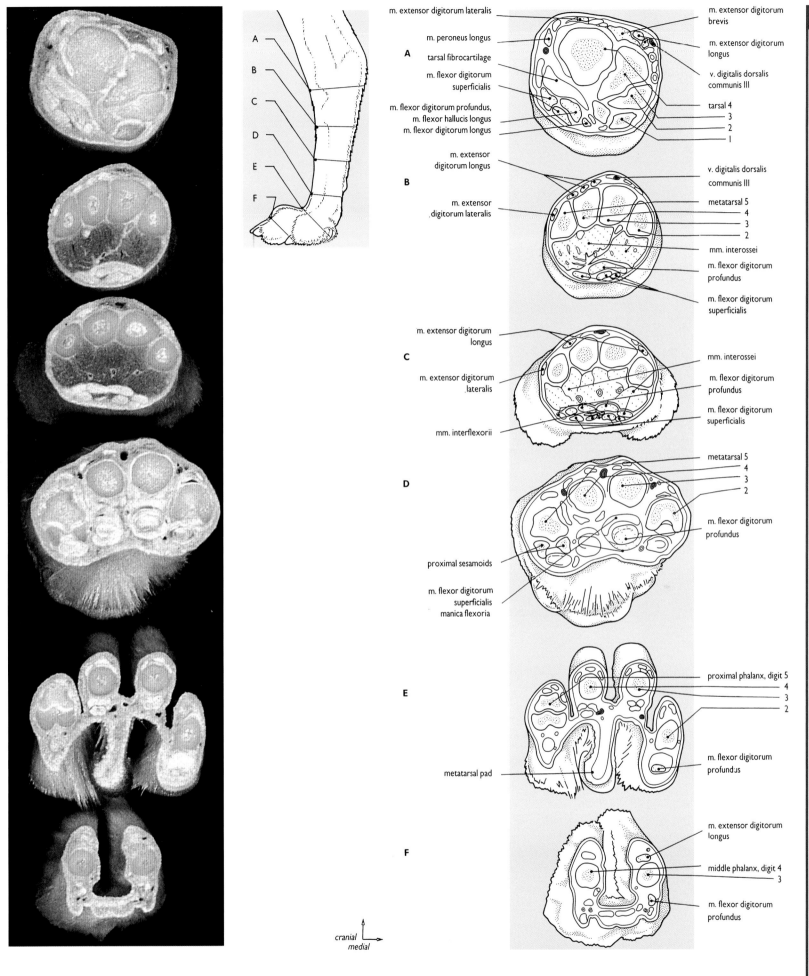

Fig. 7.87 Transverse sections through the left tarsus and pes at the levels indicated in the accompanying drawing: view of proximal surfaces of sections.

8. THE PELVIS

Clinically, the pelvis is an important region as it contains the rectum, anal sacs, prostate and male accessory organs, female reproductive tract and part of the urinary tract. For the purposes of this chapter, we have placed the reproductive tracts and urinary tract together in the pelvis.

More time is spent in veterinary practice dealing with the anal glands than any other small area of the body. These anal sacs lie between the internal and external sphincter muscles and are normally emptied when passing motion or on demand to mark out territory. The sac accumulates secretion from glands within their walls and this then passes to the exterior via ducts opening at the periphery of the anal orifice. These ducts can be cannulated. They may require simple emptying when they are full and causing irritation; irrigation, cleaning and filling with antibiotics/cortisone cream when impacted; may need complete removal if they are a persistent source of problem (taking care not to damage the anus and innervation to the anus). In some instances when the process has reached anal furunculosis (blind-ending tracts) the whole anal region has to be cleaned, tracts dissected and a repair made. This is almost a specific condition of German Shepherd dogs and may have immunological causes. Surgery is now often discouraged and treatment is largely via medication (ciclosporin and others).

We have already talked about two of the three hernias (dogs also have scrotal and hiatal hernias in the diaphragm) that dogs may suffer (inguinal and umbilical). A third and much more difficult to repair is the perineal hernia which is seen clinically as a bulge on one or both sides of the anus and can be felt per rectum. A swelling develops subcutaneously as the abdominal and pelvic contents (usually bladder) are forced by intra-abdominal pressure further into the pelvis. In older dogs, the levator ani and coccygeus which form the structure of the pelvic diaphragm which lies either side of the rectum weaken as the muscles atrophy with age. They offer support during the contractions of defecation. The rectum then deviates to the side of the breakdown during attempts to defecate. To repair this damage the sacro-tuberous ligament is used as the anchor point for the muscles of the pelvic diaphragm (levator and coccygeus), but care must be taken not to entrap the ischiatic nerve in the repair. The initial incisions are made vertically to the side of the anus over the site of the repair. Do not forget the use of the rectum for temperature taking.

Rectal prolapse is fortunately rare in the dog. It is often dealt with by a simple purse string type of suture with or without debridement of the devitalized tissue.

The prostate is usually within the pelvic canal but in older dogs there is relocation into the abdomen and here it is accessible for surgery, although this is probably problematic, via a caudal midline ventral abdominal incision. It becomes progressively larger with age under the influence of testicular androgens and the concurrent influence of oestrogen.

The male urethra may be blocked by stones (urinary calculi) at the proximal part of the ventral groove in the os penis and here it is a simple matter to incise over the urethra and remove the stone. In some cases with persistent problems, a new opening for the urethra can be made directly to the skin ventral to the anus, thereby removing the threat of urethral blockage at the proximal penis.

Surgery of the penis is sometimes carried out to remove the problem of an infected prepuce and paraphimosis or phimosis.

In cases of trauma and road traffic accidents complete penile removal may be required.

Castration is another routine operation carried out in dogs to reduce aggression and if done in later life probably has little effect, and is a relatively simple operation. It is sometimes more difficult when carried out in dogs for the removal of testicular tumors and in some complete scrotal ablation is required when tumors involve the scrotum.

In dogs with a retained testicle, this must be removed to prevent intra-abdominal neoplasia. A para-penile incision on the side of the retained testicle can be made but an inguinal or midline incision is usually made. It often requires ligation of the superficial epigastric vein if a para-penile incision is made and then the penis can be reflected and a normal midline incision made through linea alba. You can find the *vasa deferentia* as white, wire-like threads divergent from the neck of the bladder. Gentle traction on these will usually bring the retained testicle(s) into view from abdomen or inguinal canal.

In the bitch, it is rarely necessary to remove the ventral wall of the vagina which has become prolapsed. Perivalvular dermatitis and necrotic vulvitis may require episiotomy or episioplasty to repair the inflamed tissues.

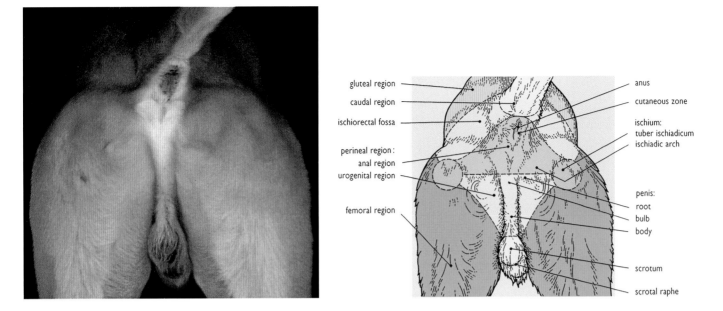

Fig. 8.1 Surface features and topographical regions of the pelvis and genitalia: caudal view. The perineal region is shown with the tail raised. It overlies the perineum, which in turn fills and closes the pelvic outlet. It corresponds to the retroperitoneal part of the pelvis and includes muscles and fibrous structures surrounding the anal canal and the termination of the urogenital tracts. The superficial boundary is the skin covering the ischiorectal fossa and extending down to the scrotum below. A horizontal line joining the ischiatic tuberosities separates an anal from a urogenital triangle.

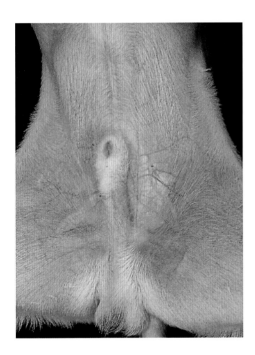

Fig. 8.2 Surface features of the prepuce: ventral view (1). The prepuce is shown completely enclosing the glans penis. The tubular sheath has a normal hairy outer layer continuous with the skin of the abdominal wall and thighs.

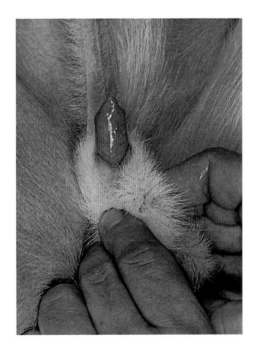

Fig. 8.3 Surface features of the prepuce: ventral view (2). The glans penis is protruded through the preputial orifice and the prepuce is rolled back, opening out the preputial cavity.

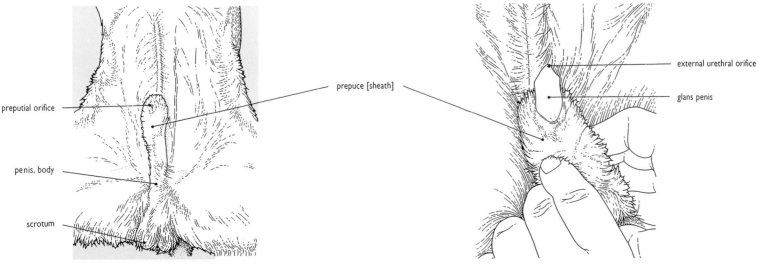

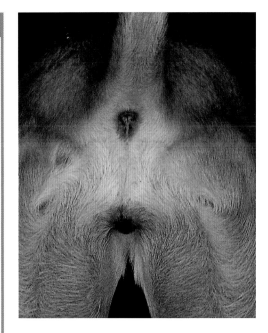

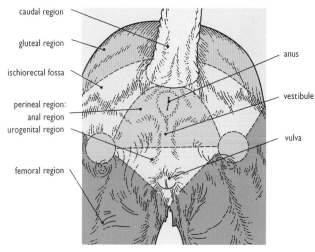

caudal region

gluteal region

ischiorectal fossa

perineal region:
anal region
urogenital region

femoral region

anus

vestibule

vulva

Fig. 8.4 Surface features and topographical regions of the pelvis and genitalia of the bitch: caudal view. The perineal region of the bitch is shown with the tail raised. Its overall disposition is much like that of the male. The urogenital triangle (also known as the pudendum or pudendal region) incorporates the only visible component of the external genitalia, the vulva positioned below the ischiatic arch. The vestibule connecting vulva with vagina may be up to 5 cm in length.

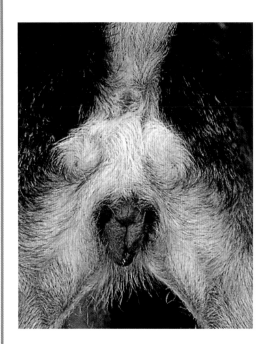

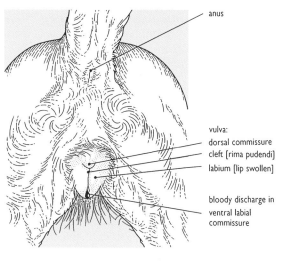

anus

vulva:
dorsal commissure
cleft [rima pudendi]
labium [lip swollen]

bloody discharge in
ventral labial
commissure

Fig. 8.5 Surface features of the genitalia of a bitch in oestrus: caudal view. The genitalia of a bitch in heat are shown with the tail raised. The vulva is enlarged and its lips congested and swollen. A blood-tinged discharge from the vulva is also typical of the bitch in heat.

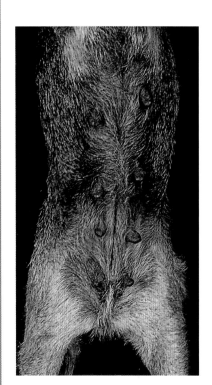

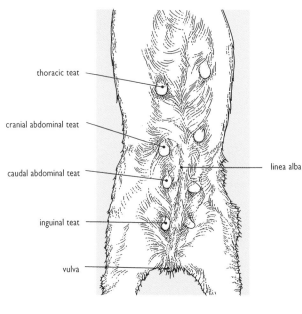

thoracic teat

cranial abdominal teat

caudal abdominal teat

inguinal teat

vulva

linea alba

Fig. 8.6 Surface features of the abdomen of a multiparous bitch: ventral view. This multiparous Border Terrier bitch displays two rows of teats. In maiden bitches the teats will be less pronounced. Four pairs are normal for this small breed although 5 pairs would be common in most breeds and very occasionally 6 pairs are present.

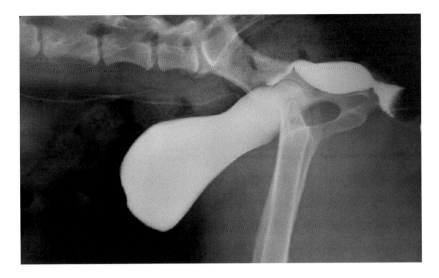

Fig. 8.7 Radiograph of the pelvis: lateral view, male dog. The urethra has been highlighted with water-soluble iodine-containing contrast medium. Air has been introduced into the bladder.

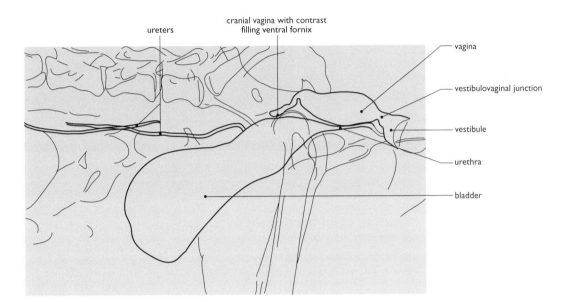

ureters

cranial vagina with contrast filling ventral fornix

vagina

vestibulovaginal junction

vestibule

urethra

bladder

bladder containing air and positive contrast

prostatic urethra

membranous urethra

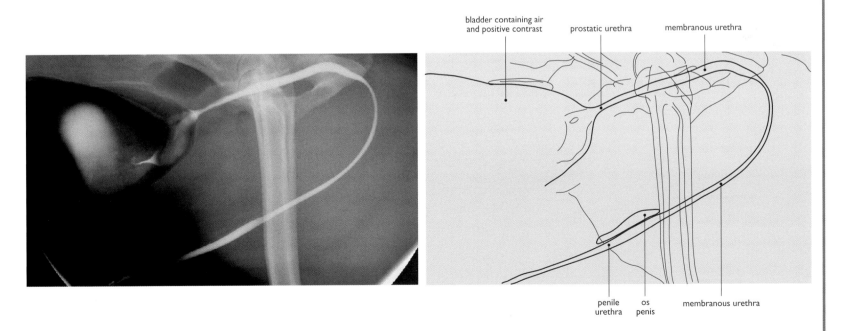

penile urethra

os penis

membranous urethra

Fig. 8.8 Radiograph of the pelvis: lateral view, female dog. Water-soluble iodine-containing contrast medium has been infused into the vestibule, vagina, urethra and bladder. There is also some contrast medium present in the ureters.

8

Fig. 8.9 Pelvic cavity and sacrotuberous ligament: left dorsolateral view. This is a slightly different view of Fig. 7.20, looking down into the pelvis through the greater ischiatic notch and onto the hip joint. The lumbosacral trunk is clearly exposed in this view leaving the pelvis to be continued as the ischiatic nerve. Caudal to the sacrotuberous ligament the coccygeal muscle and the external anal sphincter muscle form the medial boundary of the ischiorectal fossa (see Fig. 8.66). The internal obturator muscle forming the floor and lateral wall of the fossa leaves the pelvis and its tendon is visible on the gemelli muscles beneath the ischiatic nerve. Immediately cranial to it the hip joint capsule has been exposed and the articularis coxae muscle lies on its surface. The retractor penis muscle and the bulbospongiosus muscle are both exposed on the root of the penis (see Fig. 8.44).

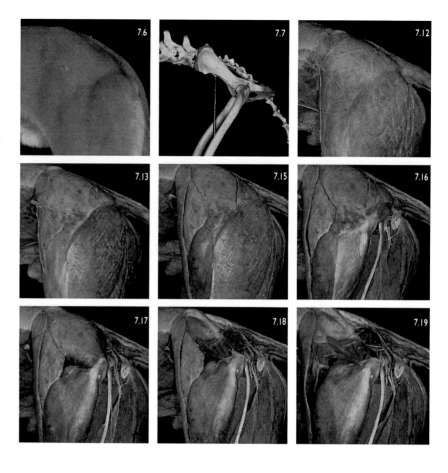

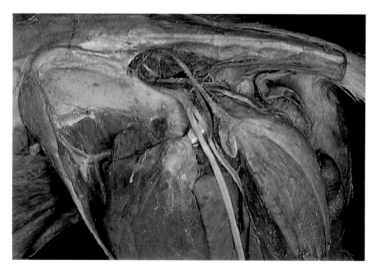

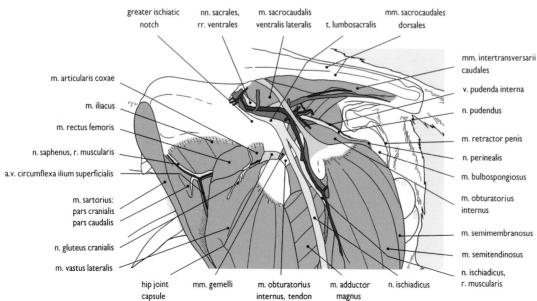

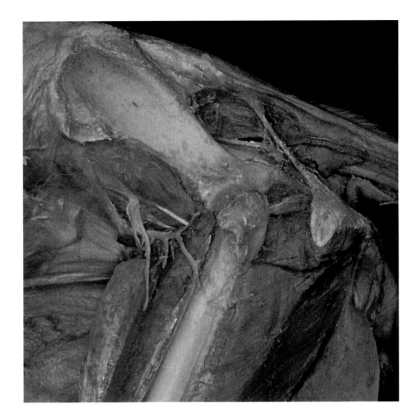

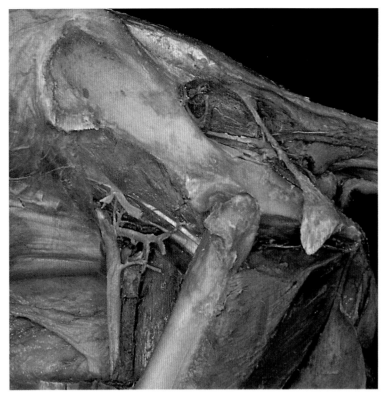

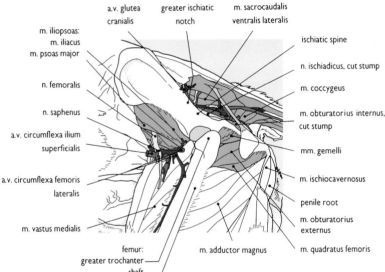

a.v. glutea cranialis   greater ischiatic notch   m. sacrocaudalis ventralis lateralis

m. iliopsoas:
m. iliacus
m. psoas major

n. femoralis

n. saphenus

a.v. circumflexa ilium superficialis

a.v. circumflexa femoris lateralis

m. vastus medialis

femur:
greater trochanter
shaft

m. adductor magnus

ischiatic spine

n. ischiadicus, cut stump

m. coccygeus

m. obturatorius internus, cut stump

mm. gemelli

m. ischiocavernosus

penile root

m. obturatorius externus

m. quadratus femoris

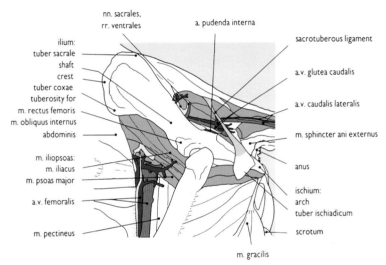

nn. sacrales, rr. ventrales   a. pudenda interna

ilium:
tuber sacrale
shaft
crest
tuber coxae
tuberosity for
m. rectus femoris
m. obliquus internus abdominis

m. iliopsoas:
m. iliacus
m. psoas major

a.v. femoralis

m. pectineus

m. gracilis

sacrotuberous ligament

a.v. glutea caudalis

a.v. caudalis lateralis

m. sphincter ani externus

anus

ischium:
arch
tuber ischiadicum

scrotum

Fig. 8.10 Pelvic bone, hip joint and muscles of the small pelvic association: left lateral view (1). The sartorius, vastus lateralis and rectus femoris muscles have been removed from the cranial surface of the thigh, exposing the medial vastus and iliopsoas muscles with the femoral nerve passing through the latter. Also exposed are the ramifications in the thigh of the superficial circumflex iliac and lateral circumflex femoral vessels. Caudal to the hip joint the ischiatic nerve, the caudal gluteal vessels, the semimembranosus and semitendinosus muscles are all removed. The internal and external obturator muscles, the gemelli and quadratus femoris muscles are visible converging onto the caudal surface of the greater femoral trochanter in the neighborhood of the trochanteric fossa.

Fig. 8.11 Pelvic bone, hip joint and muscles of the small pelvic association: left lateral view (2). Removal of the medial vastus muscle from the front thigh exposes the iliopsoas and pectineus muscles with the femoral vessels running down the thigh cranial to the latter muscle. Although the femoral nerve is largely removed its saphenous branch remains in position in relation to the femoral vessels. Caudal to the hip joint the internal obturator tendon has been removed along with the underlying gemelli muscles. Only the external obturator and quadratus femoris muscles remain of the small pelvic association. Removal of the semimembranosus and semitendinosus completes removal of the 'hamstring' muscles and exposes the adductor and gracilis muscles of the inner thigh and the ischiocavernosus muscle of the penile root.

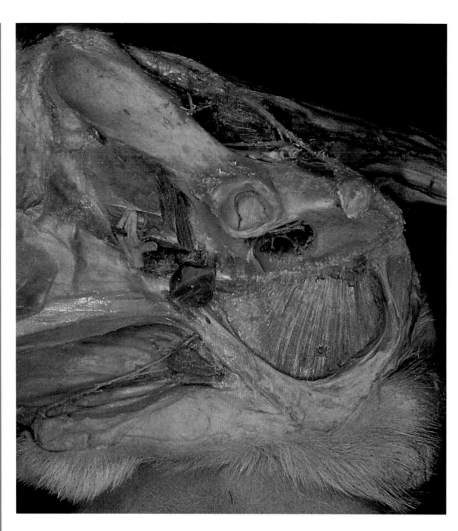

Fig. 8.12 Pelvic bone, external genitalia and inguinal region after removal of the hindlimb: left lateral view. The remains of the hindlimb have been removed by severing the pectineus and iliopsoas muscles (their cut surfaces are clearly exposed); completely removing adductor, gracilis, quadratus femoris and external obturator muscles from their pelvic attachments; and disarticulating the hip joint following severance of its fibrous capsule and internal ligament of the femoral head. The femoral vessels and saphenous nerve are also severed cranial to the pectineus muscle. The bony pelvic wall and floor formed from the pelvic bone are now exposed and extending ventrally from the pelvic symphysis is the midline symphyseal tendon onto which the bulk of the adductor muscles attached. The internal obturator muscle is visible through the obturator foramen and the remnants of the obturator nerve and vessels are exposed. The external genitalia remain completely intact although a small amount of penile skin is removed. The vaginal process extends caudally onto the lateral surface of the penis; superficial inguinal lymph nodes and external pudendal vessels lie in the superficial abdominal fascia cranial to it. Preputial and penile fascia also merge with abdominal and femoral fascia in the fold of the groin and medial side of the thigh.

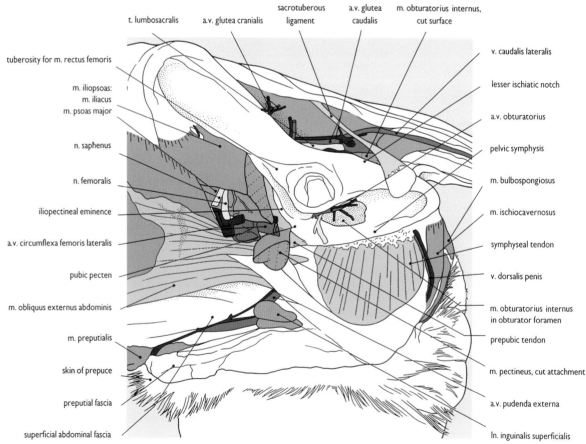

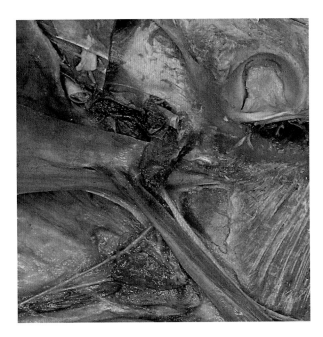

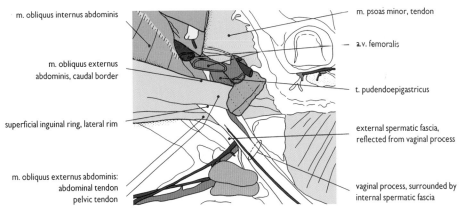

m. obliquus internus abdominis

m. obliquus externus abdominis, caudal border

superficial inguinal ring, lateral rim

m. obliquus externus abdominis:
abdominal tendon
pelvic tendon

m. psoas minor, tendon

a.v. femoralis

t. pudendoepigastricus

external spermatic fascia,
reflected from vaginal process

vaginal process, surrounded by
internal spermatic fascia

Fig. 8.13 Inguinal canal (1). External abdominal oblique muscle and superficial inguinal ring: left lateral view. This is a closer view of the inguinal region of a dog and begins a sequence of inguinal canal dissections (see Figs 8.53–8.57 for a ventral sequence in a bitch). Abdominal fascia has been cleared to expose the superficial inguinal ring, and reflection of spermatic fascia has exposed the vaginal process. The femoral vessels are cut back to expose the caudal border of the external oblique muscle.

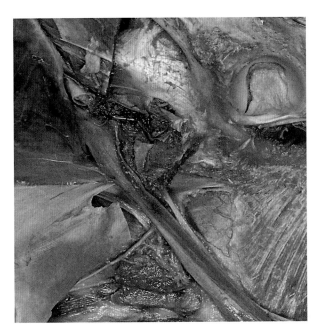

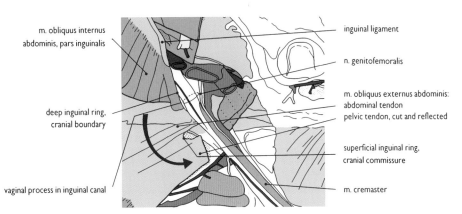

m. obliquus internus
abdominis, pars inguinalis

deep inguinal ring,
cranial boundary

vaginal process in inguinal canal

inguinal ligament

n. genitofemoralis

m. obliquus externus abdominis:
abdominal tendon
pelvic tendon, cut and reflected

superficial inguinal ring,
cranial commissure

m. cremaster

Fig. 8.14 Inguinal canal (2). Internal abdominal oblique muscle, deep and superficial inguinal rings: left lateral view. The pelvic tendon of the external oblique muscle has been cut close to its merger with the pectineus tendon, and the whole aponeurosis is reflected ventrally, destroying the superficial inguinal ring and the lateral and ventral walls of the inguinal canal. The poorly defined deep inguinal ring is located at the point where the vaginal process crosses the caudal border of the internal abdominal oblique muscle.

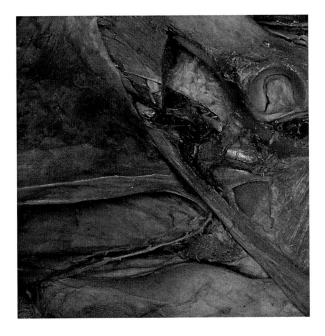

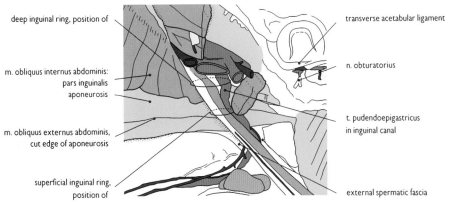

deep inguinal ring, position of

m. obliquus internus abdominis:
pars inguinalis
aponeurosis

m. obliquus externus abdominis,
cut edge of aponeurosis

superficial inguinal ring,
position of

transverse acetabular ligament

n. obturatorius

t. pudendoepigastricus
in inguinal canal

external spermatic fascia

Fig. 8.15 Inguinal canal (3). Internal abdominal oblique muscle, spermatic fascia and cremaster muscle: left lateral view. The reflected part of the external oblique has been removed and the line of the cut edge of the tendon is visible on the rectus abdominis muscle where it contributes to the rectus sheath (see Chapter 6). The approximate positions of the inguinal rings, and therefore the extent of the inguinal canal, are shown.

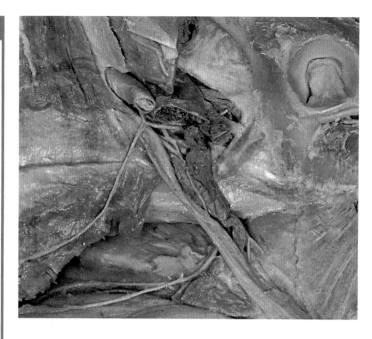

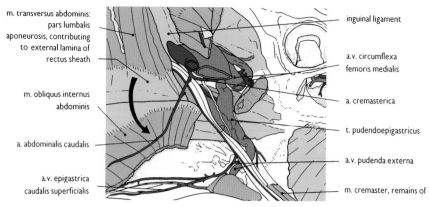

Fig. 8.16 Inguinal canal (4). Vaginal process, pudendoepigastric trunk and genitofemoral nerve: left lateral view. The internal oblique muscle has been dissected away from its origin on the inguinal ligament and is reflected ventrally. The cremaster muscle derived from the internal oblique is also removed from the fascia surrounding the vaginal process.

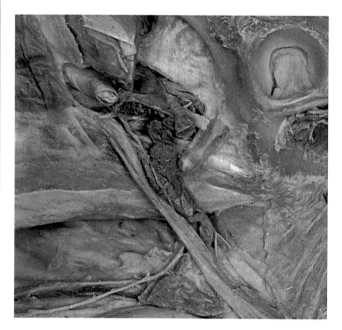

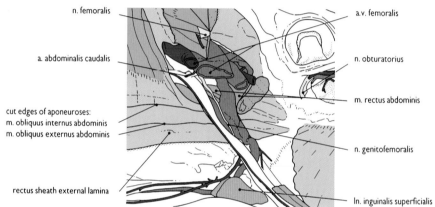

Fig. 8.17 Inguinal canal (5). Transverse abdominal and rectus abdominis muscles: left lateral view. The reflected part of the internal oblique has been removed and the line of the cut edge of its tendon is visible on the surface of the rectus abdominis parallel to that of the external oblique where both contribute to the rectus sheath. The transverse abdominal muscle also contributes to the superficial layer of the rectus sheath.

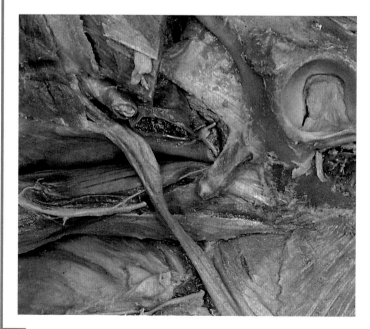

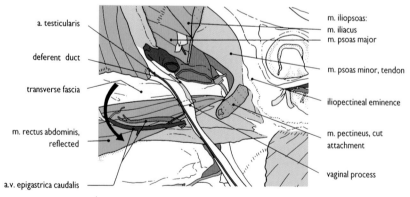

Fig. 8.18 Inguinal canal (6). Vaginal process, testicular artery and deferent duct: left lateral view. The transverse abdominal muscle has been cut through on a line with the dorsal edge of the rectus abdominis allowing the rectus to be reflected ventrally away from the abdominal wall, totally destroying what remains of the inguinal canal. Transverse fascia lines the abdomen and here forms the internal layer of the rectus sheath (see Chapter 6).

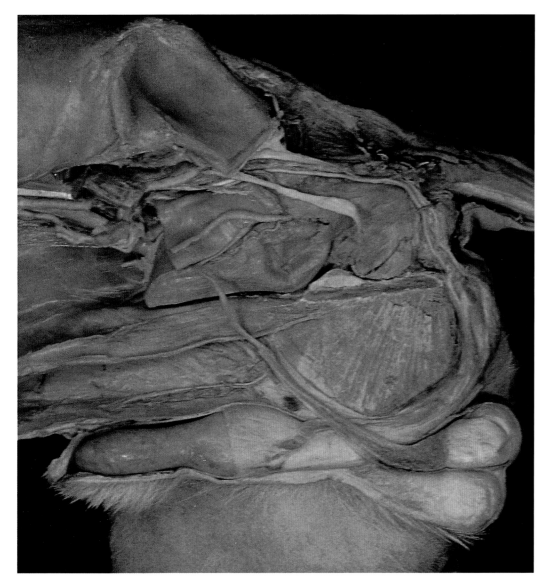

Fig. 8.19 Pelvic cavity after removal of the pelvic bone: left lateral view. The abdominal wall has been removed and the iliopsoas muscle and external iliac vessels have been cut back into the abdominal roof. The pelvic bone of the left side was removed by sawing through the pelvic symphysis and through the iliac shaft ventral to the sacroiliac joint. The coccygeus muscle was severed from its iliac attachment and the left crus of the penis and left ischiocavernosus muscle were severed at their attachments to the ischiatic arch. The sacrotuberous ligament was cut through at its sacral attachment and removed with the pelvic bone. The internal obturator muscle, attached to the pelvic surface of the pelvic bone, has also been removed. The pelvic cavity is opened from the left side and the levator ani muscle of the pelvic diaphragm is left in position after its origin from the pelvic bone was severed on pelvic bone removal. The preputial cavity has been opened by removal of the left half of the prepuce as far caudally as the preputial fornix on the bulbus glandis. The scrotum has also been opened displaying the testis and epididymis of the left side inside the cavity of the vaginal process.

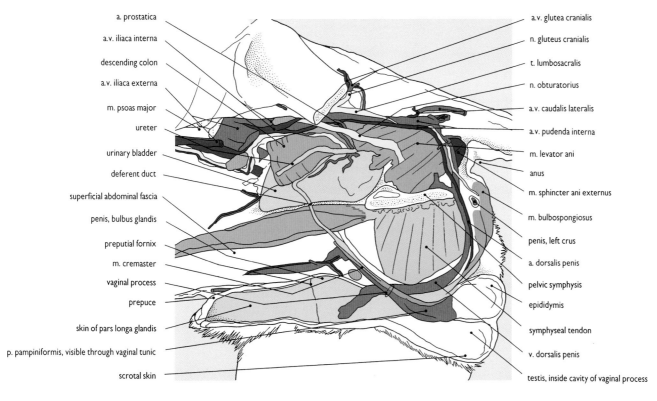

a. prostatica

a.v. iliaca interna

descending colon

a.v. iliaca externa

m. psoas major

ureter

urinary bladder

deferent duct

superficial abdominal fascia

penis, bulbus glandis

preputial fornix

m. cremaster

vaginal process

prepuce

skin of pars longa glandis

p. pampiniformis, visible through vaginal tunic

scrotal skin

a.v. glutea cranialis

n. gluteus cranialis

t. lumbosacralis

n. obturatorius

a.v. caudalis lateralis

a.v. pudenda interna

m. levator ani

anus

m. sphincter ani externus

m. bulbospongiosus

penis, left crus

a. dorsalis penis

pelvic symphysis

epididymis

symphyseal tendon

v. dorsalis penis

testis, inside cavity of vaginal process

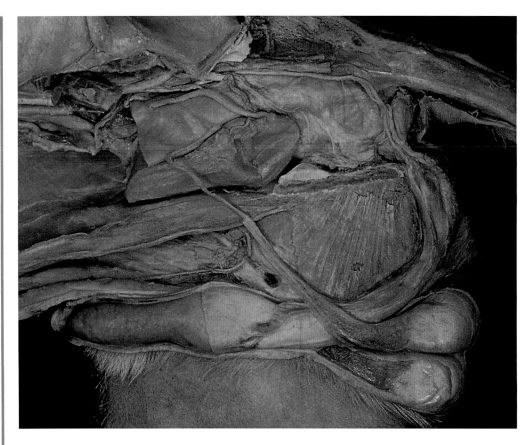

Fig. 8.20 Pelvic viscera (1) after removal of the levator ani muscle: left lateral view. Removal of the levator ani muscle and trimming of the obturator nerve and lumbosacral trunk has begun visceral exposure in the more cranial peritoneal part of the pelvic cavity. Loose pelvic and perineal fascia still obscures detail in the more caudal retroperitoneal part of the cavity underlying the perineum. The main continuation of the internal pudendal vessels as dorsal penile vessels is now clear. The origin of the dorsal penile vein in the bulbus glandis is visible, and the superficial vein of the glans is cut through in the prepuce dorsal to the pars longa glandis.

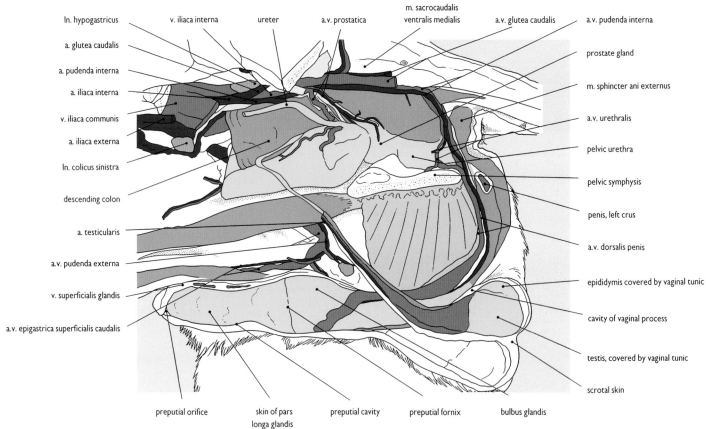

ln. hypogastricus
a. glutea caudalis
a. pudenda interna
a. iliaca interna
v. iliaca communis
a. iliaca externa
ln. colicus sinistra
descending colon
a. testicularis
a.v. pudenda externa
v. superficialis glandis
a.v. epigastrica superficialis caudalis

v. iliaca interna
ureter
a.v. prostatica
m. sacrocaudalis ventralis medialis
a.v. glutea caudalis
a.v. pudenda interna

prostate gland
m. sphincter ani externus
a.v. urethralis
pelvic urethra
pelvic symphysis
penis, left crus
a.v. dorsalis penis
epididymis covered by vaginal tunic
cavity of vaginal process
testis, covered by vaginal tunic
scrotal skin

preputial orifice
skin of pars longa glandis
preputial cavity
preputial fornix
bulbus glandis

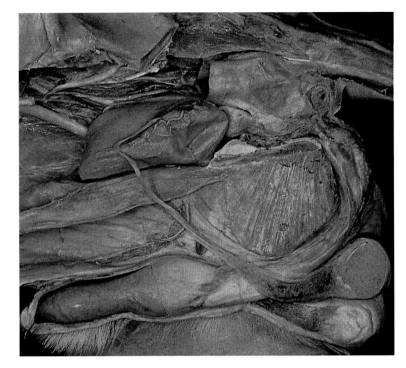

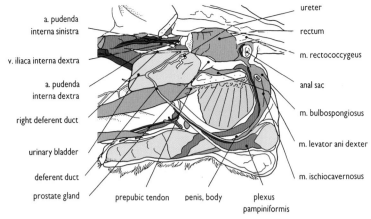

Fig. 8.21 Pelvic viscera (2). Prostate gland and anal sac after removal of the external anal sphincter muscle: left lateral view. The internal iliac vessels have been removed along with considerable amounts of pelvic and perineal fascia and the external anal sphincter muscle. The anal sac has been exposed with the rectococcygeus muscle lying dorsal to it. The rectum at the cranial end of the pelvis has been removed, exposing the apposition of left and right deferent ducts on the dorsum of the neck of the bladder.

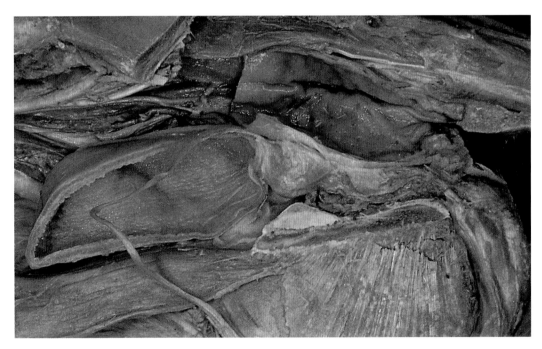

Fig. 8.22 Pelvic viscera (3). Interior of the bladder and rectum and the anal canal: left lateral view. The left half of the bladder, rectum and anal canal have been removed, displaying their interiors. In the anal canal columns are apparent and the opening of the anal sac of the right side is visible at the anocutaneous line. In the cranial part of the pelvis a pelvic nerve is exposed on the levator ani muscle of the right side.

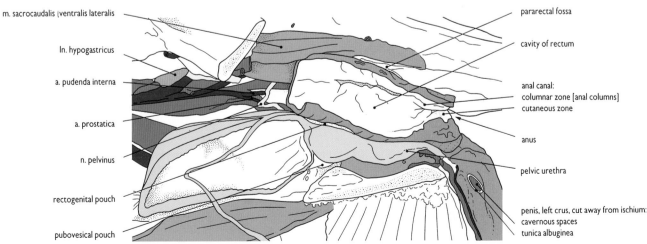

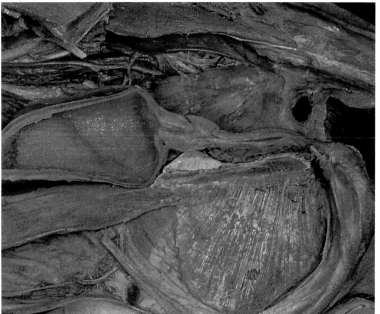

Fig. 8.23 Pelvic viscera (4). Bladder, prostate gland and pelvic urethra in sagittal section: left medial view. The rectum has been removed and the pelvic urethra and prostate gland are sectioned in the midline. The levator ani of the right side is exposed following rectal removal and its nerve supply is displayed. The anal sac of the right side is opened following removal of the internal anal sphincter muscle with the anal canal. The sac contains accumulated secretion from the surrounding anal glands. The prostate gland completely surrounds the prostatic urethra and a urethral muscle surrounds the remaining part of the pelvic urethra.

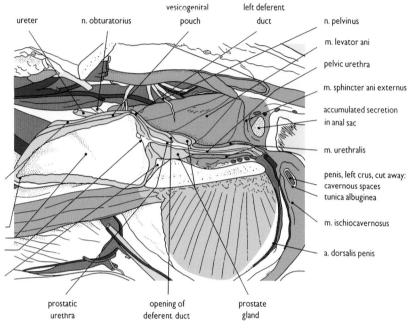

ureter — n. obturatorius — vesicogenital pouch — left deferent duct — n. pelvinus — m. levator ani — pelvic urethra — m. sphincter ani externus — accumulated secretion in anal sac — m. urethralis — penis, left crus, cut away: cavernous spaces tunica albuginea — m. ischiocavernosus — a. dorsalis penis

right deferent duct — urinary bladder: apex, body, neck — pubovesical pouch

prostatic urethra — opening of deferent duct — prostate gland

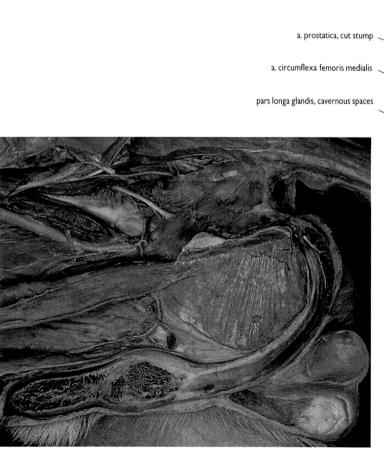

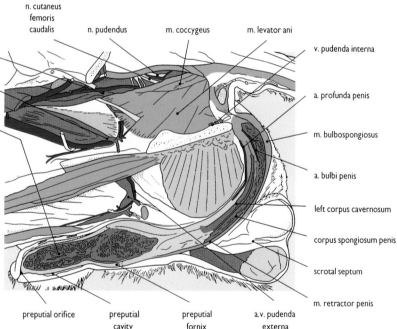

n. cutaneus femoris caudalis — n. pudendus — m. coccygeus — m. levator ani — v. pudenda interna

a. prostatica, cut stump — a. circumflexa femoris medialis — pars longa glandis, cavernous spaces — a. profunda penis — m. bulbospongiosus — a. bulbi penis — left corpus cavernosum — corpus spongiosum penis — scrotal septum — m. retractor penis

preputial orifice — preputial cavity — preputial fornix — a.v. pudenda externa

Fig. 8.24 Pelvic wall of the right side in medial view (1) and the penis in parasagittal section. The bladder, prostate gland and pelvic urethra have been removed and the pelvic diaphragm of the right side is exposed; the coccygeus muscle is visible dorsal to the levator ani. The remains of the vaginal process and testis of the left side have been removed and the penis sectioned parasagittally to the left of its midline. The corpus cavernosum and corpus spongiosum are opened in the root and body and the cavernous tissue of the bulbus glandis and pars longa glandis is visible.

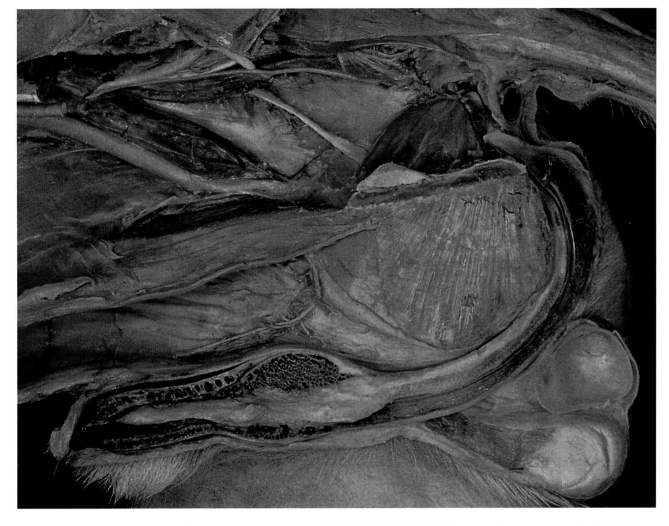

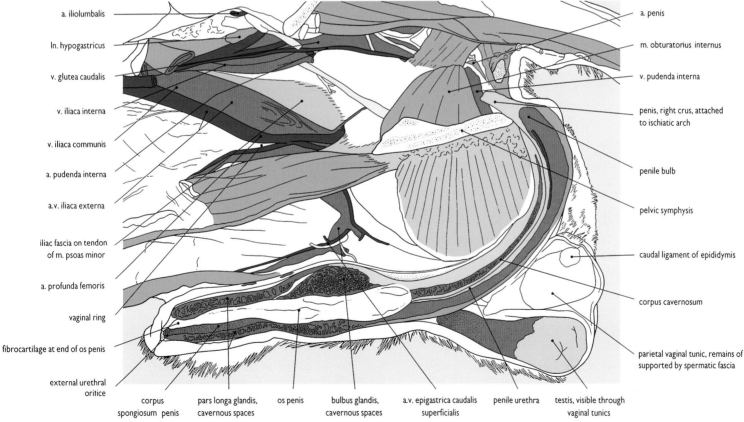

a. iliolumbalis

ln. hypogastricus

v. glutea caudalis

v. iliaca interna

v. iliaca communis

a. pudenda interna

a.v. iliaca externa

iliac fascia on tendon
of m. psoas minor

a. profunda femoris

vaginal ring

fibrocartilage at end of os penis

external urethral
oritice

a. penis

m. obturatorius internus

v. pudenda interna

penis, right crus, attached
to ischiatic arch

penile bulb

pelvic symphysis

caudal ligament of epididymis

corpus cavernosum

parietal vaginal tunic, remains of
supported by spermatic fascia

corpus
spongiosum penis

pars longa glandis,
cavernous spaces

os penis

bulbus glandis,
cavernous spaces

a.v. epigastrica caudalis
superficialis

penile urethra

testis, visible through
vaginal tunics

Fig. 8.25 Pelvic wall of the right side in medial view (2) and the penis in sagittal section. Removal of the levator ani muscle has exposed the internal obturator and coccygeus muscles of the right side. Sagittal sectioning of the penis exposes much of its internal anatomy, especially the extent of the os penis in the glans and the disposition of cavernous tissues of the bulbus and pars longa glandis (see Fig. 8.26 for further details of penile anatomy). At the pelvic outlet the right crus of the penis is exposed at its attachment to the ischiatic arch caudal to a prominent internal pudendal vein. Cranial to the pelvic inlet, in the right abdominal wall, the deep femoral artery is displayed with its branching in the neighborhood of the vaginal ring.

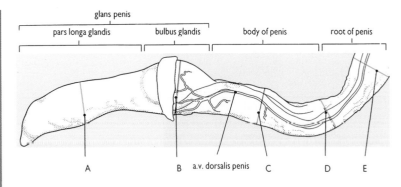

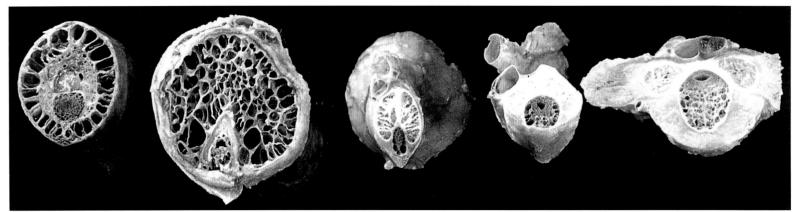

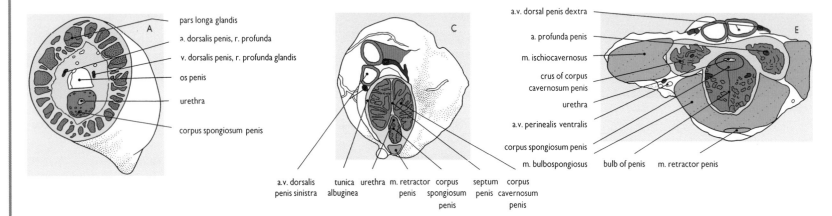

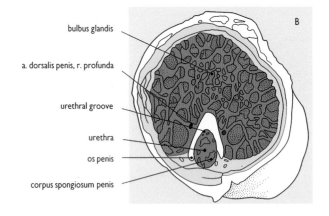

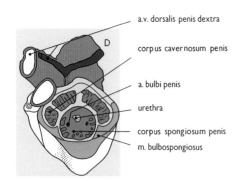

Fig. 8.26 The structure of the penis in transverse section: caudal views of sections. The accompanying sketch of the penis shows the levels at which the sections were taken. Section E through the penile root demonstrates the crura of the penis based on the diverging corpora cavernosa with their associated ischiocavernosus muscles, and the penile bulb expansion of the corpus spongiosum covered by the bulbospongiosus muscle. These structures are particularly well displayed in Fig. 8.44. Sections D and C are both through the penile body, the corpora cavernosa having come together in the midline only separated by a fibrous septum. In the body of the penis the corpus spongiosum surrounding the urethra remains a fairly restricted component underlain by the penile retractor muscle. Sections B and A through the penile glans show the os penis (penile bone) as a continuation of the corpora cavernosa with the corpus spongiosum and urethra running in a 'gutter' on its underside. The full extent of the penile bone is shown in Fig. 8.25. The remaining spongy tissue of the glans develops from the corpus spongiosum and comes to surround it and os penis as the globular bulb of the glans (B) and the elongated pars longa of the glans (A).

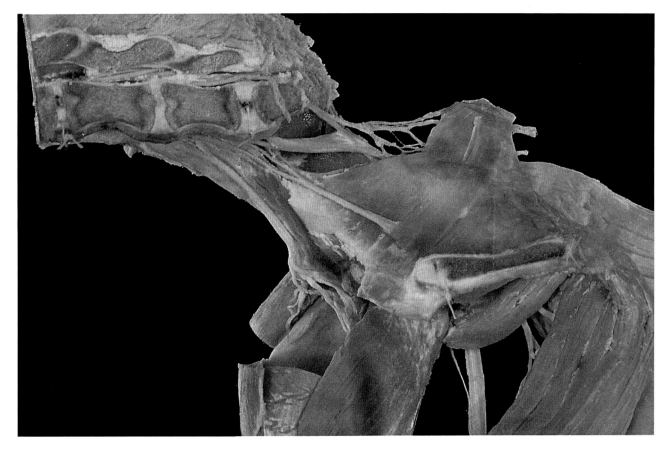

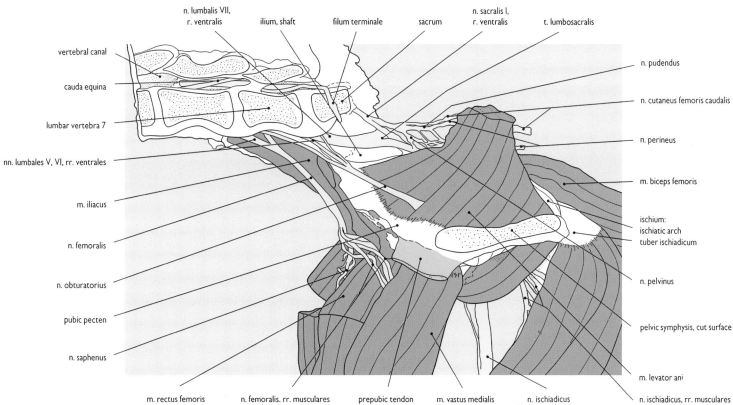

n. lumbalis VII, r. ventralis	ilium, shaft	filum terminale	sacrum	n. sacralis I, r. ventralis	t. lumbosacralis

vertebral canal

cauda equina

lumbar vertebra 7

nn. lumbales V, VI, rr. ventrales

m. iliacus

n. femoralis

n. obturatorius

pubic pecten

n. saphenus

n. pudendus

n. cutaneus femoris caudalis

n. perineus

m. biceps femoris

ischium:
ischiatic arch
tuber ischiadicum

n. pelvinus

pelvic symphysis, cut surface

m. levator ani

n. ischiadicus, rr. musculares

m. rectus femoris   n. femoralis. rr. musculares   prepubic tendon   m. vastus medialis   n. ischiadicus

Fig. 8.27 Pelvic wall of the right side (3). Lumbosacral plexus and nerves to the pelvis and hindlimb: medial view. This dissection gives an overall picture of the nerves to the hindlimb and pelvis arising from the lumbosacral plexus and lying in the pelvic wall. The vertebral column has been sectioned in the midline but the caudal part of the sacrum and the caudal vertebrae have been removed completely. Contributions from lumbar nerves 5, 6 and 7, and from sacral nerve 1 are clearly apparent. Those nerves arising from the sacral part of the plexus have been somewhat artificially displayed along with the levator ani muscle.

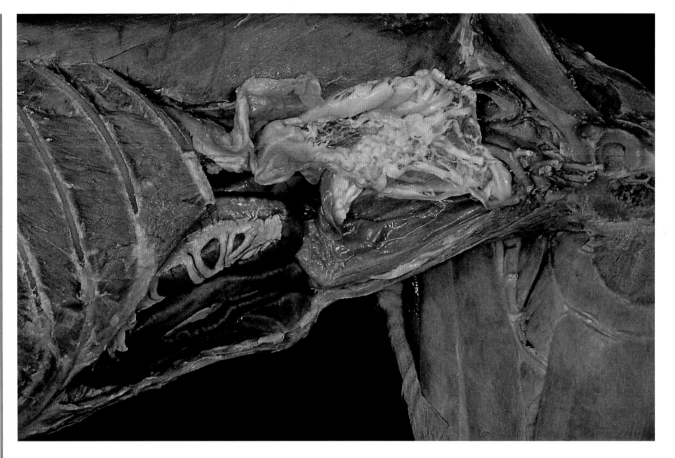

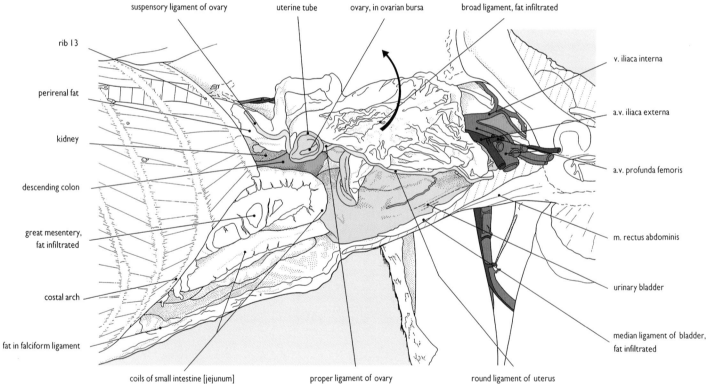

suspensory ligament of ovary   uterine tube   ovary, in ovarian bursa   broad ligament, fat infiltrated

rib 13

perirenal fat

kidney

descending colon

great mesentery,
fat infiltrated

costal arch

fat in falciform ligament

v. iliaca interna

a.v. iliaca externa

a.v. profunda femoris

m. rectus abdominis

urinary bladder

median ligament of bladder,
fat infiltrated

coils of small intestine [jejunum]   proper ligament of ovary   round ligament of uterus

Fig. 8.28 Reproductive tract of the bitch (1). Left uterine horn and broad ligament: left lateral view. The abdominal wall of the left side has been removed from this bitch exposing the abdominal contents from a left lateral view. The fat-infiltrated broad ligament (mesometrium) has been reflected dorsally in order to expose the ovary in its ovarian bursa, and to display the round ligament of the uterus in the edge of its own fold of mesometrium. The round ligament is traceable caudally to the inguinal region, and cranially is continued by the proper ligament of the ovary. The suspensory ligament of the ovary is visible related to the dorsolateral surface of the kidney.

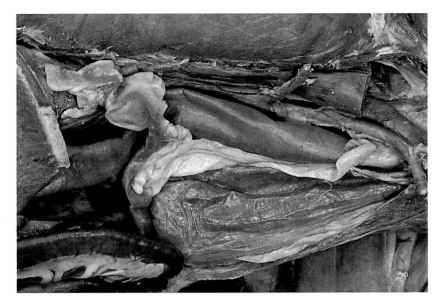

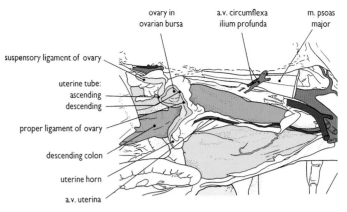

Fig. 8.29 Reproductive tract of the bitch (2). Ovary, ovarian bursa and uterine horn: left lateral view. The broad ligament has been removed, except for that part supporting the ovary, and the descending colon is exposed. The small intestine has been reflected cranioventrally to display the extent of the left uterine horn.

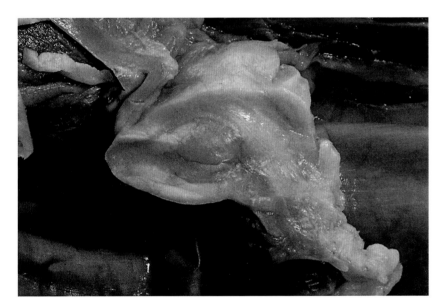

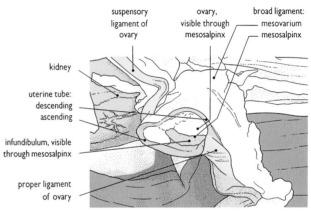

Fig. 8.30 Reproductive tract of the bitch (3). Ovary, ovarian bursa and uterine tube (1): left lateral view. This is an enlarged view of the ovary and ovarian bursa shown in Fig. 8.29. The mesosalpinx forms the lateral bursal wall and the ovary and infundibulum are visible through it.

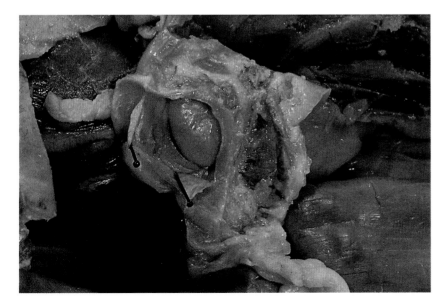

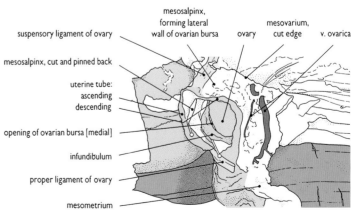

Fig. 8.31 Reproductive tract of the bitch (4). Ovary, ovarian bursa and uterine tube (2): left lateral view. The lateral wall of the ovarian bursa has been cut into and is pinned back, exposing the ovary and infundibulum of the uterine tube. Between these two in the medial wall of the bursa the opening into the bursal cavity is displayed.

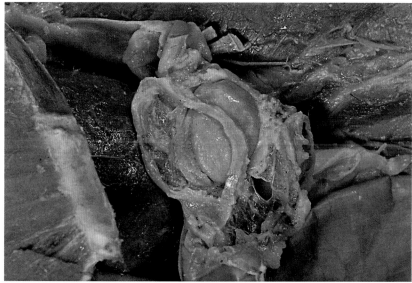

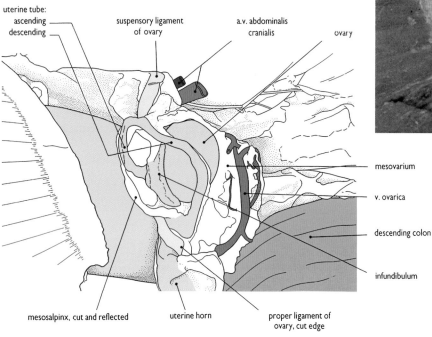

uterine tube:
ascending
descending

suspensory ligament
of ovary

a.v. abdominalis
cranialis

ovary

mesovarium

v. ovarica

descending colon

infundibulum

mesosalpinx, cut and reflected

uterine horn

proper ligament of
ovary, cut edge

Fig. 8.32 Reproductive tract of the bitch (5). Ovary, ovarian bursa and uterine tube (3): left lateral view. The wall of the ovarian bursa (mesosalpinx) has been removed bar a small part linking the ascending component of the uterine tube with the proper ovarian ligament. The uterine tube is exposed and the ovary is completely uncovered. Some mesovarium is left intact attached to the ovary with elements of the ovarian vein displayed in it.

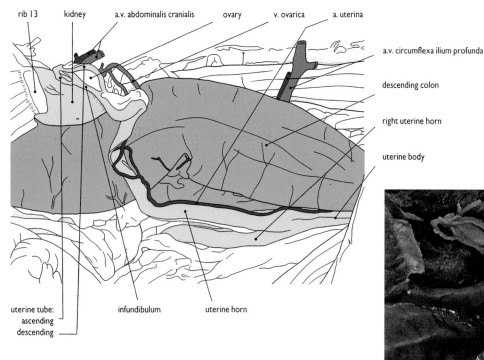

rib 13

kidney

a.v. abdominalis cranialis

ovary

v. ovarica

a. uterina

a.v. circumflexa ilium profunda

descending colon

right uterine horn

uterine body

uterine tube:
ascending
descending

infundibulum

uterine horn

Fig. 8.33 Reproductive tract of the bitch (6). Ovary and uterus: left lateral view. The remaining parts of the broad ligament have been removed and the ovary and uterine tube are outlined. The ovarian vein is left in place after mesovarial removal; the uterine artery is left after mesometrial removal. Both uterine horns are now visible and the uterine body is apparent ventral to the descending colon.

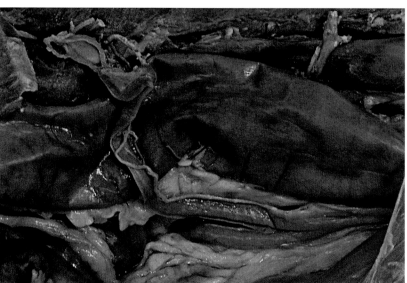

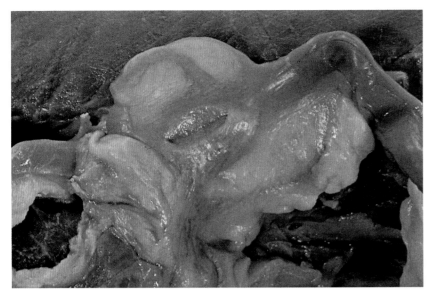

Fig. 8.34 Reproductive tract of the bitch (7). Left ovary and ovarian bursa reflected dorsally: left lateral view. The ovary and ovarian bursa have been reflected dorsally so that the medial surface of the bursa is exposed. The bursal opening is visible and the infundibulum with its finger-like fimbriae is visible through the bursal opening.

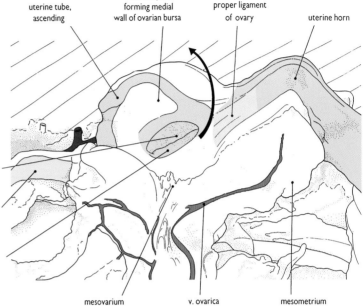

uterine tube, ascending

mesosalpinx, forming medial wall of ovarian bursa

proper ligament of ovary

uterine horn

infundibulum with fimbriae visible in bursa

suspensory ligament of ovary

ovarian bursa, opening

mesovarium

v. ovarica

mesometrium

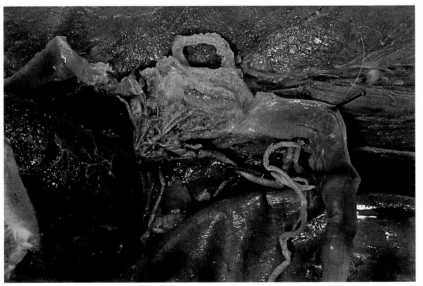

Fig. 8.35 Reproductive tract of the bitch (8). Left ovarian bursa after removal of the ovary and dorsal reflection: left lateral view. The ovary, mesosalpinx and mesovarium have been removed, exposing the complete uterine tube and extensive ramifications of the ovarian vein. The somewhat tortuous uterine artery is also left in association with the left uterine horn.

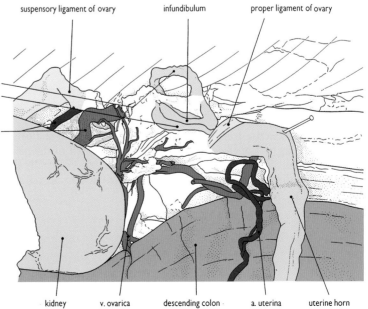

suspensory ligament of ovary

infundibulum

proper ligament of ovary

uterine tube:
ascending
descending

a.v. abdominalis
cranialis

kidney

v. ovarica

descending colon

a. uterina

uterine horn

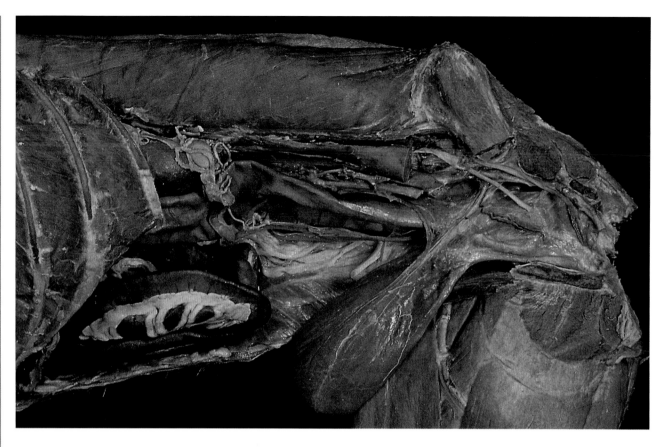

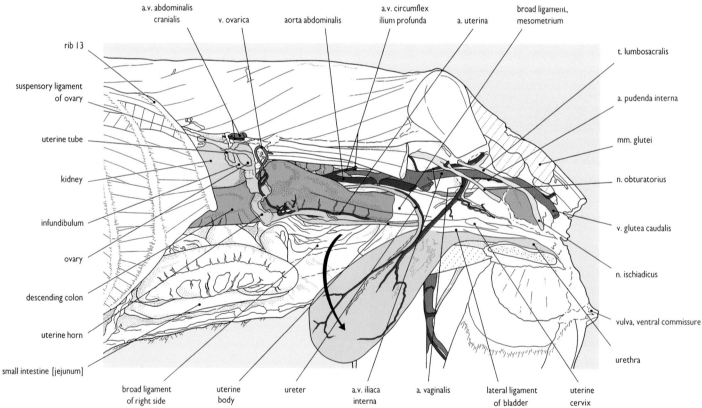

rib 13

suspensory ligament
of ovary

uterine tube

kidney

infundibulum

ovary

descending colon

uterine horn

small intestine [jejunum]

a.v. abdominalis
cranialis

v. ovarica

aorta abdominalis

a.v. circumflex
ilium profunda

a. uterina

broad ligament,
mesometrium

t. lumbosacralis

a. pudenda interna

mm. glutei

n. obturatorius

v. glutea caudalis

n. ischiadicus

vulva, ventral commissure

urethra

broad ligament
of right side

uterine
body

ureter

a.v. iliaca
interna

a. vaginalis

lateral ligament
of bladder

uterine
cervix

Fig. 8.36 Reproductive tract of the bitch (9) in the abdomen and pelvis: left lateral view. The pelvic bone has been removed from this bitch in the same manner as that of the dog (Fig. 8.19). The left half of the pelvic diaphragm has been removed and the iliopsoas muscle cut back into the abdominal roof. The urinary bladder has been reflected ventrally out of the body cavity. The dissection specimen used for this and the next four pictures had already been partially dissected; the tail was cut off at its roots and the entire caudodorsal vestibular wall was removed.

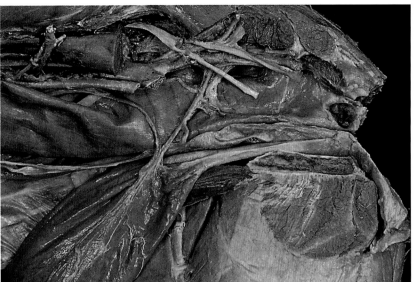

Fig. 8.37 Pelvic viscera of the bitch (1). After removal of the pelvic bone and pelvic diaphragm: left lateral view. The lateral bladder ligament and fat and fascia have been removed from the pelvis, exposing the rectum, vagina and urethra. The external anal sphincter has been removed from the anal canal and the anal sac has been opened, revealing accumulated secretion from the anal glands.

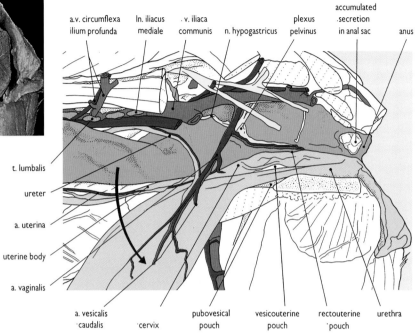

Fig. 8.38 Pelvic viscera of the bitch (2). Interior of the rectum, vagina and urethra: left lateral view. The rectum and anal canal, the vagina and the urethra are all sectioned in the midline. With the removal of the caudal wall of the vestibule, the vagina and external urethral orifice 'appear' to open on the surface immediately below the anus.

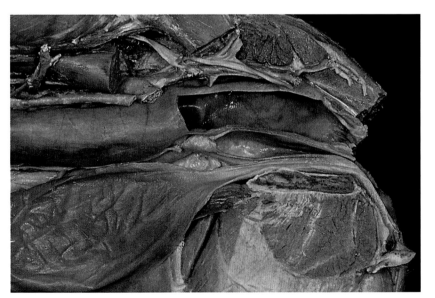

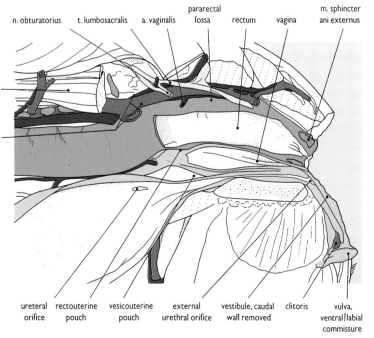

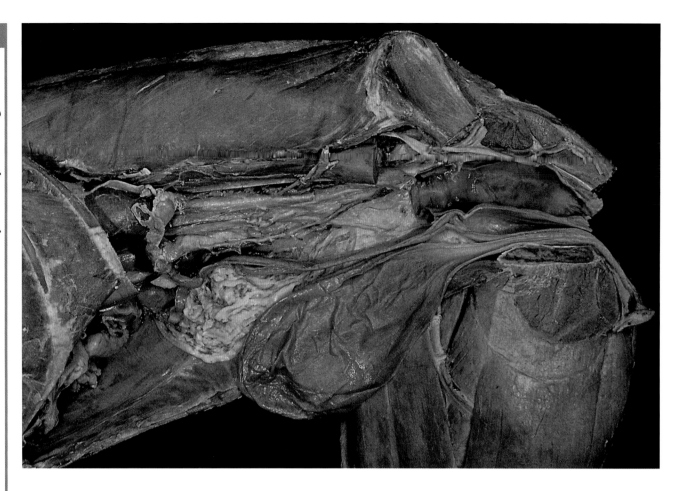

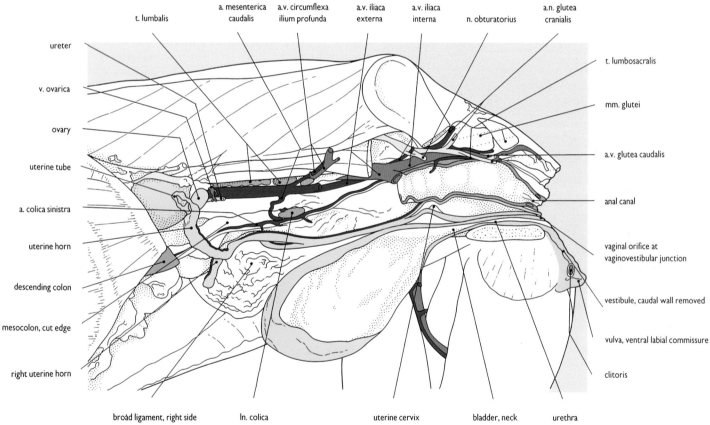

t. lumbalis | a. mesenterica caudalis | a.v. circumflexa ilium profunda | a.v. iliaca externa | a.v. iliaca interna | n. obturatorius | a.n. glutea cranialis

ureter

v. ovarica

ovary

uterine tube

a. colica sinistra

uterine horn

descending colon

mesocolon, cut edge

right uterine horn

t. lumbosacralis

mm. glutei

a.v. glutea caudalis

anal canal

vaginal orifice at vaginovestibular junction

vestibule, caudal wall removed

vulva, ventral labial commissure

clitoris

broad ligament, right side | ln. colica | uterine cervix | bladder, neck | urethra

Fig. 8.39 Reproductive tract of the bitch (10): left lateral view. The remains of the small intestine and most of the descending colon have been removed, although much of the mesocolon has been left in position. The left colic artery and caudal mesenteric artery have therefore been preserved and a colic lymph node is displayed. The ureter has been removed except for a stump at the cranial end of the abdomen close to the ovarian vein. Both uterine horns are now displayed and the uterine cervix is opened.

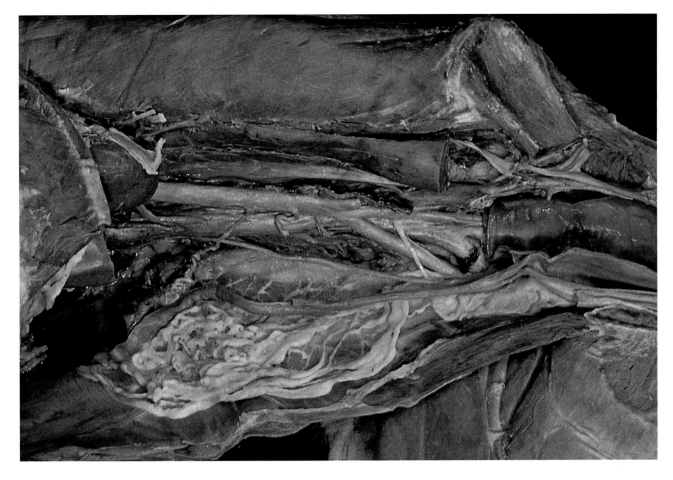

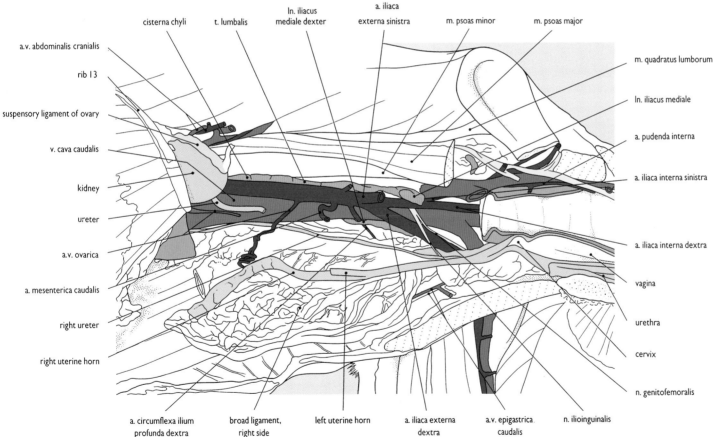

cisterna chyli   t. lumbalis   ln. iliacus
mediale dexter

a. iliaca
externa sinistra   m. psoas minor   m. psoas major

a.v. abdominalis cranialis

rib 13

suspensory ligament of ovary

v. cava caudalis

kidney

ureter

a.v. ovarica

a. mesenterica caudalis

right ureter

right uterine horn

m. quadratus lumborum

ln. iliacus mediale

a. pudenda interna

a. iliaca interna sinistra

a. iliaca interna dextra

vagina

urethra

cervix

n. genitofemoralis

a. circumflexa ilium
profunda dextra   broad ligament,
right side   left uterine horn   a. iliaca externa
dextra   a.v. epigastrica
caudalis   n. ilioinguinalis

Fig. 8.40 Reproductive tract of the bitch (11). Uterine horn and broad ligament of the right side: ventromedial view. The urinary bladder has been removed, as has the mesocolon and fat and fascia from the abdominal roof. This view is from a ventromedial aspect and looks up into the abdominal roof onto both abdominal aorta and caudal vena cava. Removal of the deep circumflex iliac vessels has exposed the lumbar lymph trunk of the left side, somewhat swollen, and clearly linking a medial iliac lymph node caudally with the cisterna chyli cranially. A large medial iliac lymph node is also visible on the right side, as are both ilioinguinal and genitofemoral nerves.

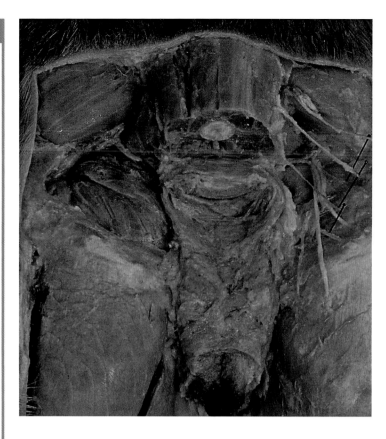

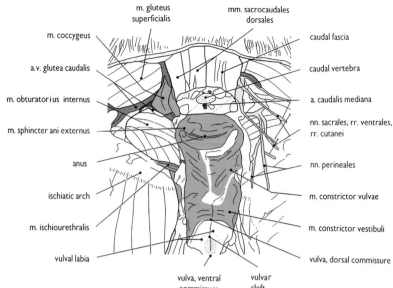

Fig. 8.41 External genitalia of the bitch (1). External anal sphincter and constrictor muscles: caudal view. The skin and superficial fascia have been removed from the pelvic outlet (perineum), and quantities of fat have been taken out of the ischiorectal fossae. The tail has been cut through at its root immediately dorsal to the anus. On the right side a number of cutaneous nerves have been pinned out after freeing from the fat in the ischiorectal fossa.

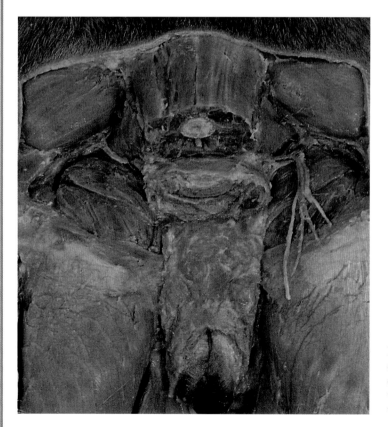

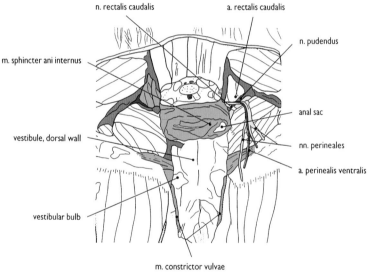

Fig. 8.42 External genitalia of the bitch (2). Anal glands and vestibular bulbs: caudal view. Part of the external anal sphincter muscle has been removed, exposing the anal sac of the right side. The constrictor muscles of the vestibule and vulva have also been removed from the dorsocaudal wall of the vestibule and the vestibular bulbs are exposed on either side.

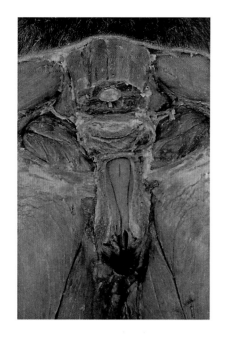

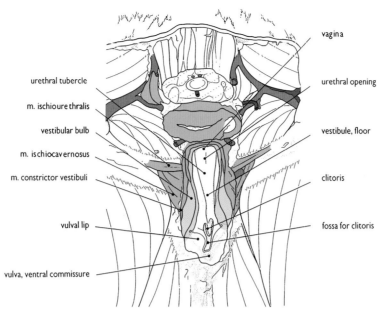

vagina

urethral tubercle

m. ischioure thralis

vestibular bulb

m. ischiocavernosus

m. constrictor vestibuli

vulval lip

vulva, ventral commissure

urethral opening

vestibule, floor

clitoris

fossa for clitoris

Fig. 8.43 External genitalia of the bitch (3). Vestibule and vulva: caudal view. The dorsocaudal wall of the vestibule, including the dorsal commissure of the vulva, has been removed as far proximally as the vaginal opening into the vestibule immediately ventral to the anal canal. Distal to this opening the external urethral orifice is apparent, while just within the ventral vulval commissure the clitoris is housed within a marked clitoral fossa.

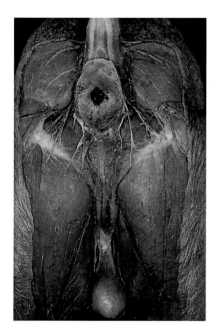

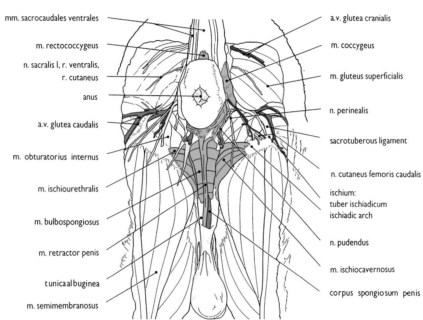

mm. sacrocaudales ventrales

m. rectococcygeus

n. sacralis l, r. ventralis, r. cutaneus

anus

a.v. glutea caudalis

m. obturatorius internus

m. ischiourethralis

m. bulbospongiosus

m. retractor penis

t unica al buginea

m. semimembranosus

a.v. glutea cranialis

m. coccygeus

m. gluteus superficialis

n. perinealis

sacrotuberous ligament

n. cutaneus femoris caudalis

ischium:
tuber ischiadicum
ischiadic arch

n. pudendus

m. ischiocavernosus

corpus spongiosum penis

Fig. 8.44 External genitalia (1). Penile root and nerves of the perineum: caudal view. The skin and superficial fascia have been removed from the rump, ischiorectal fossa, perineum and caudal thigh of both left and right sides. A number of cutaneous nerves and blood vessels have been retained and are spread out in their approximate arrangement in life. The muscles associated with the penis are particularly well displayed in this specimen.

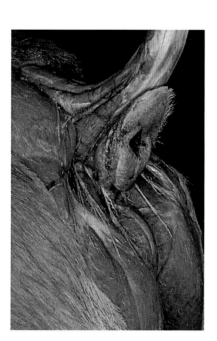

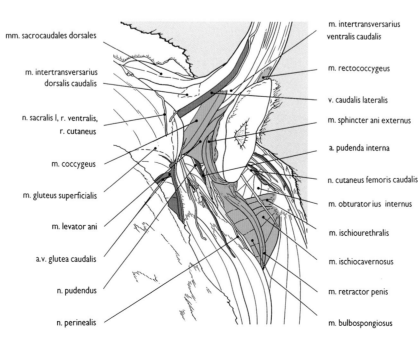

mm. sacrocaudales dorsales

m. intertransversarius dorsalis caudalis

n. sacralis l, r. ventralis, r. cutaneus

m. coccygeus

m. gluteus superficialis

m. levator ani

a.v. glutea caudalis

n. pudendus

n. perinealis

m. intertransversarius ventralis caudalis

m. rectococcygeus

v. caudalis lateralis

m. sphincter ani externus

a. pudenda interna

n. cutaneus femoris caudalis

m. obturatorius internus

m. ischiourethralis

m. ischiocavernosus

m. retractor penis

m. bulbospongiosus

Fig. 8.45 External genitalia (2). Penile root and nerves of the perineum: caudolateral view. This is a view of the previous dissection from a slightly different angle. It shows the terminations on the tail of both coccygeus and levator ani muscles and the association of the latter with the external anal sphincter. This view also shows the pudendal nerve more clearly accompanying the internal pudendal artery.

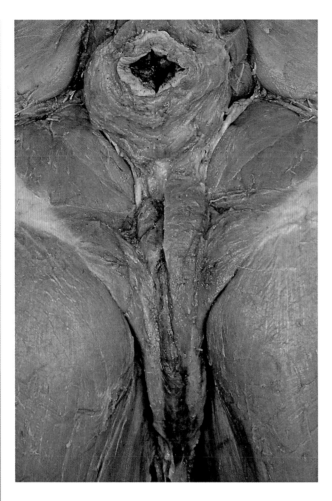

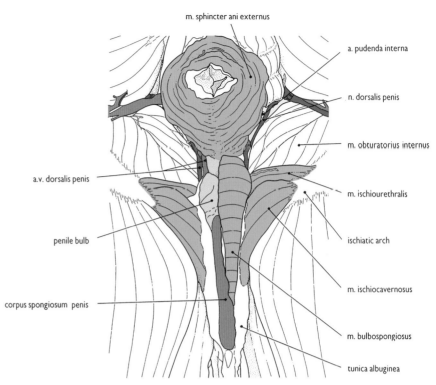

m. sphincter ani externus

a. pudenda interna

n. dorsalis penis

m. obturatorius internus

a.v. dorsalis penis

m. ischiourethralis

penile bulb

ischiatic arch

m. ischiocavernosus

corpus spongiosum penis

m. bulbospongiosus

tunica albuginea

Fig. 8.46 External genitalia (3). Penile bulb and dorsal penile vessels: caudal view. The retractor penis muscle has been removed and the bulbospongiosus muscle of the left side has also been cut away. The penile bulb and, more distally, the corpus spongiosum penis are uncovered on the left side. Dorsal penile vessels enter the penis as the major continuations of the internal pudendal vessels.

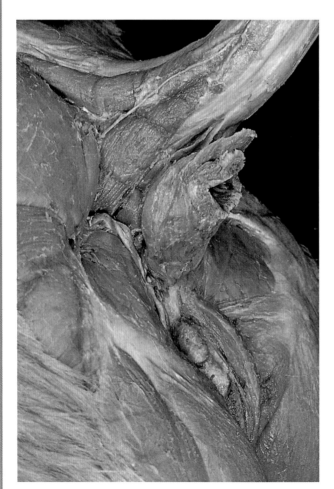

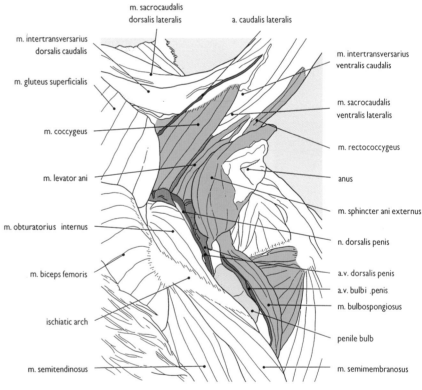

m. sacrocaudalis dorsalis lateralis

a. caudalis lateralis

m. intertransversarius dorsalis caudalis

m. intertransversarius ventralis caudalis

m. gluteus superficialis

m. sacrocaudalis ventralis lateralis

m. coccygeus

m. rectococcygeus

m. levator ani

anus

m. obturatorius internus

m. sphincter ani externus

n. dorsalis penis

m. biceps femoris

a.v. dorsalis penis

a.v. bulbi .penis

m. bulbospongiosus

ischiatic arch

penile bulb

m. semitendinosus

m. semimembranosus

Fig. 8.47 External genitalia (4). Penile bulb and dorsal penile vessels: caudolateral view. This is a view of the previous dissection but from a slightly different angle. The levator ani muscle association with the external anal sphincter muscle is now clearly displayed, and the rectococcygeus muscle is visible entering the tail dorsal to the anal sphincter muscle. The dorsal penile vessels are clearly displayed, accompanied in this view by the dorsal penile nerve.

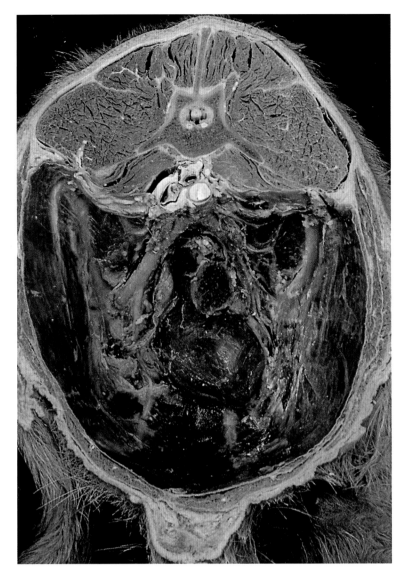

Fig. 8.48 Caudal abdominal cavity and pelvic inlet: cranial view. The abdomen has been sectioned through the caudal lumbar region and the abdominal organs have been removed.

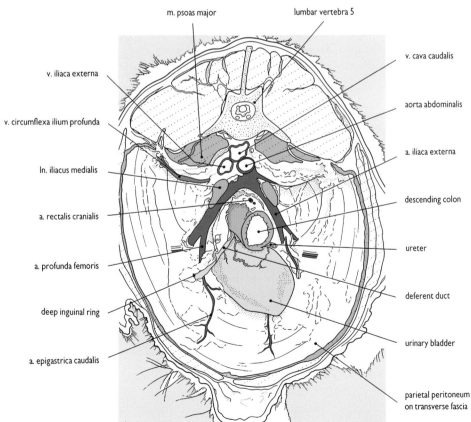

m. psoas major

lumbar vertebra 5

v. iliaca externa

v. circumflexa ilium profunda

ln. iliacus medialis

a. rectalis cranialis

a. profunda femoris

deep inguinal ring

a. epigastrica caudalis

v. cava caudalis

aorta abdominalis

a. iliaca externa

descending colon

ureter

deferent duct

urinary bladder

parietal peritoneum
on transverse fascia

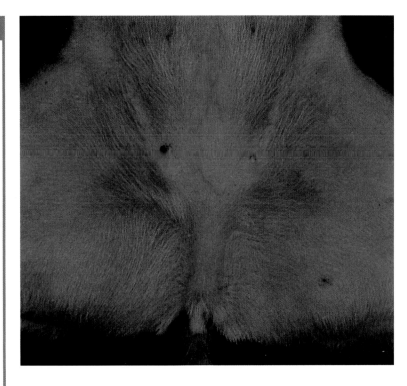

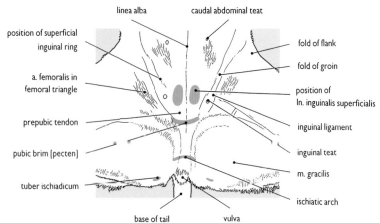

Fig. 8.49 Surface features of the pelvis and inner thigh of the bitch: ventral view. The few bony features that are generally palpable on the undersurface of the pelvis and inner side of the thigh are indicated in this figure. These points correspond to those colored green on the bones illustrated below (Fig. 8.50). Figures 7.1 and 9.1 show the surface of the pelvis from lateral and dorsal views, and from behind in Figs 8.1 and 8.4, and should be compared with this figure to obtain an overall view of the surface anatomy of the pelvis.

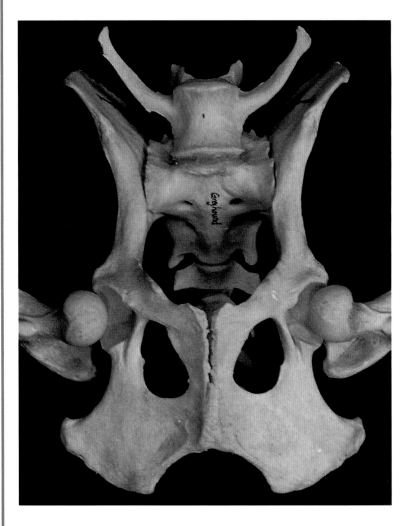

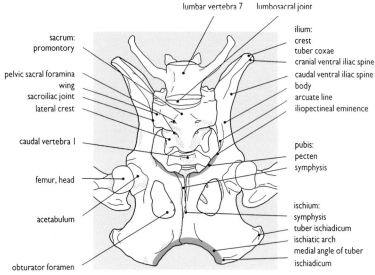

Fig. 8.50 Skeleton of the pelvis and thighs: ventral view. The few palpable features shown in the surface view above (Fig. 8.49) are colored green on this skeleton for reference. The pelvic skeleton is also shown in Figs 7.6 and 9.2 from lateral and dorsal views, and in Fig. 7.4 from a caudal view. The fairly complete bony pelvic floor is to be compared with roof and walls, which are primarily muscular and ligamentous.

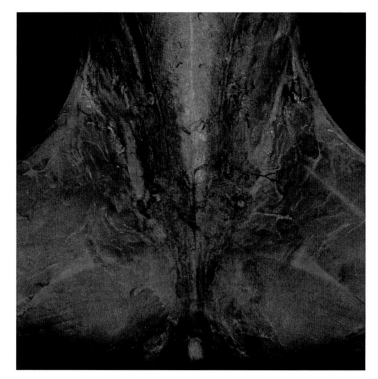

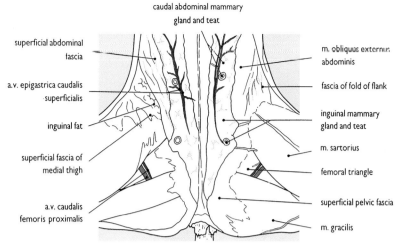

caudal abdominal mammary
gland and teat

superficial abdominal
fascia

a.v. epigastrica caudalis
superficialis

inguinal fat

superficial fascia of
medial thigh

a.v. caudalis
femoris proximalis

m. obliquus externus
abdominis

fascia of fold of flank

inguinal mammary
gland and teat

m. sartorius

femoral triangle

superficial pelvic fascia

m. gracilis

Fig. 8.51 Superficial fascia of the inguinal regions, pelvis and inner thighs of the bitch: ventral view. The skin has been removed displaying the superficial fascia, a thick, somewhat featureless subcutaneous covering infiltrated with fat and which contains the considerable caudal abdominal and inguinal mammary glands.

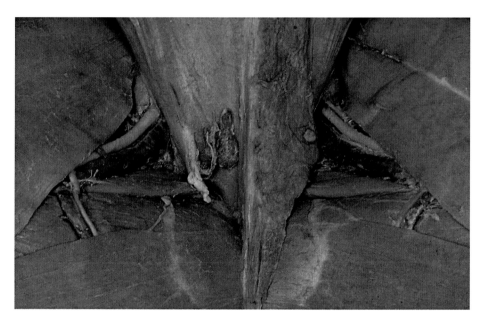

Fig. 8.52 Femoral triangle, vaginal process and superficial inguinal ring of the right side of the bitch: ventral view. The superficial fat and fascia of the right side has been cleaned away from the inside of the thigh and the mammary glands are removed from the underside of the belly and pelvis. Exposed by this are: the femoral vessels in the femoral triangle, a small fat-filled vaginal process projecting through the superficial inguinal ring of the external oblique aponeurosis, caudal superficial epigastric vessels, genitofemoral nerve, and a prominent superficial inguinal lymph node (compare with Fig. 8.23 of the intact male canal with traversing structures).

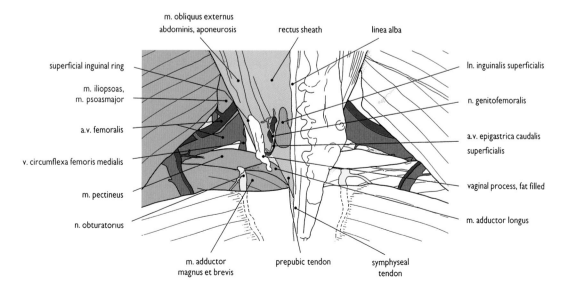

m. obliquus externus
abdominis, aponeurosis

rectus sheath

linea alba

superficial inguinal ring

m. iliopsoas,
m. psoasmajor

a.v. femoralis

v. circumflexa femoris medialis

m. pectineus

n. obturatorius

ln. inguinalis superficialis

n. genitofemoralis

a.v. epigastrica caudalis
superficialis

vaginal process, fat filled

m. adductor longus

m. adductor
magnus et brevis

prepubic tendon

symphyseal
tendon

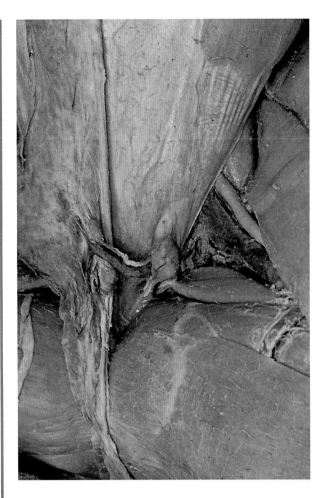

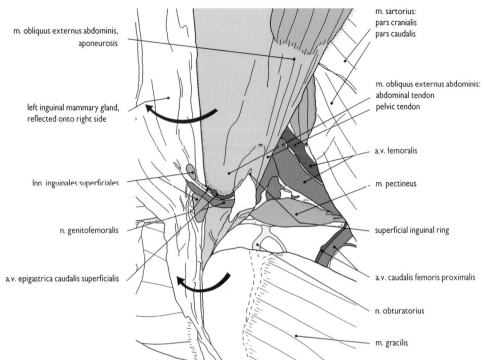

m. obliquus externus abdominis, aponeurosis

left inguinal mammary gland, reflected onto right side

lnn. inguinales superficiales

n. genitofemoralis

a.v. epigastrica caudalis superficialis

m. sartorius: pars cranialis pars caudalis

m. obliquus externus abdominis: abdominal tendon pelvic tendon

a.v. femoralis

m. pectineus

superficial inguinal ring

a.v. caudalis femoris proximalis

n. obturatorius

m. gracilis

Fig. 8.53 Vaginal process, external pudendal vessels and superficial inguinal lymph nodes of the left side of the bitch: ventral view. The inguinal mammary gland of the left side has been reflected onto the right side of the pelvis exposing a picture much like that of Fig. 8.52 on the previous page of the right side. However, there are two superficial inguinal lymph nodes on this side. The fat-filled vaginal process can also be seen through the external abdominal oblique aponeurosis inside the inguinal canal cranial to the superficial inguinal ring.

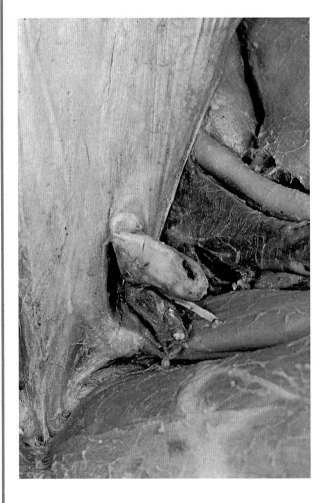

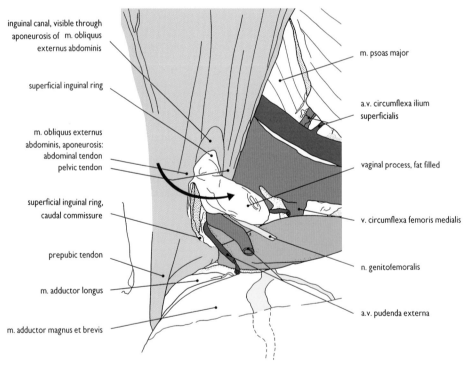

inguinal canal, visible through aponeurosis of m. obliquus externus abdominis

superficial inguinal ring

m. obliquus externus abdominis, aponeurosis: abdominal tendon pelvic tendon

superficial inguinal ring, caudal commissure

prepubic tendon

m. adductor longus

m. adductor magnus et brevis

m. psoas major

a.v. circumflexa ilium superficialis

vaginal process, fat filled

v. circumflexa femoris medialis

n. genitofemoralis

a.v. pudenda externa

Fig. 8.54 Inguinal canal of the left side of the bitch (1). Superficial inguinal ring: ventral view. The inguinal mammary gland and superficial inguinal lymph nodes have been removed and the genitofemoral nerve and pudendal vessels have been severed. These latter structures and the vaginal process are all reflected laterally and pinned to the pectineus muscle on the inside of the thigh. The abdominal tendon of the external oblique is displayed forming the medial border of the superficial inguinal ring.

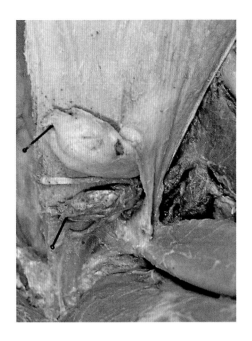

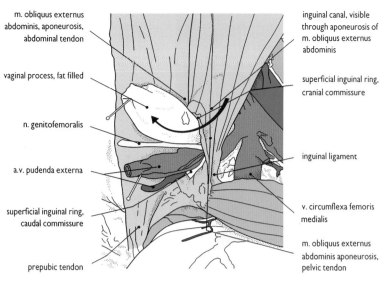

m. obliquus externus abdominis, aponeurosis, abdominal tendon

vaginal process, fat filled

n. genitofemoralis

a.v. pudenda externa

superficial inguinal ring, caudal commissure

prepubic tendon

inguinal canal, visible through aponeurosis of m. obliquus externus abdominis

superficial inguinal ring, cranial commissure

inguinal ligament

v. circumflexa femoris medialis

m. obliquus externus abdominis aponeurosis, pelvic tendon

Fig. 8.55 Inguinal canal of the left side of the bitch (2). Pelvic tendon of the external abdominal oblique muscle: ventral view. The vaginal process, pudendal vessels and genitofemoral nerve are in this picture reflected medially in order to expose the pelvic tendon of the external oblique which forms the lateral border of the superficial inguinal ring and much of the lateral wall of the inguinal canal.

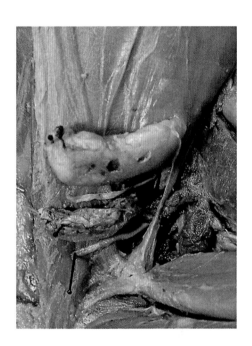

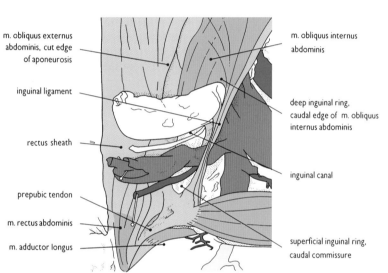

m. obliquus externus abdominis, cut edge of aponeurosis

inguinal ligament

rectus sheath

prepubic tendon

m. rectus abdominis

m. adductor longus

m. obliquus internus abdominis

deep inguinal ring, caudal edge of m. obliquus internus abdominis

inguinal canal

superficial inguinal ring, caudal commissure

Fig. 8.56 Inguinal canal of the left side of the bitch (3). Inguinal ligament and internal abdominal oblique muscle: ventral view. The external oblique muscle has been removed, destroying the superficial inguinal ring and the lateral and ventral walls of the inguinal canal. The deep inguinal ring is indicated at the caudal edge of the internal oblique muscle and the inguinal ligament is intact.

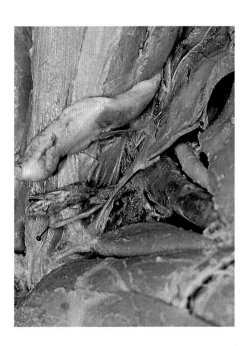

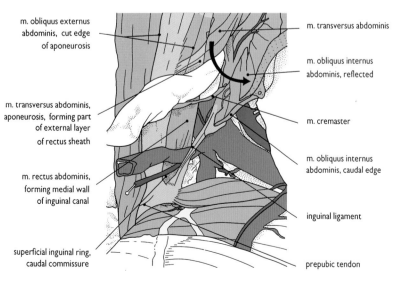

m. obliquus externus abdominis, cut edge of aponeurosis

m. transversus abdominis, aponeurosis, forming part of external layer of rectus sheath

m. rectus abdominis, forming medial wall of inguinal canal

superficial inguinal ring, caudal commissure

m. transversus abdominis

m. obliquus internus abdominis, reflected

m. cremaster

m. obliquus internus abdominis, caudal edge

inguinal ligament

prepubic tendon

Fig. 8.57 Inguinal canal of the left side of the bitch (4). Cremaster muscle and rectus abdominis muscle: ventral view. The internal abdominal oblique muscle has been cut through and reflected laterally, destroying the deep inguinal ring but demonstrating the attachment of the muscle to the inguinal ligament. From the internal face of the internal oblique a small cremaster muscle runs out through the inguinal canal.

411

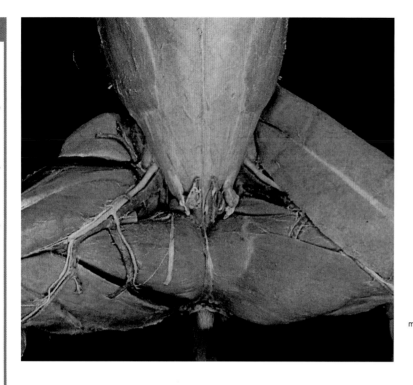

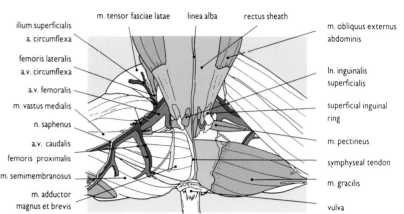

m. tensor fasciae latae   linea alba   rectus sheath

ilium superficialis

a. circumflexa
femoris lateralis

a.v. circumflexa

a.v. femoralis

m. vastus medialis

n. saphenus

a.v. caudalis
femoris proximalis

m. semimembranosus

m. adductor
magnus et brevis

m. obliquus externus
abdominis

ln. inguinalis
superficialis

superficial inguinal
ring

m. pectineus

symphyseal tendon

m. gracilis

vulva

Fig. 8.58 Femoral triangle of the right side of the bitch following removal of the sartorius, pectineus and gracilis muscles: ventral view. The femoral triangles of both sides have been cleaned of fat and fascia to display the femoral vessels, and the triangle of the right side has also had its cranial and caudal boundaries removed (sartorius and pectineus respectively). Consequently medial and lateral circumflex vessels are exposed and the saphenous component of the femoral nerve. Removal of the gracilis muscle from the inside of the right thigh has left its motor branch from the obturator nerve in place and has exposed proximal caudal femoral vessels.

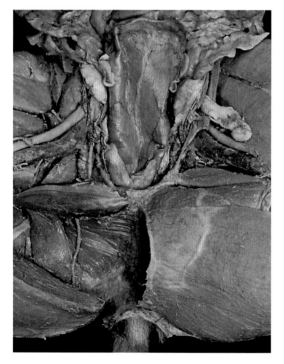

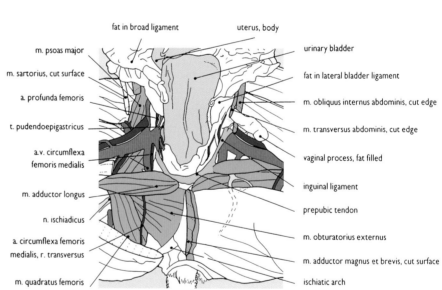

fat in broad ligament   uterus, body

m. psoas major

m. sartorius, cut surface

a. profunda femoris

t. pudendoepigastricus

a.v. circumflexa
femoris medialis

m. adductor longus

n. ischiadicus

a. circumflexa femoris
medialis, r. transversus

m. quadratus femoris

urinary bladder

fat in lateral bladder ligament

m. obliquus internus abdominis, cut edge

m. transversus abdominis, cut edge

vaginal process, fat filled

inguinal ligament

prepubic tendon

m. obturatorius externus

m. adductor magnus et brevis, cut surface

ischiatic arch

Fig. 8.59 Pelvic inlet and pelvic floor of the bitch after removal of the abdominal wall and great adductor muscle of the right side: ventral view. The muscular abdominal wall has been removed, leaving the inguinal ligament intact on the left side and the prepubic tendon applied to the cranial border of the pubic bones ventrally. On the right side the continuity of the external iliac and femoral vessels is apparent.

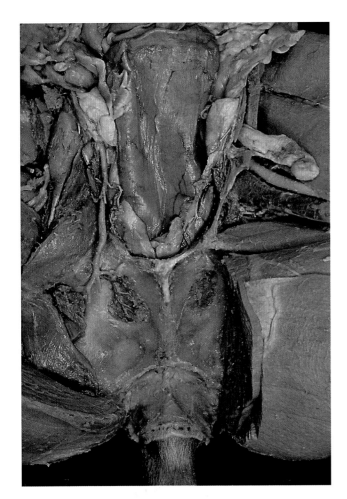

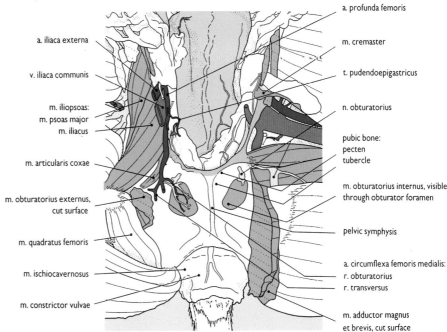

a. profunda femoris

a. iliaca externa

m. cremaster

v. iliaca communis

t. pudendoepigastricus

m. iliopsoas:
m. psoas major
m. iliacus

n. obturatorius

m. articularis coxae

pubic bone:
pecten
tubercle

m. obturatorius externus,
cut surface

m. obturatorius internus, visible
through obturator foramen

m. quadratus femoris

pelvic symphysis

m. ischiocavernosus

a. circumflexa femoris medialis:
r. obturatorius
r. transversus

m. constrictor vulvae

m. adductor magnus
et brevis, cut surface

Fig. 8.60 Prepubic tendon, pelvic symphysis and bones of the pelvic floor of the bitch: ventral view. Removal of the long adductor and external obturator muscles has exposed the pelvic bone of the right side. Through the obturator foramen the internal obturator muscle is visible. On the left side muscle has also been cleared from the underside of the pelvis; the entire pelvic symphysis and the ischiatic arch are now exposed. On the right side removal of the femoral vessels has allowed exposure of the deep femoral artery with its pudendoepigastric and medial circumflex femoral branches.

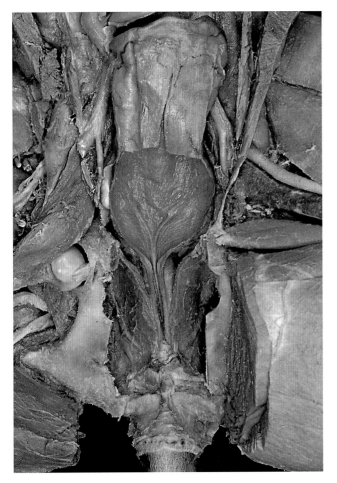

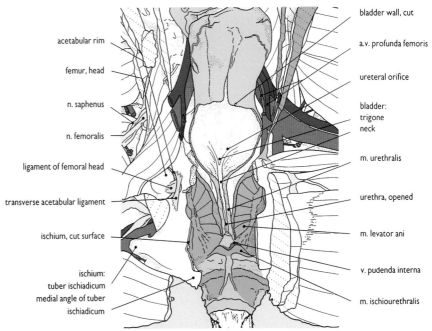

bladder wall, cut

acetabular rim

a.v. profunda femoris

femur, head

ureteral orifice

n. saphenus

bladder:
trigone
neck

n. femoralis

ligament of femoral head

m. urethralis

transverse acetabular ligament

urethra, opened

ischium, cut surface

m. levator ani

ischium:
tuber ischiadicum
medial angle of tuber
ischiadicum

v. pudenda interna

m. ischiourethralis

Fig. 8.61 Pelvic cavity and pelvic diaphragm of the bitch after removal of the bony pelvic floor: ventral view. The pubic and ischiadic bones of both sides have been sawn through cranial and caudal to the obturator foramina and the bony pelvic floor removed. The internal obturator and levator ani muscles of both sides were cut from their attachments and the internal obturator muscles were removed as far laterally as the bony removal exposing the levator ani muscles. Part of the ventral wall of the bladder has been removed and the urethra, exposed between the levator ani muscles, is also opened ventrally. Ureteral openings and the bladder trigone converge on the neck of the bladder in the dorsal bladder wall.

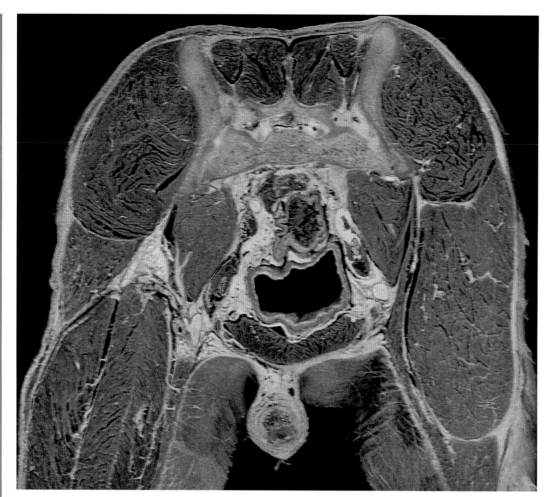

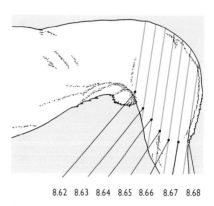

8.62 8.63 8.64 8.65 8.66 8.67 8.68

Fig. 8.62 Transverse section (1) through the sacroiliac joints, descending colon, bladder and vascular lacunae: cranial view. This and the following six sections were made at approximately the levels shown in the accompanying sketch, and all are viewed from the cranial aspect. They continue the sequence of transverse sections through the abdomen (Chapter 6). Because of the obliquity of the pelvic inlet the pelvic floor is not cut through until section three is reached.

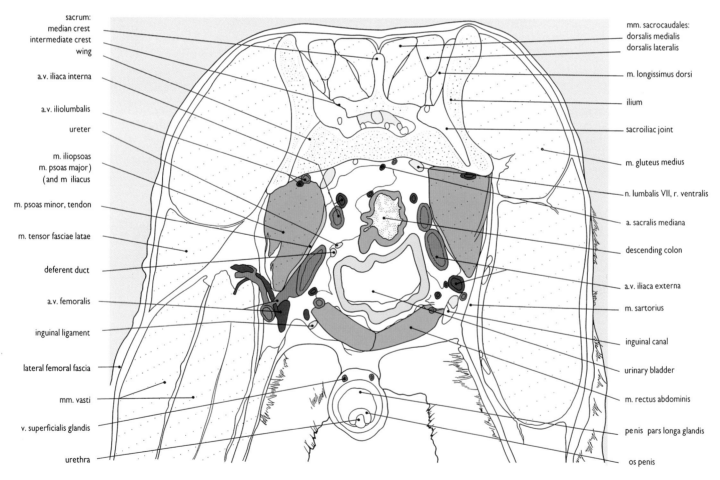

sacrum:
median crest
intermediate crest
wing

a.v. iliaca interna

a.v. iliolumbalis

ureter

m. iliopsoas
m. psoas major)
(and m iliacus

m. psoas minor, tendon

m. tensor fasciae latae

deferent duct

a.v. femoralis

inguinal ligament

lateral femoral fascia

mm. vasti

v. superficialis glandis

urethra

mm. sacrocaudales:
dorsalis medialis
dorsalis lateralis

m. longissimus dorsi

ilium

sacroiliac joint

m. gluteus medius

n. lumbalis VII, r. ventralis

a. sacralis mediana

descending colon

a.v. iliaca externa

m. sartorius

inguinal canal

urinary bladder

m. rectus abdominis

penis pars longa glandis

os penis

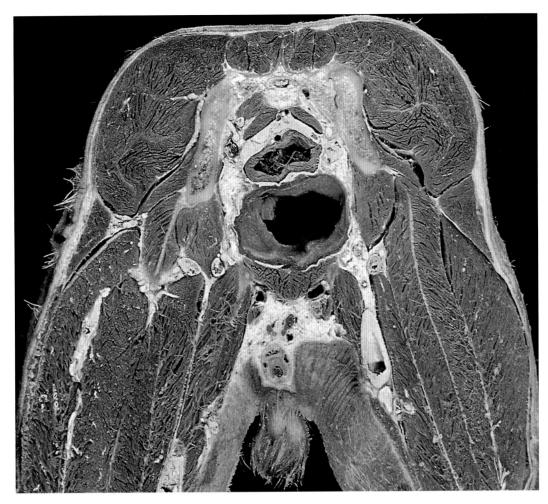

Fig. 8.63 Transverse section (2) through the iliac shafts, bladder, femoral vessels and penis: cranial view. This section is immediately cranial to the pubic pecten and includes the pectineus muscles on either side entering the thighs. The bladder and rectum fill the body cavity at this level and the iliacus muscles on either side form an important limiting partition ventral to the iliac shafts and dorsal to the rectus abdominis muscles. Ventral to the rectus muscles in the superficial fascia between the thighs external pudendal vessels and the spermatic cords in vaginal processes are visible on both sides against the pectineus muscles. Dorsal to the sectioned penis, superficial inguinal lymph nodes are visible.

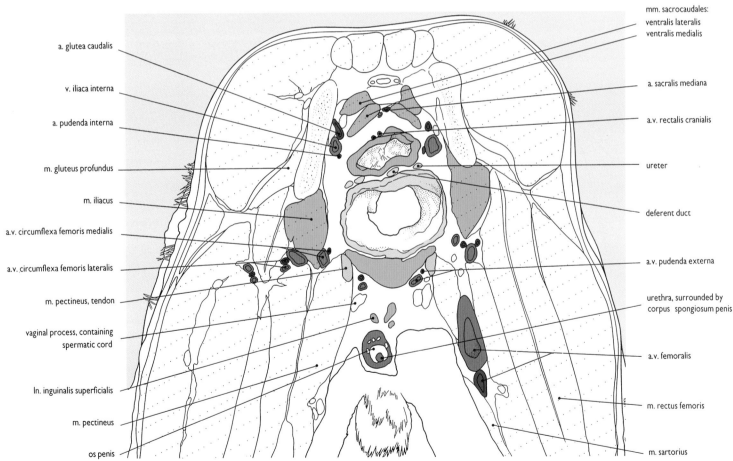

a. glutea caudalis

v. iliaca interna

a. pudenda interna

m. gluteus profundus

m. iliacus

a.v. circumflexa femoris medialis

a.v. circumflexa femoris lateralis

m. pectineus, tendon

vaginal process, containing spermatic cord

ln. inguinalis superficialis

m. pectineus

os penis

mm. sacrocaudales:
ventralis lateralis
ventralis medialis

a. sacralis mediana

a.v. rectalis cranialis

ureter

deferent duct

a.v. pudenda externa

urethra, surrounded by corpus spongiosum penis

a.v. femoralis

m. rectus femoris

m. sartorius

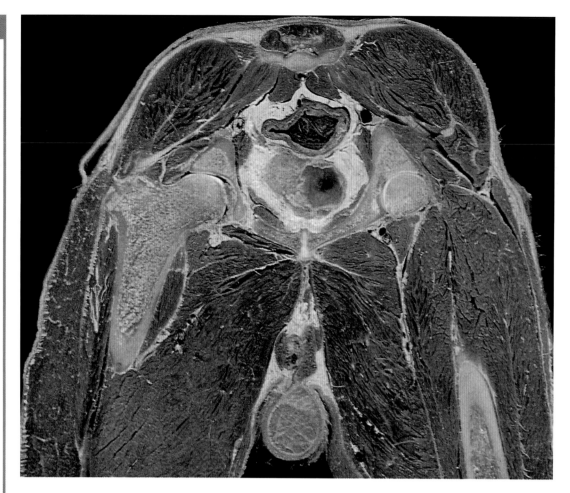

Fig. 8.64 Transverse section (3) through the hip joints, bladder neck, penis and scrotum: cranial view. This section passes through the entire pelvis, cutting the pubic bones immediately caudal to the pecten. The section also passes through the hip joints and on the right side the ligament of the femoral head is demonstrated to advantage. Dorsolaterally the pelvic wall at this level is formed from the piriform muscle in the greater ischiatic notch. Blue latex which has escaped from the venous system is found within the pelvic cavity in all of these sections and conveniently demonstrates the various peritoneal 'excavations' between the pelvic viscera. Between the thighs the vaginal processes with contained spermatic cords flank the penile body.

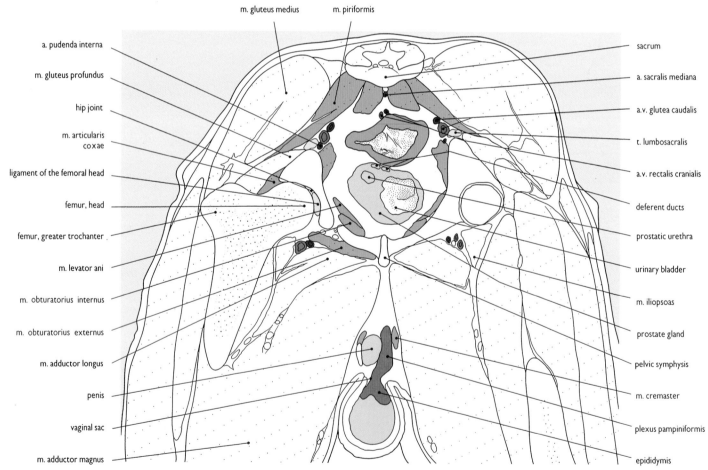

m. gluteus medius

m. piriformis

a. pudenda interna

m. gluteus profundus

hip joint

m. articularis coxae

ligament of the femoral head

femur, head

femur, greater trochanter

m. levator ani

m. obturatorius internus

m. obturatorius externus

m. adductor longus

penis

vaginal sac

m. adductor magnus

sacrum

a. sacralis mediana

a.v. glutea caudalis

t. lumbosacralis

a.v. rectalis cranialis

deferent ducts

prostatic urethra

urinary bladder

m. iliopsoas

prostate gland

pelvic symphysis

m. cremaster

plexus pampiniformis

epididymis

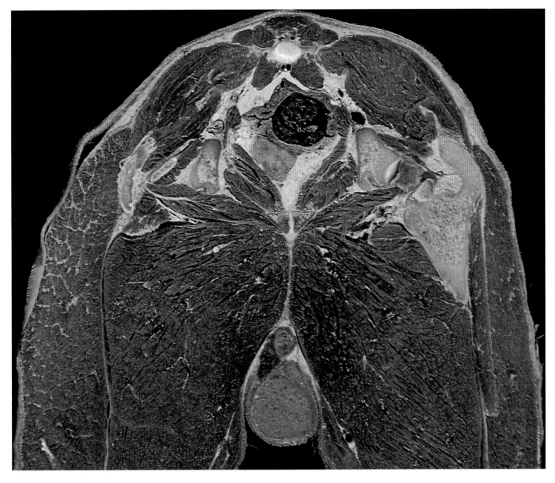

Fig. 8.65 Transverse section (4) through caudal vertebra 1, obturator foramina, prostate gland, penis and scrotum: cranial view. This section passes through the obturator foramina in the pelvic floor; both internal and external obturator muscles are clearly displayed. In the pelvic cavity the pelvic diaphragm of levator ani and coccygeus muscles flanks the pelvic viscera, of which the prostate gland is apparent. It lies predominantly on the dorsal surface of the urethra. Lateral to the pelvic diaphragm the caudal gluteal vessels are visible in the lesser ischiatic notch. The symphyseal tendon extends ventrally from the pelvic symphysis and the adductor muscles attach to it.

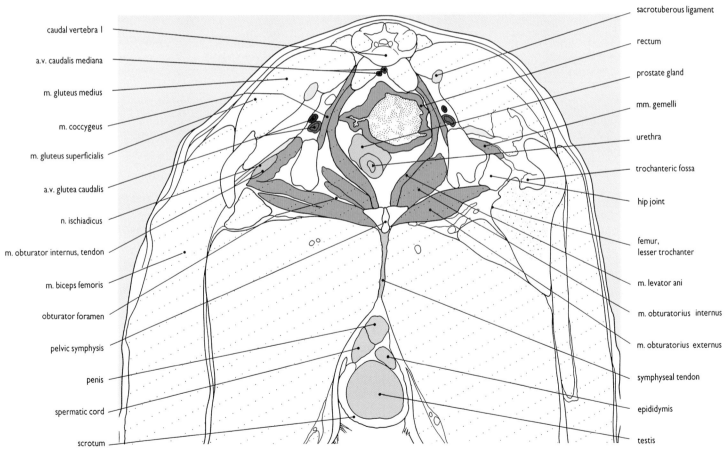

caudal vertebra 1

a.v. caudalis mediana

m. gluteus medius

m. coccygeus

m. gluteus superficialis

a.v. glutea caudalis

n. ischiadicus

m. obturator internus, tendon

m. biceps femoris

obturator foramen

pelvic symphysis

penis

spermatic cord

scrotum

sacrotuberous ligament

rectum

prostate gland

mm. gemelli

urethra

trochanteric fossa

hip joint

femur,
lesser trochanter

m. levator ani

m. obturatorius internus

m. obturatorius externus

symphyseal tendon

epididymis

testis

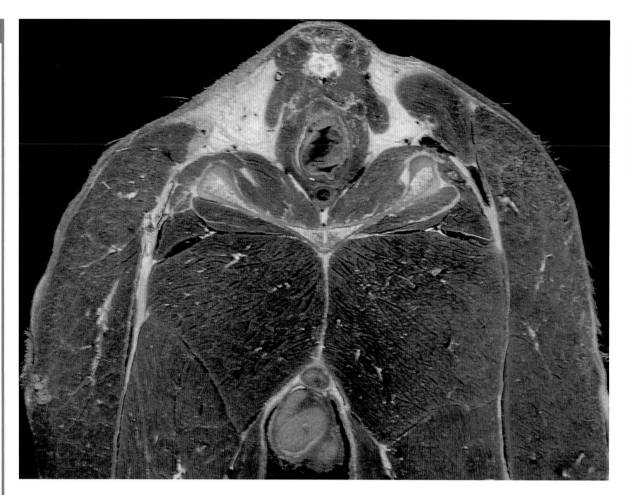

Fig. 8.66 Transverse section (5) through the ischiatic arch, pelvic diaphragm and ischiorectal fossae: cranial view. This section demonstrates the importance of the pelvic diaphragm in confining the terminal part of the rectum and anal canal. It forms the medial boundary of the ischiorectal fossa which is normally fat-filled.

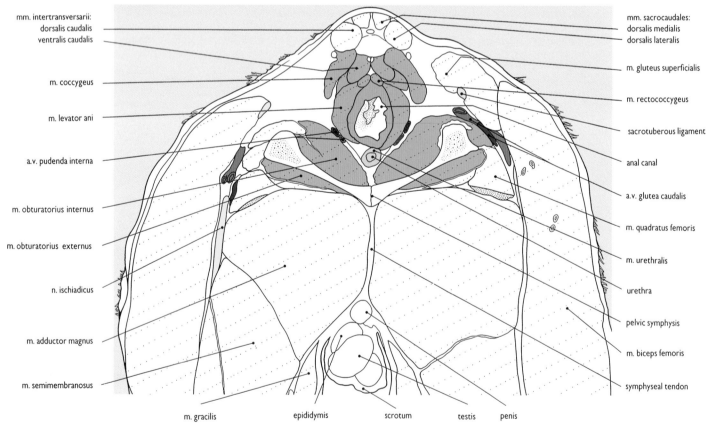

mm. intertransversarii:
dorsalis caudalis
ventralis caudalis

m. coccygeus

m. levator ani

a.v. pudenda interna

m. obturatorius internus

m. obturatorius externus

n. ischiadicus

m. adductor magnus

m. semimembranosus

mm. sacrocaudales:
dorsalis medialis
dorsalis lateralis

m. gluteus superficialis

m. rectococcygeus

sacrotuberous ligament

anal canal

a.v. glutea caudalis

m. quadratus femoris

m. urethralis

urethra

pelvic symphysis

m. biceps femoris

symphyseal tendon

m. gracilis   epididymis   scrotum   testis   penis

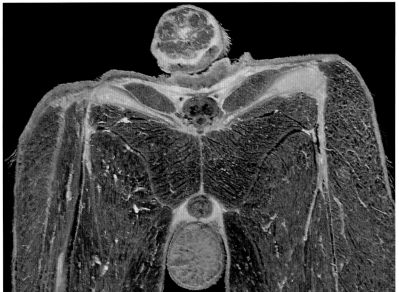

Fig. 8.67 Transverse section (6) through the root of the tail and the ischiatic tuberosities: cranial view. This section passes through the ischiatic arch on either side of the midline at the point at which the urethra is entering the urethral bulb, immediately proximal to the penile root.

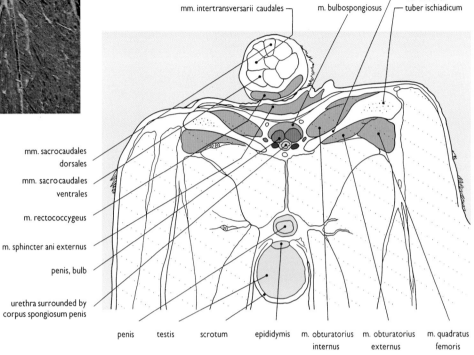

mm. intertransversarii caudales

m. bulbospongiosus

ischium:
ischiatic arch
tuber ischiadicum

mm. sacrocaudales dorsales

mm. sacrocaudales ventrales

m. rectococcygeus

m. sphincter ani externus

penis, bulb

urethra surrounded by corpus spongiosum penis

penis   testis   scrotum   epididymis   m. obturatorius internus   m. obturatorius externus   m. quadratus femoris

Fig. 8.68 Transverse section (7) through the root of the penis and base of the tail: cranial view. This section passes through the root of the penis and exposes both ischiocavernosus and bulbospongiosus muscles, and opens the urethral bulb in the midline.

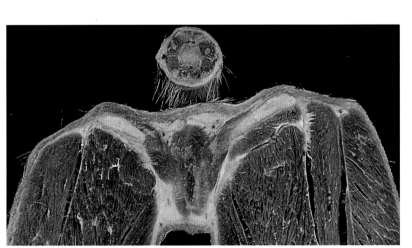

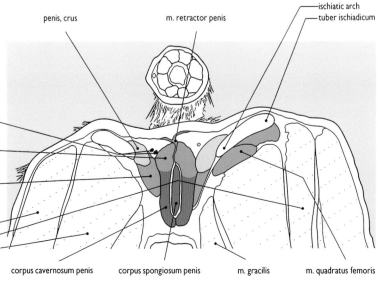

penis, crus

m. retractor penis

ischium:
ischiatic arch
tuber ischiadicum

a.v. penis

m. bulbospongiosus

m. ischiocavernosus

hamstring muscles:
m. biceps femoris
m. semitendinosus
m. semimembranosus

corpus cavernosum penis   corpus spongiosum penis   m. gracilis   m. quadratus femoris

9. THE VERTEBRAL COLUMN

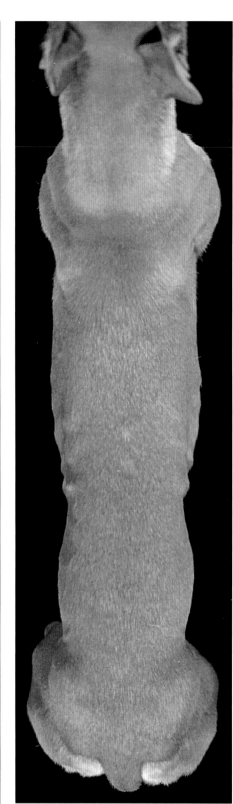

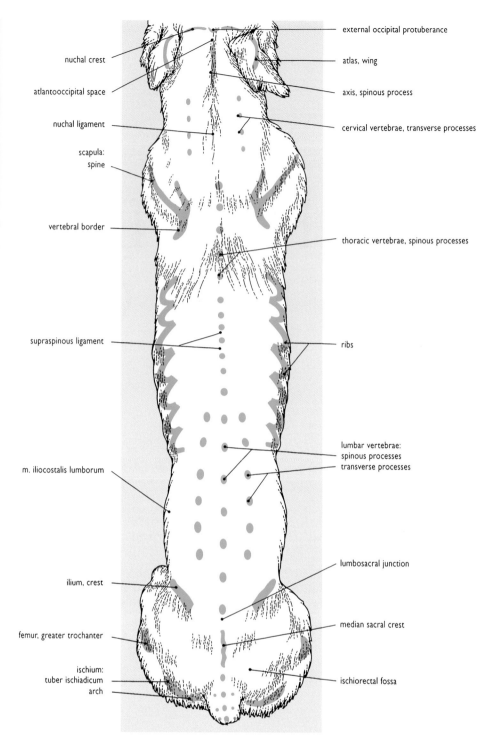

nuchal crest

atlantooccipital space

nuchal ligament

scapula:
spine

vertebral border

supraspinous ligament

m. iliocostalis lumborum

ilium, crest

femur, greater trochanter

ischium:
tuber ischiadicum
arch

external occipital protuberance

atlas, wing

axis, spinous process

cervical vertebrae, transverse processes

thoracic vertebrae, spinous processes

ribs

lumbar vertebrae:
spinous processes
transverse processes

lumbosacral junction

median sacral crest

ischiorectal fossa

Fig. 9.1 Surface features of the neck, trunk and tail: dorsal view. The palpable bony 'landmarks' of the vertebral column and adjoining bones are shown in this figure. For comparable lateral views see Figs 3.1, 5.1, 6.1 and 7.6.

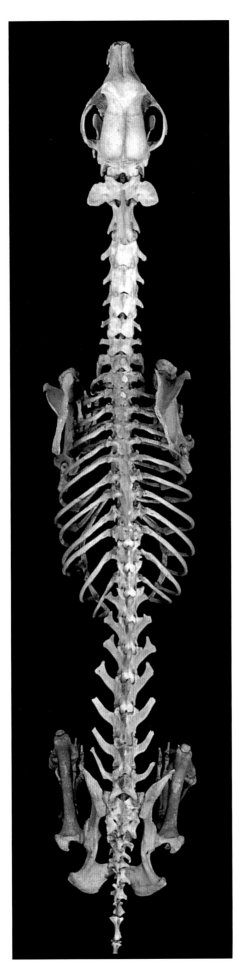

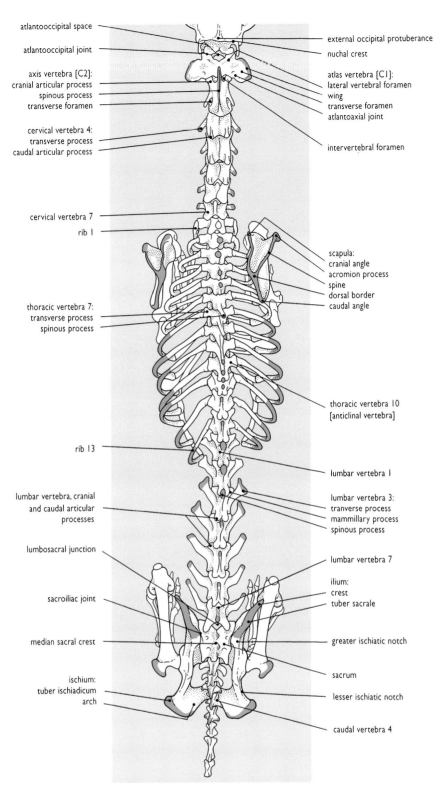

atlantooccipital space

atlantooccipital joint

axis vertebra [C2]:
cranial articular process
spinous process
transverse foramen

cervical vertebra 4:
transverse process
caudal articular process

cervical vertebra 7

rib 1

thoracic vertebra 7:
transverse process
spinous process

rib 13

lumbar vertebra, cranial
and caudal articular
processes

lumbosacral junction

sacroiliac joint

median sacral crest

ischium:
tuber ischiadicum
arch

external occipital protuberance

nuchal crest

atlas vertebra [C1]:
lateral vertebral foramen
wing
transverse foramen
atlantoaxial joint

intervertebral foramen

scapula:
cranial angle
acromion process
spine
dorsal border
caudal angle

thoracic vertebra 10
[anticlinal vertebra]

lumbar vertebra 1

lumbar vertebra 3:
tranverse process
mammillary process
spinous process

lumbar vertebra 7

ilium:
crest
tuber sacrale

greater ischiatic notch

sacrum

lesser ischiatic notch

caudal vertebra 4

Fig. 9.2 Axial skeleton: dorsal view. The palpable bony features shown in the surface view are colored green for reference. Other bony features of the vertebral column are normally impalpable through the overlying dorsal (epaxial) musculature, especially in the neck and lumbar region. For comparable lateral views of the skeleton see Figs 3.2, 5.2, 6.2 and 7.7.

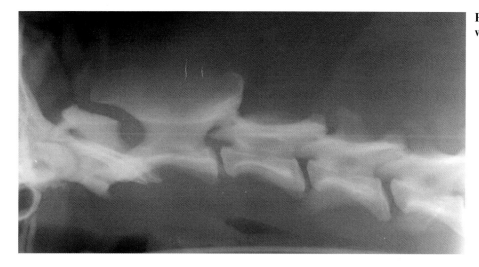

Fig. 9.3 Radiograph of the cranial cervical spine: lateral view. The intervertebral disc spaces can be clearly seen.

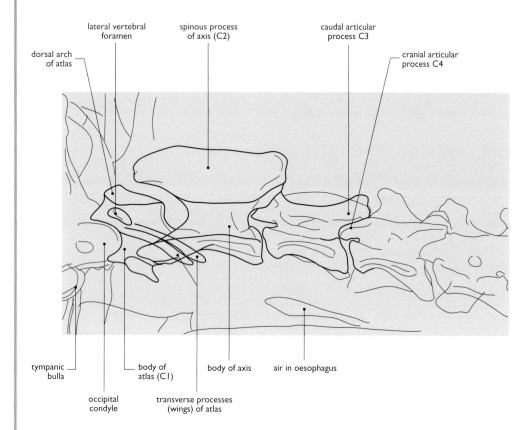

lateral vertebral
foramen

spinous process
of axis (C2)

caudal articular
process C3

cranial articular
process C4

dorsal arch
of atlas

tympanic
bulla

body of
atlas (CI)

body of axis

air in oesophagus

occipital
condyle

transverse processes
(wings) of atlas

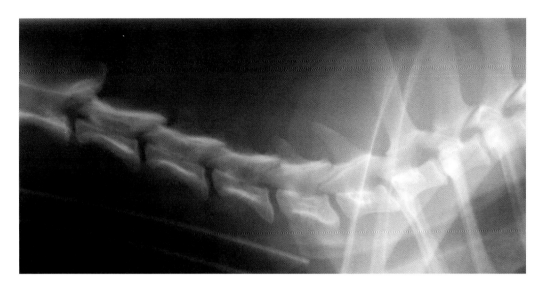

Fig. 9.4 Radiograph of the caudal cervical spine: lateral view. The large transverse processes of the sixth cervical vertebra are visible.

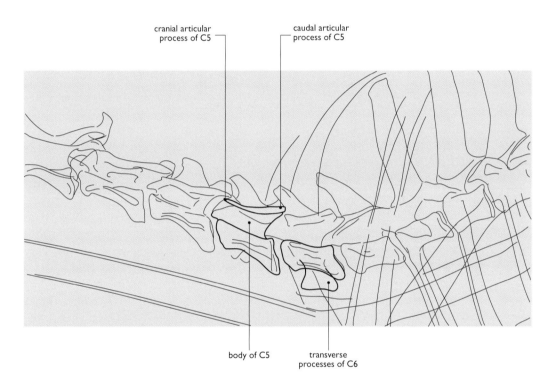

cranial articular
process of C5

caudal articular
process of C5

body of C5

transverse
processes of C6

Veterinary Anatomy: The Dog and Cat

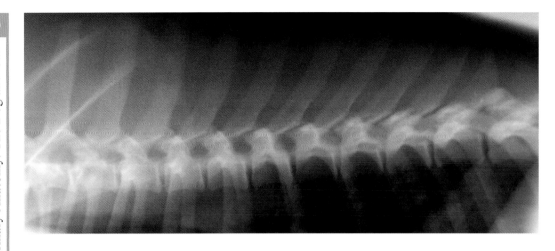

Fig. 9.5 Radiograph of the thoracic spine: lateral view. The intervertebral synovial articulations are orientated in the dorsal plane cranial to the anticlinal vertebra.

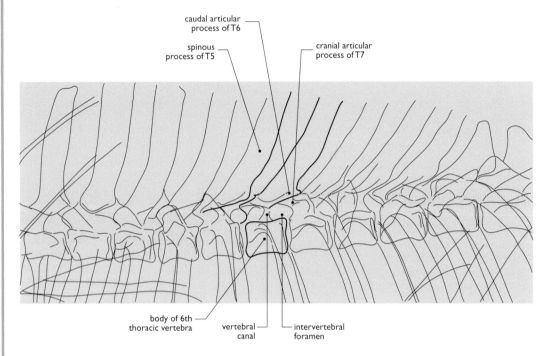

caudal articular process of T6

spinous process of T5

cranial articular process of T7

body of 6th thoracic vertebra

vertebral canal

intervertebral foramen

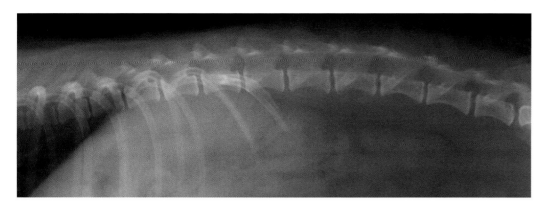

Fig. 9.6 Radiograph of the thoracolumbar junction: lateral view, anatomic variant. The first lumbar vertebra has elongated and enlarged transverse processes, described as vestigial ribs. A vertebra at the edge of a section of the vertebral column may take on some characteristics of the adjacent section. In this case, this would be described as thoracalization of the first lumbar vertebra.

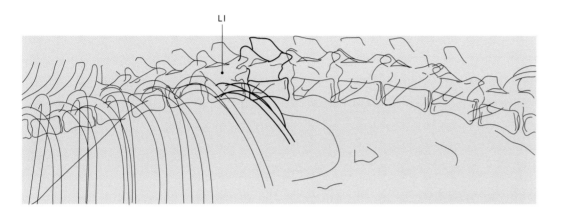

LI

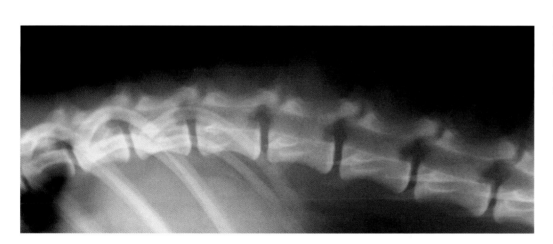

Fig. 9.7 Radiograph of the thoracolumbar junction: lateral view. The intervertebral synovial articulations are orientated in the sagittal plane from the anticlinal vertebra caudally (compare with Figure 9.5).

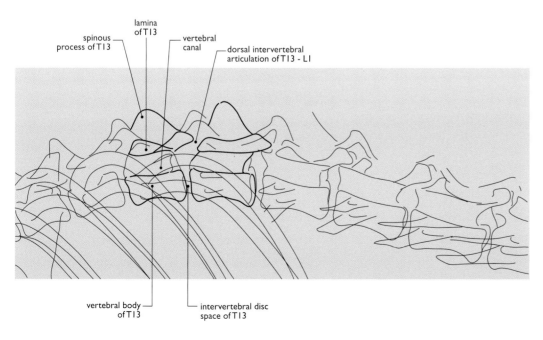

spinous process of T13 — lamina of T13 — vertebral canal — dorsal intervertebral articulation of T13 - L1

vertebral body of T13 — intervertebral disc space of T13

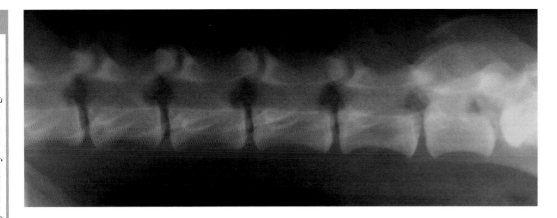

Fig. 9.8 Radiograph of the lumbar spine: lateral view. The large intervertebral foramina can be clearly seen.

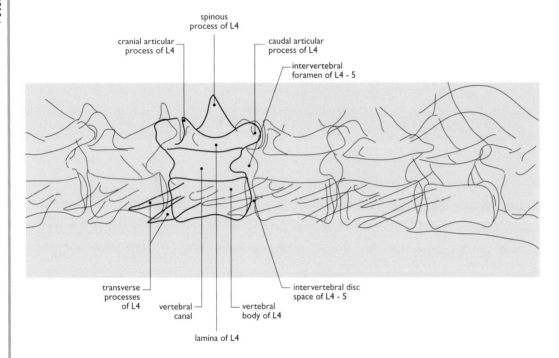

cranial articular
process of L4

spinous
process of L4

caudal articular
process of L4

intervertebral
foramen of L4 - 5

transverse
processes
of L4

vertebral
canal

vertebral
body of L4

intervertebral disc
space of L4 - 5

lamina of L4

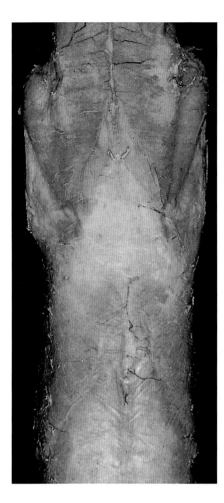
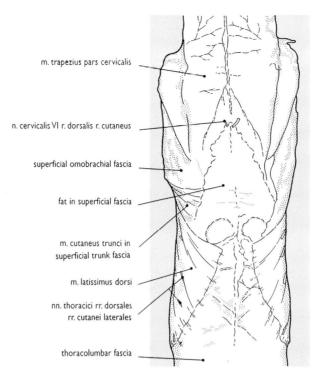

m. trapezius pars cervicalis

n. cervicalis VI r. dorsalis r. cutaneus

superficial omobrachial fascia

fat in superficial fascia

m. cutaneus trunci in
superficial trunk fascia

m. latissimus dorsi

nn. thoracici rr. dorsales
rr. cutanei laterales

thoracolumbar fascia

Fig. 9.9 Superficial structures of the caudal end of the neck and thoracic vertebral region: dorsal view. The loose superficial fascia is variably infiltrated with fat and contains the cutaneous muscle of the trunk. Lateral cutaneous branches from the dorsal rami of thoracic nerves are apparent in the dorsolateral thorax. Comparable views from the lateral aspect are shown in Figs 3.6 and 5.7.

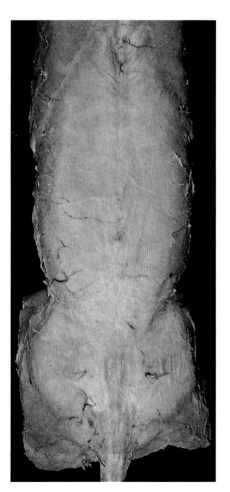
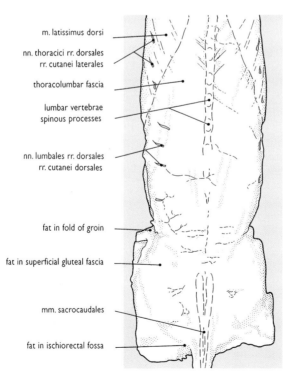

m. latissimus dorsi

nn. thoracici rr. dorsales
rr. cutanei laterales

thoracolumbar fascia

lumbar vertebrae
spinous processes

nn. lumbales rr. dorsales
rr. cutanei dorsales

fat in fold of groin

fat in superficial gluteal fascia

mm. sacrocaudales

fat in ischiorectal fossa

Fig. 9.10 Superficial structures of the lumbar and pelvic regions and the root of the tail: dorsal view. Fat is quite extensively infiltrated into the lumbar and gluteal fascia and is present in the fold of the flank and ischiorectal fossa. Comparable views from a lateral aspect are shown in Figs 6.11 and 7.11.

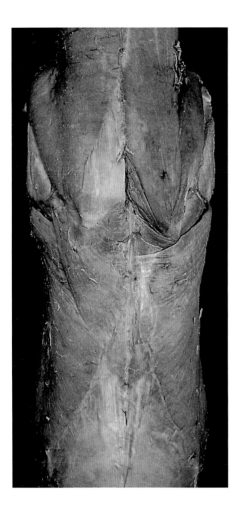

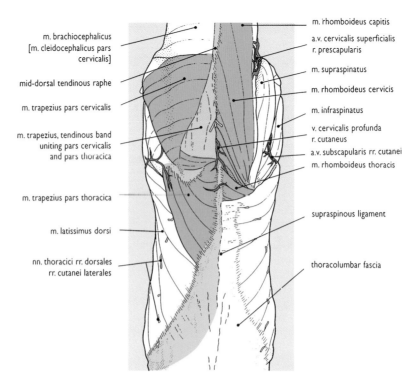

m. brachiocephalicus
[m. cleidocephalicus pars
cervicalis]

mid-dorsal tendinous raphe

m. trapezius pars cervicalis

m. trapezius, tendinous band
uniting pars cervicalis
and pars thoracica

m. trapezius pars thoracica

m. latissimus dorsi

nn. thoracici rr. dorsales
rr. cutanei laterales

m. rhomboideus capitis

a.v. cervicalis superficialis
r. prescapularis

m. supraspinatus

m. rhomboideus cervicis

m. infraspinatus

v. cervicalis profunda
r. cutaneus

a.v. subscapularis rr. cutanei

m. rhomboideus thoracis

supraspinous ligament

thoracolumbar fascia

Fig. 9.11 Superficial muscles of the caudal end of the neck and the thoracic vertebral region: dorsal view. The superficial fascia has been cleaned from the surface to expose superficial extrinsic limb muscles on the left side. These are not covered externally by the deep thoracolumbar fascia which is continued internal to them on the surface of the epaxial musculature. On the right side the cleidocervical component of the brachiocephalic and the trapezius muscles have been removed to expose the rhomboid muscle in the interscapular region. For comparable views from the lateral aspect see Figs 5.9 and 5.10.

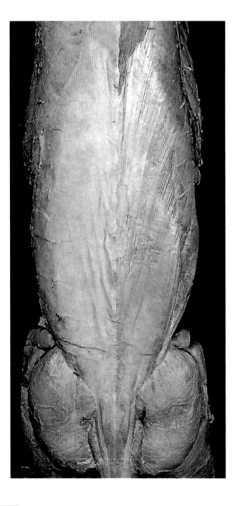

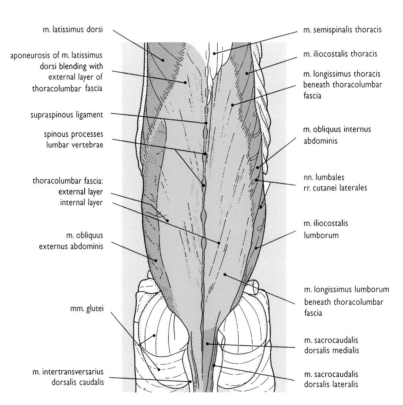

m. latissimus dorsi

aponeurosis of m. latissimus
dorsi blending with
external layer of
thoracolumbar fascia

supraspinous ligament

spinous processes
lumbar vertebrae

thoracolumbar fascia:
external layer
internal layer

m. obliquus
externus abdominis

mm. glutei

m. intertransversarius
dorsalis caudalis

m. semispinalis thoracis

m. iliocostalis thoracis

m. longissimus thoracis
beneath thoracolumbar
fascia

m. obliquus internus
abdominis

nn. lumbales
rr. cutanei laterales

m. iliocostalis
lumborum

m. longissimus lumborum
beneath thoracolumbar
fascia

m. sacrocaudalis
dorsalis medialis

m. sacrocaudalis
dorsalis lateralis

Fig. 9.12 Superficial muscles of the lumbar and pelvic regions and the root of the tail: dorsal view. Cleaning of superficial fascia from the surface has exposed the superficial muscles to some extent, although the dense thoracolumbar fascia obscures detail of the underlying epaxial muscles. On the right side the external layer of thoracolumbar fascia has been removed along with the latissimus dorsi and external abdominal oblique muscles, exposing an internal layer of fascia closely applied to the muscles. For comparable views from the lateral aspect see Figs 6.14, 6.15 and 7.15.

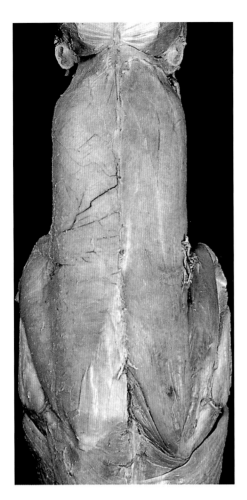

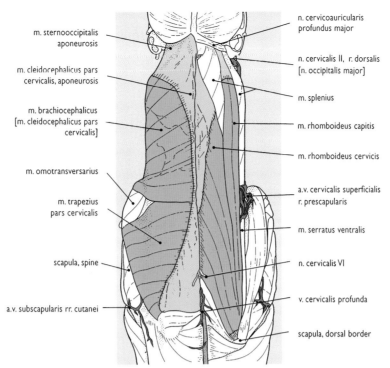

m. sternooccipitalis aponeurosis

m. cleidocephalicus pars cervicalis, aponeurosis

m. brachiocephalicus [m. cleidocephalicus pars cervicalis]

m. omotransversarius

m. trapezius pars cervicalis

scapula, spine

a.v. subscapularis rr. cutanei

n. cervicoauricularis profundus major

n. cervicalis II, r. dorsalis [n. occipitalis major]

m. splenius

m. rhomboideus capitis

m. rhomboideus cervicis

a.v. cervicalis superficialis r. prescapularis

m. serratus ventralis

n. cervicalis VI

v. cervicalis profunda

scapula, dorsal border

Fig. 9.13 Superficial muscles of the neck and interscapular region: dorsal view. The superficial fascia has been cleaned from the left side of the neck and shoulder to expose the superficial muscles. This removal also included the platysma muscle (see Figs 3.6 and 3.7) and the muscles of the auricular cartilages (see Figs 2.41–2.45). On the right side removal of the cleidocervical component of the brachiocephalic muscle and the cervical trapezius has exposed the extent of the cervical and capital parts of the rhomboid muscle. Comparable views of the neck from a lateral aspect are given in Figs 3.13 and 3.15.

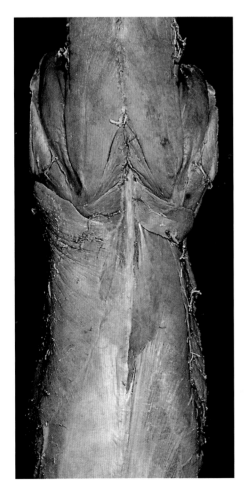

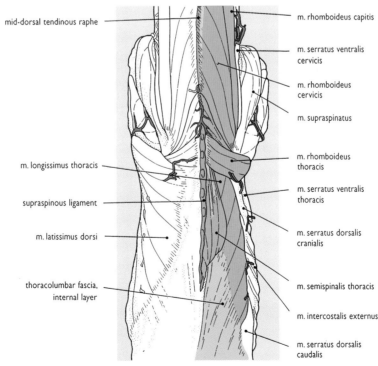

mid-dorsal tendinous raphe

m. longissimus thoracis

supraspinous ligament

m. latissimus dorsi

thoracolumbar fascia, internal layer

m. rhomboideus capitis

m. serratus ventralis cervicis

m. rhomboideus cervicis

m. supraspinatus

m. rhomboideus thoracis

m. serratus ventralis thoracis

m. serratus dorsalis cranialis

m. semispinalis thoracis

m. intercostalis externus

m. serratus dorsalis caudalis

Fig. 9.14 Rhomboid and thoracic epaxial muscles after removal of the trapezius and latissimus dorsi muscles: dorsal view. Removal of the latissimus dorsi muscle on the right side completes the exposure of the thoracic component of the rhomboid muscle in the interscapular region. The thoracolumbar fascia is continued cranially on the surface of the epaxial muscles beneath the thoracic rhomboid; through it the combined spinal and semispinal muscle of the thorax and the thoracic longissimus are visible. A comparable view from the lateral aspect is given in Fig. 5.10 in which the deep thoracolumbar fascia between the attachments of the dorsal serrate muscles has been removed.

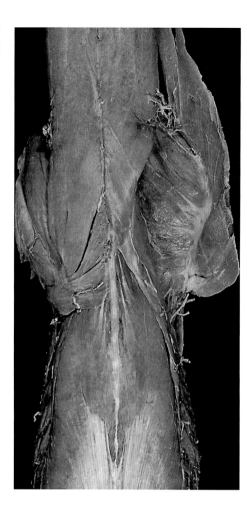

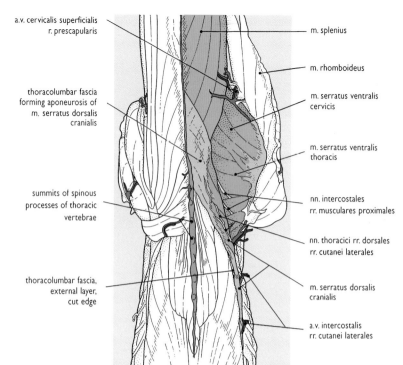

a.v. cervicalis superficialis
r. prescapularis

thoracolumbar fascia
forming aponeurosis of
m. serratus dorsalis
cranialis

summits of spinous
processes of thoracic
vertebrae

thoracolumbar fascia,
external layer,
cut edge

m. splenius

m. rhomboideus

m. serratus ventralis
cervicis

m. serratus ventralis
thoracis

nn. intercostales
rr. musculares proximales

nn. thoracici rr. dorsales
rr. cutanei laterales

m. serratus dorsalis
cranialis

a.v. intercostalis
rr. cutanei laterales

Fig. 9.15 Ventral serrate muscle after transection of the rhomboid muscle and lateral displacement of the scapula: dorsal view. The rhomboid muscle of the right side has been severed and the upper end of the scapula has been rotated laterally to expose the cervical and thoracic parts of the ventral serrate muscle converging on the serrated face of the scapula. The ventral serrate muscle is also shown in lateral view in Fig. 4.16 with the forelimb still in place, and in Fig. 5.11 with the forelimb removed. The cranial continuation of the thoracolumbar fascia exposed provides attachment for the cranial dorsal serrate and the splenius muscle.

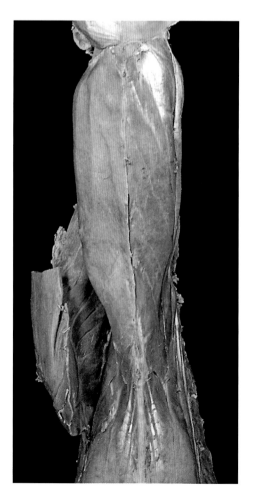

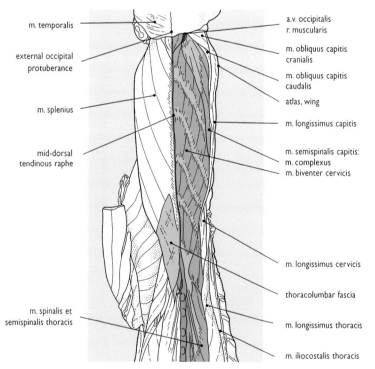

m. temporalis

external occipital
protuberance

m. splenius

mid-dorsal
tendinous raphe

m. spinalis et
semispinalis thoracis

a.v. occipitalis
r. muscularis

m. obliquus capitis
cranialis

m. obliquus capitis
caudalis

atlas, wing

m. longissimus capitis

m. semispinalis capitis:
m. complexus
m. biventer cervicis

m. longissimus cervicis

thoracolumbar fascia

m. longissimus thoracis

m. iliocostalis thoracis

Fig. 9.16 Epaxial muscles of the neck and cranial end of the thorax. (1) Splenius and semispinalis capitis muscles: dorsal view. Severance of the rhomboid muscle and scapular displacement on the left side has exposed the entire splenius muscle in the neck originating from the thoracolumbar fascia at the cranial end of the thorax. Splenius muscle removal on the right side exposes the combined spinal and semispinal muscle of the thorax and its prominent bipartite continuation in the neck as the semispinal component of the head.

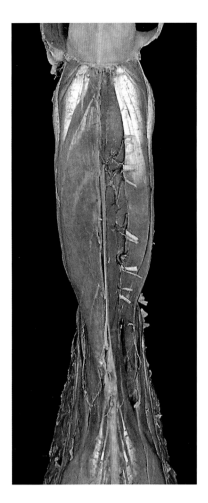

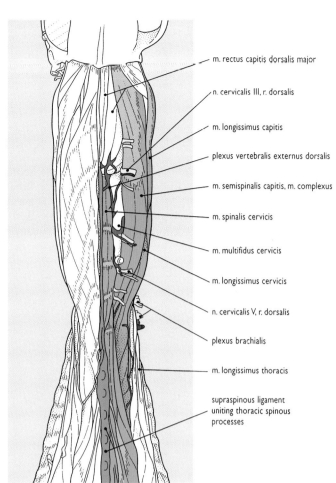

m. rectus capitis dorsalis major

n. cervicalis III, r. dorsalis

m. longissimus capitis

plexus vertebralis externus dorsalis

m. semispinalis capitis, m. complexus

m. spinalis cervicis

m. multifidus cervicis

m. longissimus cervicis

n. cervicalis V, r. dorsalis

plexus brachialis

m. longissimus thoracis

supraspinous ligament
uniting thoracic spinous
processes

Fig. 9.17 Epaxial muscles of the neck and cranial end of the thorax. (2) Spinalis cervicis and semispinalis capitis muscles and dorsal rami of cervical spinal nerves: dorsal view. Removal of the biventer cervicis muscle on the right side has exposed the underlying complexus component and muscular ramifications of the dorsal rami of cervical nerves. Also exposed are the spinalis components in the neck bordering the nuchal ligament in the midline, and the longissimus components forming the lateral boundary. The continuity of longissimus muscles through the thorax and neck is now clearly demonstrated. A comparable view from the lateral aspect is seen in Fig. 3.18.

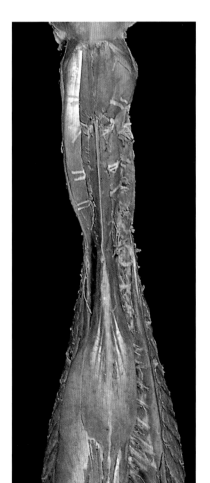

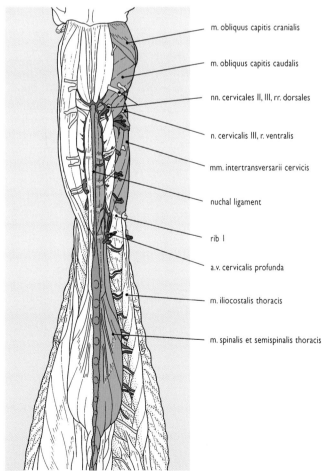

m. obliquus capitis cranialis

m. obliquus capitis caudalis

nn. cervicales II, III, rr. dorsales

n. cervicalis III, r. ventralis

mm. intertransversarii cervicis

nuchal ligament

rib I

a.v. cervicalis profunda

m. iliocostalis thoracis

m. spinalis et semispinalis thoracis

Fig. 9.18 Epaxial muscles of the neck and cranial end of the thorax. (3) Intertransverse, multifidus and spinalis muscles: dorsal view. Removal of the complexus and longissimus muscles on the right side displays the prominent and complex intertransverse muscles in the neck, with their continuations as oblique muscles on the atlas/axis complex. Intertransverse muscles are barely represented in the thorax and lumbar regions but are prominent in the tail. The rectus capitis dorsalis muscle towards the dorsal midline is a continuation of the interspinal muscles as yet uncovered. A comparable view from the lateral aspect is seen in Fig. 3.19.

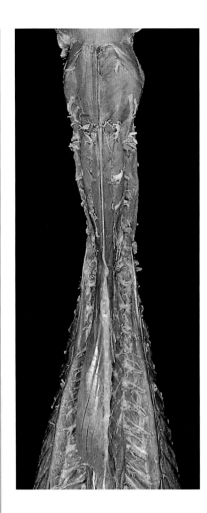
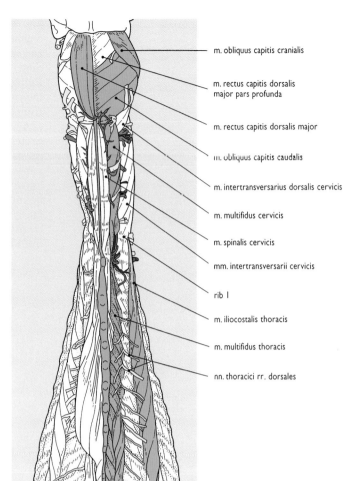

m. obliquus capitis cranialis

m. rectus capitis dorsalis major pars profunda

m. rectus capitis dorsalis major

m. obliquus capitis caudalis

m. intertransversarius dorsalis cervicis

m. multifidus cervicis

m. spinalis cervicis

mm. intertransversarii cervicis

rib I

m. iliocostalis thoracis

m. multifidus thoracis

nn. thoracici rr. dorsales

Fig. 9.19 Epaxial muscles of the neck and cranial end of the thorax. (4) Special muscles of the atlanto-occipital complex: dorsal view. The rectus capitis dorsalis major muscle, in place on the left side, is removed from the right, exposing the capital oblique muscles and the deep component of the rectus capitis dorsalis. Removal of the spinalis and semispinalis component in the thorax displays the thoracic multifidus muscles and muscular ramifications of the dorsal rami of thoracic nerves. Comparable lateral views of the neck are shown in Fig. 3.20, and of the thorax in Fig. 5.40.

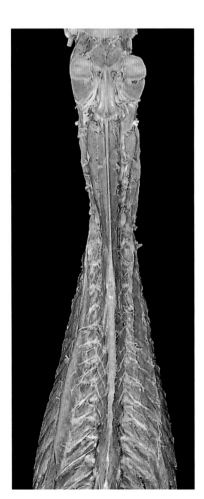
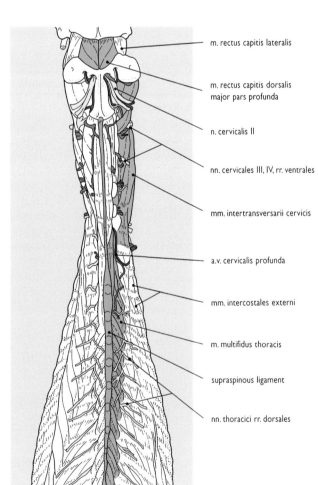

m. rectus capitis lateralis

m. rectus capitis dorsalis major pars profunda

n. cervicalis II

nn. cervicales III, IV, rr. ventrales

mm. intertransversarii cervicis

a.v. cervicalis profunda

mm. intercostales externi

m. multifidus thoracis

supraspinous ligament

nn. thoracici rr. dorsales

Fig. 9.20 Epaxial muscles of the neck and cranial end of the thorax. (5) The atlanto-occipital complex and nuchal ligament: dorsal view. Oblique and rectus capitis dorsalis muscles have been removed from both sides except for the deep part of the rectus capitis dorsalis in the atlanto-occipital space. The multifidus muscles in the neck and some components of the cervical intertransverse muscles have been removed, leaving the more ventral intertransverse muscles in place with the stumps of ventral rami of cervical spinal nerves crossing them. Comparable lateral views of the neck are shown in Figs 3.21 and 3.22.

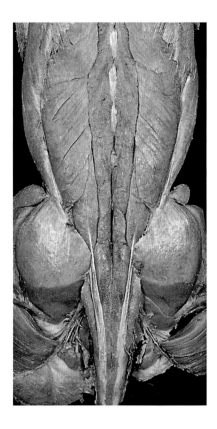

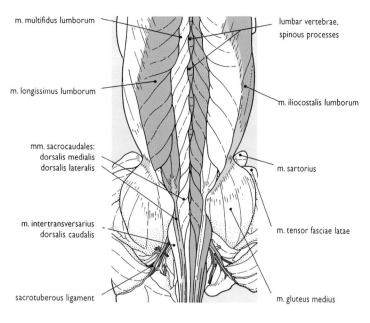

m. multifidus lumborum

m. longissimus lumborum

mm. sacrocaudales:
dorsalis medialis
dorsalis lateralis

m. intertransversarius
dorsalis caudalis

sacrotuberous ligament

lumbar vertebrae,
spinous processes

m. iliocostalis lumborum

m. sartorius

m. tensor fasciae latae

m. gluteus medius

Fig. 9.21 Epaxial muscles of the lumbar and sacral regions and root of the tail. (1) After removal of the deep fascia: dorsal view. Removal of the thoracolumbar, sacral, caudal and gluteal fascia, and the superficial gluteal muscles, displays the epaxial muscles. The continuity of both multifidus and longissimus components into the base of the tail as dorsal sacrocaudal muscles is clearly apparent. Intertransverse caudal musculature is visible after removal of the superficial gluteal muscles. A comparable view of the rump and ischiorectal fossa from the lateral aspect is seen in Fig. 7.17.

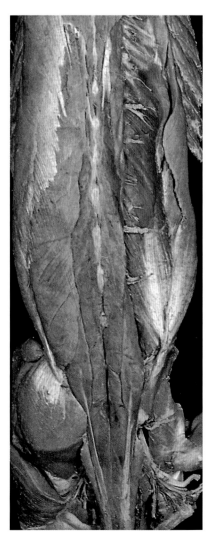

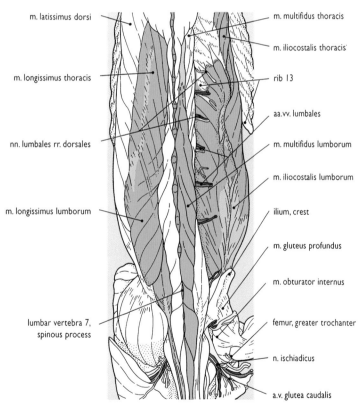

m. latissimus dorsi

m. longissimus thoracis

nn. lumbales rr. dorsales

m. longissimus lumborum

lumbar vertebra 7,
spinous process

m. multifidus thoracis

m. iliocostalis thoracis

rib 13

aa.vv. lumbales

m. multifidus lumborum

m. iliocostalis lumborum

ilium, crest

m. gluteus profundus

m. obturator internus

femur, greater trochanter

n. ischiadicus

a.v. glutea caudalis

Fig. 9.22 Epaxial muscles of the lumbar and sacral regions and the root of the tail. (2) After removal of the longissimus and gluteal musculature: dorsal view. The thoracic and lumbar longissimus has been removed from the right side although the continuation into the tail (dorsal lateral sacrocaudal muscle) remains. The iliocostal muscle is exposed laterally together with muscular ramifications from dorsal rami of lumbar nerves and branches from lumbar vessels. Removal of the gluteal muscles of the right side allows clearer delineation of the root of the tail. As in the neck prominent intertransverse muscles characterize the tail. For a comparable lateral view see Fig. 7.19.

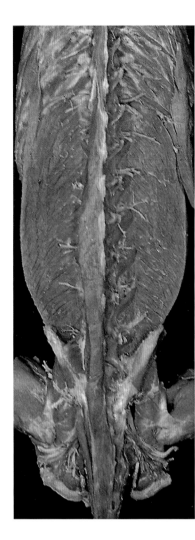

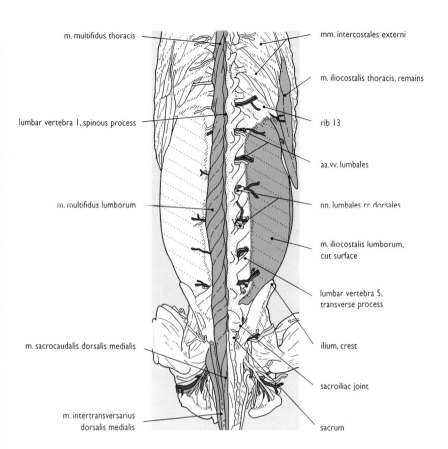

m. multifidus thoracis

mm. intercostales externi

m. iliocostalis thoracis, remains

lumbar vertebra I, spinous process

rib 13

aa.vv. lumbales

m. multifidus lumborum

nn. lumbales rr. dorsales

m. iliocostalis lumborum, cut surface

lumbar vertebra 5, transverse process

m. sacrocaudalis dorsalis medialis

ilium, crest

sacroiliac joint

m. intertransversarius dorsalis medialis

sacrum

Fig. 9.23 Lumbar and sacral regions of the vertebral column and the root of the tail: dorsal view. The lumbar multifidus muscles and the dorsal sacrocaudal muscles have been removed from the right side, exposing the lumbar vertebrae and dorsal sacral surface with the sacroiliac joint. The iliocostal muscle has been almost completely removed, although some of its bulk bulging below the tips of the lumbar transverse processes has been left in place to provide stability for the specimen.

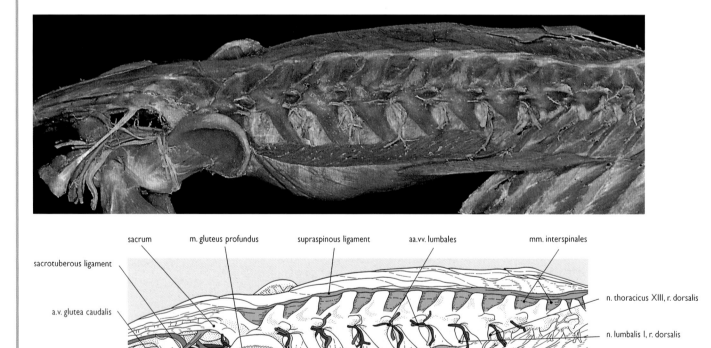

sacrum

m. gluteus profundus

supraspinous ligament

aa.vv. lumbales

mm. interspinales

sacrotuberous ligament

n. thoracicus XIII, r. dorsalis

a.v. glutea caudalis

n. lumbalis I, r. dorsalis

n. ischiadicus

rib 13

n. gluteus cranialis

m. iliocostalis lumborum

Fig. 9.24 Lumbar and sacral regions of the vertebral column and the root of the tail: lateral view. This lateral view of Fig. 9.23 shows the lumbar region cleaned of epaxial muscle except for the most ventral part of the iliocostal. The muscular ramifications of the dorsal rami of lumbar nerves are still apparent, accompanied by muscular branches from lumbar vessels.

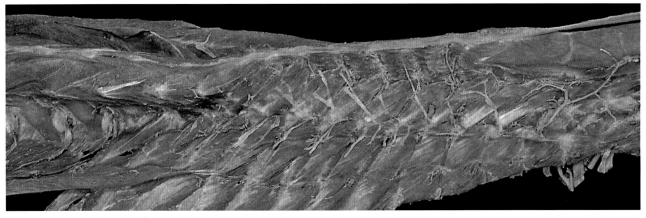

m. multifidus lumborum   nn. thoracici rr. dorsales   mm. interspinales   m. multifidus thoracis   supraspinous ligament   nuchal ligament

m. longissimus lumborum

m. iliocostalis lumborum

rib 13   mm. levatores costarum   mm. intercostales externi   rib I   m. multifidus cervicis

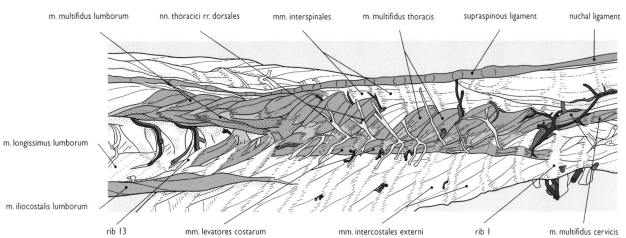

Fig. 9.25 Epaxial muscles of the thorax. (1) After removal of longissimus and iliocostal muscles: lateral view. All that remains of the thoracic epaxial musculature are multifidus and interspinal muscles. The multifidus ('long rotator' muscles) are overlain by extensive ramifications of the dorsal rami of thoracic spinal nerves. Iliocostal muscle removal at the extreme lateral boundary of the epaxial muscles also exposes the rib levator muscles – dorsal continuations of the external intercostals. A comparable view, also from the lateral aspect, is shown in Fig. 5.40.

lumbar vertebra:
mammillary process
spinous process
transverse process
accessory process

mm. rotatores   mm. interspinales   a.v. cervicalis profunda

n. lumbalis I, r. dorsalis

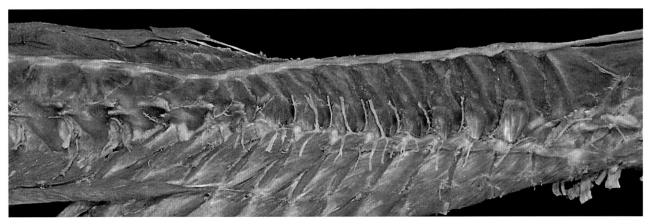

n. thoracicus XIII, r. dorsalis   nn. thoracici rr. dorsales   mm. levatores costarum

Fig. 9.26 Epaxial muscles of the thorax. (2) Rotator and interspinal muscles: lateral view. The 'long rotator' components of the thoracic multifidus muscle have been removed to expose the shorter and more vertically oriented rotator muscles and the rib levator muscles. Interspinal muscles and the longitudinal supraspinous ligament are clearly displayed.

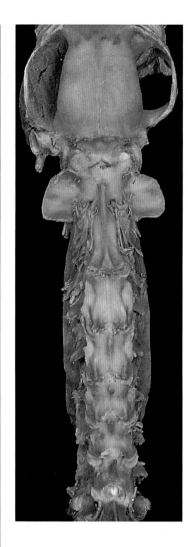

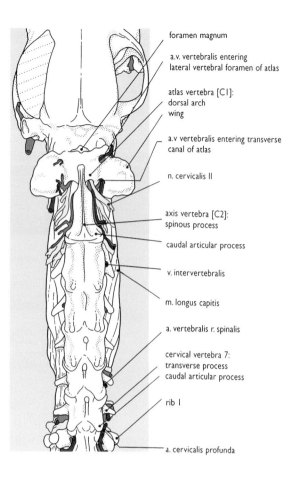

foramen magnum

a.v. vertebralis entering
lateral vertebral foramen of atlas

atlas vertebra [C1]:
dorsal arch
wing

a.v vertebralis entering transverse
canal of atlas

n. cervicalis II

axis vertebra [C2]:
spinous process

caudal articular process

v. intervertebralis

m. longus capitis

a. vertebralis r. spinalis

cervical vertebra 7:
transverse process
caudal articular process

rib I

a. cervicalis profunda

Fig. 9.27 Cervical region of the vertebral column after removal of the epaxial musculature: dorsal view. All of the epaxial muscle has been removed from the neck to give a complete view of the cervical vertebrae. The passage of the vertebral artery through the transverse canal of the atlas has been retained on the right side with the continuation of the artery entering the vertebral canal through the lateral vertebral foramen in the dorsal arch. The complete passage of the vertebral artery is shown in Figs 3.21–3.23 and Fig. 3.26, in which the lateral wall of the transverse canal had been removed from all cervical vertebrae.

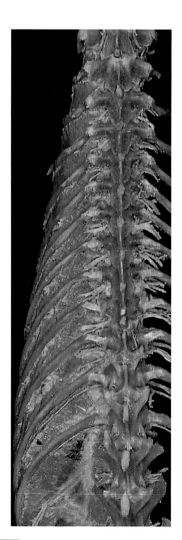

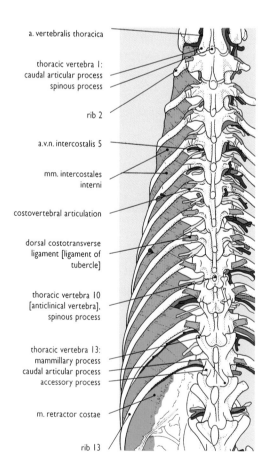

a. vertebralis thoracica

thoracic vertebra 1:
caudal articular process
spinous process

rib 2

a.v.n. intercostalis 5

mm. intercostales
interni

costovertebral articulation

dorsal costotransverse
ligament [ligament of
tubercle]

thoracic vertebra 10
[anticlinical vertebra],
spinous process

thoracic vertebra 13:
mammillary process
caudal articular process
accessory process

m. retractor costae

rib 13

Fig. 9.28 Thoracic region of the vertebral column, intercostal nerves and blood vessels: dorsal view. All of the epaxial musculature has been removed from the thorax along with the intercostal musculature from the right side. The internal intercostal muscles remain in place on the left side. Intercostal 'triads' of artery, vein and nerve are apparent in the upper ends of the intercostal spaces (see also Figs 5.18 and 5.23 of the thorax in lateral view).

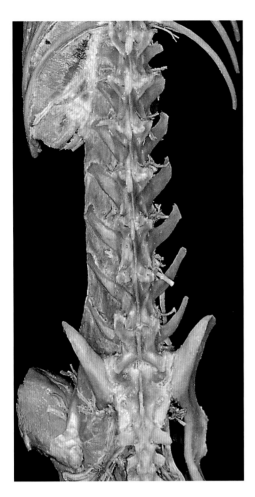
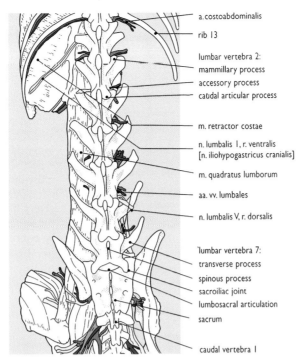

Fig. 9.29 Lumbar, sacral and caudal regions of the vertebral column after removal of the epaxial muscles: dorsal view. All of the epaxial musculature has been removed from the lumbar region and the root of the tail to give a complete view of the vertebrae in this region. Also shown on the left side are the nerves and blood vessels leaving the pelvic cavity through the lesser ischiatic foramen beneath the sacrotuberous ligament en route for the hindlimb (shown in lateral view in Figs 7.16–7.19 and Fig. 8.9).

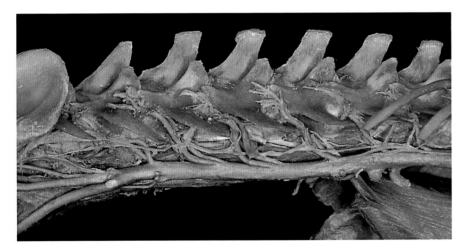

Fig. 9.30 Lumbar region of the vertebral column, lumbar vessels and lumbar sympathetic nerve trunk: lateral view. Removal of the iliocostalis lumborum of the epaxial musculature and the quadratus lumborum and psoas muscles of the subvertebral hypaxial musculature exposes the full length of the abdominal aorta. Lumbar arteries are clearly apparent, as are the sympathetic trunk and its communicating rami with the ventral rami of lumbar spinal nerves.

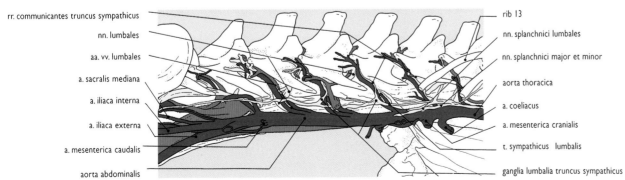

439

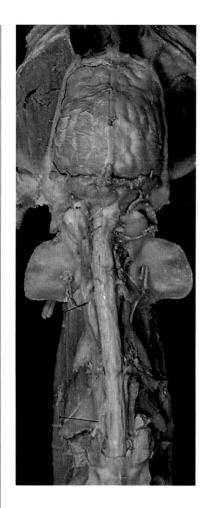

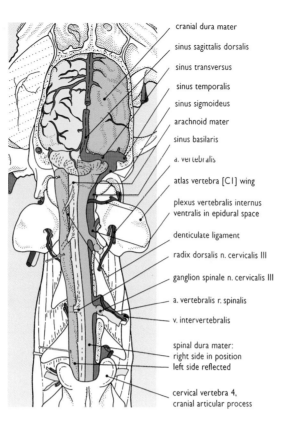

cranial dura mater
sinus sagittalis dorsalis
sinus transversus
sinus temporalis
sinus sigmoideus
arachnoid mater
sinus basilaris
a. vertebralis
atlas vertebra [CI] wing
plexus vertebralis internus
ventralis in epidural space
denticulate ligament
radix dorsalis n. cervicalis III
ganglion spinale n. cervicalis III
a. vertebralis r. spinalis
v. intervertebralis
spinal dura mater:
right side in position
left side reflected
cervical vertebra 4,
cranial articular process

Fig. 9.31 Spinal cord and spinal meninges in situ. (1) Cranial cervical region: dorsal view. The calvarium of the skull has been removed along with the dorsal arch of the atlas and the arches and spinous processes of the axis and third cervical vertebra, opening the cranial cavity and the vertebral canal. The brain, cranial meninges and dural venous sinuses have been considered elsewhere (Figs 2.117 and 2.118). In the spinal canal the dura has been cut through longitudinally in the dorsal midline and the left half is reflected to display dorsal nerve roots entering their individual dural 'tubes' and a component of the denticulate ligament. On the right side the vertebral artery has been retained entering the epidural space in the spinal canal and disappearing beneath the cord to be continued as the ventral spinal and basilar arteries (see Figs 2.111 and 2.124).

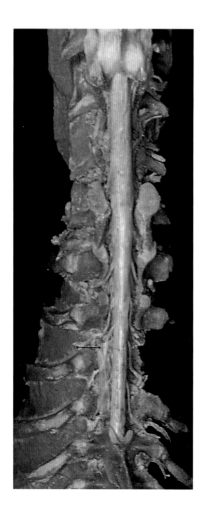

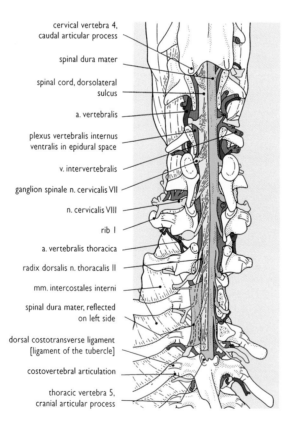

cervical vertebra 4,
caudal articular process
spinal dura mater
spinal cord, dorsolateral
sulcus
a. vertebralis
plexus vertebralis internus
ventralis in epidural space
v. intervertebralis
ganglion spinale n. cervicalis VII
n. cervicalis VIII
rib I
a. vertebralis thoracica
radix dorsalis n. thoracalis II
mm. intercostales interni
spinal dura mater, reflected
on left side
dorsal costotransverse ligament
[ligament of the tubercle]
costovertebral articulation
thoracic vertebra 5,
cranial articular process

Fig. 9.32 Spinal cord and spinal meninges in situ. (2) Cervicothoracic junction: dorsal view. This section of spinal cord shows the cervical enlargement associated with forelimb innervation lying within vertebral segments C5–C7. The progressive lengthening of spinal nerve roots inside the epidural space is also evident: at C6 the roots pass at more or less right angles from their origin on the cord to their exit through the intervertebral foramen; at T3 and T4 the nerve roots travel caudally within the spinal canal for some distance prior to their exit. In this more caudal region the spinal dura mater has been reflected from the cord on the left side and a component of the denticulate ligament is exposed.

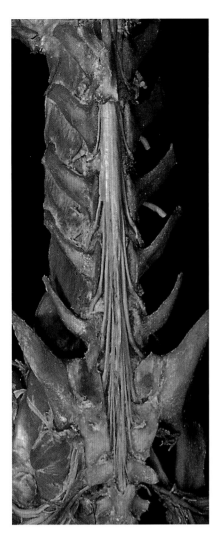

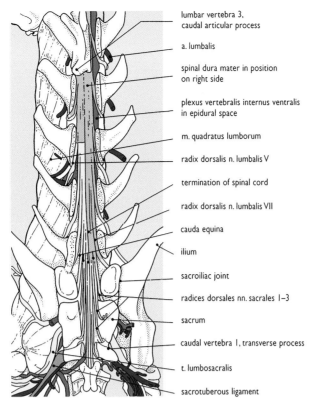

lumbar vertebra 3,
caudal articular process

a. lumbalis

spinal dura mater in position
on right side

plexus vertebralis internus ventralis
in epidural space

m. quadratus lumborum

radix dorsalis n. lumbalis V

termination of spinal cord

radix dorsalis n. lumbalis VII

cauda equina

ilium

sacroiliac joint

radices dorsales nn. sacrales I–3

sacrum

caudal vertebra I, transverse process

t. lumbosacralis

sacrotuberous ligament

Fig. 9.33 Spinal cord and spinal meninges in situ. (3) Lumbar region and cauda equina: dorsal view. The lumbar enlargement of the spinal cord associated with innervation to the hindlimbs is located within lumbar vertebral segments 3–5. Beyond this the cord narrows rapidly and actually terminates at lumbar vertebra 7, only being continued by a strand of non-nervous tissue. Flanking the caudal end of the cord and this filum terminale are the roots of sacral and caudal spinal nerves producing the cauda equina.

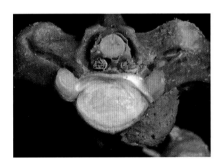

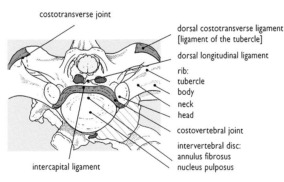

costotransverse joint

dorsal costotransverse ligament [ligament of the tubercle]

dorsal longitudinal ligament

rib:
tubercle
body
neck
head

costovertebral joint

intervertebral disc:
annulus fibrosus
nucleus pulposus

intercapital ligament

Fig. 9.34 Ligaments of the vertebral column. (1) Intercapital ligament: cranial view. The vertebral column and spinal cord have been severed by cutting through between thoracic vertebrae 2 and 3. The sectioned intervertebral disc displays an outer fibrocartilaginous component surrounding a centrally placed pulpy nucleus. An intercapital ligament uniting the heads of the ribs across the dorsum of a disc is present between the heads of ribs 2 to 10.

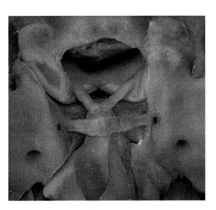

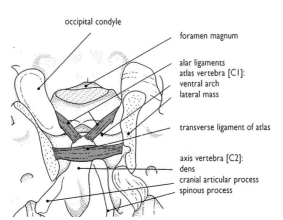

occipital condyle

foramen magnum

alar ligaments
atlas vertebra [C1]:
ventral arch
lateral mass

transverse ligament of atlas

axis vertebra [C2]:
dens
cranial articular process
spinous process

Fig. 9.35 Ligaments of the vertebral column. (2) Atlantoaxial ligaments: dorsal view. The dorsal arch of the atlas has been removed and the spinal cord, spinal meninges and vertebral venous plexuses cleared from the vertebral canal to expose the ligaments associated with the dens (odontoid process) of the axis where it forms the atlantoaxial joint.

10. THE CAT: COMPARATIVE ASPECTS

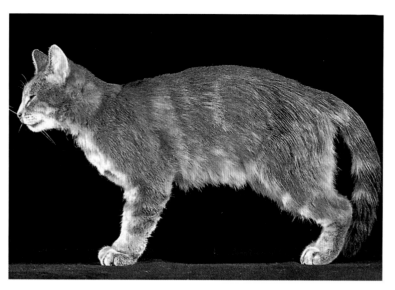

Fig. 10.1 Surface features of the cat: left lateral view. The cat differs from the dog in a number of ways (see Fig. 1.1), although most are differences in shape and proportion. Rather than attempting a comprehensive coverage of gross feline anatomy, which is beyond the scope of this book, the few significant gross anatomical differences are illustrated in this chapter. The most obvious of these differences ascertainable on surface examination are: (i) shortened face with greater development of the vibrissae on the muzzle and an absence of vibrissae from below the chin; (ii) elliptical pupil in the eye which can be almost completely closed up in bright light to a practically vertical slit; (iii) tooth reduction to a purely sectorial dentition with relatively longer and stronger canines designed for stabbing, a considerable post-canine space, and carnassials the most scissor-like of the carnivores, (iv) short, curved and pointed claws which are retractile; (v) short, caudally-directed penis with prepuce opening close to the scrotum.

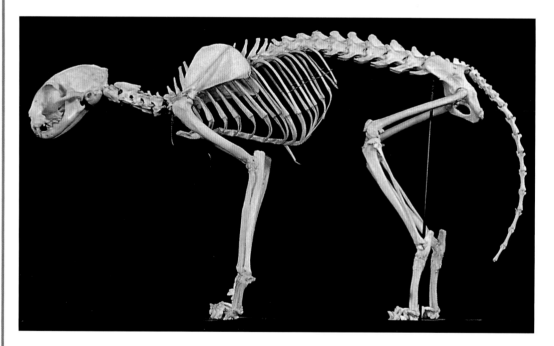

Fig. 10.2 Skeleton of the cat: left lateral view. Skeletal pictures and radiographs are used to demonstrate the osteology of the cat. Of immediate significance is the close overall similarity to the dog, although the bones generally are built to a more delicate plan. A skeletal picture does provide a clear indication of the difference in posture between the two animals (compare with Fig. 1.2).

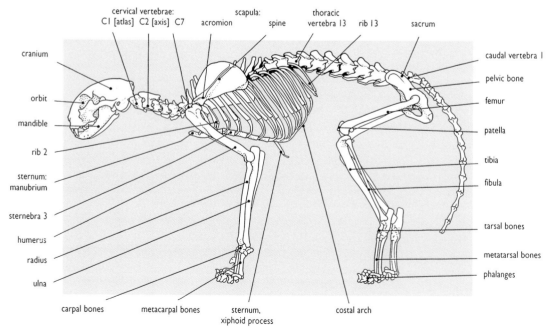

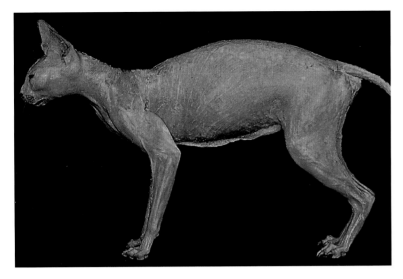

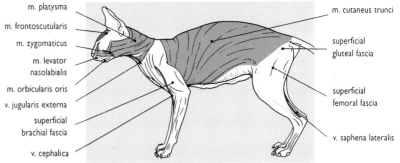

Fig. 10.3 Superficial structures and cutaneous muscles: left lateral view. The skin has been removed revealing the superficial fascia comparable in extent to that in the dog (see Figs 2.24, 3.6, 4.10, 4.50, 5.6, 6.11, 7.11, 7.42, 9.9 and 9.10). The cutaneous muscle of the trunk is greater in extent in the cat, clearly originating from the rump and sacral region and possibly from the base of the tail.

Fig. 10.4 Superficial musculature: left lateral view. Superficial fascia and the cutaneous muscle contained within it have been removed, exposing superficial musculature. The remains of lateral cutaneous branches from the dorsal rami of thoracic nerves and from intercostal nerves (ventral rami of thoracic nerves) emerge through the trunk muscles dorsolaterally and laterally respectively.

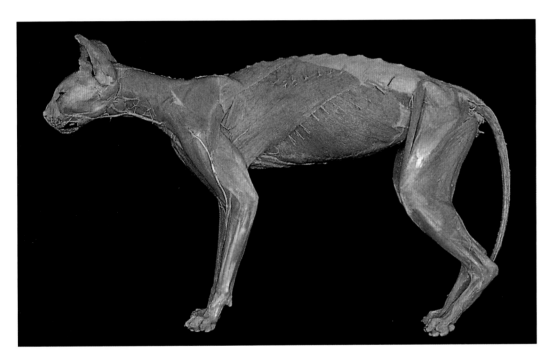

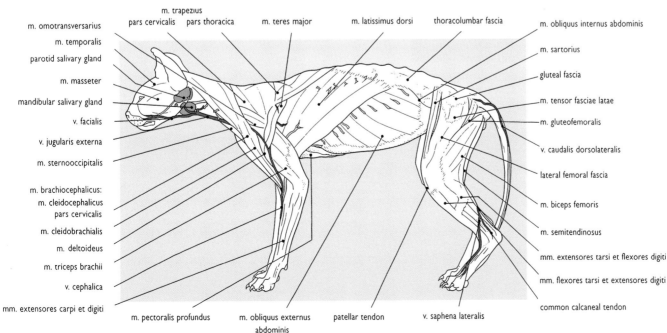

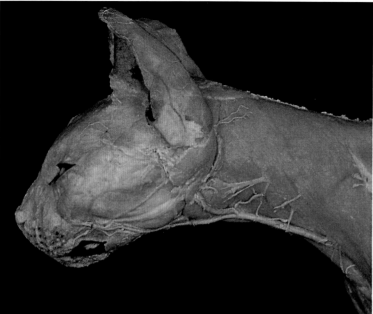

Fig. 10.5 Superficial structures of the head and neck: left lateral view. The head has been skinned and most of the cutaneous musculature has been removed except that on the muzzle (compare with Figs 2.27–2.30 of the dog). Apart from differences in shape and proportion other visible differences include a molar salivary gland, a more pronounced structure than the buccal glands of the dog (Fig. 2.38). An additional, and large, superficial parotid lymph node is present caudal to the parotid gland. NB Lymph nodes in the cat generally are relatively larger than those in the dog.

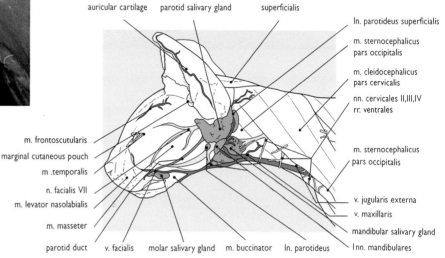

Fig. 10.6 Skeleton of the head and cranial end of the neck: left lateral view. The skull displays a number of differences from the dog (Fig. 2.2). The facial length is reduced in relation to the cranium, brought about primarily by jaw shortening. The dentition is reduced and purely sectorial (shearing), lacking any molar tooth grinding capacity; suppression/reduction in size of the premolar teeth also produces a considerable post-canine space. The enlarged orbit has a practically complete bony margin and faces more rostrally, giving cats the most highly developed binocular vision of all carnivores. An external sagittal crest is short and restricted to the caudal part of the cranium, while the tympanic bulla containing the middle ear cavity is noticeably larger.

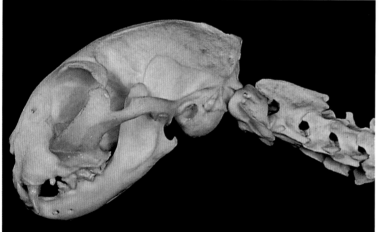

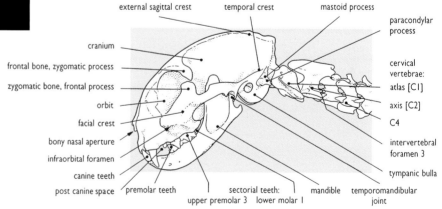

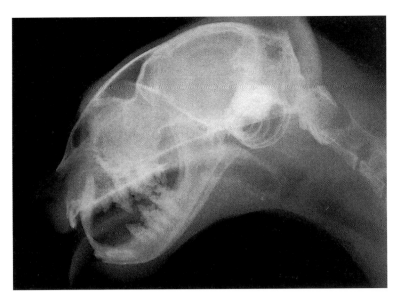

Fig. 10.7 Radiograph of the head and cranial end of the neck: lateral view. The major radiographic features of the head are shown in this picture and in Fig. 10.17. As with radiographs of the dog head (Figs 2.4 and 2.6) detailed internal osteology is omitted, emphasis is placed on identifying the main features and those differing from the dog. The large relative size of the cranial cavity is apparent and the single cavity of the frontal sinus. The dental arches and tooth roots are visible through the jaw bones but few soft features are discernible, although the pharynx and trachea are apparent from the air contained within them (see Fig. 2.7).

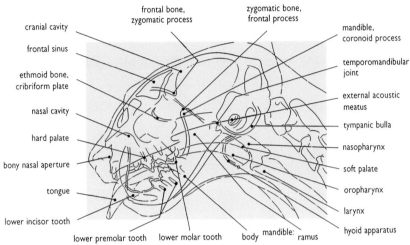

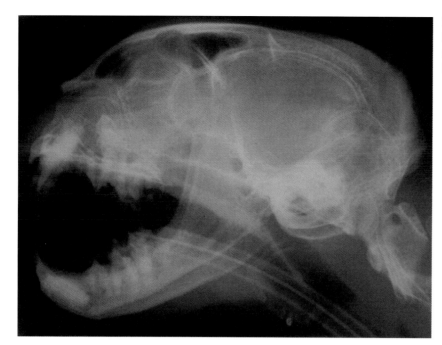

Fig. 10.8 Radiograph of the head: lateral view, brachycephalic breed. The frontal and nasal bones are more domed in this breed and there is flaring of the ethmoturbinates and shortening of the nasal chambers.

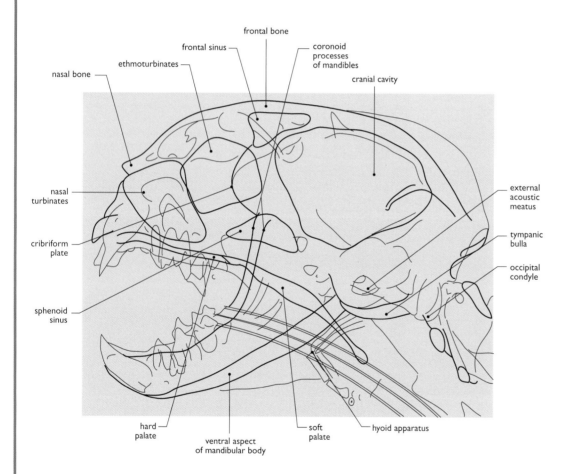

nasal bone

ethmoturbinates

frontal sinus

frontal bone

coronoid processes of mandibles

cranial cavity

nasal turbinates

cribriform plate

sphenoid sinus

external acoustic meatus

tympanic bulla

occipital condyle

hard palate

ventral aspect of mandibular body

soft palate

hyoid apparatus

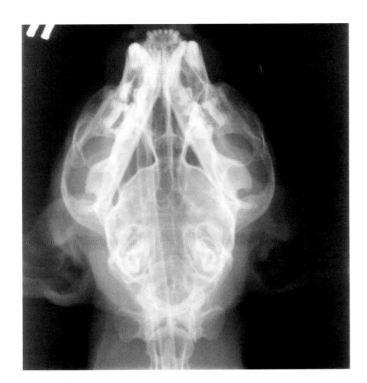

Fig. 10.9 Radiograph of the head: ventrodorsal view. The large zygomatic arches can be seen.

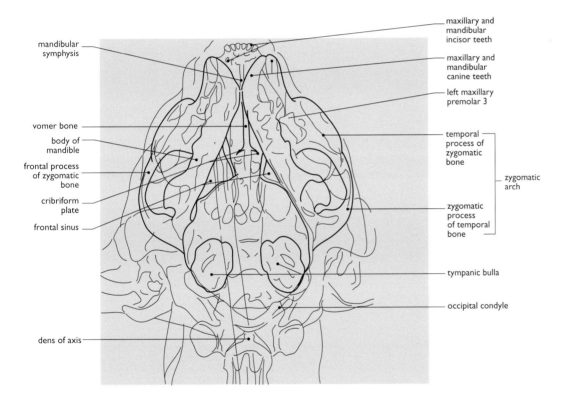

mandibular
symphysis

maxillary and
mandibular
incisor teeth

maxillary and
mandibular
canine teeth

left maxillary
premolar 3

vomer bone

body of
mandible

frontal process
of zygomatic
bone

cribriform
plate

frontal sinus

temporal
process of
zygomatic
bone

zygomatic
arch

zygomatic
process
of temporal
bone

tympanic bulla

occipital condyle

dens of axis

Veterinary Anatomy: The Dog and Cat

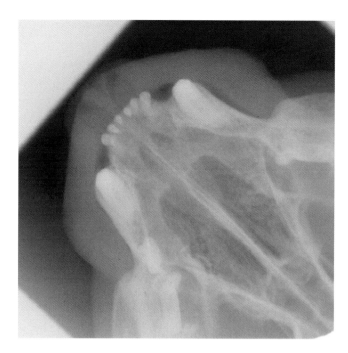

Fig. 10.10 Radiograph of the maxilla and nasal chambers: dorsoventral intraoral view. The tooth roots appear foreshortened in this view as they are angled relative to the x-ray beam. The two nasal chambers can be seen without superimposition. Some premolars and molars have been lost.

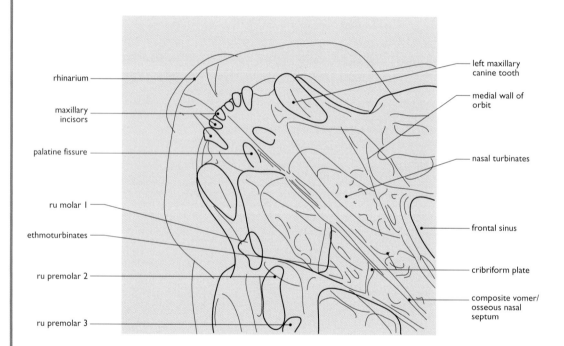

rhinarium

maxillary incisors

palatine fissure

ru molar 1

ethmoturbinates

ru premolar 2

ru premolar 3

left maxillary canine tooth

medial wall of orbit

nasal turbinates

frontal sinus

cribriform plate

composite vomer/ osseous nasal septum

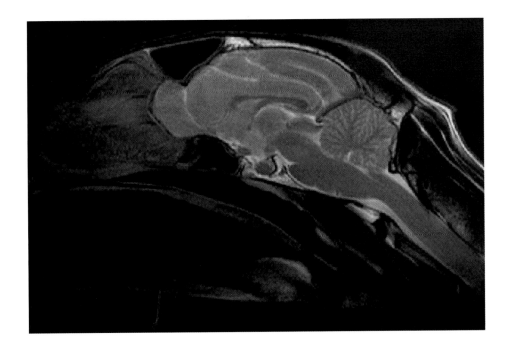

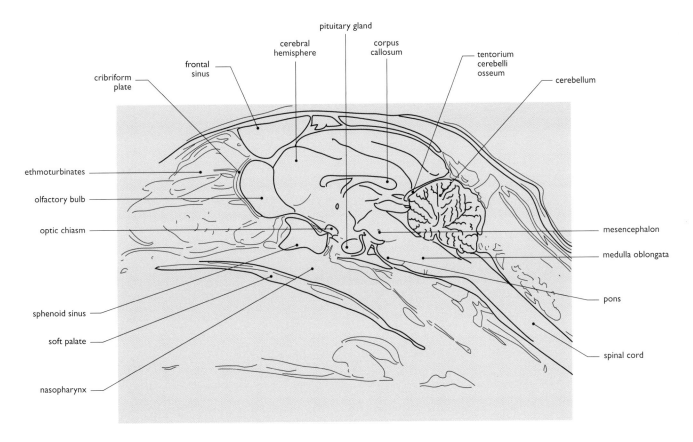

Fig. 10.11 Magnetic resonance image of the head: sagittal plane, midline, T$_2$ weighted image.

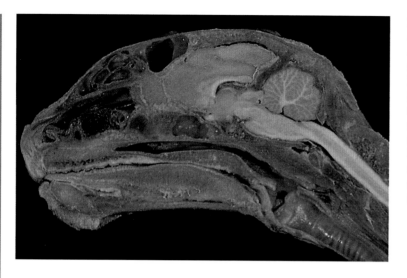

Fig. 10.12 Head and cranial end of the neck in median section: medial view of the right half. The difference in shape and proportion are again apparent in this view of the head comparable to Fig. 2.87 of the dog. A sphenoid sinus is a considerably larger cavity than in the dog skull and lies ventral to an olfactory bulb of the brain, which is relatively much smaller in the cat. The olfactory epithelium in the fundus of the nasal cavity is also less extensive than in the dog, having only half as many olfactory receptors. The larynx displays a somewhat more simple structure with a less pronounced vestibular fold and a barely discernible laryngeal ventricle. Although not visible here, the arytenoid cartilage is also simplified, lacking the corniculate and cuneiform processes of the dog (see Fig. 2.91). The most significant difference in the neck is the absence of a nuchal ligament in the cat.

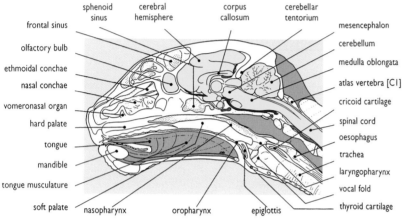

Labels (left):
frontal sinus
olfactory bulb
ethmoidal conchae
nasal conchae
vomeronasal organ
hard palate
tongue
mandible
tongue musculature
soft palate
nasopharynx
oropharynx
epiglottis

Labels (top):
sphenoid sinus
cerebral hemisphere
corpus callosum
cerebellar tentorium

Labels (right):
mesencephalon
cerebellum
medulla oblongata
atlas vertebra [CI]
cricoid cartilage
spinal cord
oesophagus
trachea
laryngopharynx
vocal fold
thyroid cartilage

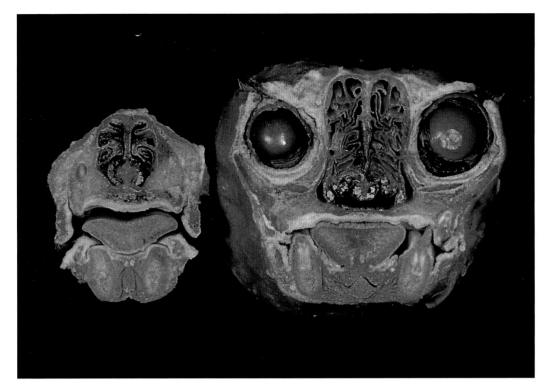

Fig. 10.13 Head in transverse section: (1) Through the nasal region: caudal view; **(2) Through the orbits:** rostral view. The accompanying sketch of the head in outline shows the approximate levels at which these and the next two sections were taken. The head used for sectioning had already been skinned. In the section through the rostral end of the nasal cavity the vomeronasal organs are apparent (compare with Fig. 2.139 of the dog). The highly vascular nature of the submucosal tissue in the ventral part of the nasal cavity is apparent in this and the section on the right. This second section can be compared with Fig. 2.142 of the dog and shows the relatively greater size of the eyes in the cat. They are also greater in size in relation to the nasal cavity. A cat uses its eyes in combination with the muzzle vibrissae to interpret the environment much as a dog does using its sense of smell.

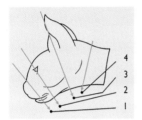

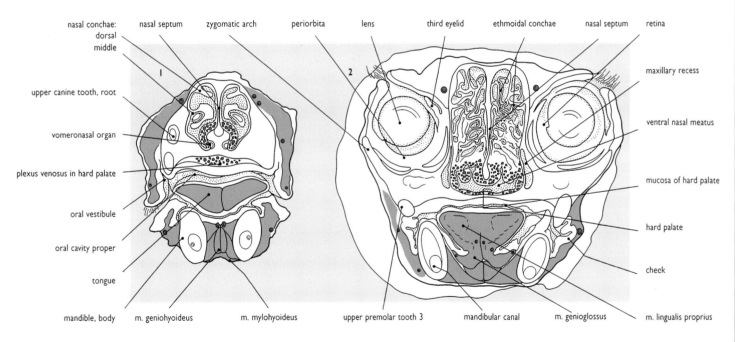

nasal conchae:
dorsal
middle

nasal septum

zygomatic arch

periorbita

lens

third eyelid

ethmoidal conchae

nasal septum

retina

upper canine tooth, root

maxillary recess

vomeronasal organ

ventral nasal meatus

plexus venosus in hard palate

mucosa of hard palate

oral vestibule

hard palate

oral cavity proper

check

tongue

mandible, body

m. geniohyoideus

m. mylohyoideus

upper premolar tooth 3

mandibular canal

m. genioglossus

m. lingualis proprius

Veterinary Anatomy: The Dog and Cat

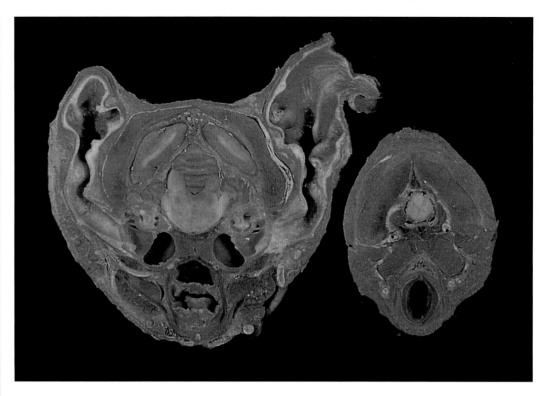

Fig. 10.14 Head in transverse section: (3) Through the auditory regions: rostral view; **(4) Through the larynx and cranial end of the neck:** cranial view. The section on the left passes through the auditory meatuses which open into the prominent cavities of the middle ear on both sides. The septum subdividing the cavity into two chambers is also apparent, a feature not present in the dog. Ventrally the section passes through the soft palate and caudal end of the oropharynx immediately rostral to the larynx. The oral surface of the epiglottis is apparent. The section on the right passes through the infraglottic cavity of the larynx surrounded by the cricoid cartilage. At this level the entry into the esophagus is directly dorsal to the larynx. Compare with sections Figs 2.145 and 3.37 of the dog.

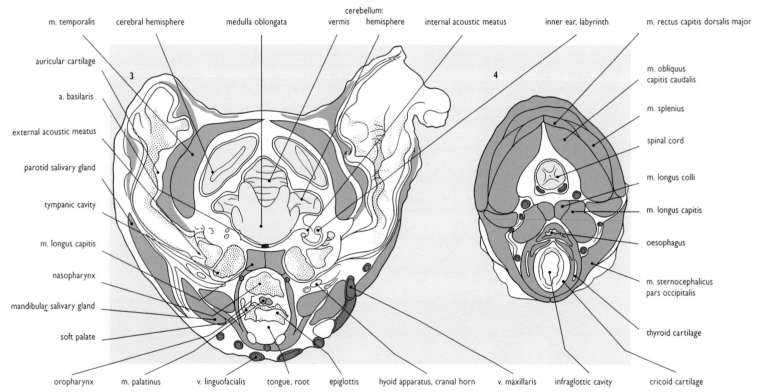

m. temporalis — cerebral hemisphere — medulla oblongata — cerebellum: vermis — hemisphere — internal acoustic meatus — inner ear, labyrinth — m. rectus capitis dorsalis major

auricular cartilage

m. obliquus capitis caudalis

a. basilaris

m. splenius

external acoustic meatus

spinal cord

parotid salivary gland

m. longus colli

tympanic cavity

m. longus capitis

m. longus capitis

oesophagus

nasopharynx

mandibular salivary gland

m. sternocephalicus pars occipitalis

soft palate

thyroid cartilage

oropharynx — m. palatinus — v. linguofacialis — tongue, root — epiglottis — hyoid apparatus, cranial horn — v. maxillaris — infraglottic cavity — cricoid cartilage

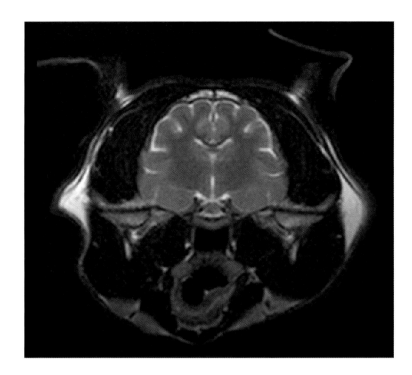

Fig. 10.15 Magnetic resonance image of the head: transverse plane, at the level of the pituitary, T$_2$ weighted image.

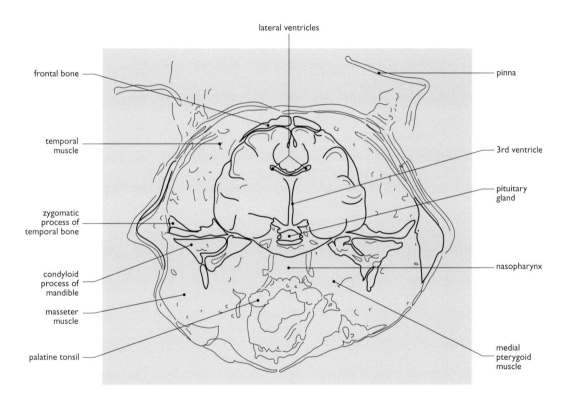

lateral ventricles

frontal bone

pinna

temporal muscle

3rd ventricle

pituitary gland

zygomatic process of temporal bone

condyloid process of mandible

nasopharynx

masseter muscle

palatine tonsil

medial pterygoid muscle

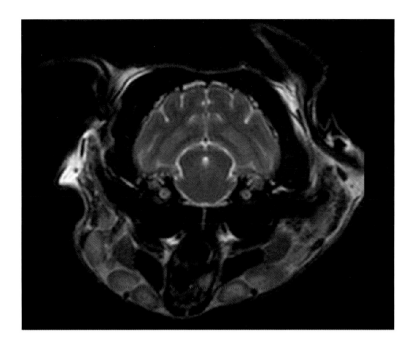

Fig. 10.16 Magnetic resonance image of the head: transverse plane, at the level of the tympanic bullae, T₂ weighted image.

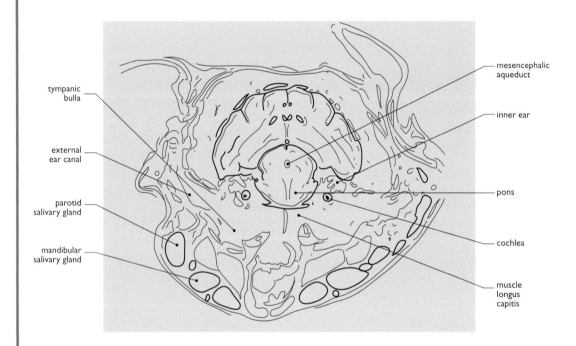

mesencephalic
aqueduct

tympanic
bulla

inner ear

external
ear canal

parotid
salivary gland

pons

cochlea

mandibular
salivary gland

muscle
longus
capitis

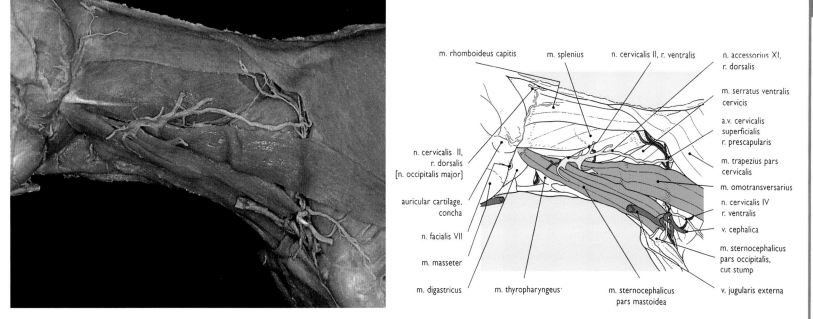

m. rhomboideus capitis   m. splenius   n. cervicalis II, r. ventralis   n. accessorius XI, r. dorsalis

m. serratus ventralis cervicis

a.v. cervicalis superficialis r. prescapularis

m. trapezius pars cervicalis

n. cervicalis II, r. dorsalis [n. occipitalis major]

m. omotransversarius

auricular cartilage, concha

n. cervicalis IV r. ventralis

v. cephalica

n. facialis VII

m. sternocephalicus pars occipitalis, cut stump

m. masseter

m. digastricus   m. thyropharyngeus   m. sternocephalicus pars mastoidea   v. jugularis externa

Fig. 10.17 Neck after removal of the cleidocervical and sterno-occipital muscles: left lateral view. The sterno-occipital component of the sternocephalic muscle has been removed, along with the external jugular vein and the mandibular and parotid salivary glands. The strap-like cleidomastoid and sternomastoid components of overlying muscles are left in place ventral to and paralleling the omotransverse muscle. The structures exposed are essentially similar to those shown in Fig. 3.13 of the dog.

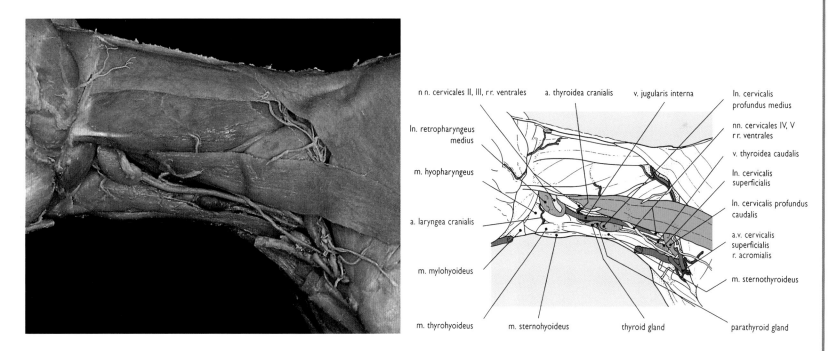

n n. cervicales II, III, r r. ventrales   a. thyroidea cranialis   v. jugularis interna   ln. cervicalis profundus medius

nn. cervicales IV, V r r. ventrales

ln. retropharyngeus medius

v. thyroidea caudalis

m. hyopharyngeus

ln. cervicalis superficialis

ln. cervicalis profundus caudalis

a. laryngea cranialis

a.v. cervicalis superficialis r. acromialis

m. mylohyoideus

m. sternothyroideus

m. thyrohyoideus   m. sternohyoideus   thyroid gland   parathyroid gland

Fig. 10.18 Thyroid gland and lymph nodes of the neck: left lateral view. Removal of the mastoid components of both brachiocephalic and sternocephalic muscles exposes the 'visceral' compartment of the neck. Medial retropharyngeal and superficial cervical lymph nodes are evident, and in addition a prominent deep cervical node is displayed midway down the neck, not evident in the dog (see Figs 3.14 and 3.16). Craniomedial to this lymph node the thyroid gland is just visible with a noticeable parathyroid component (see Fig. 3.20). The internal jugular vein is also exposed, a significantly larger vessel than its counterpart in the dog.

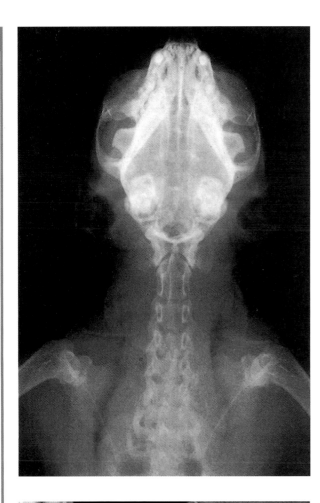

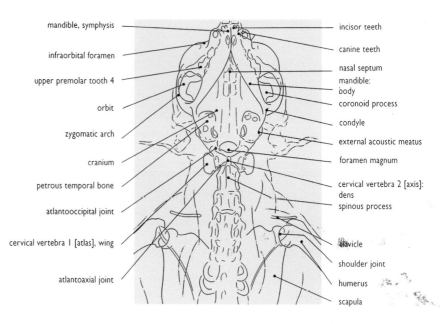

mandible, symphysis — incisor teeth

infraorbital foramen — canine teeth

upper premolar tooth 4 — nasal septum

orbit — mandible:
body
coronoid process

zygomatic arch — condyle

cranium — external acoustic meatus

petrous temporal bone — foramen magnum

atlantooccipital joint — cervical vertebra 2 [axis]:
dens
spinous process

cervical vertebra I [atlas], wing — clavicle

shoulder joint

atlantoaxial joint — humerus

scapula

Fig. 10.19 Radiograph of the head, neck and shoulders: ventrodorsal view. The more rounded, bulbous nature of the skull is shown in this view, and the shortened jaws with temporomandibular joints displaying pronounced retroarticular and articular processes. It is comparable with Fig. 2.6 of the dog. The clavicle is a transversely orientated rod with its lateral extremity approximately 1 cm cranial to the greater tubercle of the humerus. It is free in the musculature subdividing the brachiocephalic muscle, although situated on a line connecting sternal manubrium with hamate process of the acromion.

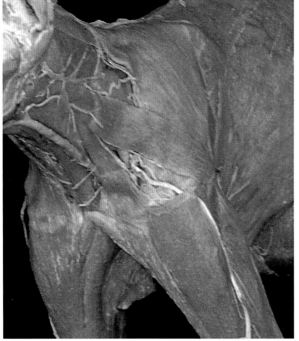

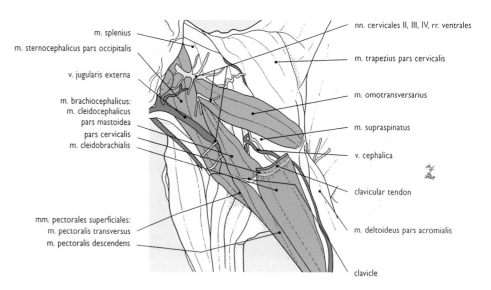

m. splenius — nn. cervicales II, III, IV, rr. ventrales

m. sternocephalicus pars occipitalis — m. trapezius pars cervicalis

v. jugularis externa — m. omotransversarius

m. brachiocephalicus:
m. cleidocephalicus
pars mastoidea
pars cervicalis — m. supraspinatus
m. cleidobrachialis

v. cephalica

clavicular tendon

mm. pectorales superficiales:
m. pectoralis transversus — m. deltoideus pars acromialis
m. pectoralis descendens

clavicle

Fig. 10.20 Neck after removal of the cleidocervical muscle: craniolateral view. The cleidocervical component of the brachiocephalic muscle has been removed to give a view comparable to Fig. 3.9 of the dog. The clavicle is exposed, as is the cephalic vein connection with the external jugular vein (an omobrachial vein is absent in the cat). The cleidobrachial and superficial pectoral muscles are displayed; unlike the dog both extend into the forearm. The presence of a clavicle means that a jugular (supraclavicular) fossa is not bordered by pectoral musculature as in the dog.

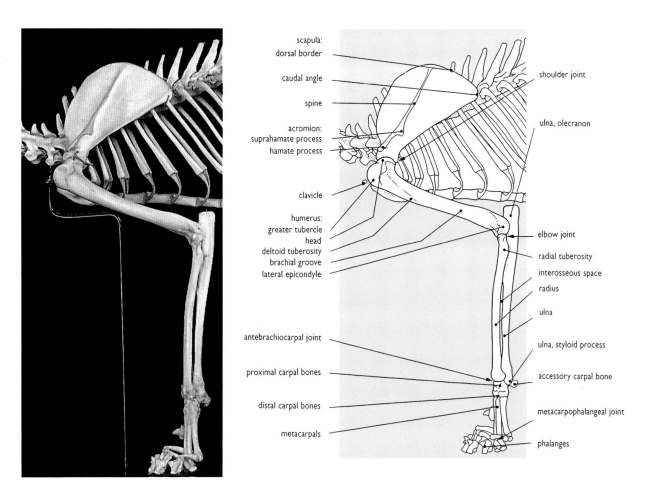

scapula:
dorsal border

caudal angle

spine

acromion:
suprahamate process
hamate process

clavicle

humerus:
greater tubercle
head
deltoid tuberosity
brachial groove
lateral epicondyle

antebrachiocarpal joint

proximal carpal bones

distal carpal bones

metacarpals

shoulder joint

ulna, olecranon

elbow joint

radial tuberosity

interosseous space

radius

ulna

ulna, styloid process

accessory carpal bone

metacarpophalangeal joint

phalanges

Fig. 10.21 Skeleton of the forelimb: left lateral view. Several differences are apparent in this view in comparison with the dog (Figs 4.8 and 4.47). In addition to the more slender overall nature of the bones, the scapula has a slight tuber projecting caudally from its spine and the acromion is enlarged with hamate and suprahamate processes. At the elbow the olecranon of the ulna forming the point of the elbow is shorter and truncated. A supracondylar foramen is present in the humerus for the passage of the brachial artery and median nerve (see Figs 10.29 and 10.30), although a supratrochlear foramen present in the humerus of the dog is absent in the cat. The accessory carpal bone is not as prominent a structure as in the dog.

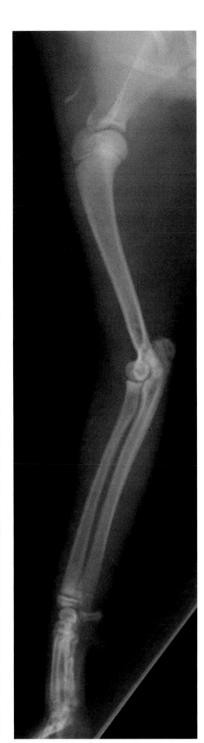

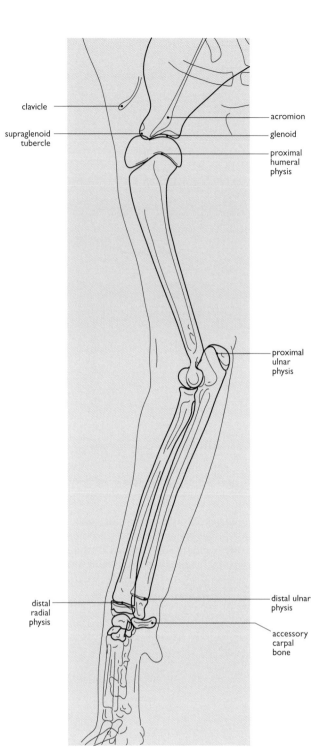

clavicle

acromion

supraglenoid tubercle

glenoid

proximal humeral physis

proximal ulnar physis

distal radial physis

distal ulnar physis

accessory carpal bone

Fig. 10.22 Radiograph of the forelimb: lateral view, 6 months old. Open physes are visible at the proximal humerus, proximal and distal radius and ulna, and distal metacarpal bones.

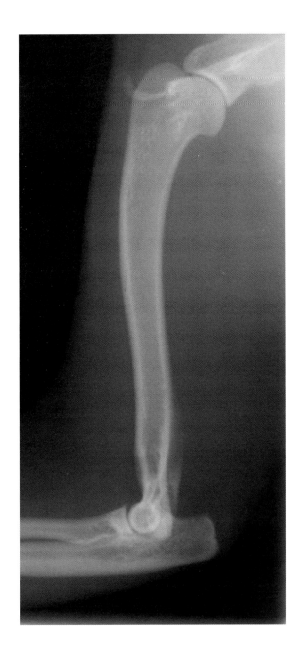

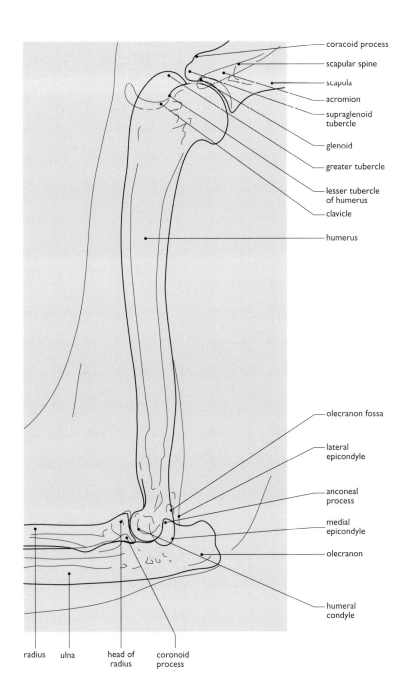

coracoid process
scapular spine
scapula
acromion
supraglenoid tubercle
glenoid
greater tubercle
lesser tubercle of humerus
clavicle
humerus

olecranon fossa
lateral epicondyle
anconeal process
medial epicondyle
olecranon
humeral condyle

radius   ulna   head of radius   coronoid process

Fig. 10.23 Radiograph of the brachium: lateral view. The clavicle can be seen partially superimposed on the proximal humerus.

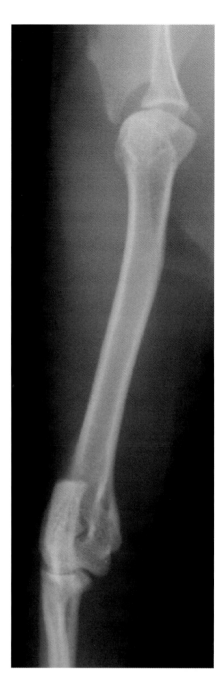

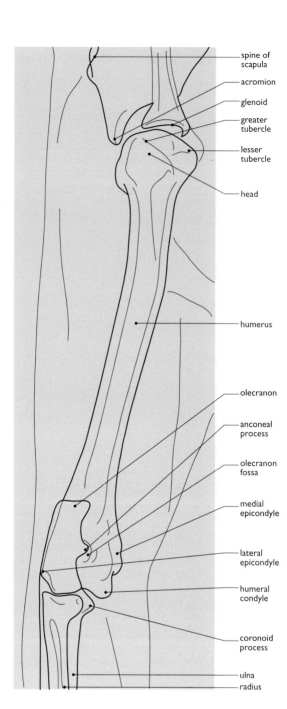

spine of
scapula

acromion

glenoid

greater
tubercle

lesser
tubercle

head

humerus

olecranon

anconeal
process

olecranon
fossa

medial
epicondyle

lateral
epicondyle

humeral
condyle

coronoid
process

ulna

radius

Fig. 10.24 Radiograph of the brachium: craniocaudal view.

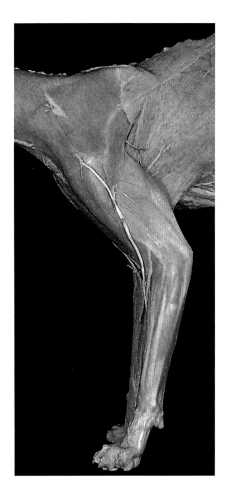

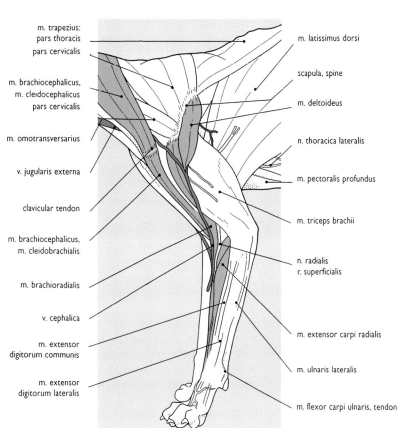

m. trapezius:
pars thoracis
pars cervicalis

m. brachiocephalicus,
m. cleidocephalicus
pars cervicalis

m. omotransversarius

v. jugularis externa

clavicular tendon

m. brachiocephalicus,
m. cleidobrachialis

m. brachioradialis

v. cephalica

m. extensor
digitorum communis

m. extensor
digitorum lateralis

m. latissimus dorsi

scapula, spine

m. deltoideus

n. thoracica lateralis

m. pectoralis profundus

m. triceps brachii

n. radialis
r. superficialis

m. extensor carpi radialis

m. ulnaris lateralis

m. flexor carpi ulnaris, tendon

Fig. 10.25 Superficial musculature of the forelimb: left lateral view. Superficial fascia has been cleaned from the limb to expose superficial limb muscles much as in Figs 4.12, 4.51 and 4.82 of the dog. At the shoulder region the absence of a superficial omobrachial venous connection between cephalic vein and external jugular vein is apparent, and the subdivision of the deltoid muscle into spinal and acromial parts is evident. A considerably more prominent brachioradialis muscle is visible more distally in the arm and the radial carpal extensor muscle is a bipartite structure.

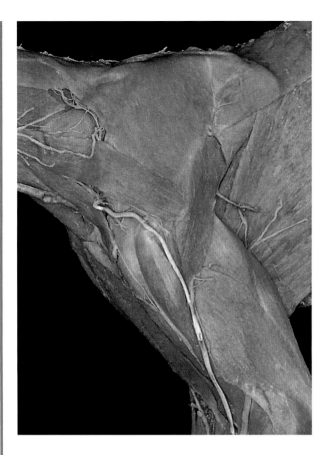

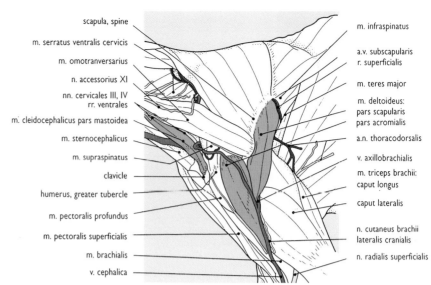

scapula, spine
m. serratus ventralis cervicis
m. omotransversarius
n. accessorius XI
nn. cervicales III, IV
rr. ventrales
m. cleidocephalicus pars mastoidea
m. sternocephalicus
m. supraspinatus
clavicle
humerus, greater tubercle
m. pectoralis profundus
m. pectoralis superficialis
m. brachialis
v. cephalica

m. infraspinatus
a.v. subscapularis
r. superficialis
m. teres major
m. deltoideus:
pars scapularis
pars acromialis
a.n. thoracodorsalis
v. axillobrachialis
m. triceps brachii:
caput longus
caput lateralis
n. cutaneus brachii
lateralis cranialis
n. radialis superficialis

Fig. 10.26 Shoulder and brachium after removal of the brachiocephalic muscle: left lateral view. Brachiocephalic muscle removal has exposed the cephalic vein continuation to the external jugular vein at the base of the neck. The lateral cranial cutaneous brachial nerve (from the axillary) appears caudal to the bipartite deltoid muscle with the axillobrachial vein, and accompanies the cephalic vein in the arm. At the elbow the superficial branch of the radial nerve appears on the brachial muscle and accompanies the brachioradialis muscle into the forearm. Compare this view with Figs 4.12 and 4.13 of the dog.

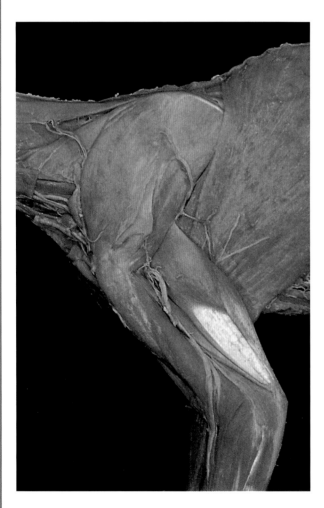

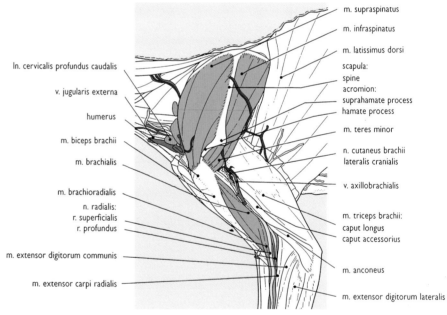

ln. cervicalis profundus caudalis
v. jugularis externa
humerus
m. biceps brachii
m. brachialis
m. brachioradialis
n. radialis:
r. superficialis
r. profundus
m. extensor digitorum communis
m. extensor carpi radialis

m. supraspinatus
m. infraspinatus
m. latissimus dorsi
scapula:
spine
acromion:
suprahamate process
hamate process
m. teres minor
n. cutaneus brachii
lateralis cranialis
v. axillobrachialis
m. triceps brachii:
caput longus
caput accessorius
m. anconeus
m. extensor digitorum lateralis

Fig. 10.27 Shoulder and brachium after removal of the deltoid muscle: left lateral view. In addition to deltoid removal, the trapezius, omotransverse and lateral head of the triceps muscles have also been removed to expose the intrinsic forelimb musculature around the shoulder joint. The subdivision of the acromion process is evident. Cranial to the shoulder a caudal deep cervical lymph node and the superficial cervical nodes are visible. Proximal to the elbow joint removal of the lateral head of the triceps muscle exposes the origin of the brachioradialis muscle and the subdivision of the radial nerve. Compare this view with Figs 4.14 and 4.15 of the dog.

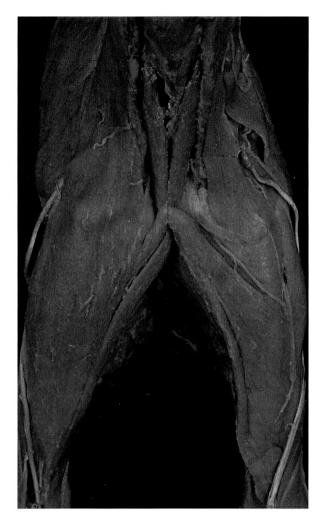

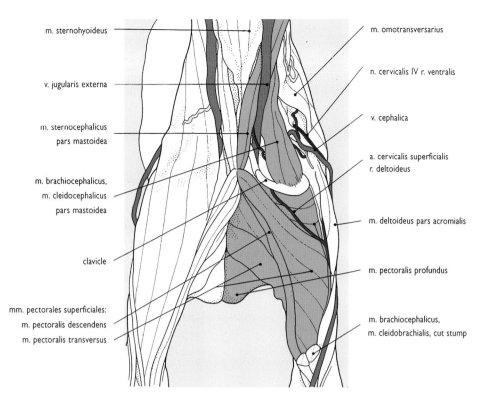

m. sternohyoideus

m. omotransversarius

v. jugularis externa

n. cervicalis IV r. ventralis

m. sternocephalicus
pars mastoidea

v. cephalica

a. cervicalis superficialis
r. deltoideus

m. brachiocephalicus,
m. cleidocephalicus
pars mastoidea

m. deltoideus pars acromialis

clavicle

m. pectoralis profundus

mm. pectorales superficiales:
m. pectoralis descendens
m. pectoralis transversus

m. brachiocephalicus,
m. cleidobrachialis, cut stump

Fig. 10.28 Shoulder and brachium with clavicle exposed: cranial view. The clavicle and cleidomastoid component of the brachiocephalic muscle remain in place after removal of the cervical and brachial components. The sternocephalic muscle is displayed in the midline and the superficial and deep pectoral attachments to the humerus are exposed. More distally in the arm the continuations of cleidobrachial and superficial pectoral muscles onto the forearm have been left in place. Compare this view with Figs 4.21 and 4.23 of the dog.

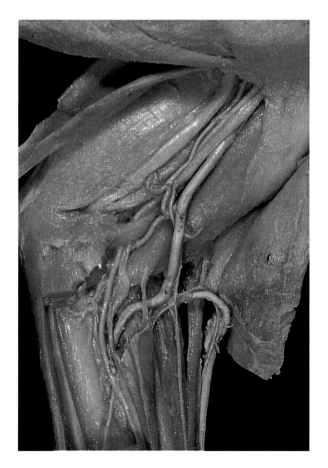

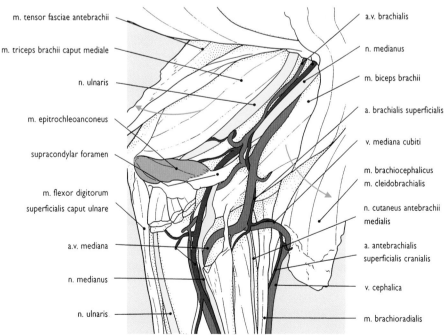

m. tensor fasciae antebrachii

a.v. brachialis

m. triceps brachii caput mediale

n. medianus

n. ulnaris

m. biceps brachii

a. brachialis superficialis

m. epitrochleoanconeus

supracondylar foramen

v. mediana cubiti

m. brachiocephalicus
m. cleidobrachialis

m. flexor digitorum
superficialis caput ulnare

n. cutaneus antebrachii
medialis

a.v. mediana

a. antebrachialis
superficialis cranialis

n. medianus

v. cephalica

n. ulnaris

m. brachioradialis

Fig. 10.29 Brachial artery and median nerve at the elbow region of the left forelimb: medial view. The tensor muscle of the antebrachial fascia has been reflected caudodorsally; the cleidobrachial and superficial pectoral muscles craniodorsally. The passage of the brachial artery and median nerve through the supracondylar foramen of the humerus and the epitrochleoanconeus muscle are displayed. Removal of forearm flexor muscles from the medial epicondyle has exposed the median and ulnar nerves and brachial/median artery into the forearm. Compare with Fig. 4.61 of the dog.

465

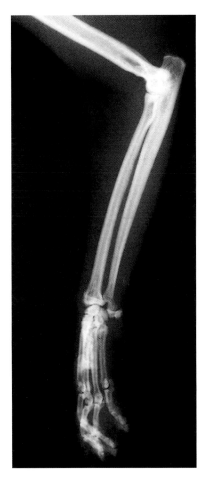

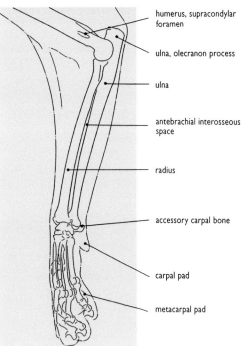

humerus, supracondylar foramen

ulna, olecranon process

ulna

antebrachial interosseous space

radius

accessory carpal bone

carpal pad

metacarpal pad

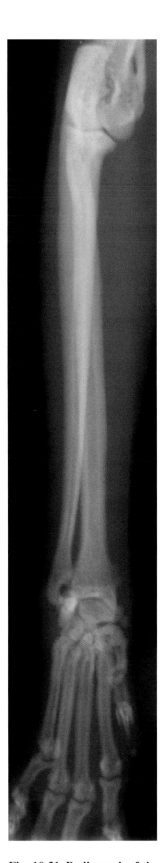

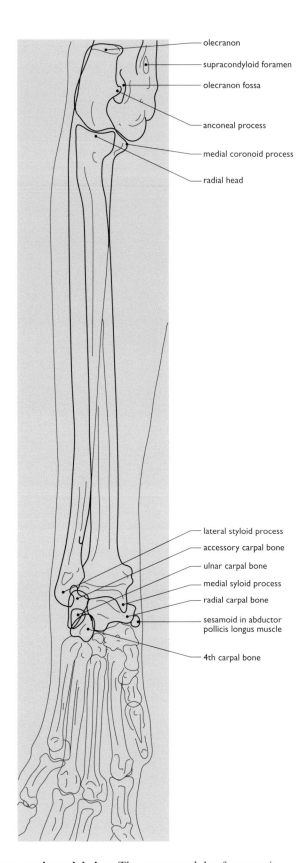

olecranon

supracondyloid foramen

olecranon fossa

anconeal process

medial coronoid process

radial head

lateral styloid process

accessory carpal bone

ulnar carpal bone

medial syloid process

radial carpal bone

sesamoid in abductor pollicis longus muscle

4th carpal bone

Fig. 10.31 Radiograph of the antebrachium: craniocaudal view. The supracondylar foramen is visible on the medial aspect of the distal humerus.

Fig. 10.30 Radiograph of the antebrachium and paw of the left forelimb: craniolateral view. The supracondylar foramen in the humerus is visible and the somewhat wider spacing of the forearm bones to produce a noticeably wider interosseous space indicative of the greater range of forearm/forepaw mobility in the cat. Forepaw osteology is closely comparable with the dog (Figs 4.6 and 4.80).

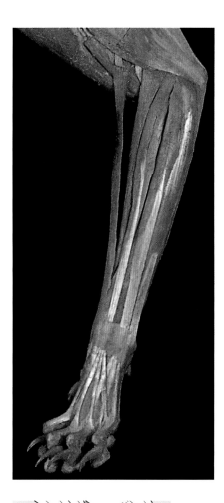

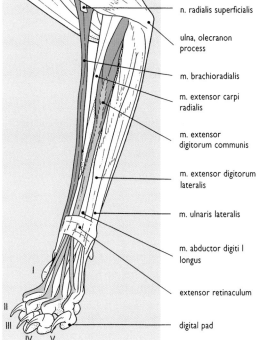

n. radialis superficialis

ulna, olecranon
process

m. brachioradialis

m. extensor carpi
radialis

m. extensor
digitorum communis

m. extensor digitorum
lateralis

m. ulnaris lateralis

m. abductor digiti I
longus

extensor retinaculum

digital pad

I
II
III
IV   V

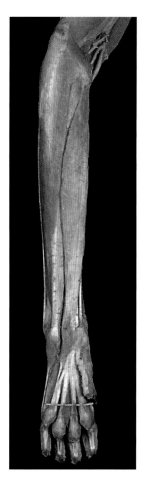

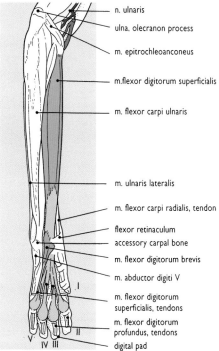

n. ulnaris

ulna, olecranon process

m. epitrochleoanconeus

m. flexor digitorum superficialis

m. flexor carpi ulnaris

m. ulnaris lateralis

m. flexor carpi radialis, tendon

flexor retinaculum

accessory carpal bone

m. flexor digitorum brevis

m. abductor digiti V

m. flexor digitorum
superficialis, tendons

m. flexor digitorum
profundus, tendons

digital pad

I

V   IV III II

Fig. 10.32 Musculature of the antebrachium and paw of the left forelimb: craniolateral view. Superficial fascia, vessels and nerves and the sleeve of deep antebrachial fascia have been removed to display the extensor muscles of the carpus and digits on the craniolateral aspect of the forearm. At the carpus the extensor retinaculum has been left in place. Compare with Figs 4.52 and 4.83 of the dog.

Fig. 10.33 Musculature of the antebrachium and paw of the left forelimb: caudal view. The flexor muscles are displayed after partial removal of the flexor retinaculum. The short digital flexor muscle, poorly represented in the dog in which it lies deep to the superficial digital flexor tendon, arises from the superficial digital flexor muscle and from the flexor retinaculum. Compare with Figs 4.55 and 4.86 in the dog.

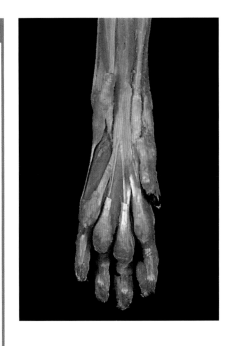

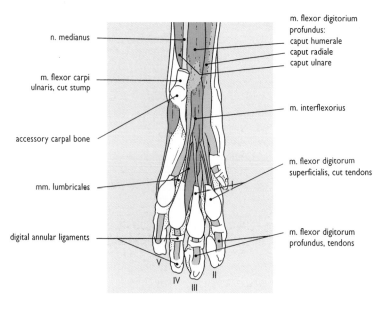

n. medianus

m. flexor carpi
ulnaris, cut stump

accessory carpal bone

mm. lumbricales

digital annular ligaments

m. flexor digitorium
profundus:
caput humerale
caput radiale
caput ulnare

m. interflexorius

m. flexor digitorum
superficialis, cut tendons

m. flexor digitorum
profundus, tendons

V
IV
III
II

Fig. 10.34 Musculature of the left forepaw: palmar view. Radial and ulnar carpal flexors and the superficial digital flexor have been removed, along with the flexor retinaculum, to expose the deep digital flexor muscle. The interflexorius muscle (radial head of the superficial digital flexor) has tendons extending to digits 2, 3 and 4. The fleshy lumbrical muscles, also arising from the deep digital flexor tendon, are apparent between the diverging tendons of the interflexorius. Compare with Fig. 4.88 of the dog.

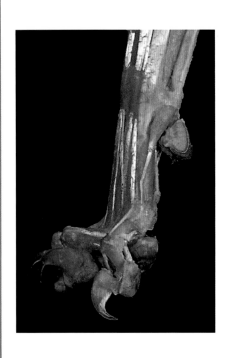

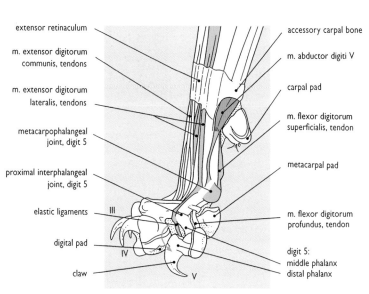

extensor retinaculum

m. extensor digitorum
communis, tendons

m. extensor digitorum
lateralis, tendons

metacarpophalangeal
joint, digit 5

proximal interphalangeal
joint, digit 5

elastic ligaments

digital pad

claw

accessory carpal bone

m. abductor digiti V

carpal pad

m. flexor digitorum
superficialis, tendon

metacarpal pad

m. flexor digitorum
profundus, tendon

digit 5:
middle phalanx
distal phalanx

III
IV
V

Fig. 10.35 Left forepaw: lateral view. Clearance of fascia and superficial vessels has exposed the tendons of the digital flexor and extensor muscles to digit 5. Markedly curved and pointed claws are shown after clearance of their enclosing cutaneous sheaths. In contrast to the dog the distal interphalangeal joints are so arranged that when retracted the claw on its distal phalanx is swivelled back to lie alongside the middle phalanx by tension in elastic ligaments. The claw on digit 5 is pinned to display the elastic ligaments. Compare with Fig. 4.83 of the dog.

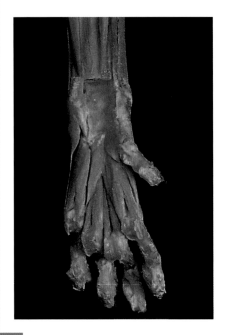

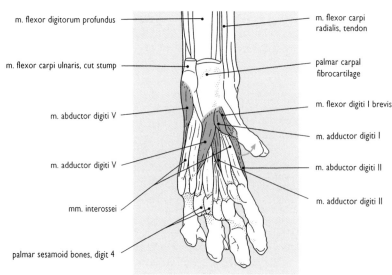

m. flexor digitorum profundus

m. flexor carpi ulnaris, cut stump

m. abductor digiti V

m. adductor digiti V

mm. interossei

palmar sesamoid bones, digit 4

m. flexor carpi
radialis, tendon

palmar carpal
fibrocartilage

m. flexor digiti I brevis

m. adductor digiti I

m. abductor digiti II

m. adductor digiti II

Fig. 10.36 Intrinsic musculature of the left forepaw: palmar view. Removal of the deep flexor muscle tendon exposes the intrinsic musculature of the paw (see Fig. 4.88). Adductor and abductor muscles are associated with both digits 2 and 5. The abductor of the second digit has no representation in the dog; the remaining ones are more substantial muscles than in the dog. The small first digit also has short flexor and adductor muscles.

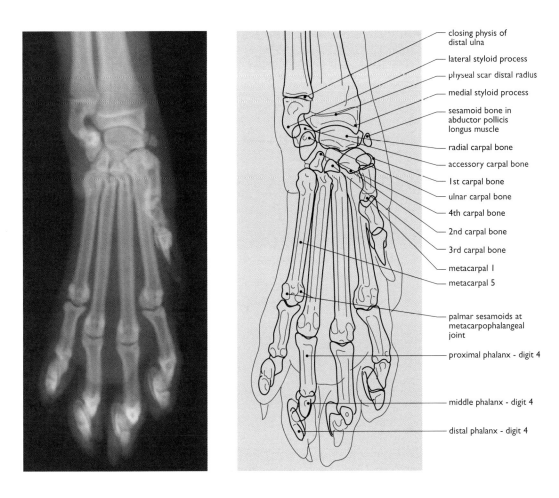

closing physis of distal ulna
lateral styloid process
physeal scar distal radius
medial styloid process
sesamoid bone in abductor pollicis longus muscle
radial carpal bone
accessory carpal bone
1st carpal bone
ulnar carpal bone
4th carpal bone
2nd carpal bone
3rd carpal bone
metacarpal 1
metacarpal 5
palmar sesamoids at metacarpophalangeal joint
proximal phalanx - digit 4
middle phalanx - digit 4
distal phalanx - digit 4

Fig. 10.37 Radiograph of the forepaw: dorsopalmar view. The distal ulnar physis is open.

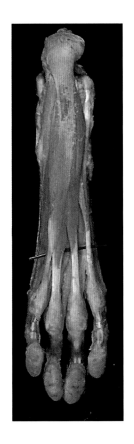

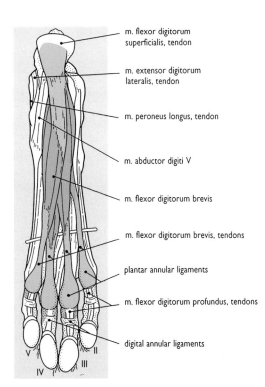

m. flexor digitorum superficialis, tendon
m. extensor digitorum lateralis, tendon
m. peroneus longus, tendon
m. abductor digiti V
m. flexor digitorum brevis
m. flexor digitorum brevis, tendons
plantar annular ligaments
m. flexor digitorum profundus, tendons
digital annular ligaments

Fig. 10.38 Musculature of the left hindpaw: plantar view (1). Removal of the plantar fascia and superficial vessels and nerves reveals the short digital flexor muscle not evident in the dog (see Fig. 7.81). This arises from the superficial digital flexor tendon and forms its direct continuation into the digits. A piece of wire has been inserted beneath its four tendons to distinguish them more clearly from underlying tendons.

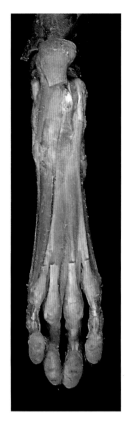

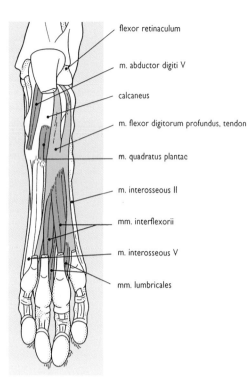

flexor retinaculum

m. abductor digiti V

calcaneus

m. flexor digitorum profundus, tendon

m. quadratus plantae

m. interosseous II

mm. interflexorii

m. interosseous V

mm. lumbricales

Fig. 10.39 Musculature of the left hindpaw: plantar view (2). Removal of the short digital flexor muscle exposes the deep digital flexor tendon with prominent interflexorius muscles on its ventral surface. Compare with Fig. 7.85 of the dog. Fleshy lumbrical muscles appear distally between the diverging flexor tendons. The quadratus plantae muscle, somewhat more substantial than in the dog, is visible beneath the deep flexor tendon to which it attaches.

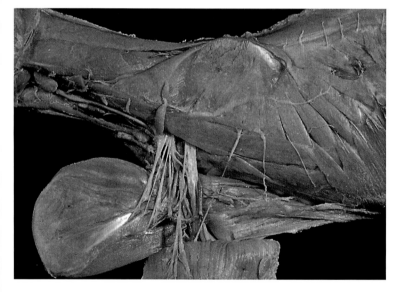

Fig. 10.40 Brachial plexus and axillary structures after lateral reflection of the scapula: left lateral view. The ventral serrate muscle has been severed from the serrated face of the scapula to allow the scapula to be reflected laterally, opening the axilla from above and giving a view comparable with Fig. 4.19 of the dog. The major nerves derived from the brachial plexus are displayed in addition to the axillary vessels and lymph nodes. An especially large accessory axillary node, of variable presence in the dog, is present in the axilla caudally, and a deep cervical node cranially at the boundary with the neck.

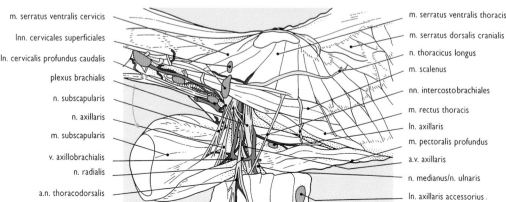

m. serratus ventralis cervicis

lnn. cervicales superficiales

ln. cervicalis profundus caudalis

plexus brachialis

n. subscapularis

n. axillaris

m. subscapularis

v. axillobrachialis

n. radialis

a.n. thoracodorsalis

m. serratus ventralis thoracis

m. serratus dorsalis cranialis

n. thoracicus longus

m. scalenus

nn. intercostobrachiales

m. rectus thoracis

ln. axillaris

m. pectoralis profundus

a.v. axillaris

n. medianus/n. ulnaris

ln. axillaris accessorius .

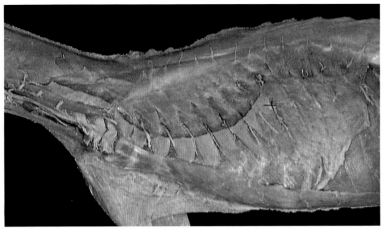

Fig. 10.41 Superficial musculature of the thorax after removal of the forelimb: left lateral view. The forelimb has been removed by severing the nerves and vessels crossing the axilla and cutting through the pectoral musculature at its origin from the sternum. Subsequently the scalene and ventral serrate muscles have been removed, except for the terminal serrations of the latter attaching to the cervical vertebrae and ribs. More caudally removal of the external abdominal oblique muscle displays the ribcage back to the costal arch with its intercostal musculature (compare with Figs 5.12 and 5.13 of the dog). The dorsal serrate muscle is well developed in comparison with the dog, especially its caudal component.

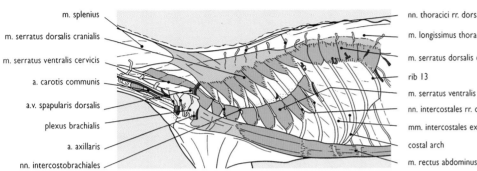

m. splenius
m. serratus dorsalis cranialis
m. serratus ventralis cervicis
a. carotis communis
a.v. spapularis dorsalis
plexus brachialis
a. axillaris
nn. intercostobrachiales

nn. thoracici rr. dorsales rr. cutanei laterales
m. longissimus thoracis
m. serratus dorsalis caudalis
rib 13
m. serratus ventralis thoracis
nn. intercostales rr. cutanei laterales
mm. intercostales externi
costal arch
m. rectus abdominus

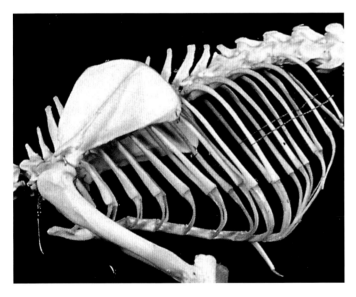

Fig. 10.42 Skeleton of the thorax: left lateral view. The overall shape of the thorax is slightly different from the dog (Fig. 5.2) being shallower and relatively longer, although extensive breed variations are encountered in the dog. In more detailed anatomy there are few significant differences between cat and dog except for a more prominent manubrium of the sternum and a longer and narrower xiphoid cartilage.

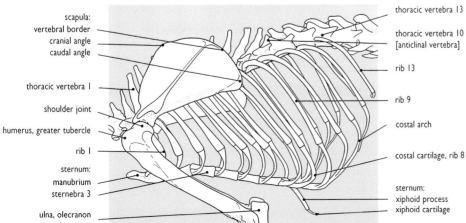

scapula:
vertebral border
cranial angle
caudal angle
thoracic vertebra 1
shoulder joint
humerus, greater tubercle
rib 1
sternum:
manubrium
sternebra 3
ulna, olecranon

thoracic vertebra 13
thoracic vertebra 10 [anticlinal vertebra]
rib 13
rib 9
costal arch
costal cartilage, rib 8
sternum:
xiphoid process
xiphoid cartilage

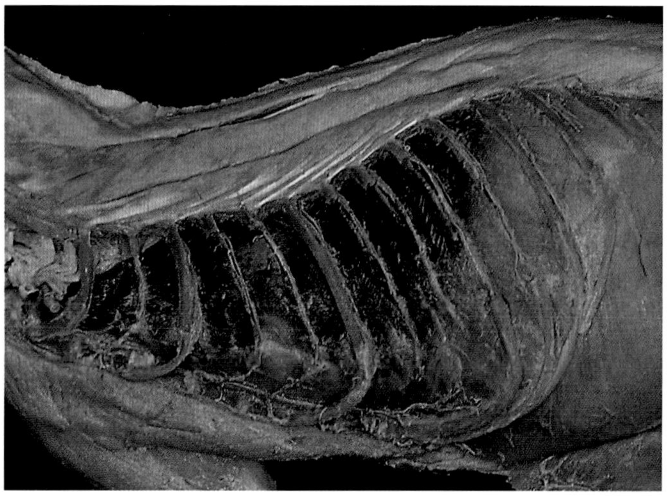

Fig. 10.43 Endothoracic fascia and transverse thoracic muscle: left lateral view. Intercostal musculature has been removed along with several of the ribs but leaving the endothoracic fascia and transverse thoracic muscle intact. Compare this view with Fig. 5.18 of the dog – especially where ribs have been removed the intercostal artery and nerve are displayed in the fascia. Intercostal nerves 9 to 12 and the costoabdominal nerve are continued into the abdominal wall on the surface of the transverse abdominal muscle. The interdigitating fibers of the costal component of the diaphragm and the transverse abdominal muscle internal to the costal arch indicate the approximate position of the costodiaphragmatic line of pleural reflection (broken green line). The internal thoracic artery, with some of its ventral intercostal and perforating branches, is displayed on the undersurface of the transverse thoracic muscle.

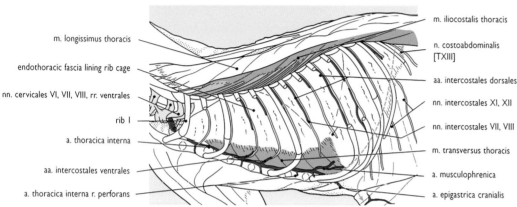

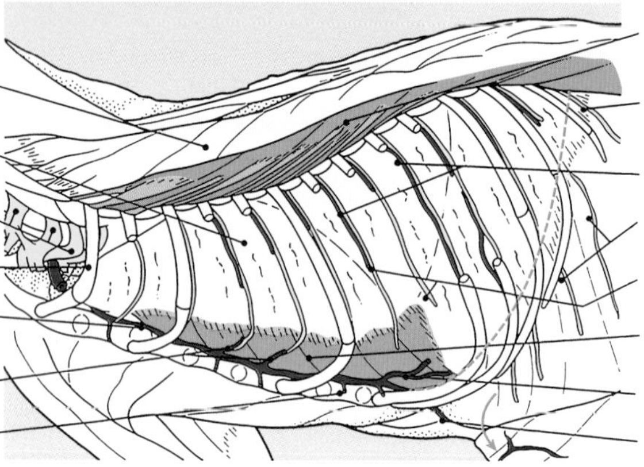
m. longissimus thoracis
endothoracic fascia lining rib cage
nn. cervicales VI, VII, VIII, rr. ventrales
rib I
a. thoracica interna
aa. intercostales ventrales
a. thoracica interna r. perforans
m. iliocostalis thoracis
n. costoabdominalis
[TXIII]
aa. intercostales dorsales
nn. intercostales XI, XII
nn. intercostales VII, VIII
m. transversus thoracis
a. musculophrenica
a. epigastrica cranialis

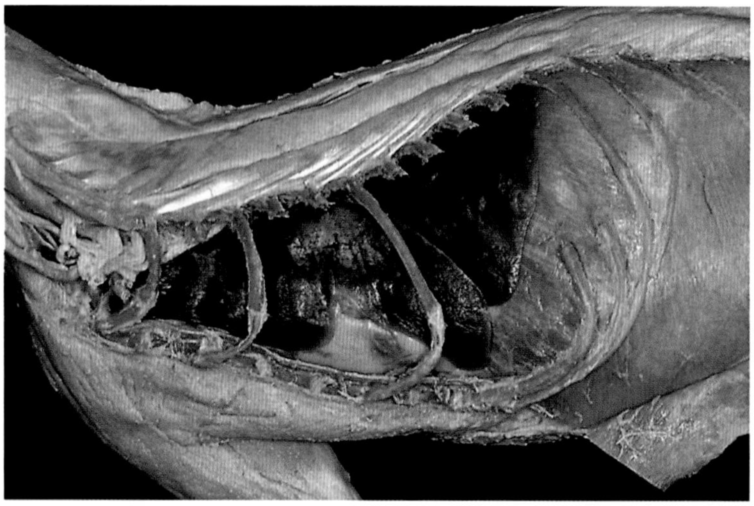

Fig. 10.44 Thoracic viscera in situ: left lateral view. The endothoracic fascia and intercostal vessels and nerves have been removed, leaving ribs 1, 3 and 6 in place to show the costal relationships of the viscera. Compare this view with Fig. 5.21 of the dog. A cardiac notch of some dimension is present on this left side although not in the dog. The approximate position that the basal (caudal) border of the lung would occupy after normal expiration is shown by a broken line on the drawing; the position of the costodiaphragmatic line of pleural reflection is shown by the broken green line adjacent to the costal arch.

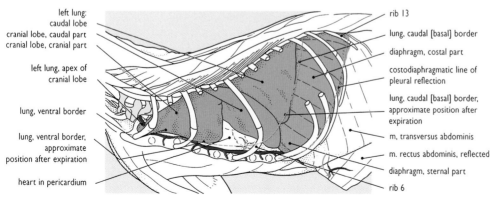

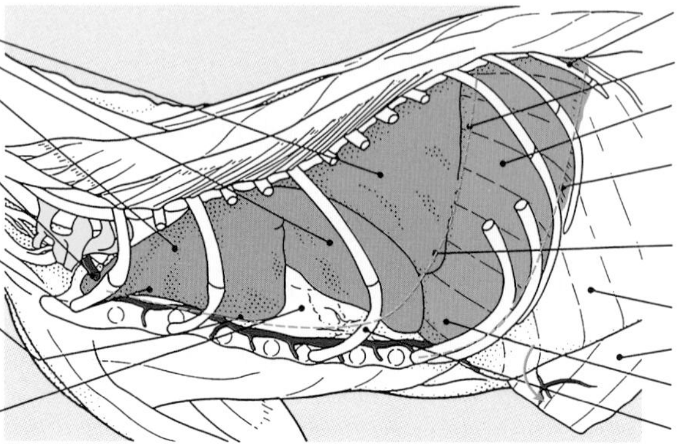
left lung:
caudal lobe
cranial lobe, caudal part
cranial lobe, cranial part
left lung, apex of
cranial lobe
lung, ventral border
lung, ventral border,
approximate
position after expiration
heart in pericardium
rib 13
lung, caudal [basal] border
diaphragm, costal part
costodiaphragmatic line of
pleural reflection
lung, caudal [basal] border,
approximate position after
expiration
m, transversus abdominis
m. rectus abdominis, reflected
diaphragm, sternal part
rib 6

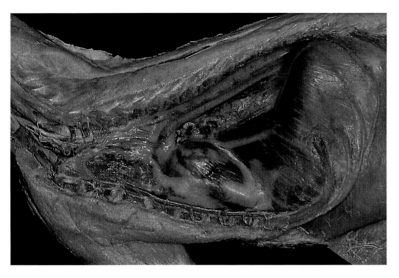

Fig. 10.45 Mediastinum after removal of the left lung: left lateral view. Most of the ribcage and the lung have been removed to give a view comparable to Fig. 5.28 of the dog. The glistening layer of mediastinal pleura forms the left lateral boundary of the mediastinum but is incomplete where it reflected around the root of the lung. The root structures are visible where they were sectioned on lung removal. Considerable quantities of subpleural fat are present obscuring mediastinal viscera, although significant remnants of the thymus gland are clearly apparent in the cranial mediastinum. An internal thoracic artery, not a mediastinal structure, is displayed in relation to the sternum with a very small sternal lymph node cranial to it at the lower end of intercostal space 2.

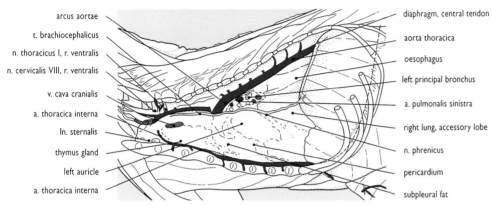

arcus aortae
t. brachiocephalicus
n. thoracicus I, r. ventralis
n. cervicalis VIII, r. ventralis
v. cava cranialis
a. thoracica interna
ln. sternalis
thymus gland
left auricle
a. thoracica interna

diaphragm, central tendon
aorta thoracica
oesophagus
left principal bronchus
a. pulmonalis sinistra
right lung, accessory lobe
n. phrenicus
pericardium
subpleural fat

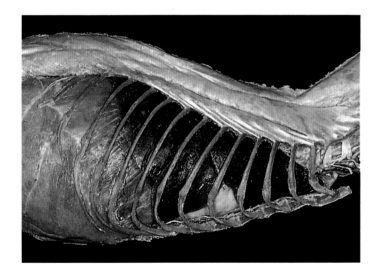

Fig. 10.46 Ribcage and lung in situ: right lateral view. The intercostal spaces of the right side of the thorax have been cleared, including the transverse thoracic muscle, to obtain a view comparable to Fig. 5.27 of the dog. The right lung displays a considerable cardiac notch between cranial and middle lobes. As on the left side, broken lines on the drawing indicate the approximate position of the basal (caudal) border of the lung after normal expiration, and the costodiaphragmatic line of pleural reflection (green).

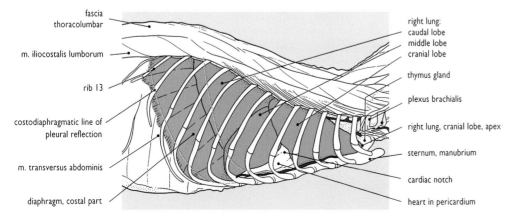

fascia thoracolumbar
m. iliocostalis lumborum
rib 13
costodiaphragmatic line of pleural reflection
m. transversus abdominis
diaphragm, costal part

right lung:
caudal lobe
middle lobe
cranial lobe
thymus gland
plexus brachialis
right lung, cranial lobe, apex
sternum, manubrium
cardiac notch
heart in pericardium

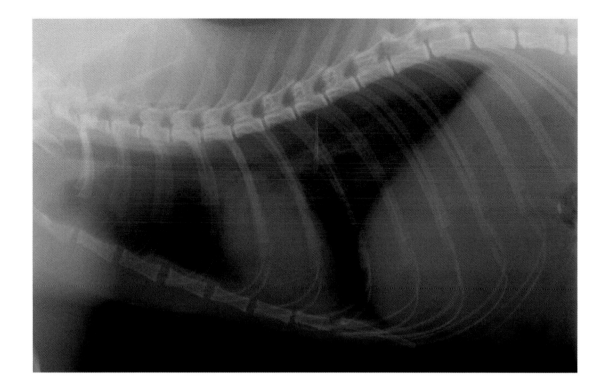

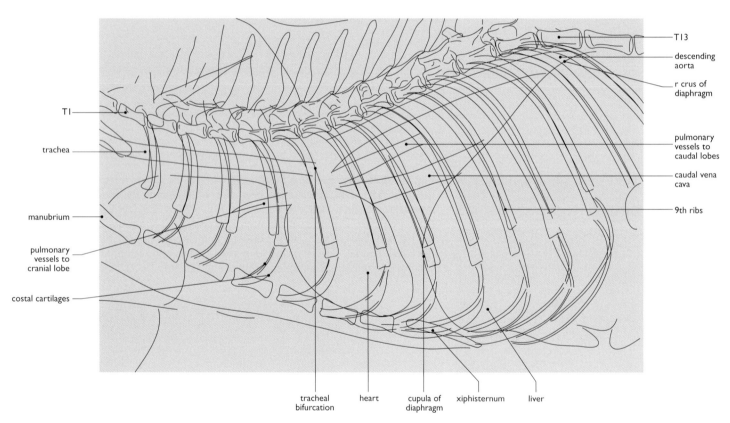

T13

descending aorta

r crus of diaphragm

T1

trachea

pulmonary vessels to caudal lobes

caudal vena cava

manubrium

9th ribs

pulmonary vessels to cranial lobe

costal cartilages

tracheal bifurcation

heart

cupula of diaphragm

xiphisternum

liver

Fig. 10.47 Radiograph of the thorax: lateral view. Air within its lumen highlights the trachea. The heart is clearly visible and has a slightly more horizontal orientation from that of the dog. The lungs can be seen by virtue of their air content. The majority of other structures are soft tissue and mediastinal and so cannot be clearly distinguished from one another.

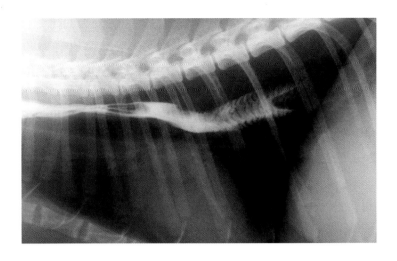

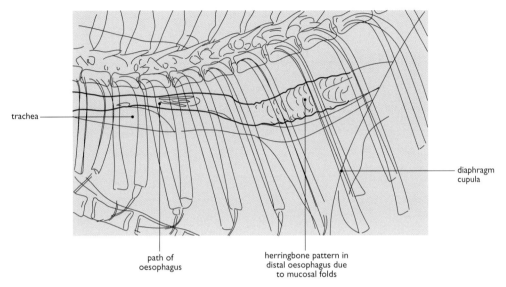

trachea

diaphragm
cupula

path of
oesophagus

herringbone pattern in
distal oesophagus due
to mucosal folds

Fig. 10.48 Radiograph of the thorax: lateral view, immediately following oral administration of barium. The mucosal surface of the esophagus is highlighted. The mucosa has a longitudinal pattern cranially and a more herringbone or transverse pattern caudally. This change represents alterations in mucosal folds and an increase in the proportion of smooth muscle within the wall.

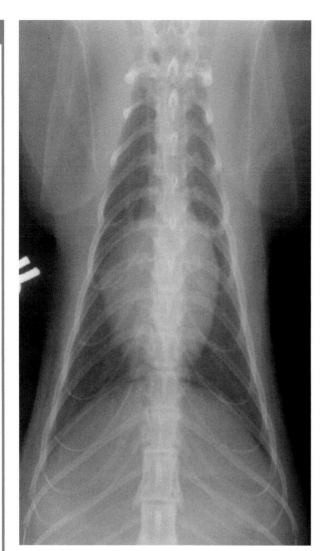
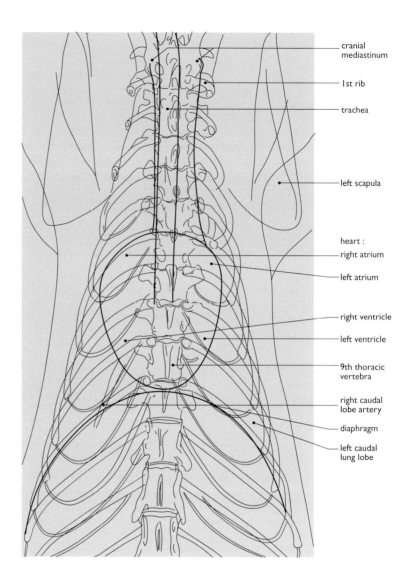

cranial
mediastinum

1st rib

trachea

left scapula

heart :
right atrium

left atrium

right ventricle

left ventricle

9th thoracic
vertebra

right caudal
lobe artery

diaphragm

left caudal
lung lobe

Fig. 10.49 Radiograph of the thorax: dorsoventral view. Only the lungs and the heart can be easily appreciated in this view as other structures are mediastinal and thus superimposed on the spine and sternum.

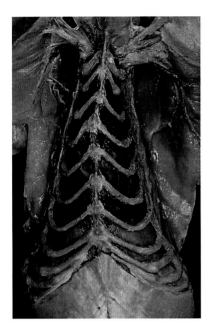

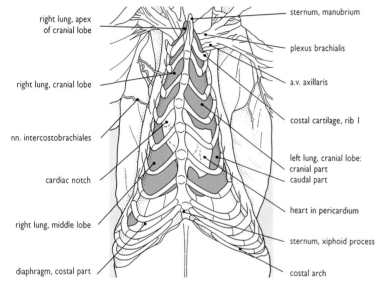

right lung, apex of cranial lobe

right lung, cranial lobe

nn. intercostobrachiales

cardiac notch

right lung, middle lobe

diaphragm, costal part

sternum, manubrium

plexus brachialis

a.v. axillaris

costal cartilage, rib I

left lung, cranial lobe:
cranial part
caudal part

heart in pericardium

sternum, xiphoid process

costal arch

Fig. 10.50 Ribcage and thoracic viscera in situ: ventral view. Intercostal and transverse thoracic musculature has been cleared from the lower ends of the intercostal spaces to give a view comparable to Fig. 5.70 of the dog. With the animal in dorsal recumbency the ribcage overall is distorted somewhat with the caudal ribs being pulled caudally. Consequently the position of the heart and lungs in relation to the ribs differs slightly from the relationship in the normal standing posture.

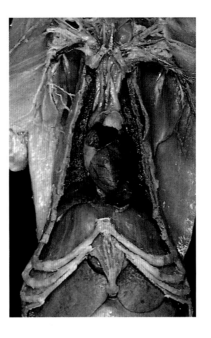

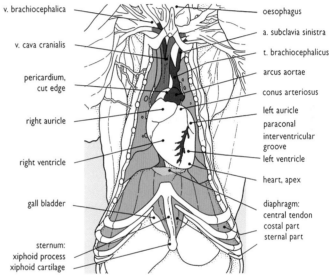

v. brachiocephalica

v. cava cranialis

pericardium,
cut edge

right auricle

right ventricle

gall bladder

sternum:
xiphoid process
xiphoid cartilage

oesophagus

a. subclavia sinistra

t. brachiocephalicus

arcus aortae

conus arteriosus

left auricle

paraconal
interventricular
groove

left ventricle

heart, apex

diaphragm:
central tendon
costal part
sternal part

Fig. 10.51 Heart and great vessels in situ: ventral view. The lower ends of ribs 2 to 8 and the sternum except for the manubrium and xiphoid have been removed. The lungs have been resected in the same horizontal plane as the ribs to expose the heart, from which the pericardium has been removed. In this view, comparable to Fig. 5.71 of the dog, the more 'horizontal' positioning of the heart is evident with more of the right auricle and aortic arch visible. Pronounced sternal fibers of the diaphragm project back onto the xiphoid process.

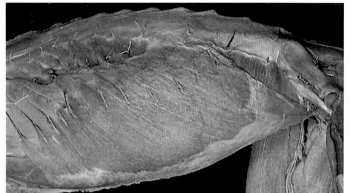

Fig. 10.52 Abdominal wall musculature. (1) External abdominal oblique muscle: left lateral view. Skin and superficial fascia have been removed exposing the external abdominal oblique muscle and its aponeurosis where it contributes to the external layer of the rectus sheath. This view is comparable to Fig. 6.14 of the dog. In this spayed queen the inguinal canal is inadequately represented; however, the canal is essentially of the same construction as in the bitch illustrated in Figs 8.53 to 8.57.

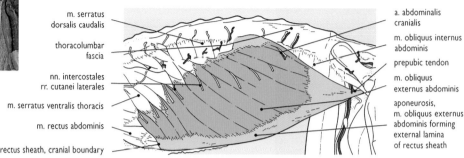

Fig. 10.53 Abdominal wall musculature. (2) Internal abdominal oblique muscle: left lateral view. The external oblique and practically all of its aponeurosis of attachment has been removed, exposing the internal abdominal oblique with its aponeurotic contribution to the rectus sheath, a view comparable to Fig. 6.15 of the dog. The position of the costodiaphragmatic line of pleural reflection is indicated by the broken green line on the ribcage cranial to the costal arch, denoting the effective boundary between thoracic and abdominal cavities on the surface.

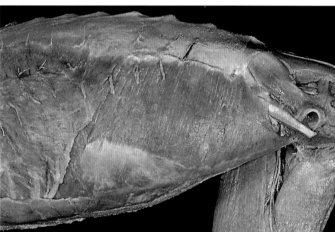

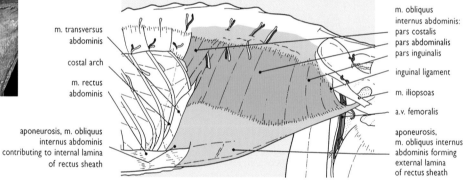

Fig. 10.54 Abdominal wall musculature. (3) Transverse abdominal and rectus muscles: left lateral view. Removal of the internal oblique and its aponeurosis exposes the transverse abdominal and rectus muscles in a view comparable to Fig. 6.19 of the dog. As in the dog the transverse abdominal aponeurosis contributes to the external layer of the rectus sheath in the caudal abdomen, the internal layer being composed solely of transversalis fascia. The position of the costodiaphragmatic line of pleural reflection shows that the pleural cavity extended slightly caudal to rib 13, bounded laterally by the costal part of the internal abdominal oblique muscle.

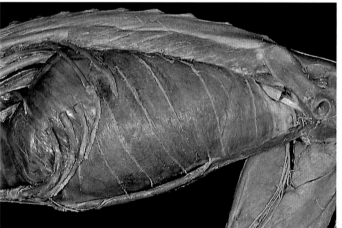

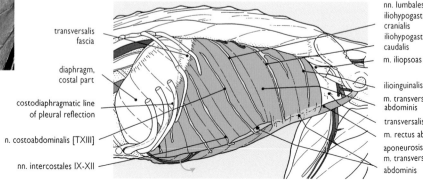

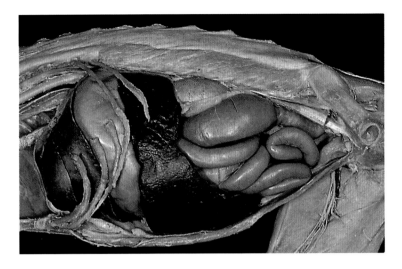

Fig. 10.55 Abdominal viscera in situ: left lateral view. The left abdominal wall and left half of the diaphragm have been removed and the fat-infiltrated greater omentum severed from its attachments to the stomach and spleen and removed from the surface of the intestines to give a view comparable to Fig. 6.24 of the dog. The spleen is considerably larger than would normally be expected – a possible 'normal' outline is shown by the broken line on the surface of the spleen. A similarly enlarged spleen was seen in the dog used for sectioning of the abdomen (Figs 6.95–6.97).

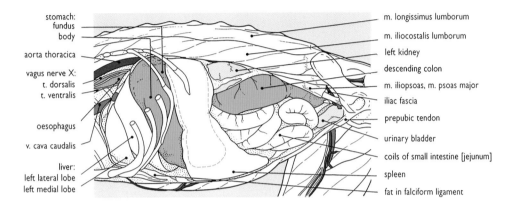

stomach:
fundus
body
aorta thoracica
vagus nerve X:
t. dorsalis
t. ventralis
oesophagus
v. cava caudalis
liver:
left lateral lobe
left medial lobe

m. longissimus lumborum
m. iliocostalis lumborum
left kidney
descending colon
m. iliopsoas, m. psoas major
iliac fascia
prepubic tendon
urinary bladder
coils of small intestine [jejunum]
spleen
fat in falciform ligament

Veterinary Anatomy: The Dog and Cat

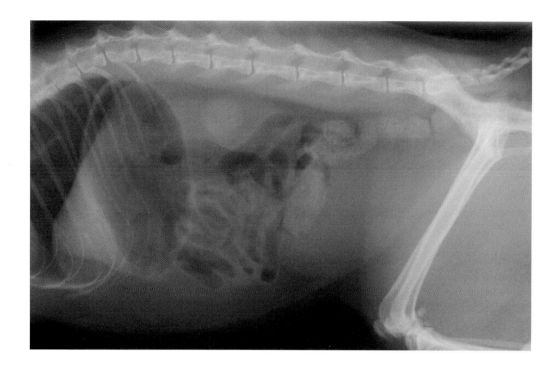

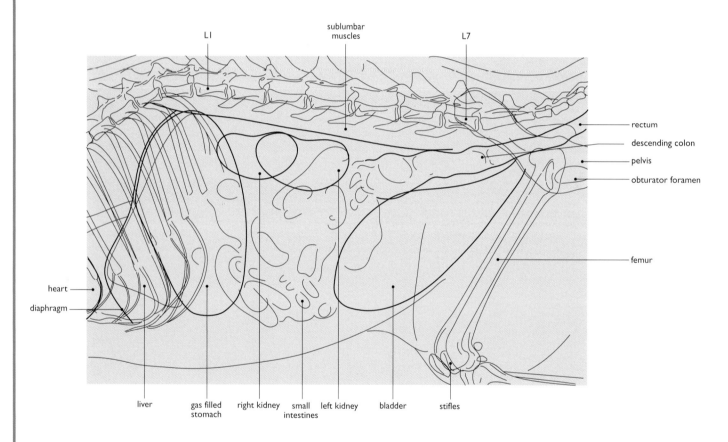

sublumbar
muscles

LI
L7

heart
diaphragm

liver
gas filled
stomach
right kidney
small
intestines
left kidney
bladder
stifles

rectum
descending colon
pelvis
obturator foramen

femur

Fig. 10.56 Radiograph of the abdomen: lateral view. The smaller size and relatively larger intra-abdominal fat deposits in the cat result in greater intra-abdominal detail.

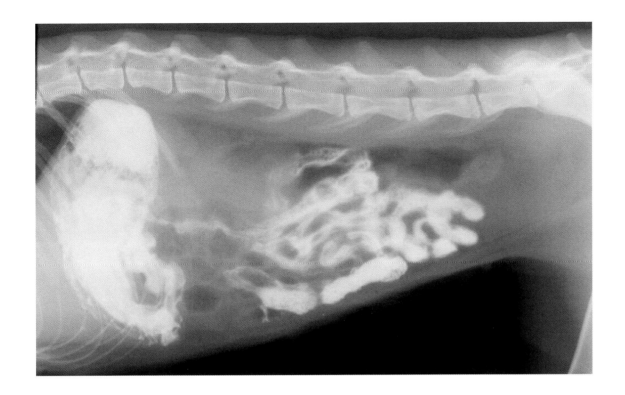

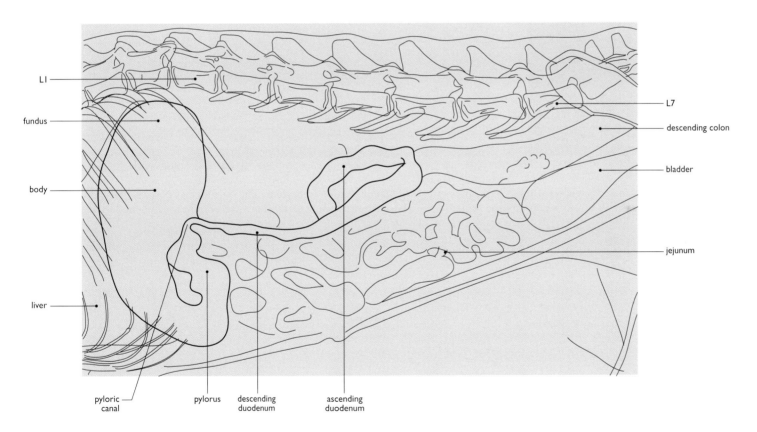

Fig. 10.57 Radiograph of the abdomen: lateral view, 30 minutes after oral administration of barium. The barium can be seen highlighting the stomach and small intestines. The small intestines occupy the center of the abdomen, extending caudally to the cranial pole of the bladder.

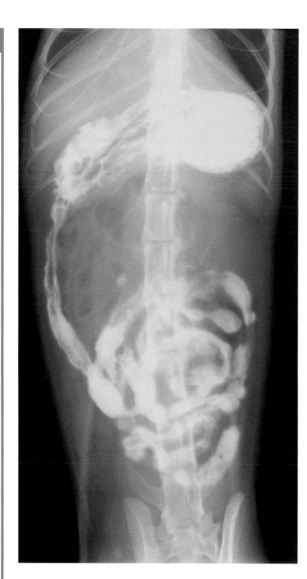
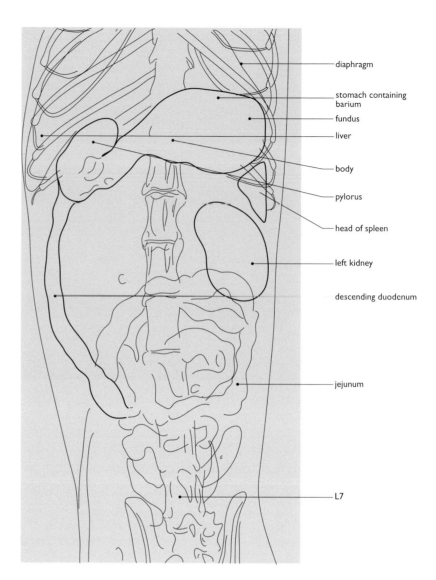

diaphragm

stomach containing barium

fundus

liver

body

pylorus

head of spleen

left kidney

descending duodenum

jejunum

L7

Fig. 10.58 Radiograph of the abdomen: ventrodorsal view, 30 minutes after oral administration of barium. The barium can be seen highlighting the stomach and small intestines. The small intestines occupy the center of the abdomen, extending caudally to the cranial pole of the bladder.

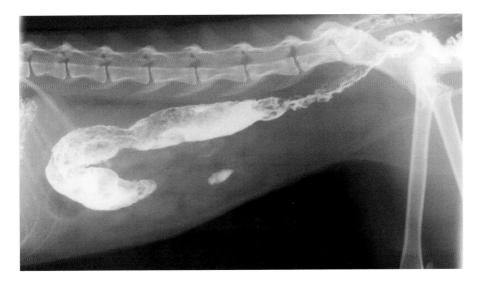

Fig. 10.59 Radiograph of the abdomen: lateral view 6 hours after oral administration of barium. The barium can be seen highlighting the rectum, colon and part of the caecum. Part of the gastric fundus is also highlighted.

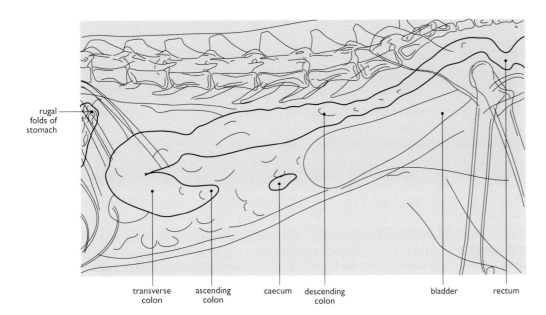

rugal folds of stomach

transverse colon   ascending colon   caecum   descending colon   bladder   rectum

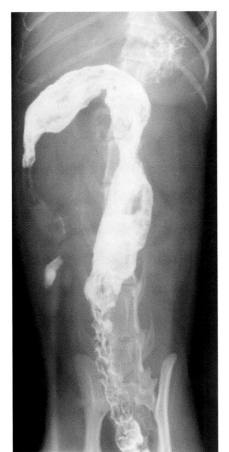

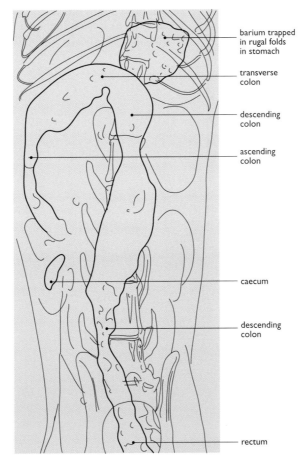

Fig. 10.60 Radiograph of the abdomen: ventrodorsal view, 6 hours after oral administration of barium. The barium can be seen highlighting the rectum, colon and part of the caecum. Part of the gastric fundus is also highlighted.

barium trapped in rugal folds in stomach

transverse colon

descending colon

ascending colon

caecum

descending colon

rectum

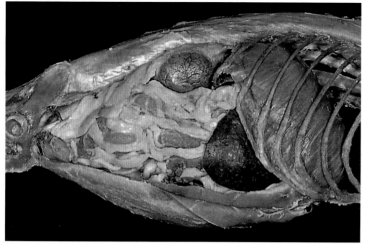

Fig. 10.61 Abdominal viscera in situ: right lateral view (1). In this view the right abdominal wall has been removed but the greater omentum is left in place covering the coils of the small intestine to give a view comparable to Fig. 6.48 of the dog. The greater omentum is extensively infiltrated with fat while other fat depots are located around the kidney, in the abdominal roof and in the abdominal floor cranially and caudally. The branched network of capsular veins is visible on the surface of the kidney through the fibrous renal capsule.

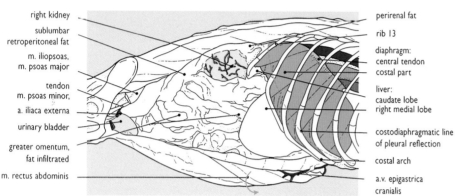

right kidney
sublumbar retroperitoneal fat
m. iliopsoas, m. psoas major
tendon m. psoas minor, a. iliaca externa
urinary bladder
greater omentum, fat infiltrated
m. rectus abdominis

perirenal fat
rib 13
diaphragm: central tendon costal part
liver: caudate lobe right medial lobe
costodiaphragmatic line of pleural reflection
costal arch
a.v. epigastrica cranialis

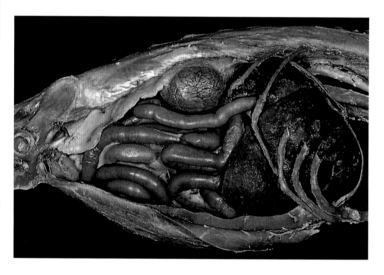

Fig. 10.62 Abdominal viscera in situ: right lateral view (2). The greater omentum and the right half of the diaphragm have been removed to expose the entire abdominal cavity in a comparable view to Fig. 6.51 of the dog. The liver is a prominent feature on this side with the descending duodenum passing caudally ventral to the right kidney. The costodiaphragmatic line of pleural reflection is indicated by the broken green line in advance of the costal arch, as it is on the previous picture. This line marks the position of the junction of thoracic and abdominal cavities on the surface.

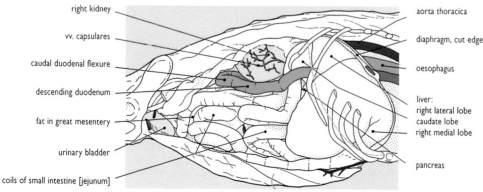

right kidney
vv. capsulares
caudal duodenal flexure
descending duodenum
fat in great mesentery
urinary bladder
coils of small intestine [jejunum]

aorta thoracica
diaphragm, cut edge
oesophagus
liver: right lateral lobe caudate lobe right medial lobe
pancreas

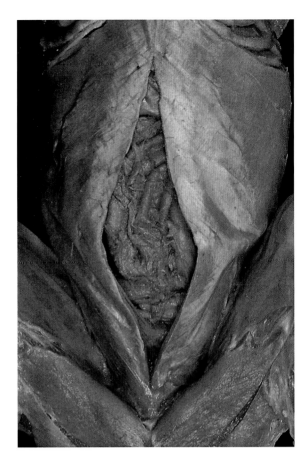

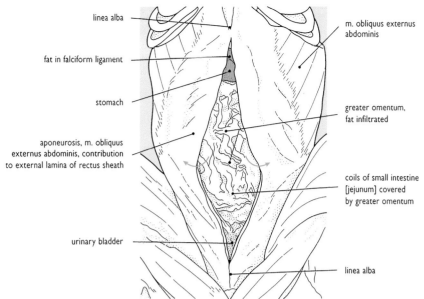

linea alba

fat in falciform ligament

stomach

aponeurosis, m. obliquus externus abdominis, contribution to external lamina of rectus sheath

urinary bladder

m. obliquus externus abdominis

greater omentum, fat infiltrated

coils of small intestine [jejunum] covered by greater omentum

linea alba

Fig. 10.63 Abdominal viscera in situ viewed through a midventral incision: ventral view. A longitudinal incision has been made along almost three-quarters of the length of the linea alba and the abdominal wall has been pulled apart to give a view somewhat comparable to Fig. 6.73 of the dog. An initial midventral opening reveals the fat-infiltrated greater omentum covering the coils of small intestine. At the cranial end of the incision the falciform ligament has been reached and the stomach in the region of the greater curvature is just visible; at the caudal end the bladder is not covered by greater omentum and is just visible.

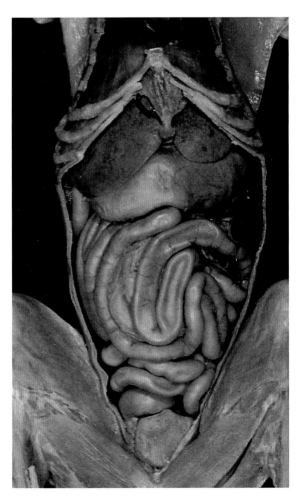

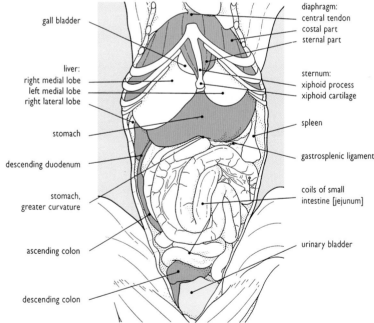

gall bladder

liver:
right medial lobe
left medial lobe
right lateral lobe

stomach

descending duodenum

stomach, greater curvature

ascending colon

descending colon

diaphragm:
central tendon
costal part
sternal part

sternum:
xiphoid process
xiphoid cartilage

spleen

gastrosplenic ligament

coils of small intestine [jejunum]

urinary bladder

Fig. 10.64 Abdominal viscera after removal of the greater omentum: ventral view. The abdominal wall has been removed and the greater omentum severed at its connection with the greater curvature of the stomach and removed. A comparable view of the dog's abdomen is shown in Fig. 6.74. The liver and stomach are prominent, although in dorsal recumbency the hardened liver does tend to project further caudally than it might in the normal standing posture so that more of it is visible beyond the costal arch in the abdominal wall. The spleen in this specimen is of a more normal size and does not reach as far ventrally as the midline.

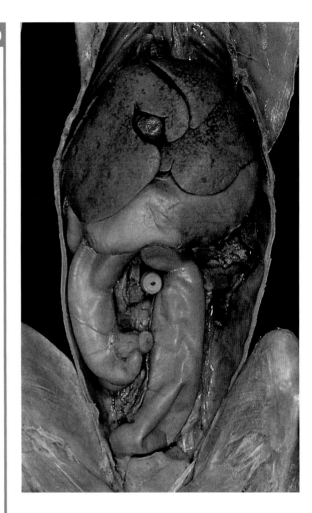

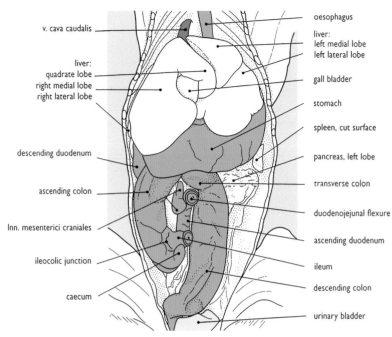

liver:
oesophagus
v. cava caudalis
left medial lobe
left lateral lobe

liver:
quadrate lobe
right medial lobe
right lateral lobe

gall bladder

stomach

spleen, cut surface

descending duodenum

pancreas, left lobe

transverse colon

ascending colon

duodenojejunal flexure

lnn. mesenterici craniales

ascending duodenum

ileocolic junction

ileum

descending colon

caecum

urinary bladder

Fig. 10.65 Abdominal viscera of the spayed queen after removal of the jejunum and ileum: ventral view. Jejunum and ileum are removed by severing the root of the mesentery and cutting the jejunum at the duodenojejunal flexure and at the ileocolic boundary. The root of the mesentery has been cleaned of fat and mesenteric lymph nodes are exposed. The small comma-shaped caecum can be compared to the larger and corkscrewed caecum of the dog (Fig. 6.75). Removal of the diaphragm and the costal arches exposes the gall bladder and the incompletely separated quadrate and right medial lobes of the liver (compare with Fig. 6.77 of the dog).

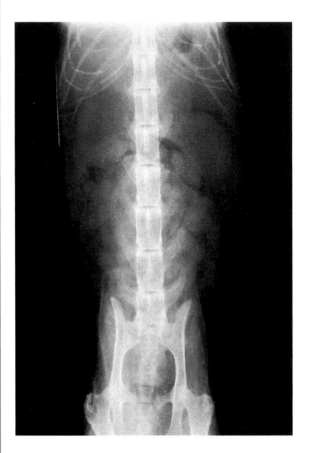

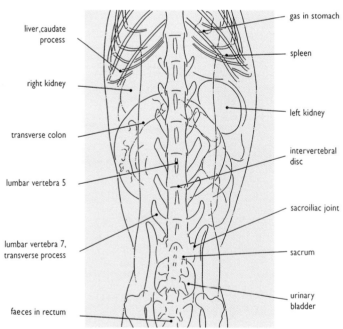

gas in stomach

liver, caudate
process

spleen

right kidney

left kidney

transverse colon

intervertebral
disc

lumbar vertebra 5

sacroiliac joint

lumbar vertebra 7,
transverse process

sacrum

urinary
bladder

faeces in rectum

Fig. 10.66 Radiograph of the abdomen: ventrodorsal view.

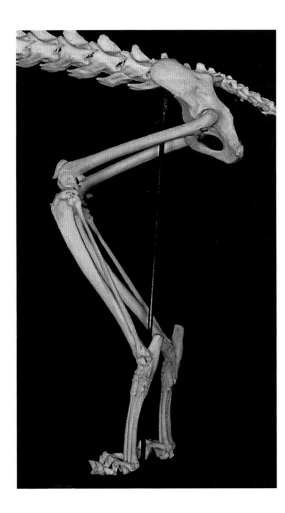

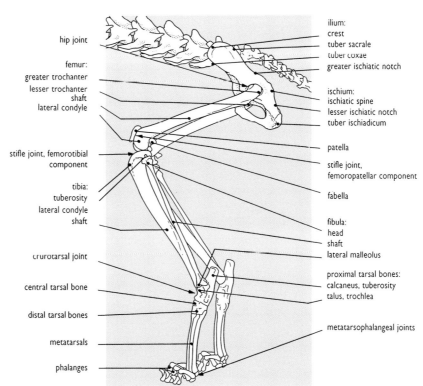

hip joint

femur:
greater trochanter
lesser trochanter
shaft
lateral condyle

stifle joint, femorotibial
component

tibia:
tuberosity
lateral condyle
shaft

crurotarsal joint

central tarsal bone

distal tarsal bones

metatarsals

phalanges

ilium:
crest
tuber sacrale
tuber coxae
greater ischiatic notch

ischium:
ischiatic spine
lesser ischiatic notch
tuber ischiadicum

patella

stifle joint,
femoropatellar component

fabella

fibula:
head
shaft
lateral malleolus

proximal tarsal bones:
calcaneus, tuberosity
talus, trochlea

metatarsophalangeal joints

Fig. 10.67 Skeleton of the hindlimb: left lateral view. As with the forelimb, the overall more slender and delicate nature of the limb bones is evident. Gross anatomical differences are not however observed. Sesamoid bones are comparable with sesamoid fabellae caudal to the stifle joint in the origin of the popliteal muscle. Much of the pelvic girdle is also illustrated in the ventrodorsal radiograph of the abdomen/pelvis (Fig. 10.66).

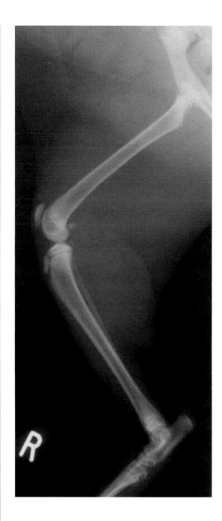

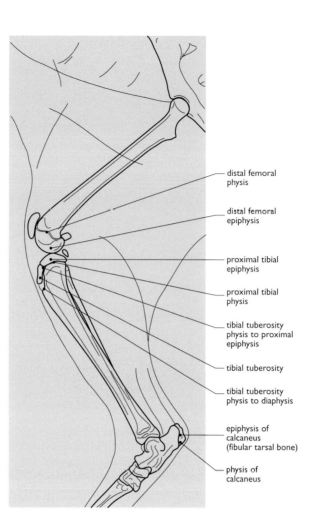

Fig. 10.68 Radiograph of the hindlimb: lateral view, 6 months old. Open physes are visible at the distal femur and proximal tibia.

distal femoral physis

distal femoral epiphysis

proximal tibial epiphysis

proximal tibial physis

tibial tuberosity physis to proximal epiphysis

tibial tuberosity

tibial tuberosity physis to diaphysis

epiphysis of calcaneus (fibular tarsal bone)

physis of calcaneus

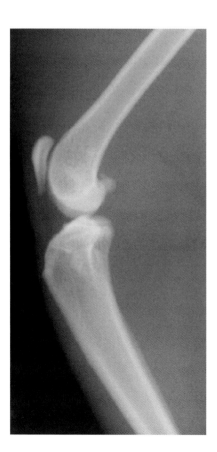

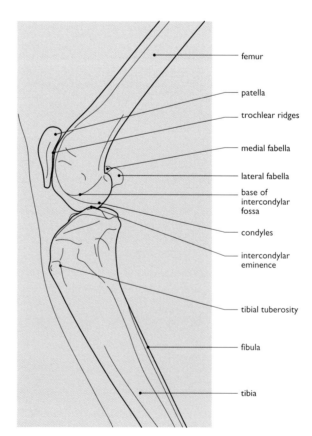

Fig. 10.69 Radiograph of the stifle: lateral view.

femur

patella

trochlear ridges

medial fabella

lateral fabella

base of intercondylar fossa

condyles

intercondylar eminence

tibial tuberosity

fibula

tibia

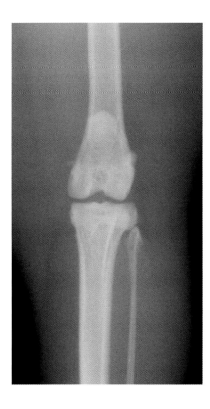

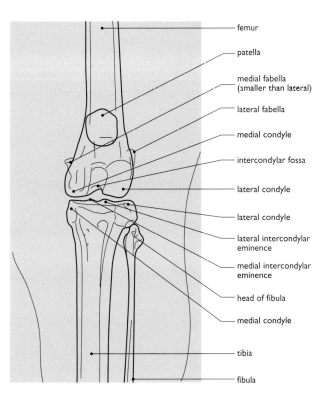

femur

patella

medial fabella
(smaller than lateral)

lateral fabella

medial condyle

intercondylar fossa

lateral condyle

lateral condyle

lateral intercondylar
eminence

medial intercondylar
eminence

head of fibula

medial condyle

tibia

fibula

Fig. 10.70 Radiograph of the stifle: craniocaudal view. The medial fabella is frequently more poorly mineralized compared with the lateral and thus appears smaller radiographically.

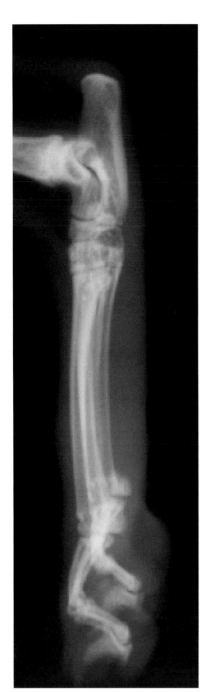

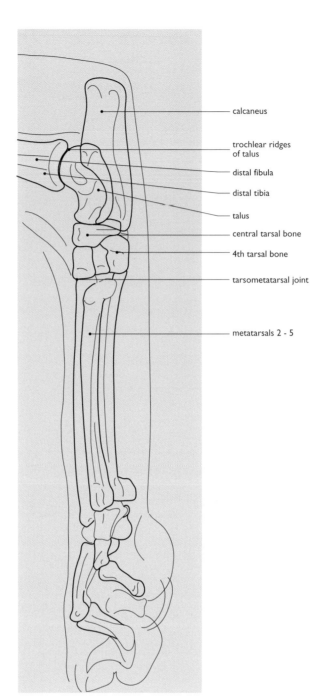

Fig. 10.71 Radiograph of the hindpaw: lateral view.

calcaneus

trochlear ridges of talus

distal fibula

distal tibia

talus

central tarsal bone

4th tarsal bone

tarsometatarsal joint

metatarsals 2 - 5

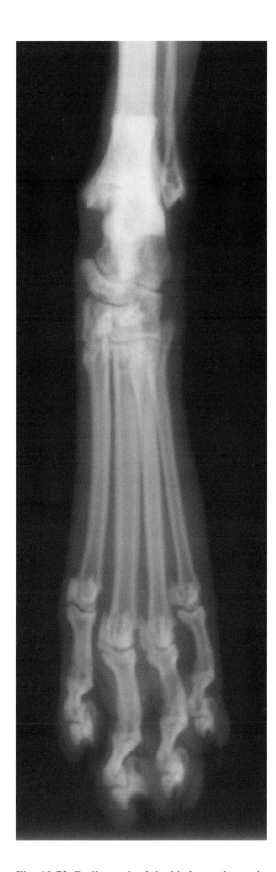
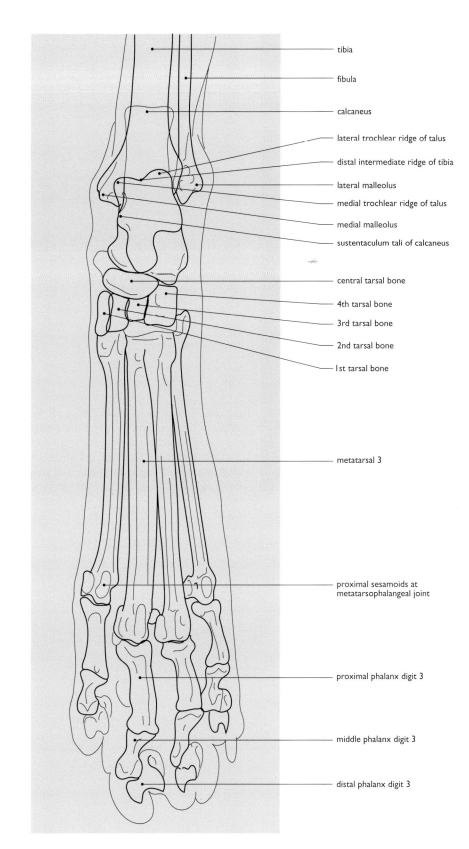

tibia

fibula

calcaneus

lateral trochlear ridge of talus

distal intermediate ridge of tibia

lateral malleolus

medial trochlear ridge of talus

medial malleolus

sustentaculum tali of calcaneus

central tarsal bone

4th tarsal bone

3rd tarsal bone

2nd tarsal bone

1st tarsal bone

metatarsal 3

proximal sesamoids at
metatarsophalangeal joint

proximal phalanx digit 3

middle phalanx digit 3

distal phalanx digit 3

Fig. 10.72 Radiograph of the hindpaw: dorsoplantar view.

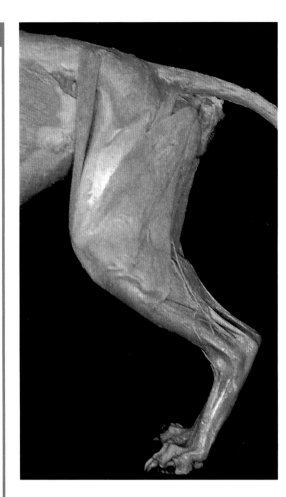

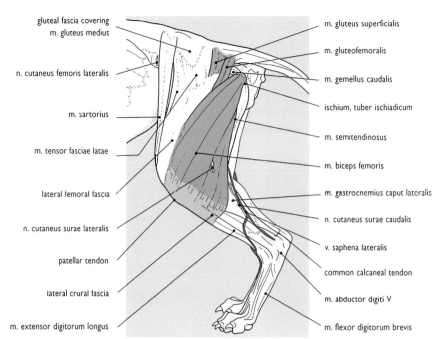

gluteal fascia covering
m. gluteus medius

n. cutaneus femoris lateralis

m. sartorius

m. tensor fasciae latae

lateral femoral fascia

n. cutaneus surae lateralis

patellar tendon

lateral crural fascia

m. extensor digitorum longus

m. gluteus superficialis

m. gluteofemoralis

m. gemellus caudalis

ischium, tuber ischiadicum

m. semitendinosus

m. biceps femoris

m. gastrocnemius caput lateralis

n. cutaneus surae caudalis

v. saphena lateralis

common calcaneal tendon

m. abductor digiti V

m. flexor digitorum brevis

Fig. 10.73 Superficial musculature of the hindlimb: left lateral view. Superficial fascia has been cleaned from the limb to expose superficial limb muscles much as in Figs 7.12, 7.44 and 7.78 of the dog. Of particular note is the gluteofemoralis muscle (cranial crural abductor) a biceps component arising from caudal vertebrae 2 and 3 and sandwiched between the biceps and the small superficial gluteal muscle. The tensor muscle of the lateral femoral fascia is quite a significant muscle, more so than in the dog.

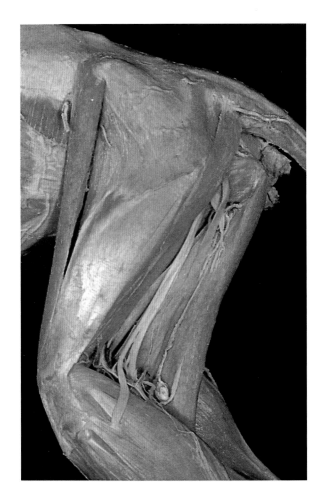

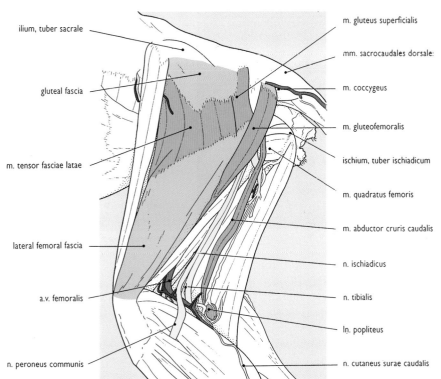

ilium, tuber sacrale

gluteal fascia

m. tensor fasciae latae

lateral femoral fascia

a.v. femoralis

n. peroneus communis

m. gluteus superficialis

mm. sacrocaudales dorsale:

m. coccygeus

m. gluteofemoralis

ischium, tuber ischiadicum

m. quadratus femoris

m. abductor cruris caudalis

n. ischiadicus

n. tibialis

ln. popliteus

n. cutaneus surae caudalis

Fig. 10.74 Hip and thigh after removal of the biceps femoris muscle: left lateral view. The biceps femoris muscle has been removed to expose the full extent of the gluteofemoralis muscle and much of the extent of the caudal crural abductor muscle. This view, comparable to Fig. 7.16 of the dog, also shows that a sacrotuberous ligament is not represented in the cat, the biceps simply originating from the ischiatic tuberosity.

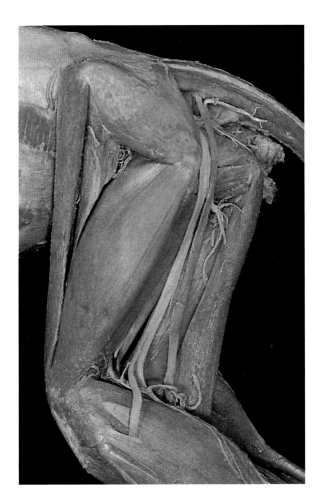

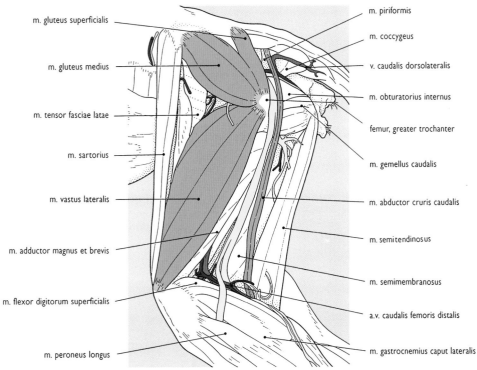

m. gluteus superficialis

m. gluteus medius

m. tensor fasciae latae

m. sartorius

m. vastus lateralis

m. adductor magnus et brevis

m. flexor digitorum superficialis

m. peroneus longus

m. piriformis

m. coccygeus

v. caudalis dorsolateralis

m. obturatorius internus

femur, greater trochanter

m. gemellus caudalis

m. abductor cruris caudalis

m. semitendinosus

m. semimembranosus

a.v. caudalis femoris distalis

m. gastrocnemius caput lateralis

Fig. 10.75 Deep musculature of the hip and thigh: left lateral view. Removal of the gluteofemoral muscle exposes the origin of the caudal crural abductor from caudal vertebrae 2 and 3. The gluteal and lateral femoral fasciae have been removed, exposing middle and superficial gluteal muscles and the lateral vastus component of the quadriceps femoris muscle. A comparable view of the hip of the dog is shown in Fig. 7.17.

Veterinary Anatomy: The Dog and Cat

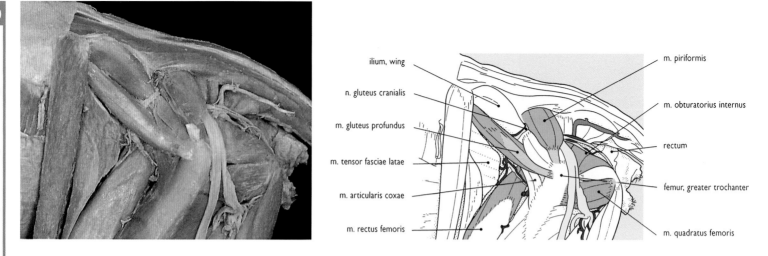

Fig. 10.76 Deep musculature of the hip (1): left lateral view. Removal of the superficial and middle gluteals and the lateral vastus muscle exposes the deep musculature of the hip joint (piriform, deep gluteal, articularis and gemellus) as well as the rectus femoris component of the quadriceps femoris muscle. A comparable view of the dog is shown in Fig. 7.18.

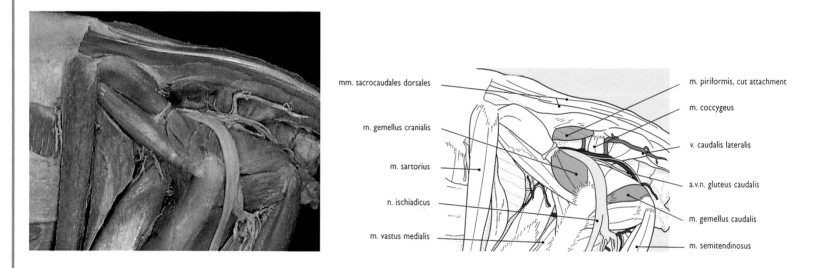

Fig. 10.77 Deep musculature of the hip (2): left lateral view. The piriform muscle is cut from its sacral attachment, displaying the emergence of the ischiadic nerve from the pelvic cavity. The considerably greater extent of the gemelli muscles contrasts with the situation in the dog (Fig. 7.19).

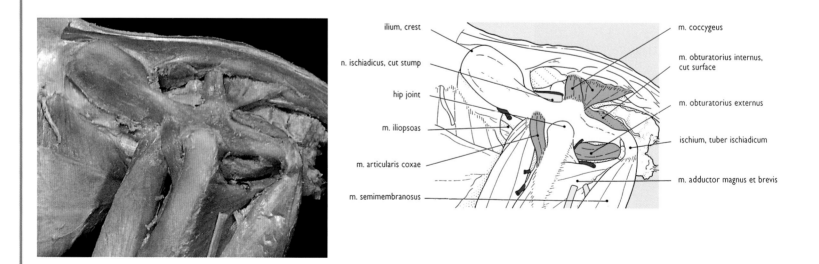

Fig. 10.78 Deep musculature of the hip (3): left lateral view. Removal of the ischiadic nerve, gemelli muscles, quadratus femoris, deep gluteal, and internal obturator muscles, exposes much of the pelvic bone, a view comparable to Fig. 7.24 of the dog. The coccygeal muscle arising from the ischiatic spine is a considerably more substantial muscle than in the dog.

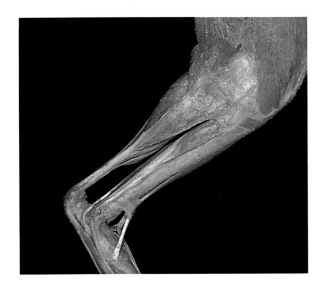

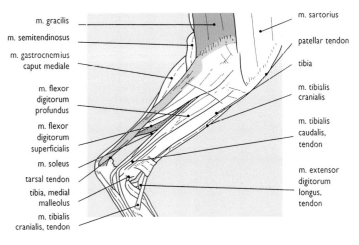

m. gracilis
m. semitendinosus
m. gastrocnemius caput mediale
m. flexor digitorum profundus
m. flexor digitorum superficialis
m. soleus
tarsal tendon
tibia, medial malleolus
m. tibialis cranialis, tendon

m. sartorius
patellar tendon
tibia
m. tibialis cranialis
m. tibialis caudalis, tendon
m. extensor digitorum longus, tendon

Fig. 10.79 Musculature of the crus and paw of the left hindlimb: medial view. Some minimal cleaning of superficial fascia and removal of superficial vessels and nerves exposes crural musculature in a view comparable to Fig. 7.45 of the dog. The tarsal tendon of the gracilis muscle and its association with the common calcaneal tendon is displayed.

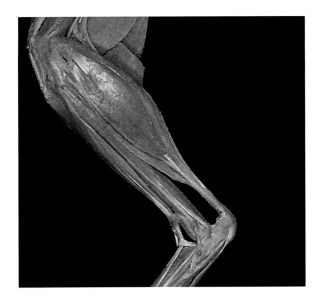

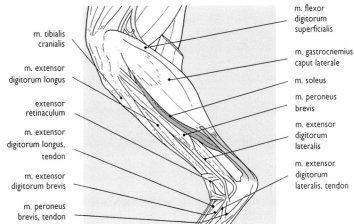

m. tibialis cranialis
m. extensor digitorum longus
extensor retinaculum
m. extensor digitorum longus, tendon
m. extensor digitorum brevis
m. peroneus brevis, tendon

m. flexor digitorum superficialis
m. gastrocnemius caput laterale
m. soleus
m. peroneus brevis
m. extensor digitorum lateralis
m. extensor digitorum lateralis, tendon

Fig. 10.80 Musculature of the crus and paw of the left hindlimb: lateral view (1). Removal of the biceps femoris muscle and the deep crural fascia exposes crural muscles in a view comparable to Figs 7.44 and 7.49 of the dog. The soleus muscle, not represented in the dog, appears between the long peroneal and the lateral head of the gastrocnemius with its tendon joining with the common calcaneal tendon.

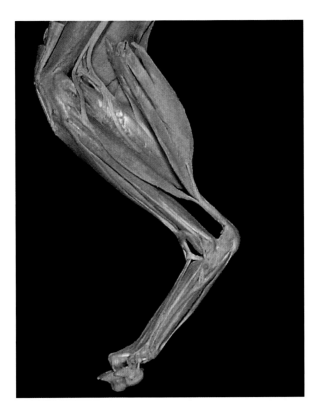

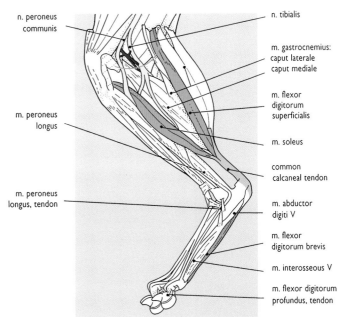

n. peroneus communis
m. peroneus longus
m. peroneus longus, tendon

n. tibialis
m. gastrocnemius: caput laterale caput mediale
m. flexor digitorum superficialis
m. soleus
common calcaneal tendon
m. abductor digiti V
m. flexor digitorum brevis
m. interosseous V
m. flexor digitorum profundus, tendon

Fig. 10.81 Musculature of the crus and paw of the left hindlimb: lateral view (2). The lateral head of the gastrocnemius muscle has been cut from the femur along with the superficial digital flexor muscle and reflected caudolaterally to expose the entire extent of the soleus and superficial digital flexor muscles, the latter blended with the lateral head of the gastrocnemius for much of its length.

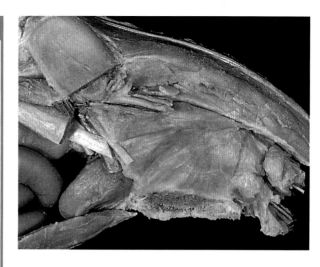

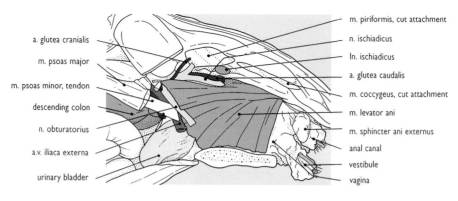

a. glutea cranialis
m. psoas major
m. psoas minor, tendon
descending colon
n. obturatorius
a.v. iliaca externa
urinary bladder

m. piriformis, cut attachment
n. ischiadicus
ln. ischiadicus
a. glutea caudalis
m. coccygeus, cut attachment
m. levator ani
m. sphincter ani externus
anal canal
vestibule
vagina

Fig. 10.82 Pelvic cavity of the queen after removal of the left pelvic bone: left lateral view. The pelvic symphysis and wing of the ilium have been sawn through and the pelvic bone removed, along with the internal obturator muscle on its internal face. The view of the pelvic cavity obtained is comparable to Fig. 8.36 of the bitch and Fig. 8.19 of the dog.

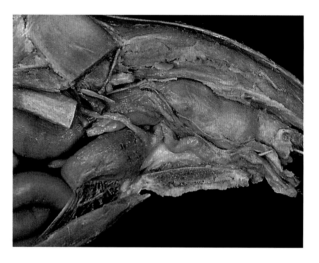

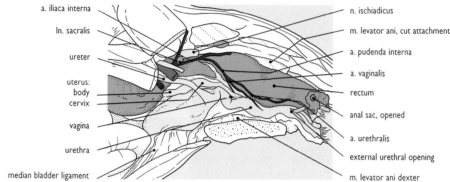

a. iliaca interna
ln. sacralis
ureter
uterus:
body
cervix
vagina
urethra
median bladder ligament

n. ischiadicus
m. levator ani, cut attachment
a. pudenda interna
a. vaginalis
rectum
anal sac, opened
a. urethralis
external urethral opening
m. levator ani dexter

Fig. 10.83 Pelvic viscera of the queen in situ: left lateral view. The levator ani muscle has been removed and some pelvic and perineal fat and fascia cleared to expose the pelvic viscera and give a comparable view to the bitch in Fig. 8.21.

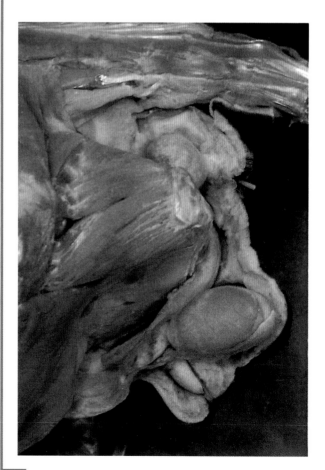

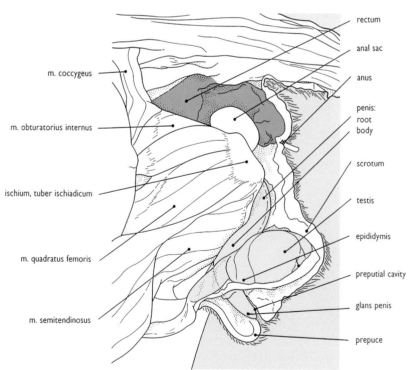

m. coccygeus
m. obturatorius internus
ischium, tuber ischiadicum
m. quadratus femoris
m. semitendinosus

rectum
anal sac
anus
penis:
root
body
scrotum
testis
epididymis
preputial cavity
glans penis
prepuce

Fig. 10.84 External genitalia of the tom cat: left lateral view. Skin and subcutaneous tissues have been removed from the left half of the pelvis and from the scrotum and penis. The left testis is exposed with epididymis and spermatic cord. The root and body of the penis are exposed with the glans penis directed caudally inside the preputial cavity.

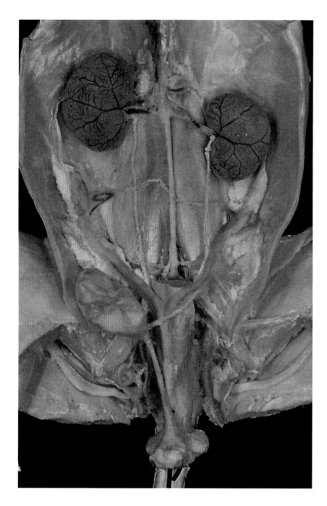

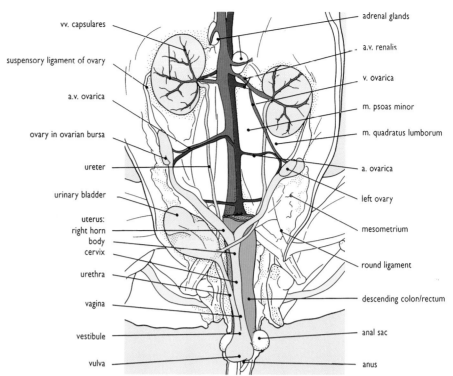

vv. capsulares — adrenal glands

suspensory ligament of ovary — a.v. renalis

a.v. ovarica — v. ovarica

ovary in ovarian bursa — m. psoas minor

— m. quadratus lumborum

ureter — a. ovarica

urinary bladder — left ovary

uterus:
right horn — mesometrium
body
cervix — round ligament

urethra

vagina — descending colon/rectum

vestibule — anal sac

vulva — anus

Fig. 10.85 Urogenital system of the queen: ventral view. The gastrointestinal tract in the abdomen has been removed and the pelvis opened by removing the midventral sections of both pelvic bones (parallel saw cuts through pubes and ischia on either side of the midline). Fat has been cleared from the left side of the abdomen and the adipose and fibrous capsules of the kidneys have been stripped off, displaying the characteristic capsular veins of the kidney. Comparable views of the bitch are seen in Figs 6.84 and 6.85.

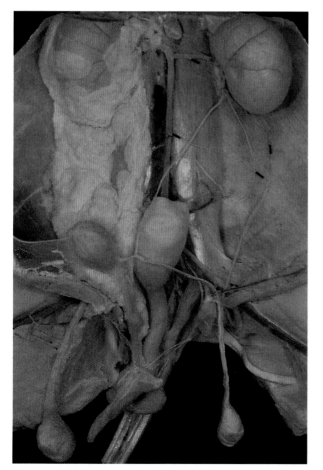

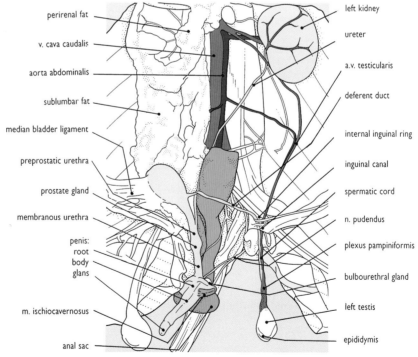

perirenal fat — left kidney

v. cava caudalis — ureter

aorta abdominalis — a.v. testicularis

sublumbar fat — deferent duct

median bladder ligament — internal inguinal ring

preprostatic urethra — inguinal canal

prostate gland — spermatic cord

membranous urethra — n. pudendus

penis:
root — plexus pampiniformis
body
glans — bulbourethral gland

m. ischiocavernosus — left testis

anal sac — epididymis

Fig. 10.86 Urogenital tract of tom cat: ventral view. The gastrointestinal tract in the abdomen has been removed and the pelvis opened by removal of the midventral region of its floor. The left penile crus and its associated ischiocavernosus muscle has been cut through and the bulbourethral gland (not represented in the dog) is visible dorsal to it. The caudally directed penis is exposed although the roughened spines on the glans surface are not in evidence.

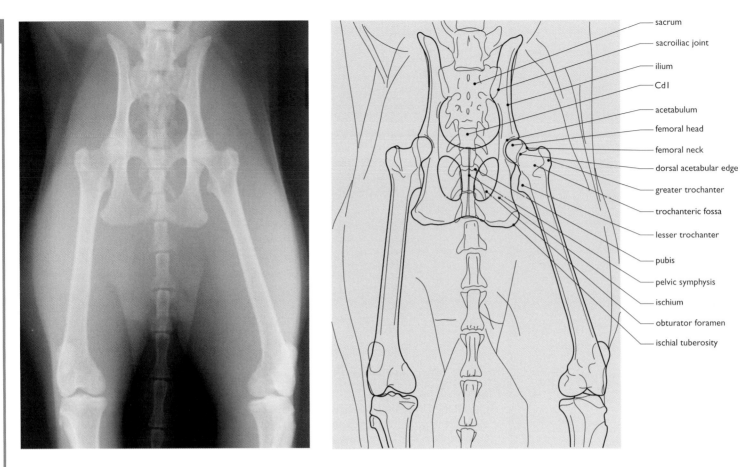

sacrum
sacroiliac joint
ilium
Cd1
acetabulum
femoral head
femoral neck
dorsal acetabular edge
greater trochanter
trochanteric fossa
lesser trochanter
pubis
pelvic symphysis
ischium
obturator foramen
ischial tuberosity

Fig. 10.87 Radiograph of the pelvis: ventrodorsal view. The acetabulum is shallower than that of the dog.

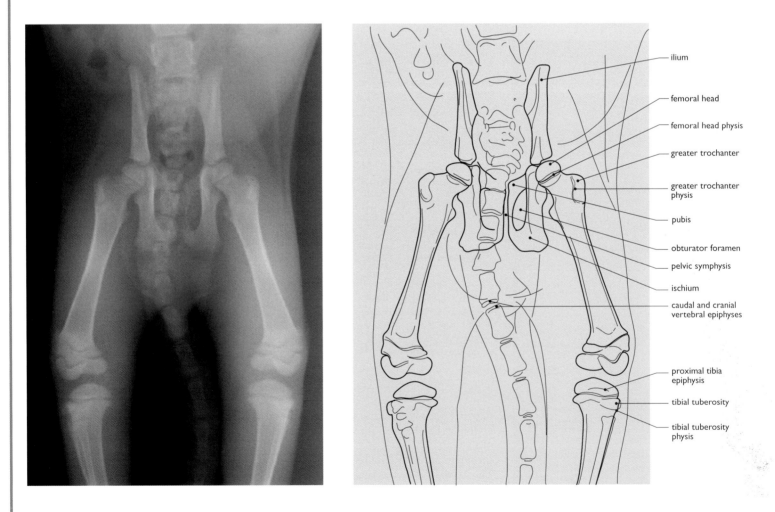

ilium
femoral head
femoral head physis
greater trochanter
greater trochanter physis
pubis
obturator foramen
pelvic symphysis
ischium
caudal and cranial vertebral epiphyses
proximal tibia epiphysis
tibial tuberosity
tibial tuberosity physis

Fig. 10.88 Radiograph of the pelvis: ventrodorsal view, 12 weeks old. The vertebrae appear relatively short. Open physes are visible at the vertebral endplates, the junction of the ilium and the pubis, the pelvic symphysis, the proximal and distal femur and the proximal tibia.

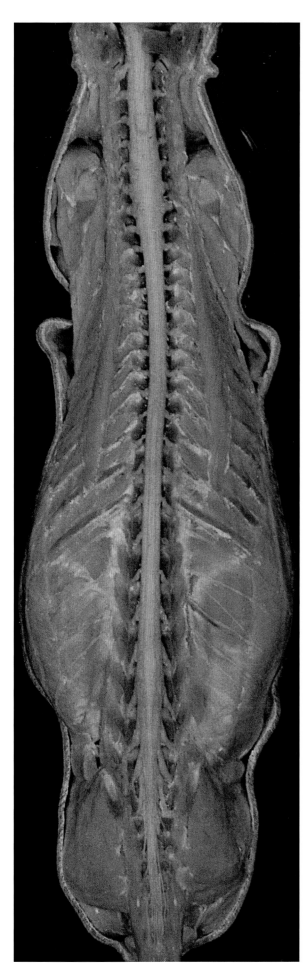

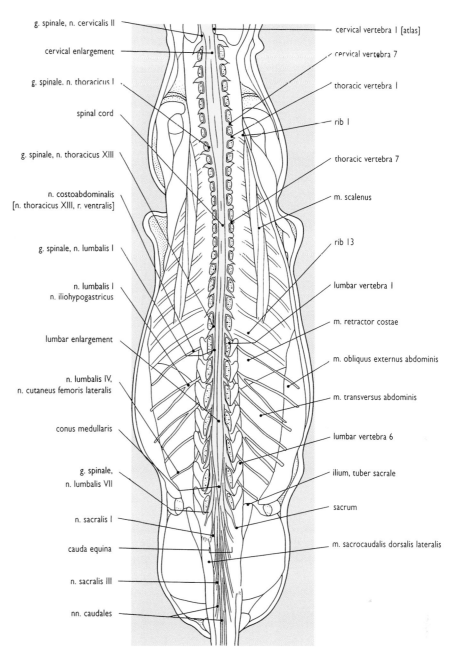

g. spinale, n. cervicalis II — cervical vertebra I [atlas]

cervical enlargement — cervical vertebra 7

g. spinale. n. thoracicus I — thoracic vertebra I

spinal cord — rib I

g. spinale, n. thoracicus XIII — thoracic vertebra 7

n. costoabdominalis [n. thoracicus XIII, r. ventralis] — m. scalenus

g. spinale, n. lumbalis I — rib 13

n. lumbalis I n. iliohypogastricus — lumbar vertebra I

lumbar enlargement — m. retractor costae

n. lumbalis IV, n. cutaneus femoris lateralis — m. obliquus externus abdominis

conus medullaris — m. transversus abdominis

g. spinale, n. lumbalis VII — lumbar vertebra 6

n. sacralis I — ilium, tuber sacrale

cauda equina — sacrum

n. sacralis III — m. sacrocaudalis dorsalis lateralis

nn. caudales

Fig. 10.89 Spinal cord in situ: dorsal view. All of the epaxial musculature has been removed and the spinal canal opened by removal of the vertebral laminae. Within the canal, blood vessels, fat and the spinal meninges were removed to expose the entire length of the spinal cord. Cervical and lumbar enlargements are noticeable associated with brachial and lumbosacral plexuses respectively. The dorsal roots of spinal nerves are displayed with dorsal root ganglia as prominent expansions. The cord actually terminates at the level of lumbar vertebra 7 in the center of the 'cauda equina' of nerve roots extending caudally into the sacral spinal canal. Compare this view with Figs 9.31–9.33 of the dog.

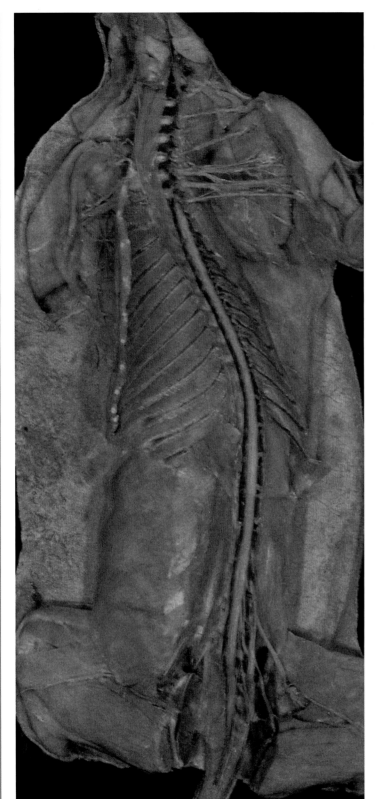

Fig. 10.90 Subvertebral musculature and spinal cord in situ: ventral view. Complete evisceration and removal of the thoracic and abdominal wall of the left side has exposed the subvertebral musculature in the neck and in the roof of the thorax and abdomen. On the right side much of the length of the left sympathetic trunk has been left in place – clearly apparent especially in thoracic and lumbar regions. Its continuation in the neck, which ran as a component of the vagosympathetic trunk close to the trachea, is also left in place. The vertebral bodies of thoracic and lumbar vertebrae and the sacrum have subsequently been removed and the spinal canal thereby opened ventrally to expose the spinal cord and spinal nerve roots. In the caudal cervical region the brachial plexus and nerves to the forelimb are displayed stretched across the opened axilla.

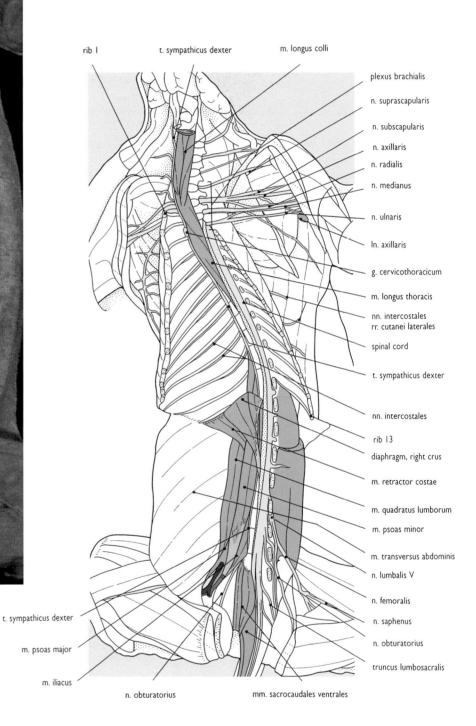

rib I — t. sympathicus dexter — m. longus colli

plexus brachialis
n. suprascapularis
n. subscapularis
n. axillaris
n. radialis
n. medianus
n. ulnaris
ln. axillaris
g. cervicothoracicum
m. longus thoracis
nn. intercostales
rr. cutanei laterales
spinal cord
t. sympathicus dexter
nn. intercostales
rib 13
diaphragm, right crus
m. retractor costae
m. quadratus lumborum
m. psoas minor
m. transversus abdominis
n. lumbalis V
n. femoralis
n. saphenus
n. obturatorius
truncus lumbosacralis

t. sympathicus dexter
m. psoas major
m. iliacus
n. obturatorius — mm. sacrocaudales ventrales

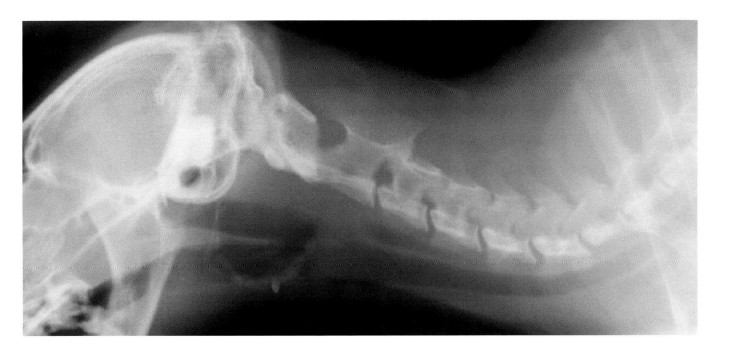

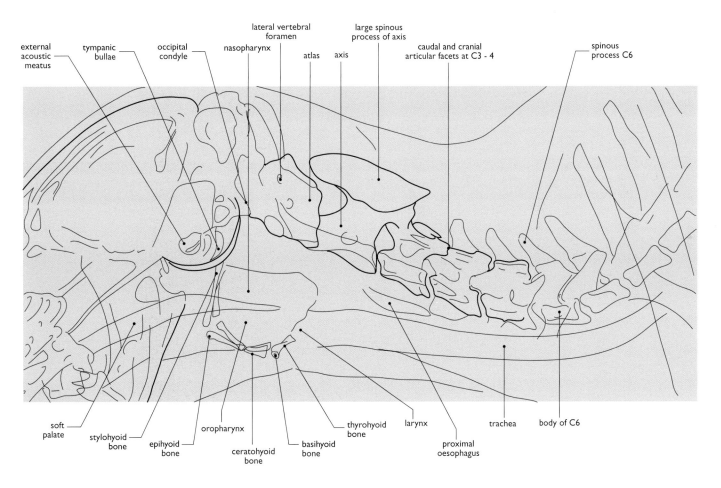

external
acoustic
meatus | tympanic
bullae | occipital
condyle | lateral vertebral
foramen
nasopharynx | atlas | axis | large spinous
process of axis | caudal and cranial
articular facets at C3 - 4 | spinous
process C6

soft
palate | stylohyoid
bone | epihyoid
bone | oropharynx | ceratohyoid
bone | basihyoid
bone | thyrohyoid
bone | larynx | proximal
oesophagus | trachea | body of C6

Fig. 10.91 Radiograph of the neck: lateral view. The vertebral canal can be seen clearly. The tympanohyoid bone is cartilaginous and so not visible radiographically. The upper esophageal sphincter is highlighted by air cranially and caudally.

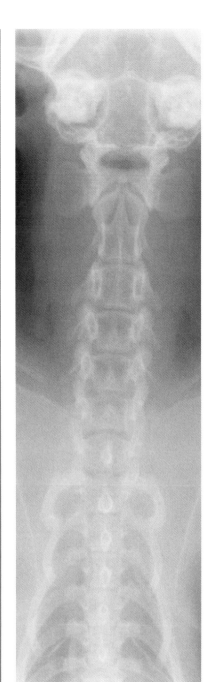

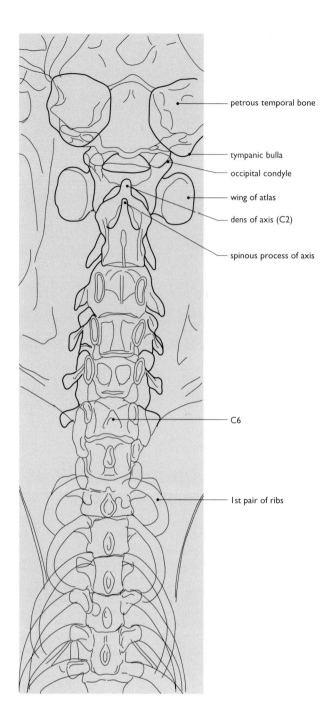

petrous temporal bone

tympanic bulla

occipital condyle

wing of atlas

dens of axis (C2)

spinous process of axis

C6

1st pair of ribs

Fig. 10.92 Radiograph of the neck: ventrodorsal view. The large wings of the atlas can be clearly seen. The clavicles are visible medial to the shoulder joints.

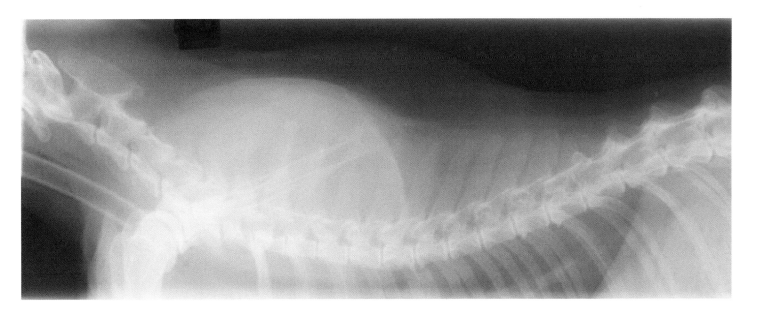

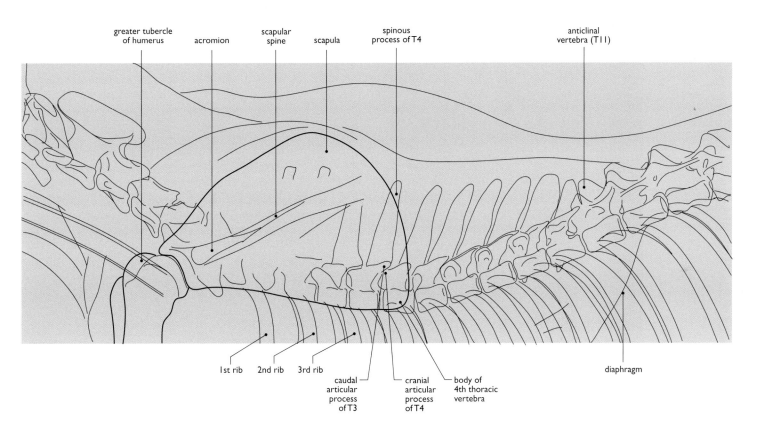

greater tubercle
of humerus

acromion

scapular
spine

scapula

spinous
process of T4

anticlinal
vertebra (T11)

1st rib   2nd rib   3rd rib

caudal
articular
process
of T3

cranial
articular
process
of T4

body of
4th thoracic
vertebra

diaphragm

Fig. 10.93 Radiograph of the thoracic spine: lateral view. The large scapula and associated shoulder muscles superimpose on the cranial thoracic spine.

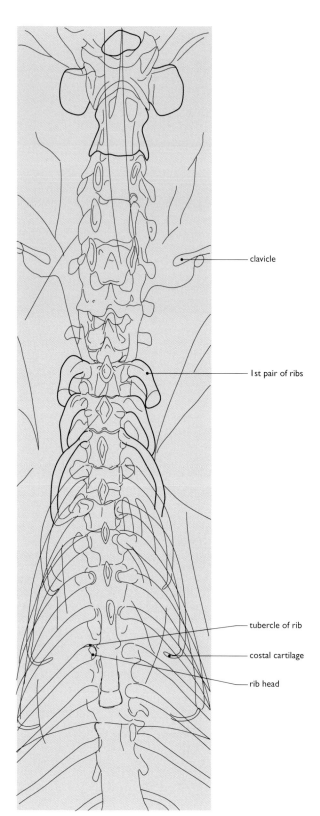

clavicle

1st pair of ribs

tubercle of rib

costal cartilage

rib head

Fig. 10.94 Radiograph of the thoracic spine: ventrodorsal view.

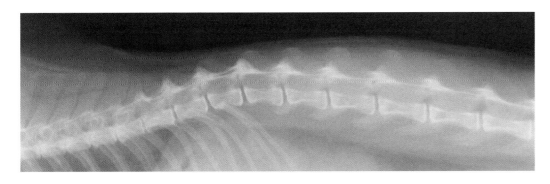

Fig. 10.95 Radiograph of the thoracolumbar junction: lateral view. The change in orientation of the synovial joints from the dorsal plane to the sagittal plane can be seen at the articulation between the 10th and 11th thoracic vertebrae. The slope of the spinous processes also changes at this point, from caudally orientated to cranially orientated. The 11th thoracic vertebra is the anticlinal vertebra in this cat.

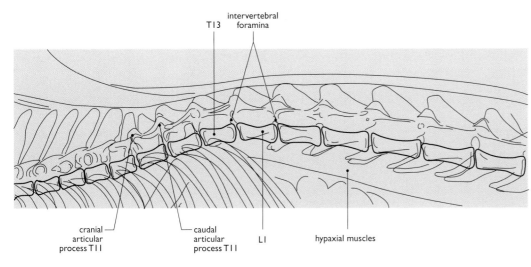

Fig. 10.96 Radiograph of the lumbar spine: lateral view.

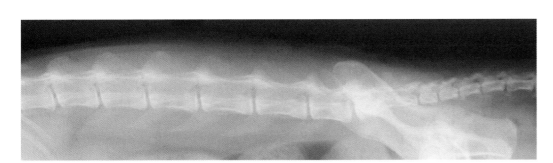

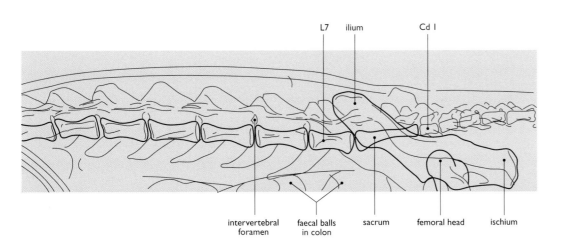

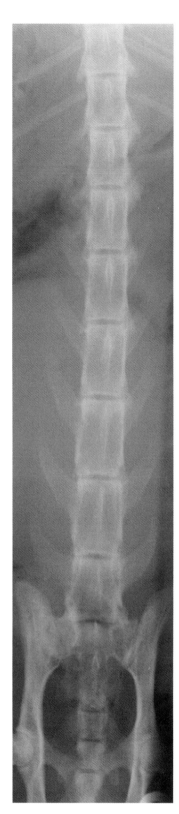

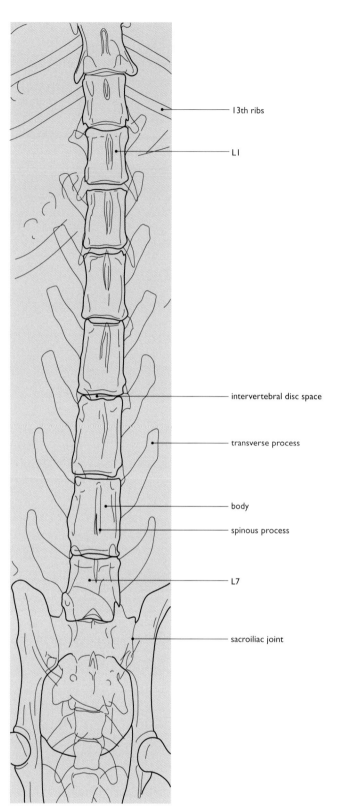

13th ribs

L1

intervertebral disc space

transverse process

body

spinous process

L7

sacroiliac joint

Fig. 10.97 Radiograph of the lumbar spine: ventrodorsal view.

SUBJECT INDEX

M